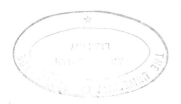

ZOONOSES

ZOONOSES

edited by

J. VAN DER HOEDEN

Israel Institute for Biological Research, Ness Ziona
Hebrew University, Hadassah Medical School, Jerusalem (Israel)

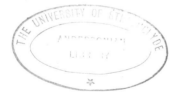

ELSEVIER PUBLISHING COMPANY

AMSTERDAM – LONDON – NEW YORK

1964

ELSEVIER PUBLISHING COMPANY
335 JAN VAN GALENSTRAAT, P.O. BOX 211, AMSTERDAM

AMERICAN ELSEVIER PUBLISHING COMPANY, INC.
52 VANDERBILT AVENUE, NEW YORK, N.Y. 10017

ELSEVIER PUBLISHING COMPANY LIMITED
RIPPLESIDE COMMERCIAL ESTATE, BARKING, ESSEX

LIBRARY OF CONGRESS CATALOG CARD NUMBER 62-18141

WITH 110 ILLUSTRATIONS AND 32 TABLES

PRINTED IN THE NETHERLANDS

LIST OF CONTRIBUTORS

Bernkopf, H., M. D. Professor of Medical Virology, Hebrew University, Hadassah Medical School, Jerusalem (Israel)

Clarenburg, A., D.V., Emeritus Head of the Laboratory for Zoonoses and Pathological Anatomy, National Institute of Public Health, Utrecht (The Netherlands)

Davies, A. M., M.D., Associate Professor of Medical Ecology, Hebrew University, Hadassah Medical School, Jerusalem (Israel)

Dekking, F., M.D., Lecturer in Medical Virology, Chief Virus Laboratory, University of Amsterdam; Amsterdam (The Netherlands)

Dinger, J. E., M.D., Emeritus Professor of Tropical Hygiene, Director of the Institute of Tropical Medicine, State University, Leiden (The Netherlands)

Donker-Voet, J., D.V.Sc., Senior Research Instructor, Institute for Veteriny Bacteriology, State University, Utrecht (The Netherlands)

Evenchik, Z., Ph.D., Department of Epidemiology, Israel Institute for Biological Research, Ness Ziona (Israel)

Frenkel, H. S., D.V.Sc., Emeritus Director National Institute for Veterinary Research, Amsterdam (The Netherlands)

Goldblum, N., Ph.D., Associate Professor of Medical Virology, Hebrew University Hadassah Medical School, Jerusalem (Israel)

Raubitschek, F., M.D., Associate Professor of Dermatology, Rothschild-Hadassah University Hospital, Chief, Medical Mycology Laboratory, Hebrew University, Jerusalem (Israel)

Ruys, A. Ch., M.D., Professor of Bacteriology, Epidemiology and Immunology; Director, Laboratory of Hygiene, University of Amsterdam (The Netherlands)

Tas, J., M.D., Clinical Associate Professor of Dermatology, Department of Dermatology and Venereology, Rothschild-Hadassah University Hospital, Hebrew University, Jerusalem (Israel)

Theodor, O., Ph.D., Associate Professor of Medical Entomology, Department of Parasitology, Hebrew University, Hadassah Medical School, Jerusalem (Israel)

Tierkel, E. S., A.B., D.V.M., M.P.H., Chief, Rabies Control Unit, Communicable Disease Center, U.S. Public Health Service, Atlanta (Ga.)

Van Riel, H., M.D., D.P.H., Professor of Public Health, Tropical Medicine, Hygiene, Health Education and Bacteriology, University of Brussels, Institute of Tropical Medicine, Antwerp (Belgium)

Van Thiel, P. H., Ph.D., Professor of Parasitology, Institute of Tropical Medicine, State University, Leiden (The Netherlands)

Van der Hoeden, J., D.V.Sc., Head, Department of Epidemiology, Israel Institute for Biological Research, Ness Ziona, Clinical Professor of Bacteriology, Hebrew University, Hadassah Medical School, Jerusalem (Israel)

Van der Schaaf, A., Professor of Bacteriology and Infectious Diseases; Director, Institute for Veterinary Bacteriology, State University, Utrecht (The Netherlands)

Witenberg, G. G., D.V.Sc., Associate Professor of Parasitology, Hebrew University, Jerusalem (Israel)

Wolff, J. W., M.D., Emeritus Professor of Tropical Hygiene, University of Amsterdam; Director, Institute of Tropical Hygiene and Geographical Pathology, Department of the Royal Tropical Institute, Amsterdam (The Netherlands)

Zidon, J., M.D., Consultant Physician, Government Hospital, Tel Hashomer (Israel)

CONTENTS

Chapter I. Bacterial Diseases

Chapter II. Rickettsial Diseases

Chapter III. Viral Diseases

A. NEUROTROPIC VIRAL DISEASES

B. ARTHROPOD-BORNE ANIMAL VIRAL DISEASES

Chapter IV. Fungal Diseases

Chapter V. Protozoal Diseases

Chapter VI. Zooparasitic diseases

A. HELMINTHOZOONOSES

Chapter VII. Diseases of man transmissible through animals

INTRODUCTION

"Zoonoses are those diseases and infections which are naturally transmitted between vertebrate animals and man".

Second Report of the Joint World Health Organization/ Food and Agriculture Organization Expert Group on Zoonoses, 1958.

Since the dawn of history the diseases of man have been compared with those of animals. It was not, however, until the discovery of the pathogenic properties of certain bacteria and other lower organisms that similarities between several communicable diseases of man and animals were properly assessed. In consequence of this, many hitherto unknown epidemiological links between human and animal diseases were revealed.

Some diseases of animals, although they are not transmitted to man, may be extremely harmful to him in an indirect way. In certain remote regions of the world, epi- and panzootics deplete domestic and game animals to such an extent, that the local population is deprived of food of animal origin, serious protein deficiency following in its wake.

Until the beginning of the present century, the animal origin of only a small number of human diseases had been recognized (mainly: rabies, cowpox, anthrax, malleus, and a few zooparasitic infections). At the present time, far more than 100 zoonoses are known. Most of those which have been recently recognized are caused by viruses or zooparasites.

Not only have more zoonoses been discerned, but their pathogenesis and epidemiology have also been elucidated. It has, in fact, become evident that the animal world is a reservoir of the agents of numerous human diseases.

Zoonoses are now among the most frequent and most dreaded risks to which mankind is exposed. This is particularly true in the tropics and sub-tropics, where arthropod vectors play a significant part in the transmission of communicable diseases.

There is ample reason to believe that most of the present infectious and parasitic diseases of the human race have originated in animals. The pathogenic organisms adapted themselves to the environment of the human body, either as parasites or commensals, these associations being eventually reversible.

References p. 5

The effects produced in both man and animals are mainly determined by the invasive capacities of the pathogen and the host's resistance to it.

Several zoonoses are almost equally harmful to man and to animals (*e.g.* anthrax, plague, rabies, bovine-type tuberculosis). Others only rarely or slightly impair animal health, but cause serious illness in man (brucellosis, Q-fever, hydatidosis). A third group includes grave epizootics, which seldom affect man (foot and mouth disease, pasteurellosis, pseudorabies). However, the seriousness of a particular zoonosis may differ considerably in various territories and at different times.

Investigations on the presence of specific antibodies in human and animal populations in given regions have shed new light on the distribution of several zoonoses. Repetition of these investigations at intervals can provide interesting information on the natural history of infectious diseases in a particular region. This is especially true of viral infections which lead to antibody production without provoking clinically perceptible damage to the host. A prolonged carrier-state without serological response may also be established.

The recently acquired data have made necessary to revise in several respects our earlier conceptions of zoonoses.

A major role in the epidemiology of zoonoses is played by wild or domestic animals, which persistently carry and excrete organisms which are potentially pathogenic to man. This may occur not only when animals have recovered from overt disease, but may also be established in host-animals which have never shown signs of illness. Reservoirs of considerable importance are formed by those animals which are fairly resistant to the pathogens, and develop a chronic carrier-state, but are not themselves clinically affected (clinically inapparent-, subclinical-, or latent infections).

Apart from nutritional and industrial zoonotic infections, most zoonoses are characterised by their focal distribution within particular geographical territories (the "landscape epidemiology" of Pavlowsky). *Ecosystems* in these localities include defined *biocenoses* (species networks), which are composed of mutually connected animal communities, combined with the local vegetable and microbial world.

When, among the vertebrate animals living in these ranges, there are hosts of potential pathogens of man, a zoonotic *nidus* is created. Frequently, arthropods and other non-vertebrate animals serve as vectors and play an important, or often necessary, part in the cycles of infection.

Under the influence of seasonally defined climatic conditions, the ecosystem is subject to repeated changes, which affect the hosts, vectors and pathogens in their habitats. Man's infringements of the natural conditions, brought about by such practices as the reclamation of waste lands, artificial irrigation or changing crops, may contribute to alterations of the environment and therefore to the propagation or abatement of zoonoses in nature.

When man becomes involved in a zoonotic nidus, it is likely that the chain of inter-animal infections will be diverted to him. When this happens no further transmission of the parasite usually occurs, so that the human host becomes an end-point of the pathogen's existence. Occasionally, however, circumstances favour inter-human transmission, for instance, in bovine-type pulmonary tuberculosis or diaplacental infection with *Listeria* or *Toxoplasma*. Even actual epidemics may develop out of an individual zoonotic infection, as may happen in secondary pulmonary plague. This situation must be differentiated from pseudo-epidemic spread appearing when numerous individuals are simultaneously exposed to the animal reservoir of a zoonotic agent (bubonic plague in a heavily rat-infested area; leptospirosis among labourers in fields swarming with rodents).

Retrograde infections, from man to animals, only exceptionally occur.

Marked differences exist in the host–parasite relationships of man having contact with infected vertebrate animals living in nature, as compared with persons keeping domestic animals in semi-natural or artificial environments. Man's repeated and intimate contact with the animals he attends, promotes the chances of the transmission of their pathogenic organisms. Under conditions prevailing in nature, man is most frequently infected along indirect routes, *e.g.* by means of soil and water contaminated with animal excretions, or through the intervention of blood-sucking arthropods.

As a rule, the clinical and pathological characteristics of a zoonosis have many points in common in both man and animals, although the localisation of the lesions, their incidence, and their degree of gravity may vary considerably. These differences are related to the species of the host, his state of immunity and the portals of entry of the pathogens, as well as to the intensity and frequency of the exposure. It is obvious, therefore, that most zoonoses occur among individuals occupationally engaged in the handling of animals, their carcasses and products (veterinary surgeons, slaughter-house personnel, raisers of livestock, milkers, workers employed in factories processing animal products, etc.). Another group of people frequently affected comprises persons who repeatedly come into contact with soil, mud or water, which are readily contaminated by animal excretions (agricultural and sewer workers, fishermen, hunters, bathers). The agents causing alimentary zoonoses (*e.g. Salmonella* and helminths) may be present in food of animal origin (milk, meat, and their products).

It is impossible to record in a single volume the enormous amount of knowledge of the zoonoses recently acquired. It has been necessary, therefore, to impose strict limitations on the choice of the facts and problems to be discussed. Only essential historical information has been included. Diagnostic and therapeutic methods and systems have not been described in detail. Most emphasis has been laid on the discussion of epidemiological problems, comparative nosology and questions of preventive medicine.

Further it has been necessary to omit all those animal diseases, the transmission of which to man has only been surmised on weak epidemiological grounds, but has not definitely been established (*e.g.* bovine actinomycosis and vesicular coital exanthema).

Diseases like equine infectious anaemia or enzootic ovine abortion, which affect man extremely rarely, and under particular conditions only, have also been omitted. Likewise, no chapter has been devoted to the relapsing fevers. The importance of animal reservoirs as sources of these human infections has not been definitely proven while, moreover, certain differences have been established between the spirochaetes encountered in rodents in an endemic area and the *Borreliae* which cause relapsing fevers in man.

In addition to the zoonoses, the agents of which are found only or chiefly in animals, there are diseases caused by organisms which frequently occur in both man and the lower animals, so that it is not possible to ascertain which are their main hosts. These diseases differ from the others just mentioned in that man can not be safeguarded merely by the eradication of the causative agents from the animal-world. Because the animals are important, or potentially important as distributors of these pathogenic organisms, some parasitic diseases, such as dracontiasis, hirudiniasis and simian malaria, have been discussed in the following pages.

Considerations of space have, unfortunately, prevented the inclusion of exhaustive lists of references, and have obliged the authors to restrict themselves to the more important publications, preferably to those of recent years.

The reader who is interested in more detailed bibliographical information, may consult the books, monographs and reviews of literature which are inserted in the List of General References and in the separate lists appearing at the end of each chapter.

Ness Ziona, October 1963. J. VAN DER HOEDEN

GENERAL REFERENCES ON ZOONOSES

ABDUSSALAM, M., Significance of ecological studies of wild animal reservoirs of zoonoses, *Bull. Wld Hlth Org.*, 21 (1959) 179.

Advances in the Control of Zoonoses, *Wld Hlth Org. Monogr. Ser.*, No. 19 (1953) 275 pp.

AUDY, J. R., The localisation of disease with special reference to zoonoses. *Trans. roy. Soc. trop. Med. Hyg.*, 52 (1958) 308.

BROUARDEL, P. and A. GILBERT, Maladies communes à l'homme et aux animaux, *Nouveau Traité de Médecine et de Thérapeutique*, IV, Paris, 1906, 428 pp.

European Seminar on Veterinary Public Health, Regional Office for Europe, World Health Organization, Copenhagen, 1957, 435 pp.

GARNHAM, P. C. C., Zoonoses or infections common to man and animals, *J. trop. Med. Hyg.*, 61 (1958) 92.

HAGAN, W. A. and others, The relation of diseases in the lower animals to human welfare, *Ann. N.Y. Acad. Sci.*, 48 (1947) 225.

HEISCH, R. B., Zoonoses as a study in ecology, *Brit. Med. J.*, 4994 (1956) 669.

HOEDEN, J. VAN DER, *De Zoonosen* (Dutch), Leyden, 1946, 444 pp.

HULL, TH. G., *Diseases Transmitted from Animals to Man*, IV ed., Springfield, 1955, 717 pp.

Joint Wld Hlth Org./FAO Expert Group on Zoonoses, *techn. Rep. Ser.*, Geneva, First Session, No. 40, 1951, 48 pp.; Second Session, No. 169, 1959, 83 pp.

KOEGEL, A., *Zoonosen*, Basel, 1951, 243 pp.

LIEBERMAN, J. and others, Animal disease and human health, *Ann. N.Y. Acad. Sci.*, 70, 1958, 485 pp.

MAKOWER, H., Biocenologic problems in immunology, *Trans. N.Y. Acad. Sci.*, 20 (1958) 765.

MEYER, K. F., Animal diseases and human welfare, *Advanc. vet. Sci.*, 1 (1953) 1.

PARNAS, J., *Antropozoonozy* (Polish), Warsaw, 1960, 319 pp.

PAWLOVSKY, Y. N., Natural nidality of disease in relation to the ecology of the zoonoses, *Wld Hlth Org. Seminar on Veterinary Public Health*, Warsaw, 1957, 30 pp.

PAWLOVSSKY, Y. N., P. A. PETRISCHEVA, D. N. ZASUKHIN and N. C. OLSUFIEV, Naturla nidi of human diseases and regional epidemiology, Abstract *Trop. Dis. Bull.*, 54 (1957) 1266.

RUDNJEV, G. P., *Zoonosy* (Russian), Moscow, 1959, 284 pp.

STAFSETH, H. J. and others, Comparative medicine in transition, *Proc. First Inst. Veterinary Public Health Practice*, Ann Arbor, Mich., 1958, 499 pp.

STEELE, J. H., Animal diseases of public health significance, *Ann. Internal Med.*, 36 (1952) 511; Veterinary Public Health, *Advanc. vet. Sci.*, 1 (1953) 329.

Wld Hlth Org. techn. Rep. Ser., Arthropod-borne Viruses (Report of a Study Group). Geneva, 1961, 68 pp.

CHAPTER I

BACTERIAL DISEASES

1

J. VAN DER HOEDEN

Tuberculosis

The majority of vertebrates are susceptible to tuberculosis, a disease of world-wide incidence. Although the name tuberculosis did not appear in literature before 1840, the disease has existed among man's forbears since the dawn of history.

Tuberculous lesions have been found in mummies of the Rameses dynasties, which are some 30 centuries old. It is said that descriptions of lung lesions given in ancient Hindu manuscripts strongly suggest that these lesions were those of pulmonary tuberculosis. Hippocrates mentioned a disease of the lungs, the course of which was similar to that of tuberculosis pulmonum, and Aristotle knew that this condition is contagious. There are several indications that tuberculosis was widespread among the populations of the ancient Greek and Roman world.

The disease has also long been known in animals. The directions laid down in the Pentateuch and Talmudic scriptures for the conduct of sacrifices and slaughter-rituals, suggest that the ancient Jews were acquainted with the tuberculous lesions in ruminants.

However, considerable time elapsed before the aetiological identity of the disease in man and animals was recognized. In sixteenth century Europe it was generally believed that the multiple tumor-like tuberculous lesions in the serous membranes of cattle (pearl disease) had a syphilitic origin and that they were due to sodomy committed by luetic persons with cows ("Lustseuche", "Gallic disease"). This explains why individuals who consumed the meat of such animals were threatened with severe punishment. This baseless belief was not discredited until the end of the eighteenth century.

In the closing years of that century some physicians expressed their conviction that there was a similarity between human "consumption" and bovine tuberculosis. At that time the bovine tuberculosis was very widespread in Europe and it is beyond doubt that bovine infections affected many human beings, youthful individuals particularly.

R. and J. Dubos established that, in the nineteenth century, approximately half of the English population was afflicted by scrofula (infection of the lymph glands and sometimes of the bones and joint surfaces) of bovine origin. They illustrated the point by quoting an instance in which all of 78 boys and 91 of the 94 girls in a work-house in Kent became affected by this lesion. A similar situation was reported from an orphanage in Berlin, in which 53% of the children were infected.

It is inevitable that, because the aetiology of the disease was not at the time known, a great many tuberculous infections of man and animals remained unidentified as such, while lesions caused by other organisms were mistaken for tuberculosis.

In 1819, Laennec tried to clarify this confusion by accurately describing the ailments which he considered to be tuberculous in nature; but much later, Virchow still regarded tuberculous lesions in the lungs and serous membranes of animals as being neoplasms, comparable with lymphosarcomatosis in human beings.

The first successful transmission of the disease to healthy rabbits was described by Klencke in 1843. After that (1865), Villemin, in a series of classical experiments, demonstrated that tuberculosis of man, as well as that of cows, can be transmitted to rabbits and guinea pigs. This result strikingly suggested that the morbid factor which caused the lesions in the human tissues was the same as that which caused the lesions in animals.

The aetiological agent was finally discovered by R. Koch in 1882. In his earliest communication he concluded that "Perlsucht" of cattle has the same aetiology as human tuberculosis and that consequently, for the sake of man's health, measures should be taken to protect him against infection by tuberculosis of bovine origin.

Better insight into the epidemiology of tuberculosis was gained from the investigations of Th. Smith (1896–1898) who taught that there were constant cultural and pathogenic differences between the bacterial strains isolated from man and those recovered from animals. This fact and also other considerations convinced Koch that his former views must be revised. At the British Congress on Tuberculosis in 1901 he expressed the belief that the human body is as strongly resistant to infection by the bovine-type of tubercle bacteria, as cattle were known to be against the human-type bacteria. Koch therefore concluded that preventive measures directed against infection of human beings with the bovine type bacteria were practically superfluous. Koch's authority was so great that his rash conclusions were accepted by the majority of physicians. The result was that many hygienic measures that had been advocated were gradually neglected and medical men lost interest in veterinary work on the control of bovine tuberculosis.

Later, however, Koch's views were strongly criticised. When the final Report of the British Commission on Tuberculosis appeared in 1911, most of the problems discussed in it had been satisfactorily worked out. In this report it was established that: ". . . the bovine tubercle bacillus has a high degree of pathogenic power to man, which is especially manifest in the early years of life, . . .", ". . . bovine animals are completely immune to the human tubercle bacillus, and adult human beings can be infected with the bovine type, even the pulmonary form of the disease in man being sometimes caused by the bovine tubercle bacillus . . .", ". . . there can be no doubt that a considerable proportion of the tuberculosis affecting children is of bovine origin, more particularly that which affects primarily the abdominal organs and the cervical glands".

The genus *Mycobacterium* (order: *Actinomycetales,* family: *Mycobacteriaceae*) includes a number of saprophytic and parasitic species. All of these are acid-fast rods, that is to say, after staining with anilin dyes they keep the colour when they are subsequently exposed to acid. They are mostly slender, straight or slightly curved rods, but are sometimes more filamentous. They are aerobic and non-motile. It has recently been shown that their metabolism is important for their differentiation.

In nature, *Mycobacteria* are found in soil and water (*e.g.* the Hay bacillus, *M. phleï*); they are often present on the skin and mucous membranes (*e.g.* the smegma bacillus), and are commonly found in milk and dairy products. Under certain favourable conditions, some of the "non-pathogenic" mycobacteria cause localized lesions and a few of these may be mentioned:

A strongly acid-fast strain can be frequently isolated from human cases of pulmonary tuberculosis; it forms bright yellow colonies. Another mycobacterium, which resembles the mammalian types of *M. tuberculosis* (*M. ulcerans*, McCallum *et al.*, 1948) causes localized chronic or subacute indolent ulceration in the cutis and subcutis of the human extremities (in Australia, North America and the Congo). The more rapidly developing *M. balnei* (Linell and Norden, 1954) has many features in common with *M. ulcerans* and is frequently encountered in Sweden as the agent of dermal ulcers on the limbs and arms, which are epidemiologically connected with swimming pools. Neither of the species just mentioned develops at temperatures above 35° and they do not cause lesions in guinea pigs, though they are pathogenic to mice and sometimes to rats.

Some pathogenic mycobacteria either grow very poorly in artificial media, or have not yet been cultivated. Examples of these are the "leprabacillus" of man (Hansen), buffaloes (Lobel) and rats (Stefansky) and the acid-fast bacteria associated with the "so-called skin-tuberculosis" (skin-lesions) of cattle (Traum).

An acid-fast organism important in veterinary practice is *M. paratuberculosis*, which causes serious chronic hypertrophic enteritis (Johne's disease) in cattle, sheep and goats.

The mycobacteria just mentioned are not aetiological factors in any zoonoses, but they are important because several of them can sensitize the host animal and can thus cause "false reactions" with tuberculin, which interfere with the control of bovine tuberculosis (see page 45).

The pathogenic mycobacteria require for their development *in vitro* nutrient media containing chicken egg, blood serum, asparagin, glycerin or other special substances. Their growth is rather slow. All types of *M. tuberculosis* are strongly resistant to desiccation and to acids and alkalis and they are relatively resistant to a number of disinfectants. Direct sunlight destroys *M. tuberculosis* rather quickly. In the shade it remains viable for 2 to 5 months or longer, depending on the temperature. The medium in which the bacteria are contained also plays a role. In large portions of sputum they were found alive after several months, but in finely divided droplets and dust particles they survived for only a number of days. In sewage, living bacteria were recovered for 100 to 200 days. The avian type *Mycobacterium tuberculosis* is even more resistant than the mammalian types. It remained alive for as long as 4 years in soil and for at least 2 years in the buried carcasses of fowl (Schalk *et al.,* 1935).

The distribution of the three types of *M. tuberculosis* is mainly correlated with that of man, bovines or birds, although many other animal species may become hosts and may be affected.

The types are determined by the cultural appearance of freshly isolated strains on solid egg-media, and by their pathogenicity for rabbits, guinea pigs and chickens. Guinea pigs are highly susceptible to infection with strains of the human and bovine-type bacteria, but in this animal the avian type causes only a local abscess.

The *human-type* of *M. tuberculosis* grows slowly, development being improved by the addition of glycerin to the medium. After a few weeks at 37° the colonies will be dry, rough, granular to warty and of a yellow-orange colour. They are strongly attached to the medium and it is difficult to homogenize them in aqueous suspension (*eugonic* growth). Intravenous injection of 0.01 mg of the culture into the bloodstream of a rabbit does not affect the general health of the animal and autopsy done several months later, reveals only few isolated regressing tubercles in the lungs and abdominal organs.

Growth of the *bovine-type* bacteria is even slower. Glycerin concentration above 0.75% hampers their development. The colourless colonies are small, flat, somewhat gleamy, with a pasty consistence and they are easily emulsified in water (*dysgonic* growth). Injection of 0.01 mg of the freshly isolated culture into the blood stream kills a rabbit within 3 to 4 weeks, and at post mortem examination it shows extreme emaciation and the organs are usually studded with tiny tubercles.

The *avian type (typus gallinaceus)* develops readily, even at temperatures above 40° into a creamy or pasty layer with soft wart-like or dome-shaped elevations each with a central indentation, especially in the presence of glycerin. The culture can be easily homogenized in water. Injection of a sufficient number of bacteria into rabbits or fowls produces either numerous tubercles, or a septicaemia without visible tubercles but characterized by the presence of an enormous number of mycobacteria scattered throughout the tissues (Yersin).

The *murine-type (M. microti, M. tuberculosis* var. *muris,* Wells, 1937) multiplies very slowly on solid egg media, growth being inhibited by glycerin. Its pathogenicity for the rabbit, guinea pig and fowl is low, but in mice it induces generalized tuberculosis.

Tubercle bacteria of the *cold-blooded type* differ considerably from mammalian- and avian-type mycobacteria.

The cultural and biological features upon which the division of the mammalian types is based are not absolutely constant. Dysgonic bovine strains subcultured on artificial media during a protracted period of time often produce a few eugonic colonies, which may gradually increase in number until finally the total culture assumes the aspect of the human-type growth. Although the virulence usually retains its high level for a long time, in some instances it declines. Strains which have altered the visible features of their growth and have become attenuated may cause confusion when an attempt is made to establish the type originally isolated from the body.

Exceptionally even the primary culture made from the animal may show an intermediate character.

Among 5,000 strains isolated from human beings, Jensen and Kiaer (1939) found that 14 showed intermediate features. In two cases of pulmonary tuberculosis, from which Jensen and Lester (1941) initially cultivated bacteria of the bovine type, isolates from the same patients taken at later dates showed a tendency towards human-type growth, pure eugonic cultures being ultimately recovered.

These examples indicate a certain degree of instability in the bovine-type strains.

The British Commission on Tuberculosis had already expressed the view that alterations of the type characteristics can suddenly appear as mutants, or can gradually develop when a new host species is infected. Because mixed infections with human- and bovine-type bacteria may occur, great caution should be exercised in concluding that bovine-type bacteria may be transformed into human-type bacteria as a result of adaptation to the metabolism of the human organism.

The fact has often been observed that bovine-type strains isolated from lupus vulgaris of man, as well as those isolated from various organs of wild animals (in Zoological Gardens) show low pathogenicity for guinea pigs and rabbits (attenuated virulence).

In an investigation conducted by the author, all 133 bovine-type strains from cattle and all 84 strains from human origin showed the characteristic type properties, whereas 2 out of 10 strains from horses developed purely eugonically in their primary cultures, and retained this feature after passages through guinea pigs and rabbits. One equine strain showed chiefly dysgonic growth with a few eugonic colonies and a fourth strain changed, after several transmissions *in vitro*, its original pure dysgonic appearance into the eugonic type of growth. It is noteworthy that the virulence to rabbits of all these ten strains of equine origin had preserved the typical "bovine character".

In contrast, Griffith observed, in strains isolated from horses, a "human-type virulence" combined with a "bovine-type cultural aspect".

As opposed to the usual high virulence of the dysgonic bovine-type strains, dysgonic human-type strains have the same low pathogenicity for rabbits as that characteristic of the human type, but they maintain their ordinary high virulence for guinea pigs.

The development and character of the disease is determined by several factors among which the following may be mentioned: the site of entrance of the organisms into the host, their type, virulence and initial number, their rate of multiplication in the host's tissues, and the sensitivity or resistance of the infected animal, which is conditioned by earlier infections.

In the majority of human cases, the relationship between the host and the parasite leads to a condition of balance which approximates to labile commensalism. When this equilibrium is disturbed by a decline of the general or local resistance, the potential parasitic capacity of the agent will be expressed in the development of pathological activity.

Whereas in brucellosis the younger host is less susceptible to infection, in tuberculosis the young host is generally more susceptible than the older one is. However, the total number of young cattle infected is considerably lower than that of the older stock. This can be explained by the fact that, contrary to what usually happens in young children, recovery from tuberculous infection in young cattle is the exception. Thornton (1952) found that the incidence of tuberculous infection among slaughter cattle in Great Britain was: 1.8% of calves, 5.9% of bullocks, 6.5% of heifers, 28.4% of bulls and 44.5% of cows.

The response to infection with a given type of *M. tuberculosis* may differ in certain breeds of the same animal species. This has been observed in rabbits, some races of which inhibit these bacteria more vigorously than other breeds do.

Gray *et al.* (1960) concluded, from observations on so-called resistant and susceptible strains of mice, that no significant difference existed in natural resistance to pulmonary infection, but that there was probably a genetically determined difference in the rate of onset of acquired immunity after infection.

It is a generally recognized fact that Zebu cattle are considerably less affected by tuberculosis than are European cattle breeds; crosses between European and Zebu cattle produce a fairly resistant breed. Indigenous races of cattle in Japan and Indonesia have the reputation of being more highly resistant to the disease than are cattle imported into those countries. As a rule, milk cows are more frequently affected than beef or labour cattle (Wilsdon, in 1937, recorded in Great Britain an incidence of 23.7% of tuberculosis among dairy cattle, and of only 2.8% among the Hereford beef race).

The higher incidence of tuberculosis in dairy cattle as compared with beef races is comprehensible, because individuals in such herds are more closely in contact and are more frequently stabled; they are also subjected to the continuous physiological strain of excessive milk production and they reach a higher average age.

Similar variations in susceptibility have been observed among different human races. Negroes, Indians, Chinese and Javanese individuals have often showed higher morbidity and mortality rates than the white population in the same regions or countries. These differences have been connected with varying ability to develop specific resistance after primary infection (Pinner, 1940). To a large extent they may, however, be attributed to the widely dissimilar ways of life and the diverse environmental conditions of the groups compared.

It is a universal experience that the incidence of bovine tuberculosis increases in proportion to the density of the cattle populations, *i.e.* to the size of the herds and the space alloted to the cattle when they are kept indoors. On pasture, the risk of infection is considerably less than it is in the barn. Abdussalam (1956), for example, found that, in Indo-Pakistan, most of the cattle and buffaloes living in the open, and scattered in small groups in the villages, were free from tuberculosis, whereas 25 % or more of the dairy herds living in the vicinity of cities were infected.

The bovine type of *M. tuberculosis* is pathogenic to a larger number of animal species than the human type is. It is especially pathogenic to cattle, goats, buffaloes, cats, rabbits, mice and voles.

It has long been thought that man and monkeys are more susceptible to infection by the human-type than by the bovine-type tubercle bacterium; but opinion on this point is no longer unanimous. The incidence of human-type or bovine-type tuberculosis and the course of the disease provoked by each of these types are markedly influenced by the different rates of exposure (density of infective agent and frequency of repeated infection) and the portals of entry (aerogenic, alimentary, dermal or via the conjunctiva or other mucous membranes). Exceptionally congenital tuberculosis occurs in calves.

When the young host has no specific immunity the infection may become generalised along the lymphatics, or less frequently, by way of the blood circulation. As a rule, in cattle of all ages, the first aërogenous infection causes a broncho-pneumonia which progresses slowly. After a long period of inactivity, a sudden flare-up may occur. In children on the other hand, the primary complex usually is non-progressive and heals

completely, although in adults it may spread by way of the bronchi.
The chief mode of infection of adult human beings and of cattle is by inhalation of minute airborne droplets of sputum or of dust particles spread
by coughing by human beings or animals with active pulmonary lesions.
The lungs are more susceptible to infection than the upper respiratory tract.

In the *cow*, the primary complex commonly consists of specific inflammatory lesions of the alveoli, bronchioli and regional lymphatic nodes.

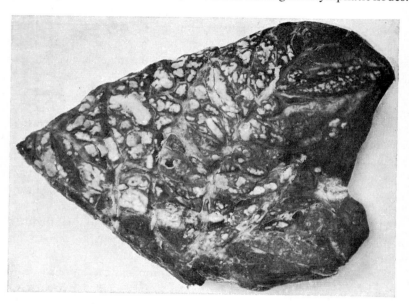

Fig. 1.   Lobular and acinous lesions with soft caseous contents in tuberculosis of the
bovine lung. (Photo: Institute for Veterinary Pathology, State University, Utrecht)

Some of these lesions may heal with fibrosis or calcification, but most
often they become necrotic. From these caseous or liquefied foci M.
tuberculosis may get into the bronchial system, thus transmitting
tubercle bacteria to various parts of the lung, where they establish new
centres of infection, the regional lymph nodes being at the same time
involved (Fig. 1).

In addition to this bronchogenous dissemination the tubercle bacteria
may be transported along the lymph vessels. In adult cattle the predominant form of tuberculosis is a chronic pneumonitis which shows a
tendency towards softening of the tissue.

Whereas in human beings in whom the primary infection has subsided, the lesions, as a rule, are located in the apical and dorsal parts of the lung, in cattle, they are chiefly found in the dorso-caudal portions.

True cavity formation, due to liquefaction of caseous tissue is rather common in man, and the dog, cat and goat, but it is not a feature of tuberculosis of cattle.

"Grape- or pearl disease", in which numerous globular nodes on the serous membranes of the chest and abdomen are found (Fig. 2), is often a feature of chronic bovine tuberculosis. It is usually the result of trans-

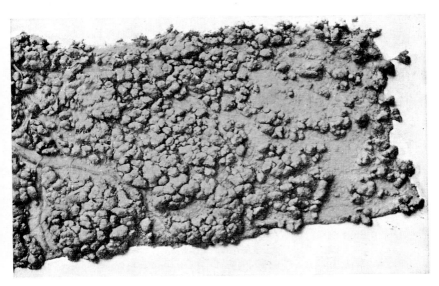

Fig. 2. "Pearl disease" of bovine omentum.
(Photo: Institute for Veterinary Pathology, State University, Utrecht)

portation of the bacteria by the lymphatics, or less frequently through the blood stream; it is seldom caused by the direct discharge into the body cavities of infectious material derived from disintegrating lesions.

Tuberculosis of the mammary glands is, as a rule, haematogenous in origin. After infection, several months may elapse before clinical changes are observed. During this interval, however, the apparently normal milk may already contain a large number of tubercle bacteria. The first noticeable sign of the infection is swelling of the affected quarter, of the udder, which acquires a firmer consistency. Subsequently the infection may develop in very different ways. The acute disseminated form, characterized by rapidly caseating and, later, sometimes calcifying, foci may result in extensive destruction, or it may acquire the aspect of diffuse mastitis caseosa. In about 75% of all cases, tuberculous mastitis has a chronic nodular or diffuse granulomatous character. Large foci some-

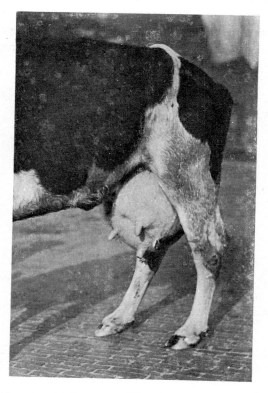

Fig. 3. Tuberculous mastitis in a cow. (Photo: Department of Internal Diseases. Veterinary Faculty, State University, Utrecht)

times soften, filling the milk sinuses with necrotic material. Diffuse tuberculous galactophoritis involves only the milk ducts. In most instances tuberculosis of the udder is restricted to only one of the quarters and also its supra-mammary lymph nodes (Fig. 3).

Several investigators observed excretion of tubercle bacteria from apparently normal milk-glands of cows which have tuberculous lesions elsewhere. In these cases the organisms had probably been conveyed by the blood stream during casual stages of bacteraemia.

In Denmark, Petersen (1948) recorded, between 1931 and 1933, among severe forms of bovine tuberculosis, 10,203 instances of lesions in the lungs, 2,064 cases of mastitis and 1,822 of metritis. Stamp observed similar high incidences of tuberculous mastitis (44%) in cases of advanced tuberculosis.

In cases of tuberculous enteritis, the site most affected is the small intestine, in which numerous minor ulcers occur. These lesions constantly liberate large numbers of *M. tuberculosis.*

Statistical data on the distribution of tuberculous lesions in the various organs of cattle will vary according to the source of the material examined. Thus, records from slaughterhouses will generally be less accurate and complete than those from veterinary research institutes. It should, more-over, be born in mind that in abattoirs the animals inspected are chiefly healthy ones, whereas research material often consists of carcasses of animals, some of which have died as a result of a chronic disease.

Table I compares the data collected from post mortem examinations in the slaughter-house and at the Institute for Pathology of the Veterinary Faculty in Utrecht (Schor-nagel, 1926).

TABLE I

FREQUENCY OF TUBERCULOUS LESIONS IN THE ORGANS OF COWS, ALL OF WHICH SHOWING PULMONARY TUBERCULOSIS

Analysis of 100 cases each

Cows	Lungs	Serous mem-branes	Liver	Intestines and mesent-eric lymph nodes	Spleen	Kidney	Uterus	Milk gland
Slaughtered	100	13	16	24	4	8	3	4
Succumbed	100	90	86	60	50	30	65	8

Only the open forms of tuberculosis disseminate the disease from cattle. The most important vehicles of the organisms leaving the animals are milk (mastitis), urine (nephritis), uterine secretion (metritis), faeces (enteritis and hepatitis) and sputum (pulmonary tuberculosis). Large quantities of contaminated sputum may be swallowed and afterwards excreted in the faeces.

Until an intensive systematic campaign was launched against the disease, the incidence of bovine tuberculosis was alarmingly high in most European countries. By these standards the overall incidence in the U.S.A., Canada and Japan has always been comparatively low. In most modern countries, the disease has markedly decreased or has even disappeared as a result of the eradication campaigns of the last decades (see page 43).

The great majority of tuberculous infections of cattle are caused by bacteria of the bovine-type. In districts in which tuberculosis has been eradicated from cattle, a "clean" herd can easily be reinfected by the sputum of human beings infected with the bovine-type of *M. tuberculosis*. Infection of cattle by the human-type bacterium has not been observed clinically. The lesions thus caused in cattle are found only at slaughter as sparse, mostly calcified tubercles; they are usually restricted to the site at which they settled in the body and in the neighbouring lymph nodes, especially in the abdomen and sometimes also in the lungs. In spite of the insignificance of these lesions, infected cattle react to the tuberculin test. When the source of infection is removed, the allergic state usually disappears within 6 to 9 months.

An illustrative epidemiological example has been given by Stenius in Finland (1938, 1941). The refuse from a tuberculosis sanatorium flowed by way of a septic tank through an outlet pipe 1250 m long, which ended in a brooklet and debouched into a small pond along the shores of which cattle grazed. The cattle, which were originally tuberculin-negative, became, after watering at the brook, tuberculin-positive. The same thing happened in cows which were deliberately given the water from the pond. It was found that the waste water was contaminated with viable tubercle bacteria of the human-type.

In bovine pathology, the avian-type infection is more important than the human-type infection. The allergy induced is stronger in response to avian than to mammalian tuberculin.

Bovine infection with the avian-type bacteria is most frequently of alimentary origin. Plum (1952), in Denmark, isolated from the lungs, mediastinal and bronchial lymph nodes of cattle, 769 strains of the bovine-type and 24 of the avian-type; from mesenterial nodes, he recorded 109 bovine type and 241 avian-type, and from the retro-pharyngeal nodes, 94 bovine- and 27 avian-type strains.

Although most avian-type infections in bovines remain localized in the lymph nodes, the illness caused may be more severe or even very serious.

An appreciable number of tuberculous abortions have been recorded in Denmark, especially by Plum (1925), who recovered avian-type strains in 6 of 151 aborting cows, isolating the organism from the mesenterial lymph nodes of the foeti. The expulsion of the foetus was due to an exudative inflammation of the uterine mucosa.

As early as 1908, O. Bang described a case of miliary avian tuberculosis in a cow. Ottosen (1944) observed ulcerative lesions in the intestines and peritoneal and pleural avian-type infection disseminated by the blood. In Holland, the author (1941) isolated 137 bovine- and 4 avian-type strains from tuberculous cows.

All of the latter had been derived from very serious cases with extensive miliary dissemination and involvement of lungs, kidneys, liver and various lymph nodes. Particularly noticeable were lobular and acinous foci in the lungs with the unusual feature of extremely dense miliary dissemination, resembling very moist catarrhal pneumonia. Numerous miliary and submiliary tubercles were present in the liver, partly perforated into the blood vessels. One cow had many isolated tubercles in various organs, like necrotic islands embedded in the tissues. Two similar cases have been described in Holland by Post and van Ulsen (1954).

Thorshaug (1947) observed a steep decline in milk yield from a dairy herd infected with avian-type tuberculosis. Several instances have been reported of long-term excretion of avian-type tubercle bacteria in the milk from outwardly normal udders.

Although *goats* are strongly susceptible to experimental infection with mammalian and avian tubercle bacteria, "spontaneous" tuberculosis in this animal seldom occurs. In German abattoirs, during a 25-year period, tuberculosis was observed in only 0.69 to 1.04% of the goats, as compared with 25.39 to 36.73% of the cows. As a cause of death, however, tuberculosis in goats is a rather important disease. Whereas in abattoirs in the Netherlands only 1 out of about 1000 goats was found to be infected, no less than 7 out of 105 goats which had died at the Veterinary Clinics, showed a serious form of tuberculosis.

Several records are available which show that, in mixed herds of cattle and goats, cross infection easily occurs. Klein (1959) found that, among the goats on a farm with a tuberculous cattle herd, 28.3% of the goats reacted to tuberculin, while on an attested farm only 1.1% reacted.

In Germany, Beller isolated from goats 28 bovine-type strains and 1 avian-type strain; in Holland the author obtained 15 strains of the bovine- and 2 of the avian-type.

References p. 48–49

While most bovine-type infections in goats are air-borne, avian-type infections are usually intestinal. Whereas in kids the disease is rapidly progressive, adult goats may partly or completely recover from the infection. Soliman *et al.* in the U.K. (1953) detected lesions in only 32 of 39 goats which gave positive tuberculin tests.

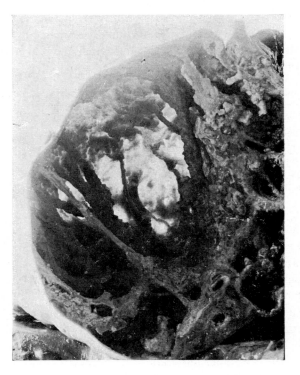

Fig. 4. Large cavern in right main lobe of goat's lung with bovine-type tuberculosis. (Photo: Institute for Veterinary Pathology, State University, Utrecht)

According to the author's (1941) experience in the Netherlands, very serious, strongly exudative processes with extensive cavity-formation in the lungs and multiple ulcers in the intestines are common in the clinical picture of tuberculous caprines (Fig. 4). This is true of both avian- and bovine-type infections. From the literature it is evident that, unlike cattle, goats respond to infection by the human-type bacteria almost as strongly as they do to the bovine-type. Tuberculous goats may be very dangerous spreaders of *M. tuberculosis* by way of the sputum, urine and faeces.

In *sheep*, tuberculosis is even rarer than it is in goats. Only 2 out of 237 autopsies of sheep which died at the Veterinary Clinics in Utrecht showed tuberculous lesions.

Out of 255,000 sheep in the Blackburn slaughter house only 2 had tuberculosis (Jowett, 1928).

All the three bacterial types have been recovered from sheep, but the bovine and the avian types predominated. In Uganda, where sheep and fowl are housed in the natives' huts, a high incidence of avian-type tuberculosis has been occasionally reported in both animals. Harshfield *et al.* (1937), examining sheep with avian-type infection, observed miliary lesions of the lungs, liver, spleen and lymph nodes. In several cases only a few rather large tubercles were found and these showed early calcification and much adjacent fibrosis.

From India, Pakistan and Egypt a fairly high incidence of bovine-type tuberculosis has been reported in *buffaloes*. There was a tendency to lung lesions and a strong tendency to caseation and softening. In contrast to cattle, calcification and pearl disease of the serous membranes are rarely observed in the buffalo.

From the Cairo slaughter house, tuberculosis has been reported in 5.4% of *camels*.

Tuberculosis of *equines* differs in several respects from the disease in other animals, its incidence being very low.

Equine tuberculosis has been recorded from European countries; it averages less than one hundredth of that found in cattle. In Germany (1941–1949), tuberculous lesions were found in 1.5% of slaughtered horses, in Denmark (1910–1932) in 0.14%, in Sweden (1921–1942) in 0.09%, in Great Britain (1943–1949) in 0.0025%, in France (1936–1941) in 0.011% and (1942–1947) 0.0053%.

The anatomical features of the lesions in tuberculosis of horses differ considerably from those of the lesions found in ruminants. Formerly this fact caused much confusion in the aetiological diagnosis. In general, equine tissues show strong resistance to tuberculosis. Some investigators claim that *M. tuberculosis* is apt to pass through the horse's lung without leaving behind any lesions that are macroscopically perceptible. Tissue regression is usually slight and calcification does not occur, proliferation being the most typical reaction. However, once the infection is established in the horse, it may provoke very serious lesions.

Thus in equines tuberculous nodules which are macroscopically of homogenous structure and resemble chronic granulation tissue or sarcoma, appear particularly in the spleen (Fig. 5), lung and lymph nodules.

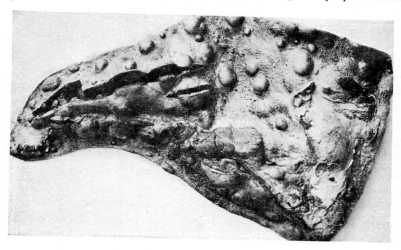

Fig. 5.   Chronic tuberculosis of horse's spleen.
(Photo: Institute for Veterinary Pathology, State University, Utrecht)

The mesenterial nodes may be exceedingly large. Compared with ruminants, the localization of the lesions in horses is strikingly different. Most remarkable is their high incidence in the spleen and bones; of the latter the vertebrae are especially involved. A frequent symptom is stiffness of the neck due to osteitis and osteomyelitis of the cervical vertebrae, which prevents the animal from taking food from the ground. Scott (1930) reported tuberculosis of the skin in 8 % of the affected horses.

As a rule, horses become infected through the alimentary tract, mostly at an early age, probably because they have been fed on untreated cow's

TABLE II

FREQUENCY OF TUBERCULOUS LESIONS OBSERVED IN THE ORGANS OF HORSES
(Schornagel, 1926)

Lung	Serous membranes	Liver	Mesenterial lymph nodes	Spleen	Kidney	Bones
55	30	22	30	90	5	44

milk. In some horses, the disease does not much impair the animal's general condition for long, the only signs of illness being gradual emaciation and stiffness. Not seldom the horse remains fit for work until shortly before it dies.

About 80 to 90% of the strains isolated from horses are of the bovine type; among the remainder, more avian- than human-type strains were found.

In contrast, however, to what has just been described, miliary lesions are sometimes produced. The author (1941) observed avian-type tuberculosis in horses with very extensive miliary dissemination all over the lungs, combined with diffuse spread in the considerably enlarged liver and numerous mycobacteria in smears of the organs.

Because tuberculosis is rare in equines and usually takes a closed form, these animals are of little or no significance in the spread of tuberculous infection to man or other animals.

Swine are highly susceptible to alimentary infection with the bovine and avian types of *M. tuberculosis* and are not uncommonly infected by the human type as well. The incidence of infection with the three types respectively varies according to the degree of exposure to infected cattle, poultry or man and according to the feeding habits of pigs. Because they are coprophagous, pigs may swallow the dung of cows contaminated with tubercle bacteria. Also, on several farms, swine live in close contact with fowl which excrete in their droppings avian-type bacteria. Not rarely farmers throw dead chickens and slaughter offal into the pig sty. Phthisical attendants may infect the hogs with their sputum, by spitting on the ground. Food containing garbage left over from the household or from a hospital has also been the source of human-type infection of pigs.

Because of the variability of local conditions, considerable differences exist in the distribution of the bacterial types (Table III).

Bovine-type and avian-type strains have been repeatedly isolated from one and the same pig.

In Norway, the occurrence of human-type infection in pigs has been utilized by the Public Health Service as a means for the detection of tuberculosis in the rural population. Fourie *et al.* (1950) described in South Africa an outbreak of subclinical tuberculous infection of pigs which was caused by the human-type bacterium.

The control of bovine tuberculosis has not only resulted in a significant

References p. 48–49

TABLE III

TYPES OF *M. tuberculosis* ISOLATED FROM SWINE

Country	Year	Total number of strains examined	Types bovine %	avian %	human %
Great Britain	1936	258	71	27	2
Holland	1941	168	66.7	33.3	0
Germany	1931	101	69.4	29.61	0.99
Sweden	1939	121	89.25	8.27	2.48
Belgium	1933	57	80.7	3.5	15.8
Denmark	1946	310	13.9	84.5	1.6
Norway	1935	67	4.5	74.6	20.9
Finland *	1935	34	29.4	0	70.6
Bornholm **	1935	102	0	100	0
North America	1925	209	5.2	88.5	6.2
Portugal	1939	50	22	2.5	75.5

* No tuberculosis in fowl.
** After total eradication of tuberculosis from cattle.

decline of the total number of tuberculous infections in swine, but has also shifted the incidence of the causative types towards avian- and human-type infections.

In 1924 the U.S. Federal meat inspectors reported tuberculous lesions in 16% of the total pig kill and this figure declined to 11% in 1929, to 9.43% in 1937 and to 2.8% in 1958. The incidence varied widely in different parts of the U.S.A.: in 1936 in the abattoir of Kansas City 4.93% of the slaughter pigs showed tuberculosis, in the abattoir of Denver the percentage was found to be 25%. As early as 1925, van Es and Martin remarked that no parallelism existed between the incidence of infection among bovines and porcines in the same localities. The reason for this became apparent when it was found that the avian-type infection was present in 88.51% of the swine which had tuberculous lymph nodes. Mixed infection of the avian and mammalian types was found in 6.22% and pure mammalian-type infection in 5.21%.

At the present time, after successful campaigns against bovine tuberculosis, avian-type tubercle bacteria are almost exclusively responsible for the disease in hogs in the U.S.A. and in several other countries.

With the exception of direct infections of young piglets due to sucking a tuberculous sow's udder, pig-to-pig transmission is extremely rare. As a rule, the most serious lesions are caused by bovine-type bacteria. In the majority of cases they enter the body by way of the alimentary tract. Starting from the primary lesions in the throat (tonsils) and abdomen (mesenterium), generalization follows along the haemato-lymphogenous routes.

Tuberculosis in swine affects essentially the lymphatic tissues. Lesions appear most frequently in the lymph nodes and the liver. As a rule there is a marked difference in the morbid processes produced by the bovine- and the avian-types of *M. tuberculosis*. The former are commonly circumscribed, with a strong tendency to early caseation, central softening and calcification, and they are apt to become encapsulated by fibrous peripheral reaction of the tissues of the organ affected. In contrast, avian-type infection is usually characterized by diffuse, homogenous, smooth formations, which strongly resemble adenomatous or sarcomatous neoplasms. Usually no true tubercles are produced. Caseation, when it is present, remains a minor feature, but calcification is more marked. There is, as a rule, no pus-like softening of the lesions and encapsulation does not occur.

Besides involving the lymphatic tissue and parenchymatous organs, tuberculosis is common in the bones, particularly the vertebrae, and from the latter meningitis may develop. Joint lesions are rather frequently observed. Sometimes the lung shows numerous, minute, pneumonia-like solid lesions which have a fatty-lustrous appearance, these lesions being partly caseous and containing cavities. In the intestines, tuberculous foci are very rarely observed, even when the contiguous lymph nodes are extensively affected.

Avian-type tubercle bacteria have been isolated several times from tissues which show no macroscopic lesions, especially from lymph nodes and even from the muscles. According to Eastwood and Griffith (1925), avian tubercle bacteria in swine have a tendency to escape from the lesions and to enter the blood stream, by which they are carried all over the body and are later found in tissues which are apparently normal.

Contrary to the prevailing belief of meat inspectors and pathologists, Feldman contended in 1938 that avian-type tubercle bacteria may provoke extensively disseminated lesions in the liver, spleen, lungs, and kidneys.

In a region of Minnesota where tuberculosis most frequently occurred among chickens, he found that avian-type bacteria were the sole aetiologic agent in 24 out of 30 swine which had been declared unfit for human consumption on account of generalized tuberculosis. Crawford, in the same year, found avian-type infection in 21, and bovine-type bacteria in 15 condemned swine slaughtered in different places in Northern Central American States.

References p. 48–49

There are several points of similarity between tuberculosis in *dogs* and in man. Both hosts are relatively resistant to the mammalian types of the tubercle bacterium, although the disease may become very serious. Open forms are frequent and in view of the intimate cohabitation between man and dog the chances of mutual transmission are great. Avian-type infection is extremely rare in dogs. In almost all the statistics, especially in those from large population centers, the human-type infection predominates over bovine-type tuberculosis in the canine (65, 70, 75, 82% recorded). This is in sharp contrast with *cats,* which, although not less often exposed to human-type contamination than dogs are, almost exclusively are infected by bovine-type bacteria. Kuwabara (1938) failed to provoke lesions in cats by infecting them with human-type bacteria. The only record of spontaneous infection of cats with this type, reported by Rabinovitsch (1921) in Berlin, is insufficiently documented and should, therefore, be regarded with due reservation. Including these doubtful cases, Verge (1945) reviewed the type-determination of strains isolated from dogs and cats in various countries, as follows (Table IV):

TABLE IV

TYPES OF *M. tuberculosis* FOUND IN DOGS AND CATS

Strains from	Total number examined	Types of bacteria			
		Bovine	Human	Atypical	Avian
Dogs	606	200 (33.1%)	392 (64.7%)	12 (2%)	2 (0.3%)
Cats	132	126 (95.4%)	6 (4.5%)	—	—

The percentage of incidence of tuberculosis among dogs and cats admitted to veterinary clinics are given in Table V:

TABLE V

Place	Years	Dogs	Cats
Berlin	1925	0.3	2
Paris	1927	5.6	13.5
Stockholm	1928–37	2.5	4.8
Utrecht	1926–44	1.03	4.66
Amsterdam and Leyden	1942–44	1.5	11
London	1940	1	3.6
Liverpool	1949	6.5	13

The disease most frequently affects the young cat and dog. Among dogs, the incidence is higher in males than in females, and some breeds seem to be more susceptible to tuberculosis than others. Direct dog-to-dog or cat-to-cat infections are very rare.

Many dogs become infected with human-type bacteria along the respiratory route, but alimentary infection by human sputum and food remains from the table is also common. Cats mostly acquire bovine-type infections through the digestive tract, most frequently by drinking unboiled milk or by eating slaughter offal.

Huitema and van Vloten (1960) cultured the murine-type of tubercle bacteria from a cat with tuberculous lesions of the lungs and mesenterial lymph nodes.

Slight infections in dogs may resolve without sequelae. The primary affection of the lungs is bronchopneumonic; it takes the form of greyish-white circumscribed, neoplasm-like nodules, in which caseous and soft material, containing numerous tubercle bacteria, appears. These nodules often perforate into the bronchi and pleural cavity, causing dissemination in the lungs and a serofibrinous exudative pleuritis. Bronchiectasis and cavities are also formed. Alimentary infection usually settles first in the tonsils, lymph nodes and Peyer's patches. The primary lesions may heal, but metastatic foci often develop elsewhere, involving the organs of the abdominal and pleural cavities and producing numerous tubercles on the thickened peritoneum and omentum.

The first lesions in cats affect the tissues of the digestive tract. From there generalization spreads rapidly throughout the body. At the beginning it has a proliferative character, which soon turns into caseation and necrosis.

Skin tuberculosis occurs more frequently in cats than in dogs. The flat ulcers have a necrotic bottom and a firm margin. These, as well as subcutaneous "tuberculous abscesses", are most often situated on the nose, lips, cheek and eyelids; they produce fistulae, from which necrotic, purulent material, very rich in tubercle bacteria, drains away. The cats lick the skin lesions and in this manner the infection may easily spread to various parts of the body (Fig. 6).

Tuberculosis of dogs, especially when lung cavities are present, may be complicated by hypertrophy of the periosteum at the distal parts of the legs (acropachy, osteopathia hypertrophica, Marie).

Among farm-bred *fur-animals* outbreaks of tuberculosis have been observed with incidences of more than 10%. The disease resembles that of cats. In silver foxes, in Germany, bovine-type infection could be traced back to feeding meat offal. The course was rapid, with generalization of the lesions. In the U.S.A., Hall and Winkel (1957) observed several cases of avian-type infection in mink fed with hog liver. The disease was characterized by swelling of the lymph-glands of the digestive tract and multiple small tubercles in the spleen and liver. *Nutria* showed high

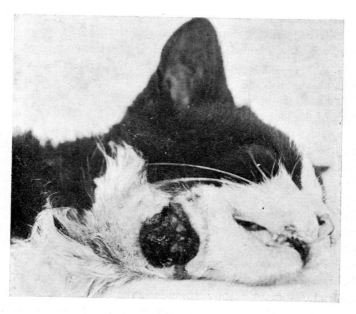

Fig. 6.   Tuberculous skin ulcer in a cat. (Photo: Department of Small animal Diseases, Veterinary Faculty, State University, Utrecht)

susceptibility to human-type tubercle bacteria, but much less to the bovine-type and none to the avian-type (Ippen, 1960).

Tuberculosis very seldom affects *animals living in the wild state.* Nevertheless, these animals remain naturally susceptible to the disease and some of those which live near to human communities may suffer from tuberculosis of very serious character.

Captive animals or those living under semi-wild conditions (in zoo-logical gardens or reservations), are not seldom infected by human sputum or by eating the meat of dead animals.

In *monkeys* tuberculosis is only observed in animals kept in captivity, where they are extremely susceptible to both types of mammalian bacteria. Unless strict precautionary measures are carried out, especially those which are designed to reduce the rate of exposure, tuberculosis usually spreads rapidly in monkey colonies in zoological gardens, and sometimes it destroys the entire monkey population.

In an American park in which the animals were kept in a semi-natural environment, Hawden found tuberculosis in 53.8% of the *bisons*, 3.7 to 6.2% of *elk*, 5.3% of *moose* and 0.83% of *mule-deer*. Schmidt (1937) examined 11,041 *wild boars* killed in Germany, and found that 1,442 had generalized tuberculosis and localized lesions were found in 3,648. This very high incidence among the omnivorous wild pigs may be related to the fact that they entered premises inhabited by man and also ate slaughter offal or viscera removed from the carcasses of hunted game, left behind in the field.

Human-type infection has been established in serious pulmonary tuberculosis of the *elephant*.

Avian-type bacteria have been isolated from *marsupials, monkeys* and *wild rabbits* in zoological gardens and the bovine-type has been commonly isolated from the *large carnivorous animals* (lion, tiger, panther, etc.), and *non-domesticated ruminants* (deer, roe, buffalo, etc.).

Despite their high susceptibility to experimental infection, spontaneous tuberculosis is very seldom observed in breeding stocks of small laboratory animals. Lindau and Jensen recorded, during a period of 8 years in the Statens Serum Institute in Copenhagen, only 1 case among about 9,000 *guinea pigs*.

The susceptibility of the organs of rodents varies greatly according to the species. In *guinea pigs*, both mammalian types produce lesions, at first chiefly in the lymph nodes and spleen, and later in the liver and lungs; macroscopic lesions are not found in the kidneys.

In *rabbits* with bovine- or avian-type infection, irrespective of the portal of entry, the course is serious, most of the lesions appearing in the lungs, pleura and kidneys. Infected test animals discharge large numbers of bacteria from fistulous skin ulcers, or in the bile, faeces and urine, and these may possibly infect animal-house attendants.

Voles are much more susceptible to bovine-type infection than *mice* and *rats*, their resistance to human- and, especially, to avian-type bacteria being high. In Great Britain 6 to 31% of field voles *(Microtus agrestis)* have been found infected with *M. tuberculosis* var. *muris*.

Tuberculosis is a wide-spread disease of various kinds of *birds*.

M. Koch and L. Rabinowitsch, examining 459 birds in the Zoological Gardens of Berlin (1907), found tuberculous lesions in 25.7% of them. In certain regions, 50% or more of the poultry farms are contaminated, the infection-rate of individual fowls being almost 100%. The infection is transmitted by food, contaminated by the droppings of the chickens. Rats may help to disseminate it among flocks. Plum (1948) established that all the rats in certain poultry houses were themselves carriers, without showing signs of the disease.

Schornagel (1926) recorded the distribution of lesions in the organs of chickens that had died from tuberculosis, and these are given in Table VI.

TABLE VI
SITE OF TUBERCULOUS LESIONS IN CHICKENS
Percentual distribution

Lung	Liver	Spleen	Kidney	Flat bones	Stomach	Intestines	Serous membranes	Ovary
48	100	90	8	20	5	100	10	8

Avian tuberculosis has a marked age incidence. Dobson did not observe tuberculin reactors in affected flocks up to the age of 6 months; at 18 months 5% reacted, at 30 months 10%, and at 42 months 20 to 30%.

The disease progresses slowly. Appetite gradually diminishes, the birds become droopy and often diarrhoea appears; the wattles and comb grow pale and shrunken; finally the animals become emaciated and many of them may die.

The primary lesions in the mucous membranes of the intestines extend into the muscular wall and progress to the subserosa, producing globular, tumor-like, firm swellings beneath the serous coat, which may protrude into the abdominal body cavity and hang down into it. (Fig. 7). The liver and spleen are usually enlarged, and show numerous lesions of different sizes. The larger lesions caseate. Tuberculosis of the joints and bones (mainly the sternum, ribs, tibia and femur) is common and often causes stiffness and lameness. As a rule, the disease develops slowly with gradual emaciation and cessation of egg-laying. In eggs of tuberculous poultry, very rarely, tubercle bacteria are found. Water-birds *(duck, goose)* may succumb from acute septicaemic tuberculosis with enormous numbers of bacteria pervading the tissues (Yersin type of disease).

Domesticated *pigeons,* and wood-pigeons also, are not infrequently infected without any known contact with tuberculous chickens. A certain

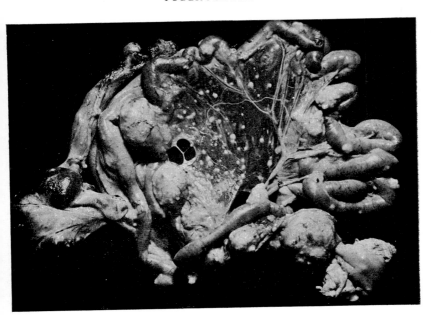

Fig. 7. Avian-type tuberculosis in the intestines of a hen.
(Photo: Institute for Veterinary Pathology, State University, Utrecht)

degree of susceptibility to bovine-type infection has been observed in pigeons and *canaries*. Avian-type tuberculosis has been found in *crows* (9 to 15%), *sparrows* (up to 40%), *starlings* (5%) and *gulls* (5%).

Warty growth on the skin and mucous membranes of the head is seen in pet *parrots* as a result of infection with the human-type bacterium. Mutual transmissions between man and parrots have been recorded (Martinaglia).

Criteria for establishing the incidence of tuberculosis in man and animals are perforce widely divergent.

Physical diagnostic methods (Röntgen, auscultation, percussion) are of little or no avail for the collection of clinical data in cattle, but meat inspection of the slaughtered animals yields a wealth of information about the presence of tuberculous lesions, thus providing a means of rounding out the overall picture.

The significance of a positive tuberculin test varies in man and bovines respectively. Whereas in the majority of reacting humans only closed or healed lesions can be found (these being to a great extent due to primary infection in early youth), most reacting cattle have open lesions and are therefore potential distributors of tubercle bacteria liable to transmit the disease to other animals or man.

It is not possible to determine the causative bacterial type from the clinical picture alone and for this reason most general statistics do not differentiate between human- and bovine-type infections.

Reliable routine determination of the bacterial types was commenced in the late twenties, when Loewenstein, Petragnani and others described simple technical methods for the isolation of pure cultures of tubercle bacteria from heavily contaminated materials, such as sputum and faeces, based upon the high resistance of the organisms to acids.

Unlike the avian-type, both mammalian types of *M. tuberculosis* can affect all the tissues and organs of the human body.

The old belief that tuberculosis in *man* caused by the bovine-type bacteria differs from human-type infection, both in its development and clinical effects, has been discarded. The relatively high incidence of localized extra-pulmonary lesions in bovine-type tuberculosis of man is not due to specific tissue affinity or lower virulence. It is more likely that it is connected with the fact that infection occurs chiefly by the alimentary route.

Table VII shows the incidence of bovine-type pulmonary and extra-pulmonary lesions in man of different ages, recorded by Holm, in Denmark, in 1946:

TABLE VII

INCIDENCE OF PULMONARY AND EXTRA-PULMONARY
TUBERCULOSIS

Age	Pulmonary	Extra-pulmonary lesions
0– 4	3.8	34.1
5– 9	3.2	28.2
10–14	1.3	16.3
15–19	3.5	17.7
20–24	3.0	12.6
25–29	3.7	16.4

Primary bovine-type infection of the digestive tract in young people usually produces non-progressing lesions restricted to the regional lymph-nodes. Evidence exists that such lesions provide a certain degree of immunity, which protects the adolescent individual from pulmonary tuberculosis. In contrast to bovine-type, the human-type bacteria, which primarily affect the more susceptible respiratory tract, are easily spread, causing serious lesions in various organs. Although it has often been stated that man possesses higher resistance to the bovine-type bacteria, and that the lesions caused by it are more frequently arrested and healed, Rich (1951) and other authorities do not agree that this view has been definitely proved. Certainly the bovine-type infection, once it has been established, is at least as pathogenic as the human-type is.

Under the environmental conditions of a heavily contaminated cowshed, coughing cows and whirling dust cause primary lung infection of the cowmen, just as human-type infection is passed on to persons in contact with phthisic patients in indoor surroundings. According to Jensen (1953), working in highly infected byres must be regarded as being far more dangerous than working in a tuberculosis hospital.

Sigurdsson (1945), in Denmark, demonstrated the presence of viable tubercle bacteria in the dust of premises in which infected cattle were housed. Bovine-type tuberculosis was much more frequent in rural patients in the age group of 15 to 30 years employed on cattle farms, than it was in persons of the same age in the same districts, who had no direct contact with cattle, although many of the latter drank unheated milk. In rural districts, 94% of the patients with bovine-type phthisis had been repeatedly exposed to strongly infected cattle during the previous 2 years. Only 3.6% of urban patients suffered from bovine-type tuberculosis as compared with 40% of rural patients.

Wiesmann (1949) reported that in the north-eastern Swiss cantons 18.8% of the children on farms with tuberculosis-free herds, reacted to tuberculin, whereas 64.3% of children living on farms with infected cattle gave positive reactions.

The similarity between human- and bovine-type tuberculosis was demonstrated by Hedvall and Magnusson (1941) in southern Sweden. Between the years 1936 and 1939, they found 67 cases of proved bovine-type tuberculosis, 26 of which were fatal. The Röntgen image and clinical course were similar to those found in human-type infection. In one family, 6 out of 7 children, living on a farm where three cows suffered from tuberculosis, developed the disease.

The hazard of air-borne transmission from cow to man is emphasized by the occurrence of primary bovine-type tuberculous conjunctivitis observed in milkers of contaminated cattle herds (Blegvad and Jensen, 1933).

When conditions are favourable, air-borne transmission of bovine-type tuberculosis from man to man may occur. The following example

observed by the author (in collaboration with de Raadt) stresses the
paramount importance of local circumstances.

3 of the 6 children of a healthy family died from rapidly developing pulmonary tuberculosis, and bovine-type tubercle bacteria were isolated from all three, as well as from
the stomach contents of a fourth child. Post mortem examinations of the three fatal
cases revealed primary tuberculosis of the lungs and regional lymph nodes with
extensive softening and perforation into the main bronchus. The initial infection
occurred in the 16-year old girl who had been, shortly before, employed as a milk-maid
on a small farm which kept heavily infected cattle. When she became ill, this girl
returned home. Constantly coughing, she shared a bed with a 15-year old sister
and a 10-year old brother, both of whom fell ill about 2 months later. All three children
died about 8 weeks after the onset of the disease. The fourth infected child had slept in
another room and remained clinically healthy, although X-ray examination showed
very suspicious patches in the hilar region. The prolonged and extremely close contact
between the eldest girl and 2 of the children gave rise to repeated massive primary
infections of the lungs in a manner more commonly associated with human-type
infection of a phthisic house mate.

The unusually rapid lethal course in these cases proved the high potential pathogenicity of the bovine-type bacterium when conditions are similar to those more
regularly encountered in "human-type" infections.

Although in regions in which infected cattle are present, many persons
who drink unheated milk become tuberculin-sensitive, the number of
those who actually develop tuberculous lesions is relatively small.
Nevertheless, the literature presents several observations which illustrate
the hazards involved.

Strempel et al. (1935), in Switzerland, established, that in the same district the incidence
of bovine-type tuberculosis was three times greater in drinkers of unboiled milk than the
human-type infection was. Wiesmann (1949), in the same country, isolated ten times
more bovine-type strains than human ones from tuberculous lesions in the throat and
neck. Prior to 1935, in Great Britain, Blacklock found bovine-type infection in 81.8%
of 108 children, most of whom lived in rural areas, with a primary complex in the
abdomen.

Non pasteurized milk and its products are the main sources of scrofula
and intestinal tuberculosis. From the primary lesions in the digestive
tract the bacteria may travel along the lymphatics through a chain of
lymph nodes to the thoracic duct and then into the blood stream, with the
resulting that systemic dissemination occurs. In this manner pulmonary
tuberculosis may arise secondarily from alimentary infection.

Griffith, carrying on the investigations of the British Royal Commission
on Tuberculosis, reported in 1914 that more than 70% of the cases of

scrofula, more than 26% of bone tuberculosis, and only 1.4% of lung tuberculosis cases, were caused by bovine-type bacteria.

In most countries an average of about 50% of the cases of cervical tuberculous adenitis (Fig. 8) were of bovine origin; the incidence was

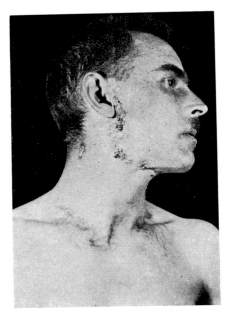

Fig. 8. Bovine-type ulcerative tuberculosis of the skin after healing of scrofulous lymph nodes. (Photo: Department of Dermatology, Medical Faculty, State University, Utrecht)

highest in childhood, and reached over 80%. Wilmot, observing 78 persons in a rural area of Northern Ireland between 1951 and 1956, found recently developed cervical lymphomas in 44.8% of the patients older than 15 years and in 34.5% of patients over the age of 25 years.

A breakdown of local resistance may bring about activation of quiescent foci.

The outstanding features of cervical adenitis are its sharp localization and the absence of constitutional symptoms (in about 95%). Besides these glandular lesions, bovine-type infection is most frequently encountered in cases of meningitis (25% or more) and skin tuberculosis (over 50%), and relatively often in osteo-arthritis and genital affections.

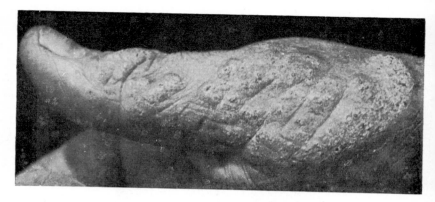

Fig. 9a

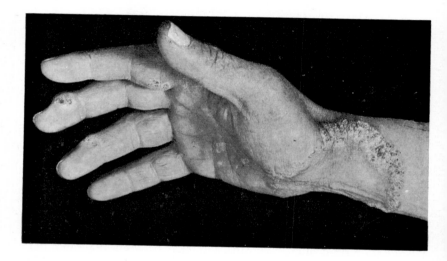

Fig. 9b

Fig. 9.   Bovine-type tuberculosis of the skin *(dermatitis verrucosa)* on the hand, (a) of a veterinary practitioner and (b) of a skinner. (Photos: Department of Dermatology, Medical Faculty, State University, Utrecht)

Bovine-type skin tuberculosis results from immediate contact of the hands with infected bovine tissues. This ailment is therefore practically always an occupational disease. The form of tuberculous skin infection most frequently in man is chronic *dermatitis verrucosa* (Fig. 9-a and -b).

Among 975 Prussian veterinarians, Jopke (1934) found 41 with bovine-type tuberculosis of the skin; among 796 Danish veterinarians, Thomsen (1937) observed 72; among 334 veterinarians in the Netherlands the author (1939) found 21 affected.

Summing up the literature, prior to 1937, on the incidence of bovine-type tuberculosis in the populations of various countries, Gervois recorded the data partly reproduced in Table VIII.

As a result of the successful campaign against tuberculosis of cattle, the incidence of human infection has greatly altered in many parts of the world. In some places, the prevailing conditions have delayed the expected decrease of the incidence.

Thus, even in 1951, McKay claimed that in the north-eastern counties of Scotland, bovine-type infections caused 35 to 40% of the human cases of nonpulmonary tuberculosis and 12.1 to 13.3% of tuberculosis of the lung. Lebele and Steinert, in 1955, found that 34% of the extra-pulmonary lesions among children in Bavaria were of bovine-type origin, 63.3% of human-type and 2.7% of both.

In Griffiths' reports the annual death rate from bovine-type infection in England and Wales was estimated to be 3,000, representing 6% of the total deaths due to tuberculosis. In 1933, Ravenel still found a death rate of 2,600 and an annual number of fresh bovine-type infections of 4,000; in 1944 Smith (1958) recorded 1,300 deaths. In 1937, Lange estimated the number of deaths from bovine-type tuberculosis in the German population at 1,000 a year, which is more than the combined figure for typhoid fever and scarlatina.

While the eradication of bovine tuberculosis is most beneficial to human health, the elimination of this serious menace is, on the other hand, connected with a certain risk. It is generally believed that the repeated ingestion or inhalation of small numbers of tubercle bacteria of animal origin provides a certain degree of natural immunity, which raises the resistance against the more dangerous air-borne infection from human sources.

Straub (1952) quoted the following illustrative experience. In regions of Scotland in which energetic veterinary control measures had been instituted in 1930, the total incidence of tuberculosis among individuals between the ages of 15 and 25 years rose until 1940 by 35%. Whereas the mortality from abdominal tuberculosis had sharply decreased, the incidence of primary air-borne infection had increased by 30%. This contrast was explained by the fact that in the preceding decade, tuberculosis had considerably decreased in livestock, and consequently only a minor fraction of the population had been stimulated to build up active resistance against the human-type infection. The interpretation of such data, however, is rather speculative and should be

TABLE VIII

PERCENTAGE OF BOVINE-TYPE INFECTIONS IN MAN IN VARIOUS LOCALIZATIONS OF TUBERCULOUS LESIONS

Country	Pulmonary	Adeno-cervical	Osteo-articular	Cutaneous and serous	Meningeal	Genito-urinary	Total	Period
England	1.46	52.1	18.4	48.5	25.2	16.6	10.4	1907–36
Scotland	5.1	70.8	39	53.8	28	23.2	20.7	1907–36
France	4		10.3		7.4		6.8	1909–37
Germany	5	28.2	4.8	23.9			10.8	1898–1936
Netherlands	6.1	28.5	15.7	20.6	16.6	0	8.7	1903–36
Denmark	4.7	48.8	18.5	34.3	24.6		13.9	1902–36
Switzerland	1.7	37.5	10.1		12.5	5.2	7.7	1932–35
Norway	0		0	5.1	0		6.5	1932–35
U.S.A.	0	36.6	27.6		6.5	6.2	11.7	1901–33
Canada	2	24.1	3.7		5.9	2.7	8	1909–36
Australia	0	61.7	0				12.1	1923–32
Japan	0	15.3	4.8	25		0	2.9	1909–36
Europe	4.4	31.6	5.2	21.6	20.2	5.2	9.38	until 1937

approached with caution, because improvements in hygienic, environmental, nutritional, social and medical conditions have all helped to diminish the incidence of both extra-pulmonary and pulmonary tuberculosis.

After bovine tuberculosis had been wiped out in Bornholm, the number of young persons who reacted to the tuberculin test and were thus relatively resistant to tuberculous infection, markedly decreased. At the same time, the incidence of primary pulmonary infection greatly increased, especially among the young adults who left the island. Because primary tuberculosis is in this age group serious, public health authorities made immunization with the Calmette-Guerin vaccine compulsory for all non-reacting individuals. In several countries in which bovine tuberculosis has disappeared, this procedure has been introduced to increase artificially the resistance of the population.

Special precautions to prevent infection with bovine-type tuberculosis are indicated for persons who are occupationally exposed to infected cattle. The incidence of primary air-borne infection of the lungs and conjunctiva is highest in cattlemen and milkers, and tuberculosis of the skin of hands and arms often attacks veterinarians, meat inspectors, slaughter house personnel, butchers and skinners. Transmission of the bovine-type infection from these persons to cattle has been observed several times.

Other animals as well as cattle, may be sources of human infection, especially dogs with the open form of pulmonary tuberculosis and cats with the ulcero-fistulous skin lesions characteristic of them. It is obvious that these animals must be promptly disposed of. Dogs and cats should not be fed with raw milk or uncooked slaughter offal. Dogs, living in the house of consumptives should not be fed with scraps from the table. The animals must be periodically examined by a veterinarian.

Feldman (1938) collected, from the literature up to 1936, 13 cases of human tuberculosis, from infancy to 57 years, in which the presence of avian-type bacteria appeared to have been reliably demonstrated. The clinical diagnoses of these cases were: submaxillary and axillary lymphadenitis, miliary patches in the lungs, fibro-cavernous tuberculosis pulmonum, malignant lymphogranuloma (Hodgkin's disease), Boeck's sarcoid and meningitis. The same author (1949) described an additional case in a $2^1/_2$-year old child with extensive involvement of the left upper lobe of the lung. Dragsted observed, between 1935 and 1949, avian-type infections in Denmark affecting 6 persons between the ages of 3 and 25 years, with healing scrofulous lesions, adenitis, abscesses in the axilla and extended active pulmonary tuberculosis with dense fibrosis and meningitis. Of all the patients described above, 4 died.

Robijns, in the Dutch province of Zeeland, recorded in 1960 a 15-months old child with pulmonary lesions, from which a strain of the avian-type tubercle bacterium was isolated by the lavage of the stomach. Among 946 school children, 4.12 % were found reacting to avian-type tuberculin, whereas, among the 96 members of the families to which these children belonged, 12 reacted with avian PPD alone and 25 with both avian- and human-type PPD.

Although tubercle bacteria have been found rarely in hen's eggs, they probably do not represent a real danger to the consumers. The chance of infection will be much greater in persons exposed to inhalation of dust contaminated with fowl's droppings. Dry cleaning of infected hen-houses and contact with pet birds with tuberculous ulcers of the skin may be especially hazardous. Present evidence, however, seems to indicate that infection with avian-type tubercle bacteria represents only a remote danger to public health.

Formerly when pasteurization had not yet been generally applied and bovine tuberculosis still largely prevailed, a great deal of the consumer's milk contained living tubercle bacteria. There was a chance that the milk from several farms might be mixed with the milk of a cow with tuberculous mastitis, or that it was polluted by excretions of cows with lesions elsewhere, e.g. urine, uterine discharge or faeces contaminated by a cow with tuberculosis pulmonum, swallowing its sputum.

In his summary of literature prior to 1937, Gervois (l.c.) recorded that the percentage of contaminated milk sold for consumption was: in the Netherlands 2, in Great Britain and Italy almost 7, in Switzerland, the U.S.A. and Germany 8.1 to 8.5, in France 10.3, in Denmark 14.3 and in Poland 22.5. These figures are strongly influenced by the conditions prevailing in the places from which the milk samples had been derived. Unsatisfactory conditions are still now and then encountered in countries which are in other respects modernised. Hofmann et al., in 1957, found living tubercle bacteria in 48 % of the unboiled milk samples in a town in Oberpfalz (Germany). However, at present viable bacteria are no longer present in the consumer's milk of most of the countries mentioned above in which pasteurization has been made compulsory by law.

In market products taken at random in the Netherlands, the author (1940) isolated bovine tubercle bacteria from 2 out of 24 specimens of farm-churned butter and from 1 out of 56 solid cheeses produced 4 weeks prior to the investigation. In dairy products prepared in the laboratory from naturally contaminated mixed milk, the survival time of the tubercle bacteria was determined. In buttermilk kept at room temperature, viable bacteria were still recovered after 32 days; in salted butter at 4° they retained full virulence for at least 151 days and a reduced number of living organisms were still present after 180 days. In fat cheeses, a year after preparation, the number and virulence of the tubercle bacteria was still unabated.

Since tuberculosis among Dutch cattle has been completely eradicated and nearly all milk is pasteurized, the above data are at present only of historical interest. They may, however, serve as an example to countries with less advanced control of the disease in livestock.

As long as the ultimate aim of total eradication has yet to be attained, compulsory pasteurization of milk for direct consumption and for the preparation of dairy products should be enforced by health authorities. The optimal recommendation is rapid heating at 85° for a short time, while the milk is allowed to flow in a thin film.

Because haematogenous dissemination of tubercle bacteria, without formation of perceptible foci, sometimes occurs in cattle with high specific resistance, it is a serious hazard to milk and meat hygiene, since it is not revealed by inspection of the live animal or its carcass.

The chance of infection from the ingestion of insufficiently heated meat is not great. When tubercle bacteria are present in muscular tissue, the number of them does not appear to be large. Organs and lymph nodes, however, may contain numerous bacteria.

Because the number of tuberculous lesions is usually limited, it is seldom necessary to condemn an entire carcass as unfit for human consumption. Standard regulations governing meat inspection enumerate the conditions which render slaughter products unsuitable for food. The main criteria for total condemnation are: acute multiple miliary tuberculosis, especially in young animals; rapidly spreading forms of the disease with caseous necrosis; a tendency to generalization; and recently developed multiple lobular pneumonic lesions. Organs or tissues in which tuberculous foci are found, or organs which are drained by recently affected lymph glands, are unfit for consumption. When the presence of tubercle bacteria cannot be established but is reasonably surmised, as in protracted generalized tuberculosis, the meat is in several countries permitted to be eaten after it has been sterilized under the supervision of the authorities.

Partial or total eradication of tuberculosis from cattle not only prevents bovine-type infection of man, but ultimately also prevents infection of horses, swine, sheep, goats, dogs and cats.

This fact is demonstrated by the following data from the Netherlands Veterinary Service (Table IX).

The almost universally applied program of controlling tuberculosis in bovines is based on the principles laid down by Bernhard Bang in 1891. These include: (1) tracing of the infected animals by clinical and bacterio-

TABLE IX

DECREASE OF TUBERCULOSIS OBSERVED IN SLAUGHTER ANIMALS EXCEPT CATTLE
IN THE NETHERLANDS
(J. M. van den Born)

Five years period	Horses	Swine *	Sheep	Goats
1950–1954	258	183,812	82	106
1955–1959	59	78,042	19	10
Decrease within five years	77%	57%	76%	91%

* The relatively slower decrease of the incidence of tuberculosis in swine is easily explained by the considerable number of avian-type infections which are not affected by the eradication measures against tuberculosis of cattle.

logical investigation and tuberculin-testing, (2) elimination or slaughter of the positively reacting animals, (3) immediate segregation of the new-born calves from the adult stock, (4) the rearing of these calves free from tuberculosis, (5) addition to the herd of non-reacting cattle only and (6) improvement of hygienic conditions. Different local circumstances dictate the variations to be introduced in the general scheme.

For many years the tuberculin test has been the cornerstone of the campaign the whole world over. Tuberculin must unite high potency with fair specificity. In several countries the purified protein derivate (P.P.D.) is preferred because it is considered the form of tuberculin that has the highest quality.

The subcutaneous reaction originally used (which measured the rise of temperature) has been replaced nearly everywhere by the easier intradermal test, which is read by determination with a caliper of local swelling of the skin.

The allergic response to tuberculin is not absolutely specific. A simple application of it does not clearly reveal the differences between bovine-, human- or avian-type infection. In order to obtain in doubtful cases more detailed aetiological information, the grade of reactivity is investigated by a comparative skin-test with mammalian and avian tuberculins injected separately on either side of the body.

The significance of the human-type infection of cattle is associated with the creation of tuberculin-sensitiveness. As a result, it is impossible to distinguish such animals from bovine-type-infected cattle, so that the "test and slaughter" eradication method often results in the sacrifice of such cattle. The official Danish reports over the period 1943–1952 (Christiansen) record 107 cases of open tuberculosis in humans who had contaminated 128 tuberculosis-free cattle herds, so that 1,100 cows were slaughtered, most of which, in fact, endangered neither man nor animals; 10.4% of 917 reinfected herds were traced to human-type contamination.

False negative results may be associated with pre-allergy in an early stage of infection, to an anergic condition in apparently healthy older animals and to asthenia due to widespread tuberculosis with breakdown of general resistance. False positive reactions occur in animals sensitized by other acid-fast organisms, as in cases of "so-called skin tuberculosis" (see page 11) and paratuberculous enteritis (Johne's disease). Unaccountable false positive reactions are observed in 0.5 to 3% of animals which do not show visible lesions at slaughter.

From the 1952 Annual Report of the Animal Health Service in Friesland (The Netherlands), it appeared that specifically reacting cows often gave negative results when they were re-examined at later dates. From the 15.5% animals still reacting, only 1.5% showed tuberculous lesions at slaughter.

In most countries the following eradication system is applied. If testing of the whole herd reveals only a few reacting animals, these are removed and the remaining cows are retested every 3 months until positive results are no longer obtained.

If the number of reactors is so large that their immediate removal does not seem to be economic, they are segregated on the farm as satisfactorily as local conditions allow. All cattle with clinical signs of infection are disposed of and replaced by non-reactors. In this manner a tuberculosis-free herd can be gradually built up.

Immediately after birth the calves are separated, and fed with milk from a tuberculosis-free herd or with pasteurized milk and they are allowed to join the "clean" section of the herd only when they have become heifers.

When a large number of cows in a herd react to tuberculin, the whole group of reactors should be removed at once; they should be replaced with cows from a tuberculosis-free stock. All "cleaned" herds must remain under the control of periodical tuberculin-testing, in order to trace possible reinfections.

Reinfections can be brought about by the sputum of attendants with open bovine- or human-type pulmonary tuberculosis, contact with cattle on neighbouring pastures, grazing on meadows sprayed or sprinkled with contaminated sewage or the effluent of slaughter houses, dairies or hospitals, and during transportation in contaminated vehicles. In view of the high resistance and long survival time of *M. tuberculosis,* chlorination must follow the biological purification of suspect sewage. After removing the manure, contaminated premises can be successfully disinfected with hot 4% solution of sodium carbonate and consecutive application of cresylic compounds.

References p. 48–49

Pastures on which an infected herd has grazed should not be used by other cattle for several months.

To complete the eradication campaign, farm personnel handling the cattle herd, as well as sheep, goats, swine, horses and poultry, should be considered as potential sources of infection, and subjected to control.

Because crowding, insufficient light and poor ventilation strongly favour the spread of infection, strict attention should be given to hygienic housing conditions. Keeping the animals in the open is most effective in preventing the transmission of tuberculosis.

In several countries in which it has been possible to enforce control measures systematically, very satisfactory results have been obtained. An adequate country-wide campaign requires close co-operation between the governmental and provincial veterinary services, agricultural organizations and dairy plants. Scientific planning and funds for the compensation of losses to farmers are essential for its ultimate success.

Classical achievements have been attained in Denmark where the campaign was launched at the beginning of the century, but was vigorously enforced only between 1935 and 1945. Whereas in 1937 not more than 26.5% of the herds were free from infection, in 1945 this number had increased to 91.1% and in 1952 it was possible to declare the country free from bovine tuberculosis. Meanwhile in the other Scandinavian countries also, and in Finland and the Netherlands, the disease has almost or completely disappeared.

In the German Federal Republic, systematic control was introduced in 1952. At that time two-thirds of the herds were infected, whereas in 1958 two-thirds were free from tuberculosis. In Great Britain the infection rate declined from about 40% in 1931 to 17–18% in 1945 and 10–12% in 1952. In October 1960, it was officially reported that tuberculosis in cattle had been virtually eradicated from England, Wales and Scotland. As from 1950, some £130 million had been spent on the scheme, mainly in indemnities to the owners.

Satisfactory results have been obtained under widely differing climatic conditions and various methods of animal husbandry.

At the start of the control program in the U.S.A., in 1917, the average incidence of bovine tuberculosis was no higher than 4.9%, although in some regions 50–75% of the cattle reacted to tuberculin. Since then the Federal-State Co-operative Plan for the Eradication of Bovine Tuberculosis has been introduced (better known as the Accredited Herd Plan of Bovine Tuberculosis Eradication). According to Ranney (1961), over 400 million tuberculin tests have been made in the U.S.A. since the start of the eradication program, and 4 million reacting animals have been sent to slaughter. By 1940, the average incidence of infection had declined to 0.46%, in 1950 it had dwindled to 0.19%, in 1952 to 0.11%. About the same level has been maintained during the following two years, with regional variations ranging from almost 0–1%. The last step towards total eradication is the most difficult, requiring the greatest efforts. The small number of infected animals still remaining constitute an extreme potential danger to the "clean" livestock, since these do not benefit from acquired specific immunity. This has clearly been demonstrated by the gradually rising percentage of reacting cattle during the following years, reaching the figure of 0.23 in 1959.

Although immunization with the Calmette-Guérin vaccine confers a reasonable amount of resistance on young calves, the procedure is very rarely applied, and, in Denmark vaccination is even forbidden by law. Because acquired resistance is not absolute, it does not prevent the infection of all treated animals. Another drawback is that B.C.G. provokes sensitivity to tuberculin, so that differentiation between infected and vaccinated non-infected cattle is difficult or impossible.

Control of tuberculosis in poultry presents problems different from those presented by cattle.

One important problem presented by poultry, which is not related to cattle, is the heavy infection rate of the soil with avian-type bacteria. Because the disease develops in poultry very slowly, open forms of tuberculosis seldom occur before the second year of life. It is therefore necessary to eliminate the older birds every year and replace them by young chickens.

The infection is traced by testing with a tuberculin derived from avian-type bacteria, which is injected into the wattle. In flocks with high infection rate, it is advisable to slaughter all of the chickens forthwith and start a new flock on another plot of land. If only a few birds are infected it may suffice to eliminate the reactors and to re-test the remainder bi-monthly with tuberculin.

Infected chicken-runs should be ploughed up and left unused for at least 1 year, before a new flock is introduced.

Several authors pointed out the presumable role played in the spread of avian tuberculosis by various wild birds, which constitute an independent reservoir of avian-type infection. This epizootiological factor should be taken into account in the control of the disease in chickens.

Therapeutic treatment of tuberculosis has taken an important step forward in recent years with the introduction of effective new drugs and surgical methods of removing the main foci of infection.

The drugs most commonly used are streptomycin, isoniazid (I.N.H.) and para-aminosalicylic acid (P.A.S.).

Despite a striking similarity of aetiology, pathogenicity and epidemiology in tuberculosis of man and animals, the valuable modern therapeutic approach has in practice benefited only man. For reasons discussed above, treatment of tuberculous animals should be discouraged. Wherever it is possible, the affected animals must be destroyed without delay.

Nothwithstanding the wide range of the animal hosts of the bovine-type tubercle bacterium, cattle are the main source of infection for man and all other susceptible animals.

Eradication of bovine tuberculosis has been successfully completed in several centers of animal industry in which formerly it had been a first rate hazard to human health and welfare. Once this has been accomplished, the leading principle should be, the maintenance of it by the exercise of the utmost vigilance in preventing the reinfection of herds which, by being "cleaned", have become highly susceptible. Periodical veterinary inspection and control of such livestock must not be on any account neglected.

REFERENCES

ABDUSSALAM, M., *Bull. Off. internat. Epizooties*, 45 (1956) 465.

BORN, J. M. v. D., *Proc. 15th internat. Vet. Congr.*, I (1953) 128.

DRAGSTED, I., *Lancet*, 257 (1949) 103.

DUBOS, R. and J. DUBOS, *The white plague*, Boston, 1952, 277 pp.

FELDMAN, W. H., *J. Am. Vet. Med. Assoc.*, 92 (1938) 681; *Ann. N.Y. Acad. Sci.*, 48 (1947) 469; *Avian tuberculosis infections*, Baltimore, 1938, 483 pp.

FELDMAN, W. H., D. W. HUTCHINSON, V. M. SCHWARTING and A. G. KARLSON, *Amer. J. Pathol.*, 25 (1949) 1183.

FOURIE, P. J. J., G. J. DE WET and G. C. v. DRIMMELEN, *J. S. Afr. Vet. Med. Assoc.*, 21 (1950) 70.

FRANCIS, J., *Tuberculosis in animals and man*, London, 1958, 357 pp.

GLOVER, R. E., *Vet. Record*, 61 (1949) 875.

GRIFFITH, A. S., *Tubercle*, 5 (1924) 569; *A system of Bacteriology*, V (1930) 198.

HALL, R. E. and F. WINKEL, *J. Amer. Vet. Med. Assoc.*, 131 (1957) 49.

HEDVALL, E. and MAGNUSSON, *Acta Med. Scand.*, 5 (1941) 135, Suppl.

HOLM, J., *Public Health Repts.*, 40 (1946) 1435.

HOEDEN, J. v. D., *Tijdschr. Diergeneesk.*, 68 (1941) 335.

HOEDEN, J. v. D. and M. F. DE RAADT, *Ned. Tijdschr. Geneesk.*, 84 (1940) 4390.

IPPEN, R., *Zentral. Bakteriol. Parasitenk.*, I. Or., 178 (1960) 195.

JENSEN, K. A., *Schweiz. Z. Pathol. Bakteriol.*, 12 (1949) 435; *W. H. Organ. Monograph.*, 1953; *Bull. W. H. Organ.*, 10 (1954) 171.

McKAY, W. M., *Vet. Record*, 63 (1951) 383.

OTTOSEN, H. E., *Skand. Vet. Tidsskr.*, 34 (1944) 1.

PETERSEN, G., *Bull. Off. internat. Epiz.*, 30 (1948) 169.

PLUM, N., *Veröff. Ser. Lab. Kgl. Tierärztl. Landb. H.*, Kopenhagen, 1925; *J. Am. Vet. Med. Assoc.*, 22 (1926) 441; *Nord. Vet. Med.*, 4 (1952) 461.

POST, R. and F. W. v. ULSEN, *Tijdschr. Diergeneesk.*, 79 (1954) 579.

RANNEY, A. F., *Diseases of the Chest*, 39 (1961) 150.

RICH, A. R., *The pathogenesis of tuberculosis*, Springfield, 1951, 1028 pp.

RITCHIE, J. N., *Advances in the Control of Zoonoses,* W.H.O. Monogr. Series, 19 (1953) 25.
SIGURDSSON, J., *Acta Tuber. Scand.,* suppl. 15 (1945).
SOLIMAN, K. N., D. H. L. ROLLINSON, N. S. BARRON and F. R. SPRATLING, *Vet. Record,* 65 (1953) 421.
STENIUS, R., *Vet. Record,* 50 (1938) 633; *Finn. Vet. Z.,* 47 (1941) 105.
THORSHAUG, K., *Norsk. Vet. Tidsskr.,* 59 (1947) 365.
VERGE, J., *Rev. Pathol. Comp.,* 45 (1945) 313.
WIESMANN, E., *Z. Tuberk.,* 6 (1949) 122.
WILMOT, T. J., E. F. JAMES and J. J. MASON BROWN, *Proc. Roy. Soc. Med.,* 50 (1957) 1057.

2

J. VAN DER HOEDEN

Pasteurellosis

The genus *Pasteurella* comprises 4 species of bacteria, 2 of which provoke serious zoonoses in human beings (plague and tularaemia) and 2 others cause important epizootic and enzootic diseases in domesticated and wild animals, only occasionally affecting man (haemorrhagic septicaemia and pseudotuberculosis).

All pasteurellae are aerobic, Gram-negative, small, short, usually ovoid rods with distinct bipolar staining *(Bac. bipolaris)*. They are relatively inactive in carbohydrate fermentation, in which no gas is produced. Their resistance to disinfectants commonly used is rather low.

The group of organisms causing haemorrhagic septicaemia in animals, *P. multocida (-septica)*, has been subdivided into varieties, adapted to the different host species. Thus the following are differentiated: *P. boviseptica, suiseptica, bubaloseptica, aviseptica, muriseptica, lepiseptica,* and others. Only recently have minor distinctions between these varieties been established.

P. multocida is a non-motile organism enveloped in a capsule to which its mucoid growth may be attributed. In addition, however, to mucoid colonies, smooth and rough colonies appear on ordinary neutral or alkaline media. The colonies produced by strains isolated from pigs are mostly mucoid, while those isolated from dogs produce this kind of colony only occasionally, and those isolated from cattle develop mucoid growth only very exceptionally (Smith, 1958).

Strains recovered from various animal species often react differently in the fermentation of particular carbohydrates and may vary in their pathogenicity to white mice. Using the haemagglutination test, Carter (1959) divided the *multocida*-group into three serological varieties. *P. pestis* differs from *P. multocida* in its ability to multiply in the presence of bile salts, its incapacity to ferment sorbitol or to produce hydrogen sulfide, as well as in a few additional minor characteristics.

Opinions are divided on the question whether the variants of *P. multocida* are transmissible from their natural host to other animal species. The organism is often found in apparently healthy animals. Smith (1955) frequently isolated it from the nose and even more often from the tonsils of dogs; Weber (1941) found pasteurellae in 75 % of the nasal cavities of cats; and Schipper (1947) recovered 14 strains from Norwegian rats, although these animals are resistant to experimental infection with *P. multocida*.

The chance of infection among farm animals is considerably heightened by a lowering of the general resistance of these animals (*e.g.* by transportation), or by weather changes. Increase of virulence, usually resulting from passage through animals, promotes the appearance of enzootic outbreaks.

Pasteurellosis in animals has a world-wide distribution and in some countries it causes considerable economic loss. The acute disease in animals characteristically takes a septicaemic course, with congestion of blood vessels, subserous and submucous haemorrhages, pneumonia and enteritis. In its subacute form, the chief features are serofibrinous and haemorrhagic lesions in the mucosae and serosae. The chronic form of the illness shows abscesses and necrotic foci in conjunction with anaemia and cachexia.

The most important diseases caused by *P. multocida* are haemorrhagic septicaemia of *cattle* ("shipping fever", "stockyard's disease"), *sheep, horses, rabbits* and several species of *wild animals* ("Wild und Rinderseuche"), enzootic pneumonia of calves, *swine* plague (fibrous pneumonia), mastitis of ewes ("blue bag") and fowl cholera, which affects a large variety of *birds*. Furthermore, *P. multocida* may be a secondary pathogenic agent in diseases of different aetiology.

Pasteurellosis has rarely been recorded in *man*. However, ample reason exists for the assumption that its incidence in human beings has been underestimated as a result of the fact that typical clinical signs are absent, the aetiological diagnosis being almost always based upon accidental laboratory findings.

Schipper, in 1947, reviewed 30 cases from the literature between 1930 and 1946, of which 21 had been bacteriologically confirmed. According to K. F. Meyer (1958) *P. multocida* was identified in 89 of 109 cases reported. In 35 patients the disease followed animal bites, 28 being caused by cats, 5 by dogs, 1 by a rabbit and 1 by a panther. The redness and swelling appearing around the indolent wound often persist for an extended period of time and in several cases abscesses, necrosis of the underlying bones and osteomyelitis developed. Lymphangitis, lymphadenitis and general symptoms, such as fever, chills, headache and insomnia, may accompany the local lesions.

Besides animal bites – especially those of cats – exposure to infected livestock may exceptionally be the cause of human pasteurellosis. 27 out of 37 pasteurellosis patients observed in the Mayo Clinics in Rochester by Olsen and Needham (1952) during almost 5 years, were either farmers or members of their family, nearly all of whom were living in rural communities.

In many cases it is impossible to establish whether the pathogenic role played by *P. multocida* is that of a primary or of a secondary invader. The organism has often been isolated from the upper respiratory tract of man without evidence of apparent damage to the tissues. *Pasteurella* strains were repeatedly recovered by Straker *et al.* (1939) from the noses and throats of two healthy veterinary students and a laboratory worker, their origin being ascribed to cattle and dogs.

In several instances of human pasteurellosis the isolated strains showed the characteristics of those generally found in cattle, pigs, dogs or cats, the patients involved usually having a history of association with such animals.

On the basis of several observations it may be assumed that trauma or change in the normal physiological conditions of the tissues will enable the pasteurellas already present to penetrate and precipitate acute infection.

The human cases of pasteurellosis recorded in literature in which *P. multocida* could be isolated include bite wounds, pneumonia, pleuritis, empyema, chronic bronchitis, bronchiectasis, septicaemia, frontal sinusitis, meningitis, abscess of the brain, peritonsillar inflammation, appendicitis, enteritis, osteomyelitis and joint affections.

With the exception of *P. pestis,* pasteurellae do not provoke haemorrhagic septicaemia in human beings, although Želigowska (1956) recorded the isolation of *P. multocida* from the blood of a fatal infection of a twelve year old girl.

The exact role of *P. multocida* in human pathology and the actual incidence of pasteurellosis as a zoonosis have not yet been fully clarified.

Reports on treatment with sulfamerazine, sulfathiazole, chlortetracycline and penicillin have been favourable. Immune serum is given to bovines as a prophylactic measure, especially before shipment. A potent vaccine (usually prepared from a buffalo strain) can confer active immunity, which lasts about a year.

REFERENCES

BARTLEY, E. O. and K. HUNTER, Lancet, 252 (1947) 908.
BYRNE, J. J., T. F. BOYD and A. K. DALY, Surg. Gynec. Obstet., 103 (156) 57.
CARTER, G. R., Amer. J. Vet. Res., 20 (1959) 173.
CAWSON, R. A. and J. M. TALBOT, J. Clin. Path., 8 (1955) 49.
COOPER, T. V. and B. MOORE, Lancet, 248 (1945) 753.
EMSON, H. E., J. Clin. Path., 10 (1957) 187.
ERICSON, C. and I. JUHLIN, Acta pathol. microbiol. scand., 46 (1959) 47.
MEYER, K. F. in R. J. DUBOIS, Bacterial and Mycotic Infections of Man, 1958, 400 pp.
NEEDHAM, G. M., Proc. Mayo Clinics, 23 (1948) 361.
OLSEN, A. M. and G. M. NEEDHAM, Amer. J. med. Sci., 224 (1952) 77.
REGAMEY, R., Les infections humaines à B. bipolaris septicus (Pasteurelloses), Bern, 1939, 126 pp.
SCHIPPER, G. L., Bull. Johns Hopk. Hosp., 81 (1947) 33.
SMITH, J. E., J. comp. Path. Therap., 65 (1955) 239; 68 (1958) 315; 69 (1959) 231.
STRAKER, E., A. B. E. HILL and R. LOVELL, Pept. Public Health. Med. Subj., London, 90. 1939.
TRUMMERT, W., H. REMKY and C. ANDERS, Münch. med. Wschr., 101 (1959) 34.

3

J. VAN DER HOEDEN

Pseudotuberculosis

Pasteurella pseudotuberculosis rodentium (Pfeiffer) closely resembles *P. pestis.*

It is differentiated from the latter by its more rapid and luxuriant growth, its ability to produce alkali in milk, its active motility at 18 to 22° (which is lost at 37°), its fermentation of rhamnose and glycerin, and its low pathogenicity for albino rats (which readily succumb to *P. pestis* infection). In contrast to *P. pseudo-tuberculosis,* which forms large opaque yellow colonies upon desoxycholate–citrate–agar medium, the growth of plague bacteria is scanty in reddish pinpoint colonies. The two organisms can further be distinguished by serological and bacteriophage tests. Differences of 0-antigenic structure enabled Thal to divide pseudotuberculosis strains into five groups, each of which is apparently linked with host preference. Some of the strains produce a thermolabile exotoxin, which is probably connected with their pathogenicity.

Besides antigens common to *P. pestis, P. pseudotuberculosis* shows co-agglutination with certain *Salmonella* strains. Guinea-pigs immunized against *P. pestis* remain susceptible to pseudotuberculosis.

According to Devignat, *P. pseudotuberculosis* is to be regarded as a mutation of *P. pestis mediaevalis* (see page 59).

Because both *P. pseudotuberculosis* and *P. pestis* affect rodents in nature, their differentiation is of major epidemiological importance in countries where plague prevails. The bacterium of pseudotuberculosis has not been recorded in the plague-endemic regions of Central Africa, China, Indo-China, Indonesia and Madagascar.

P. pseudotuberculosis can be isolated from the pus of abscesses, and during the ante-mortem stage, from the circulating blood.

Unlike guinea pigs, rabbits, white mice and certain species of birds (sparrows) which can easily be infected by feeding, white rats usually are refractory. Most often spontaneous infection occurs through the alimentary tract, less frequently by the respiratory route.

The name given to the disease was based on a superficial resemblance between its gross pathology and that of tuberculosis. However, contrary to what its name suggests *P. pseudotuberculosis* has no characteristics in common with *Mycobacterium tuberculosis.**

Pseudotuberculosis rodentium occurs chiefly in *guinea pigs*, less so in other rodents. Most affected are young and underfed animals.

Cases of pseudotuberculosis have been recorded in *cattle, horses, goats, swine, cats, rabbits, hares, foxes, monkeys, beavers, mink, nutrias, marten, chinchilla*, several *birds* (particularly in turkeys, pigeons and canaries) and *man*. The course may be either acutely septicaemic or chronic.

Post-mortem examination reveals considerably enlarged mesenteric nodules, which prove to be thickly capsulated, whitish abscesses with voluminous creamy, caseous contents. Pathological foci in the abdominal wall, omentum, liver, spleen, and occasionally in the lungs, have a similar aspect.

Human beings develop various clinical signs. A syndrome is observed which can easily be mistaken for typhoid fever. After a prodromal stage of malaise, the patient is overcome by sudden high fever, chills, general indisposition, heavy sweating, headache and gastro-enteritis. In most of these cases, the liver and spleen are palpable and tender. Acute appendicitis is often diagnosed, but at laparotomy a normal appendix is found, and in its stead, a clear serous abdominal exudate and enlarged mesenteric lymphatic nodules, single or in packets, especially in the ileocoecal angle, are perceived. Section of these nodules reveals on their surface enlarged follicles and small abscesses. Sometimes there is oedema of the serosa of the distal part of the ileum and coecum. The diagnosis can be supported by serological tests. Septicaemic and pulmonary forms of pseudotuberculosis are rarely observed.

P. pseudotuberculosis has been isolated from cases of meningitis, sinusitis, otitis media, chronic bronchitis and bronchiectasis. As in *P. multocida* infection (see page 52), it must be assumed that often the pathogenic role of the pseudotuberculosis agent is secondary.

---

* Pseudotuberculosis caused by *Corynebacterium pseudotuberculosis ovis* (Preisz-Nocard) causes caseous lymphadenitis in sheep and occasionally in goats and wild deer, ulcerative lymphangitis in horses, and a suppurative lymphangitis in cattle. Infection of human beings by this agent has not been recorded.

References p. 57

Pseudotuberculous pneumonia may take a chronic course of long duration. In cases, which develop into serious illness, death usually occurs 2 or 3 weeks after the onset of the disease. The final stage is characterized by toxaemia, stupor and jaundice.

Knapp (1958) recorded from the literature 15 cases of the septic form, 13 of which took a severe typhoidal course, with 11 deaths.

On necropsy, lesions almost identical to those found in rodents are revealed in man. The mesenteric lymph nodes, liver and spleen are enlarged and show diffuse lymphoid hyperplasia. The organs may be studded with whitish abscesses, up to 1 cm in diameter, which contain caseous tough necrotic material and are surrounded by thick capsules. Necrotic foci and ulcers have been observed in the wall of the small intestines and colon.

Most human infections follow the more benign appendicial course.

Since Knapp and Masshoff (1954) identified the aetiological nature of the enteric form of human pseudotuberculosis, it has been recognised that the incidence of the infection in Central European countries is much higher than it was previously thought to be. Thus, 117 patients between the ages of 2 and 23 years were observed by Knapp (1958) in a 3-year period, in Tübingen (Germany). The organism was isolated from the blood of 2, and from the lymphatic nodules of 13 of the patients, whereas in the remaining cases the aetiological diagnosis was based upon serological and/or histological findings.

In a study of enteric infections caused by P. pseudotuberculosis in man, Daniels (Rotterdam, 1963) described 28 cases of abdominal lymphadenitis (25 males, 3 females; ages between 5 and 24 years, with average of 11.8). No septic case was among them; the pre-operative conditions invariably suggested appendicitis. In the 17 operated patients, the appendix was normal, but extensive ileocoecal lymphadenitis was established.

Multiple cases of human infection, occurring in the same environment, are very seldom observed. According to Daniels, 5 out of 18 mentally deficient children, living together with a boy suffering from pseudotuberculosis, showed significantly rising agglutinin-titers (320–5120) for the same type of P. pseudotuberculosis.

Doubtless a larger number of cases of this infection would have been brought to light in man, had more attention been drawn to the causative organism. At any rate, human pseudotuberculosis can no longer be regarded a pathological curiosity. However, no clear insight into its epidemiology and geographic distribution has been gained, because only meagre data are as yet available. The highest incidence of infection has been noticed in children and adolescent males. Knapp's own observations, added to those earlier recorded in the literature, showed that out of 132 cases only 23 were females.

Infections have been reported from Central European countries, France, Germany, North and South America, Japan and India.

Although in some cases direct contact with animals carrying the infection could be traced, and although most of the strains isolated from man are identical with those found in animals, in many instances no plausible explanation has been found for the appearance of the disease in humans. The infection is obviously not closely connected with occupational exposure to animals.

Man to man transmission of the disease has not been reported.

Antibiotics have but limited therapeutic value. Streptomycin and oxytetracycline appear to give the most promising results.

REFERENCES

BARTLEY, E. O. and K. HUNTER, *Lancet,* 252 (1947) 908.
DANIELS, J. J. H. M., Thesis M. D., Amsterdam, 1963, pp. 194.
DEVIGNAT, R., *Bull. Wld Hlth Org.,* 4 (1951) 247; 10 (1954) 463.
DUJARDIN-BAUMETZ, E., *Rev. Path. comp.,* 38 (1938) 884; Presse méd., (1938) 43.
HÄSSIG, A., *Schweiz. med. Wschr.,* 79 (1949) 971.
KNAPP, W., *Zbl. Bakt., I. Abt. Or.,* 161 (1954) 422; *New Engl. J. Med.,* 16 (1958) 776.
KNAPP, W. and W. MASSHOFF, *Dtsch. med. Wschr.,* 79 (1954) 1266.
KNAPP, W. and W. STEUER, *Z. Immun. Forsch.,* 113 (1956) 370.
MASSHOFF, W., *Dtsch. med. Wschr.,* 78 (1953) 532.
MASSHOFF, W. and W. DÖLLE, *Virchows Arch. path. Anat.,* 323 (1953) 664.
THAL, E., *Veterinary thesis,* Stockholm, 1954, p. 69; *J. Bact.,* 69 (1955) 103.
VORTEL, V., K. JINDRÁLE and F. VÝMOLA, *Virchows Arch. path. Anat.,* 331 (1958) 631.

4

J. E. DINGER

Plague

The history of plague is the history of the domestic link between man and the house rat. Severe epidemics have been known since the most remote times. The dreadful sickness described in the Bible (1 Sam., V and VI), with which God wreaked his punishment on the Philistines for stealing the Holy Ark, was almost certainly bubonic plague.

Throughout the centuries various pandemics have ravaged Asia and Europe. The one known in history as The Great Plague started in the year 542 in the Egyptian trading center of Pelusium and spread throughout Asia and Europe. The pandemic which became known as the Black Death originated in Mesopotamia and scourged Europe from the middle of the 11th to the end of the 16th century, reaching its height in the 14th century. In 1661 plague broke out afresh in Europe, and until the middle of the 18th century there were serious local epidemics, such as the one in Marseilles in 1720. The last pandemic began in 1871 in Central Asia and, following the trade routes, spread over the entire world.

In the 20th century, epidemics of plague in Europe have remained localized. There were cases in Marseilles in 1903, 1909, 1920 and 1930; and in 1920 Paris was shaken by an epidemic among the city rag-pickers. In Asia, on the other hand, and especially in India, plague flourished continuously at the beginning of the century. In the course of the following decades a gradual decline set in, but this was interrupted in 1945–1947 by a renewed wave of epidemics in India, Burma, China, Indochina, Thailand and Indonesia. Having entered Indonesia in 1910, plague has since kept a foothold in the mountainous areas of Java.

The disease was first brought to South Africa from South America in

1899. In North America the first cases were reported at the beginning of the present century.

It is usually recorded in the literature that the plague bacillus was simultaneously identified in 1894 by Yersin and Kitasato. Many investigators, however, are of the opinion that the bacterium which Kitasato first isolated and described as being gram-positive and motile, was not the causative agent of plague (Ogata, 1897, 1955).

In older cultures of *Pasteurella pestis* and sometimes also in direct preparations from splenic and glandular fluid in cases of subacute illness, the bacillus shows marked polymorphism, manifested by larger rods which are sometimes club or seal-ring shaped or which, because of their "budding", resemble yeast cells. These "involution forms" can be induced by a 24-hour culture upon 3 % saline agar. Another characteristic is the stalactite formation in undisturbed broth culture. *P. pestis* grows best upon slightly alkaline agar (pH 7.2–7.6) at 29–30°. Bile is a selective medium for blood cultures (Kirschner, 1934). Plague bacteria have also been successfully cultured upon 12 to 14-day old chick embryos (Jawetz and Meyer, 1944). They are acid-forming with several sugars, but do not form indole, nor dissolve gelatine. The plague bacterium is readily killed by a short exposure to sunlight and dehydration. At low temperatures, however, it may remain viable for months in flea faeces. At present, three varieties of plague bacteria are differentiated.

	Glycerine fermentation	Nitrous acid formation
P. pestis orientalis	—	+
P. pestis antiqua	+	+
P. pestis mediævalis	+	—

These varieties show no specific antigenic, morphological, or cultural distinctions other than those mentioned above. It is noteworthy that *P. orientalis* is most frequently found in rats and the latter two in other wild rodents (Girard, 1954). According to Devignat (1951, 1953), *P. pestis antiqua* originated in Central Asia, whence it was carried to Asia Minor, Egypt and Africa before the Christian era. It was most probably this form of plague that spread throughout the entire Roman empire. The mediaeval variant prevailing in Europe in the 14th century, which is still found in southeast Russia, the Middle East, Mongolia and Manchuria, may have been a mutation form. The variety *P. pestis orientalis* is encountered in India, Burma and southern China.

Plague is primarily a disease of rodents, although several other mammals are also susceptible to it. Cases of infection have been recorded in *cats* (ships' cats), *monkeys, goats, deer, donkeys, camels, antelopes, kangaroos* and *bats*. The course of the disease in rodents resembles that of haemorrhagic septicaemia. At post-mortem examination swelling and haemorrhagic infiltration of the lymph glands, bloody purulent exudate in the peritoneum, pericardium and pleura, extreme splenic enlargement and a great many small necrotic foci (pseudotubercles) in the liver, lungs and spleen are all observed. Pathognomonic symptoms of the incomplete picture are: subcutaneous haemorrhages (red extremities), haemorrhagic buboes (especially submaxillary), exudate in the pleura, peritoneum and pericardium, and an enlarged spleen containing pseudotubercles.

Septicaemia is present during the entire course of the disease and plague bacteria are found in large numbers in all organs. The disease sometimes follows a chronic course, in which event the post-mortem findings are subcutaneous haemorrhages, haemorrhagic buboes, enlarged spleen and large necrotic foci in spleen, liver and lymph glands ("resolving plague"). It is then difficult to demonstrate the plague bacterium and the diagnosis can only be confirmed by means of laboratory animals.

The diagnosis of *rat* plague is established by direct demonstration of plague bacteria in the blood and organs by staining either with Giemsa or Loeffler's alkaline methylene blue, or by culture and animal test. The animal test is performed by inoculating guinea pigs under the abdominal skin; the typical symptoms of the disease develop 1 to 3 days later. A shaved and abraded area of the skin of a guinea pig is rubbed with a small amount of material freshly taken from a putrefied carcass. When the post-mortem findings are being evaluated, it must be borne in mind that a number of diseases to which rodents are susceptible bear a strong resemblance to plague (tularaemia, melioidosis, pseudotuberculosis rodentium). Diagnosis, therefore, requires bacteriological confirmation.

In *human beings* the disease adopts two main forms: bubonic plague and primary pneumonic plague. The approximate mortality rate for the two forms, if untreated, is 70–80% and 100% respectively. Other types of plague have also been distinguished, *viz.,* carbuncular plague, followed by septicaemia, and primary septicaemia which has a very swift course, death sometimes occurring within two to eight hours. Bubonic plague owes its name to the typical haemorrhagic necrotic inflammation of the lymph glands in the area in which the flea infects the patient, most often in the inguinal region, with secondary development of infections in other lymph nodes (neck, armpit, and internal glands) (Fig. 10). Necrosis of the involved tissue develops, with abscesses which frequently break down spontaneously. There is often a rapidly developing inflammation of the neighbouring connective and muscle tissue which causes extensive destruction.

When there is no rapid fatal outcome, the internal organs also become involved, with haemorrhagic necrotizing foci in the spleen, liver and kidneys. Haemorrhages are found in the mucosa of the oesophagus, stomach and intestines, with infection-foci in Peyer's patches which are sometimes surrounded by haemorrhagic areas. If the lungs are simultaneously affected, the condition is designated as a secondary pneumonia. In

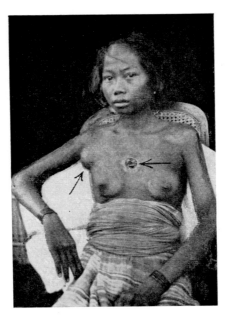

Fig. 10.   Bubonic plague.
(Photo: Deutmann; by courtesy of the Laboratory for Hygiene, University of Amsterdam)

the early stages of illness, the organ appears congested and swollen, with haemorrhagic foci spreading into the lung thereafter.

Primary pneumonic plague is characterized by an acute lobar pneumonia, which dominates the clinical picture throughout, the result being rapid death.

Carbuncular plague has the form of a rapidly developing necrosis of the skin which frequently spreads from the site of the infecting fleabites. Here, too, the prognosis is very unfavourable, because of the septicaemic spread of the plague bacteria.

Primary septicaemia has, as a rule, such a rapidly fatal course that the characteristic lesions have no opportunity to develop in the internal organs.

References p. 73

Clinical diagnosis of plague in man can be confirmed by bacteriological examination of the material in direct smears or cultures, and by using experimental animals. This material consists of blood (septicaemia), sputum (pneumonic plague), scrapings of necrotic skin (carbuncular plague) or fluid from lymph glands (bubonic plague). To obtain this fluid by puncture of a bubo, a thick hypodermic needle is used for shallow penetration of the lymph gland, because the location of the plague bacteria is usually periglandular.

If death occurs, in addition to necropsy, laboratory investigations of material taken from internal organs provide data for the diagnosis. In countries where autopsy is strongly objected to, samples obtained by puncture of the lung and spleen may supply valuable material for investigation. Lung puncture material teeming with plague bacteria is an indication of pneumonic plague; when the spleen preparation simultaneously shows only few organisms, the probability of primary pneumonic plague is great and a contact epidemic may already be under way, the early detection of which is of great epidemiological importance.

The most important reservoirs of plague are the wild rodents of the sparsely inhabited territories of the earth. According to Ricardo Jorge, this form of plague is usually called "sylvatic plague". However, where (except in California) the plague reservoir is represented by open field rodents, Hirst (1953) considers the term "campestral plague" more adequate. Although in vast areas of the world this reservoir must have existed since times immemorial, it did not attract the attention of scientific investigators until the beginning of the present century.

When plague was introduced by marine traffic into harbours of hitherto uninfected areas, the disease rapidly found a foothold among the wild rodents of the interior. In 1900, the first cases of plague were reported among the inhabitants of San Francisco and shortly thereafter it was found among the rat population of the city. In the ensuing years, plague spread among the rural ground squirrels to such an extent that in 1912 it was found in nine counties south of San Francisco. Once plague had passed the barrier of the Sierra Nevada, it spread over the entire territory west of the Rocky Mountains and in 1942 it crossed the Canadian border.

In the last few decades, many investigations of campestral plague have been conducted and these have demonstrated the existence of the disease in eastern, western and central South America, in northern China, the northern provinces of India, in central Asia, Java, Madagascar, the Soviet Union, Iran, Kurdistan, the Union of South Africa, the former Belgian Congo and Kenya (Grainger et al., 1959).

The third Report of the W.H.O. Expert Committee on Plague (1959) lists 225 species of wild rodents which were either found to be infected with *P. pestis* or were carriers of infected ectoparasites. This bacterial reservoir is composed of various kinds of hares, rabbits, cavidae, jerboas, rats, field-mice, hamsters, gerbils, voles, bandicots, squirrels, susliks, prairie dogs, marmots, chickarees and chipmunks. The principal carriers of the infection are: in Asia – the tarabagan; in South Russia – susliks; in South Africa – the gerbils; in South America – cavies; and in the United States of America – ground squirrels.

Spread of the infection in virgin regions occurs both *per continuitatem* and by migration. Both epizootics and latent chronic infections have been observed. Whether, during hibernation, the rodents or the parasitic insects remain the principal reservoir of infection, needs further elucidation. At any rate, this reservoir of wild rodents constitutes a continuous threat to man, and poses an almost insoluble problem for the control of the disease.

Direct infection of human beings occurs when the animals are hunted for commercial purposes. Much as these infections may be by their nature, sporadic in character. They carry an extreme threat, in that the plague bacterium originating in wild rodents is pneumotropic, and can secondarily cause air-borne epidemics among humans.

By far greatest hazard is the possibility of a continuous introduction of plague from the wilderness into territories inhabited by man by means of field rats and mice.

The main direct sources of infection to man are "domestic" rats, the house rat *(R. rattus* and *R. r. diardi)* and the ship's rat *(R. r. alexandrinus)*. The infection is transmitted among these rats by the fleas *Nosopsyllus fasciatus, Xenopsylla cheopis, X. braziliensis* and, to a lesser degree, *X. astia.* The number of plague bacilli increases in the proventriculus to form a mass which is regurgitated into the wound made when the flea bites a new host. The disease is usually conveyed by the flea through this regurgitation. Infection by flea faeces, passed while feeding and penetrating through a break in the host's skin, is also possible. The plague bacteria do not multiply in the tissues of the flea.

Climatic factors are very influential in the spread of plague. High temperature and saturation deficiency of the air reduce the period of infectivity, the length of the flea's life, and the larval production of the flea. This is reflected in seasonal prevalence and the phenomenon of local immunity. India provides a classic example of the former. There, plague shows an undeniable periodicity. A rise in temperature to a daily average of

28°, combined with a drop in humidity, causes an abrupt decline in incidence of the disease. For example, in Bombay the epidemic was always heaviest in the first months of the year. Between May and July, when average temperatures rise to 35°, there were only sporadic cases. By contrast, in Poona, 80 miles from Bombay, at an elevation of 2,000 feet, epidemics usually reach their height in the last months of the year and the "off-season" falls between March and May when the weather is driest.

In Java (Indonesia), which has a much more uniform climate, the seasonal prevalence is far less distinct. Nevertheless, a periodic incidence is discernible here too, running parallel with variations in the flea index.

The phenomenon of local immunity is also correlated with the nature and density of the rat flea population. In India it has long been known that there are places where plague is introduced but cannot thrive. Evidently *X. astia* is the most prevalent species in such places; where there is a great deal of plague, *X. cheopis* predominates. *X. astia* is a less efficient carrier, because it is more sensitive to high temperatures and to saturation deficiency. It also has far less affinity for man than *X. cheopis*. This type of local immunity is also encountered in Indonesia.

In Sumatra, two importations of plague occurred, one in 1905 and the other in 1918, both of which caused a limited, short-lived epidemic. After plague was imported into Java via Surabaya, and from there had travelled to Malang, it could only settle in the mountains. In Surabaya, a few cases were reported. The determining factor here is in all probability not the question of *astia–cheopis* prevalence, but the fact that the flea index of the house rat and the infectivity of the flea is appreciably lower in such low countries.

Transmission tests made by Swellengrebel and Otten showed that, in Surabaya, *X. cheopis* remained infectious for 19 days at an average temperature of 28.5° and a relative humidity rate of 64–67%; in Malang, on the other hand, with an average temperature of 23° and a relative humidity of 75–80%, the maximum duration of infectivity was 43 days. The life span of a flea with no source of food was 21 days in Malang and 7 days in Surabaya. The larval yield (*i.e.* the percentage of eggs which develop into larvae) was 60–80% in Malang, and 7–21% in Surabaya. In contrast, in Solo, which is also situated in the plains, van Steenis found a larval yield of 37–54%. This is interesting, because Solo is the only low-lying place on Java at which a severe epidemic of plague appeared.

The most important direct source of infection for man is the house rat, the rat flea acting as a vector. In general, the clinical picture is that of bubonic plague. This form of the disease – though not directly contagious from human-to-human – may nevertheless assume epidemic proportions among human populations. Because the disease causes high mortality among rats, hungry fleas will, in the absence of living animals, bite man. Bubonic plague is, therefore, not a true epidemic disease, but is actually a zoonosis with an accumulation of sporadic cases in humans, the frequency curve of which is a reflection of the epizootic among the local rats.

Whether bubonic plague can be conveyed from man to man by the human flea, *Pulex irritans,* especially in moderate and cool climates, is not yet fully agreed (Hylkema, 1922).

In India, *P. irritans* is very frequent, but no interhuman contact infections of bubonic plague have been observed. Girard (1943) caught large numbers of *Pulex irritans* in houses where there had been deaths from plague, but no plague bacteria could be shown by inoculation of guinea pigs with the crushed fleas.

In Java, where *Pulex irritans* is practically unknown, its role in the spread of plague is negligible. Swellengrebel (1953) found in Morocco 70 times as many fleas and 6 times as many lice on humans as in Java, and Blanc and Baltazard (1941) established epidemiological evidence in Morocco of *Pulex irritans* carrying the infection from human to human. They were able to demonstrate plague bacteria in the fleas of plague patients 21 days after the fleas were caught. In the opinion of these investigators, *Pulex irritans* as well as *Pediculus corporis* have at all times largely contributed to the spread of plague among human beings (Blanc, 1956). Delanoe (1922, 1932) expressed the same opinion. In French North and West Africa, where *X. cheopis* is rare and *P. irritans* is widespread, the latter would form the principal source of human infection.

The second form of human plague is the pneumonic type which is directly transmitted from man to man as an airborne infection. Thus it may cause veritable epidemics by human contacts. The origin of these epidemics is usually a case of secondary pneumonic plague in the course of zoonotic bubonic plague. Passage of *P. pestis* in persons with primary pneumonic plague enhances the virulence of the organism for humans. In India and Java, cases of primary pneumonic plague resulting from infection through rat fleas rarely occur and resultant epidemics are scarce. In general, pneumonic plague is a disease which appears more often in moderate climates and more frequently in winter than in summer. Unhygienic conditions and inadequate housing unquestionably play a large part in its development. In addition to climatological factors, the virulence of the bacteria is important. It has been found that there is more pneumonic plague among wild field rodents than among house rats. It is, therefore, accepted that the creation of variants of the plague bacteria with very high virulence and greater pneumotropism for human beings as well may here be involved. Epidemics of pneumonic plague in man caused by direct infection from wild rodents have been repeatedly described. Typical examples are the fulminating lung plague epidemics in Manchuria in 1910–1911 and 1920–1921, which resulted from infection by the tarabagan and caused 60,000 and 9,300 deaths respectively. These examples show that wild rodents are a direct and potent source of human infection.

Because of the large variety of wild rodents susceptible to plague, there are many recorded cases of occupational infection in hunters, furriers and butchers. Fleabites could not be found in all of these cases. Sources of human infection other than those originating from rodents have also been reported. A plague epidemic resulting from emergency slaughtering of camels has been described in South Russia; Yersin found plague bacteria in the meat.

The natural resistance of man to plague bacilli is limited. Of interest is the observation made by Girard and Grumbach (1958) that lepers are less susceptible to plague, and that, among the 50,000 victims of the plague epidemic in Madagascar in 1911 there were very few cases of lung tuberculosis, in spite of the fact that this disease is locally very widespread. Experiments on mice demonstrated a resistance-increasing effect of this kind.

When we enquire how plague spreads through different parts of the globe, a distinction should be made between spread over large distances and diffusion *per continuitatem* throughout the inhabited world. In the metastatic spread of plague, sea and surface traffic play an important part in that they provide transport for rats and/or fleas. Cargoes which attract rats include rice, flour, grain, peas and beans, copra, dried and salted fish, seeds of high oil content, vermicelli, coffee, capoc, paper- and wood-wool or excelsior. Plague has been repeatedly introduced into Indonesia, for example, by the importation of rice from Singapore and Rangoon. A recent epidemic on the west coast of South America was traced to the importation of burlap bags from India (Norris, 1953).

In addition to the transmission of fleas by transported goods, direct infection of house rats in harbor areas can occur. The ship rat, *R. r. alexandrinus,* is closely related to the house rat, so that contact between them is possible. The transportation of rice from the Javanese seaports of Surabaya, Semarang, Tjeribon and Djakarta has carried plague to the hinterland, where it has acquired a firm foothold in the mountain areas and whence it continued its diffusion.

In "urban" diffusion we are primarily concerned with contagion among the house rat
(*R. rattus*) population. The sewer rat, *R. norvegicus*, occurs especially in coastal areas
and *R. concolor* occurs in harbours. Other noteworthy potential vectors are the mice
Pachyura murina and *Crocidura coerulia*, which are particularly dangerous because they
may survive plague and may remain infectious for protracted periods of time. The ectoparasite carried by these animals is *X. cheopis*. These mice play no part in rural diffusion, because they do not migrate. Regarding *R. norvegicus*, this is true only for
Indonesia, because in India the sewer rat travels along the riverbanks out of the city and
it has repeatedly been shown that plague among house rats was preceded by an epizootic among *R. norvegicus*.

Diffusion from village to village can take place by means of field rats, in Java
through *R.r. brevicaudatus* and the mountain rat, *R. concolor ephippium*. *R.r. brevicaudatus* is the Javanese sawahrat; it builds its nests in the little dikes of the rice fields,
never in houses. When the grain in the fields is ripening, it finds all the food it needs on
the spot, and the rats concentrate then in maximum numbers in these fields. However,
when the fields become bare after harvesting, the rats begin to run short of food and
some of them travel to the barns and houses where they nest; they nest here all the
more easily when the house rat population has been thinned out by plague.

The same is true for *R. concolor ephippium*. These rats are infected through *X.
cheopis*, although this flea plays no part in the further spread of plague among field rats,
because it is seldom found on rats caught in the open fields. *X. cheopis* cannot resist
humidity, and its larvae do not survive in the damp nests of the field rat, whose ectoparasite is *Stivalius cognatus*, the flea which transmits the infection among them. This
flea is even more sensitive than *X. cheopis* to high temperatures and saturation deficiency, and is, therefore, not to be found in low-lying areas. It is first encountered
at an elevation of 400 to 500 m and finds optimum conditions at 800 m or higher.
Van Steenis' contention that the field rat played an important role in the diffusion
of plague in the mountainous regions of Java is supported by the observation, made
in central Java, of diffusion across mountain ranges where there had been no human
traffic. Moreover, epizootics among field rats have been observed. In this connection
it is also interesting to note that the only severe epidemic which has taken place in
a low-lying Javanese city – Solo – did not spread unto the plain. The field rat which
inhabits low-lying areas carries no fleas.

The continuous diffusion of plague over the mountainous parts of Java is
caused, not only by the field rat, but, to an important extent, by human
traffic which carries with it infected rat fleas in baggage. Although there
has as yet been no conclusive evidence of this, there are epidemiological
indications, that the so-called "small transport" has been largely instrumental in diffusion of the disease. An extensive investigation under
Swellengrebel's direction was conducted in 1912, when plague raged in
Malang. A cordon was thrown around the infected area and all travellers
and their baggage underwent an examination for fleas, with the result that
among 57,000 people, only two rat fleas were found. This figure appears

negligible, but, since in heavily populated Java the figures for such transport run into millions, the actual effect can be impressive. A single hungry, plague-infected flea deposited in a shed may start a plague epidemic among the entire local rat population.

The battle against plague comprises measures aimed at reducing the chance of infection and measures which are directed toward increasing man's specific resistance. In regions which are threatened by plague from neighbouring areas, attention should be focussed on the early detection of rat plague. Bacteriological examination of dead rats provides direct evidence. Because the affected rats withdraw to their nests, epizootics among these are frequently far advanced before the first sick rat is discovered. It is therefore important to heed indirect signs of sudden numerous deaths among house rats. This is achieved by periodic trapping; an acute drop in the density of the rat population is reflected in reduced catches and in increasing percentages of both flea carriers and the numbers of fleas found per rat ("secondary flea concentration", according to van Loghem).

As a criterion of acute increase of the flea index, Swellengrebel recommends the determination of the ratio between the number of trypanosome carriers and flea carriers. This is written T/F, a ratio which is normally $\pm$ 1, because rats are infected with *Trypanosoma lewesi* by *X. cheopis*. Because the incubation period of trypanosomiasis is 10–14 days, in the event of large-scale deaths among rats the flea index due to secondary increase will rise more rapidly than the trypanosome index, *i.e.* the ratio T/F will drop steeply.

In many underdeveloped areas medical authorities receive their first warning of plague from an increased death toll among the human population. The epizootic among the rats has by then already established itself. Plague cases among the human population are then detected by means of post-mortem examination (spleen and liver puncture of cadavers) and/or examination of patients. If bubonic plague is found, the patients must be isolated forthwith, because each of them may develop secondary pneumonic plague and may thus threaten to initiate a contact epidemic. When a patient shows symptoms of pneumonic plague, other members of the household and people who have been in close contact with the patient must also be isolated. In uncomplicated bubonic plague, isolation of the contacts is not necessary.

A large-scale campaign against plague must be directed primarily against the house rat. The most efficient form of control is the biological one, *i.e.* the *improvement of housing,* to remove the link between the house rat and man. The principle behind such measures consists in preventing the nesting of rats in dwellings. This is done by improving both material and construction of such dwellings.

Rats nest by preference in hollow bamboo, into which they gnaw through the segment walls; so bamboo should be replaced by wood wherever possible. If bamboo is used or retained, it must be whole and the two ends closed off by tin, wood or cement stoppers; vertically placed bamboo must rest on stone. Thatched roof covering must be replaced by wood or metal and clay or mud walls by stone. All dead space must be excluded from the construction or, when this is impossible, made easy to inspect. Improved housing conditions not only remove the link between man and rat, and thus between man and rat-flea, but at the same time they aim a biological blow at the rats by driving them away from the houses, making their survival difficult. In conjunction with housing, thought must be given to improving housekeeping practices; rubbish on the grounds and in the houses in which the rat conceals its nest must be removed. This manner of attack was very successful in Java. Until the outbreak of the second world war put an end to this valuable work, housing improvement had been completed in the whole of eastern and central Java and was well under way in western Java. A total of 1½ million houses had by then been improved.

In addition to dwellings, the warehouses, particularly those in which foodstuffs are stored, are veritable breeding places for rats.

Beside this time-consuming type of programme, mass vaccination of the population has provided in infected and menaced areas, an excellent method of increasing the specific resistance of the people. Extremely favourable results have been obtained with Otten's live vaccine (Tjiwidej Java strain).

In 1934 Otten tested this vaccine on a large scale with the alternate person method in two threatened subdistricts of the province of Preanger. In each house, half of the occupants were vaccinated and the other half received a placebo; a total of 37,435 people were vaccinated, the rest of the population totalling 39,483. When plague broke out, there were ten times as many deaths among the unvaccinated as among the vaccinated. Between 1935 and 1939, more than seven million people were successfully vaccinated in Java. Similar results were obtained with the live E.V. strain vaccine developed by Girard and Robic which was used on a huge scale in Madagascar.

References p. 73

The oldest and most frequently used Haffkine vaccine is a killed vaccine. It is less effective than the avirulent live vaccine and must be given in three doses, while a single dose of the live vaccine is sufficient. To maintain immunity, vaccination must be repeated annually.

It must be emphasized that mass vaccination does not replace improved housing facilities, because it is a purely repressive expedient which reduces mortality without at all affecting the source of the evil, the rat plague.

As a plague control measure, the method is not equivalent to inoculation against other diseases that are transmitted from man to man, such as smallpox, cholera and typhoid fever. Smallpox vaccination, for instance, confers collective immunity on a population, whereby even those who have not been vaccinated, benefit; in a plague area, the chance of an unvaccinated individual contracting the disease is not influenced by the vaccination situation of the population as a whole.

In many tropical countries the ultimate campaign against rat plague by housing improvement is defeated by unsurmountable economic difficulties. Wherever rat destruction must be substituted for rat eradication, the classical substances in use are: phosphorus, barium, strychnine, arsenic, scilla maritima, thallium, zelio (Bayer), or such bacteria as S. enteritidis gärtneri or S. typhi murium. In recent publications (Pollitzer, 1952; Link and Mohr, 1953), warfarin, pival, red squill, ANTU, zinc phosphide and sodium fluoroacetate (1080) have been reported upon as highly effective rodenticides.

An entirely new approach to plague control consists in the destruction of fleas by means of insecticides.

In Tumbes (Peru), an investigation of a plague epizootic among rats in 1945 showed that 27.3% of the rats and 56% of the fleas were infected. There were 40 cases of plague among the population. In three successive campaigns, the floors, the flat roofs and the spaces under the floors and between double walls, were treated with DDT powder, while sodium fluoroacetate in rat bait was used to destroy the rats themselves. As from the 4th day after the end of the campaign, there were no fresh human cases of the disease, the flea index having dropped by more than 90%, and rat plague disappeared after the second campaign (Macchiavello, 1946).

In Haifa, in 1947, a plague epidemic was successfully controlled in its early stages solely by spraying all dwellings with 5% DDT solution and treating the population with DDT powder. After 7 days, no additional human cases of plague were reported and a month later, rat plague had also disappeared altogether, the flea index having fallen from 3 to less than 1 per rat (Pollock, 1948).

This method is at present also applied in Thailand (Ebel and Thaineira, 1957). On the basis of laboratory tests, Federov (1957) recommends the elimination of rodents and ectoparasites by means of a mixed bait containing raticide and DDT.

The same method has also been used in storage sheds and chicken runs (Grouck, 1946), and recent publications (Rijckman, 1953–54) report its application in the Californian fields by spraying the burrows of ground squirrels with insecticides. A comparative study of various insecticides indicates that the new preparations heptachlor, aldrin and dieldrin yield better results than DDT.

Lastly, the important part played by international shipping in spreading plague all over the world must be mentioned. Control measures enacted in international conventions (Paris, 1903, 1912, 1926 and Washington, 1945) were replaced in 1951 by the International Sanitary Regulations of the World Health Organization which bind all participating countries, unless the contrary is declared in writing addressed to the Secretary General of the W.H.O.

One of the main provisions is the compulsory periodic deratization of ships, even though the ships have not called at plague-infected ports. The rats are extirpated by fumigation with sulphur dioxide, hydrogen cyanide gas, or cyclon B. A certificate attesting the rat-free condition of a ship is valid for 6 months. The building of rat-proof ships has been promoted as much as possible, and such ships can obtain a statement of exemption from the extirpation campaign, provided that investigation shows that they are free from rats or that the rat population is "reduced to a minimum".

Ships coming from infected ports or ships which have cases of plague on board must comply with the quarantine regulations laid down by the World Health Organization.

All the control measures mentioned have contributed to a world-wide decline of human morbidity due to plague.

The mortality rate shows an even sharper drop because death, particularly from bubonic plague, has been appreciably reduced by modern therapy (from 75 to less than 10%). The success achieved by such therapy has been reported in recent publications (Meyer, 1952; Ajl *et al.*, 1958; McCrumb *et al.*, 1953; Semenova *et al.*, 1957; Nguyen-van Ai, 1957). The drugs given are the antibiotics streptomycin, chloramphenicol, bacteriomycin, aureomycin and terramycin, the first three being the most efficacious. Pneumonic plague has been successfully treated with chloramphenicol and terramycin (McCrumb *et al.*, 1953; Mercier and McCrumb, 1952).

Although treatment with massive doses of antibiotics may indeed succeed in elimination of *P. pestis,* the patient nevertheless often dies, especially in more advanced cases, as a result of the liberation of toxins from the bacteria. It is essential, therefore, to give the antibiotics early and it is also desirable to combine them with the administration of γ-globulin from hyperimmune rabbit serum (Girard, 1953; Meyer, 1957; Semenova *et al.*, 1957). In this connection it should be mentioned that, in recent times, successful attempts have been made to obtain the toxin of *P. pestis* in purified form (Ajl *et al.*, 1958; Spivack and Kailer, 1958).

Benign cases respond to sulfonamides (sulfathiazol, sulfadiazine and sulfamerazine), which are frequently used also for the chemoprophylaxis of the contacts of pneumonic plague patients.

For the protection of severely exposed persons, vaccination and protective clothing are considered the most effective measures. Diethyl toluamide is recommended as the best flea repellent.

On the whole, the results achieved through intensive control measures and modern therapy can be regarded as most encouraging. This conclusion is reflected in the striking world-wide decline of deaths from plague during the last few years. According to Pollitzer (1951) the mortality figures for India are especially spectacular, the total deaths from plague being – between 1898 and 1938: 12,379,819, averaging 309,496 per year, and between 1939 and 1948: 217,970, averaging 21,797 per year.

Statistics of the World Health Organization recorded the following mortality figures:

in 1949:	10,801	in 1955:	163
in 1950:	7,842	in 1956:	68
in 1951:	2,481	in 1957:	16
in 1952:	1,279	in 1958:	10
in 1953:	774	in 1959:	12
in 1954:	282	in 1960:	25

Nevertheless, it is premature to draw from these figures the conclusion that plague is liable to disappear altogether within a foreseeable time. The bacterial reservoir present in wild rodents remains a potential threat, and great care should be exercised in continuously enforcing measures intended to break the link between man and either the house rat or other rodents that are potential carriers of *P. pestis*.

REFERENCES

AJL S. J. *et al.*, *J. Immunol.*, 80 (1958) 435.

BLANC, G., *Rev. Hyg. Méd. Soc.*, 4 (1956) 535.

BLANC, G. and M. BALTHAZARD, *C. R. Acad. Sci. (Paris)*, 23 (1941) 813; 849.

DELANOË, P., *Bull. Soc. Path. exot.*, 15 (1922) 39; 25 (1932) 958.

DEVIGNAT, R., *Bull. Wld Hlth Org.*, 4 (1951) 247; *Inst. roy. colonial belge, sect. Sci. nat. et Méd. Mém.*, 23 (1953) 47.

EBEL, R. E. and M. THAINEIRA, *Amer. J. trop. Med. Hyg.*, 6 (1957) 280.

FEDEROV, M. N., *Med. Parazit. (Mosk.)*, 26 (1957) 40.

GIRARD, G., *Bull. Soc. Path. exot.*, 36 (1943) 4; 46 (1953) 526; *Maroc méd.*, 33 (1954) 1016.

GIRARD, G. and F. GRUMBACH, *C. R. Soc. Biol. (Paris)*, 152 (1958) 180.

GRAINGER, W. E., R. B. HEISCH and G. S. NELSON, *J. trop. Med. Hyg.*, 42 (1959) 211.

GROUCK, H. K., *J. Econ. Entomol.*, 39 (1946) 410.

HIRST, L. F., *The conquest of plague*, Oxford, 1953, 478 pp.

HYLKEMA, B., *Ned. T. Geneesk.*, 66 (1922) 1375.

JAWETZ, E. and K. F. MEYER, *Amer. J. Path.*, 20 (1944) 457.

KIRSCHNER, L., *Geneesk. T. Ned.-Ind.*, 74 (1934) 1141.

LINK, V. B. and C. O. MOHR, *Bull. Wld Hlth Org.*, 9 (1953) 585.

MACHIAVELLO, A., *Amer. J. publ. Hlth*, 36 (1946) 842.

McCRUMB, F. R., A. LARSON and K. F. MEYER, *J. infect. Dis.*, 92 (1953) 273; *Amer. J. Med.*, 14 (1953) 284.

MERCIER, S. and F. R. McCRUMB, *Med. trop.*, 12 (1952) 693; 698.

MEYER, K. F., S. F. QUAN, F. R. McCRUMB and A. LARSON, *Ann. N.Y. Acad. Sci.*, 55 (1952) 1228.

MEYER, K. F., *Pub. Hlth Rep. (Wash.)*, 72 (1957) 705.

NGUYEN-VAN AI, *Bull. Soc. Path. exot.*, 50 (1957) 8.

NORRIS, E. W., L. B. SCHNEIDER, L. J. MANCHETT, C. E. KOHLER and W. F. BUREN, *Pub. Hlth Rep. (Wash.)*, 68 (1953) 802.

OGATA, N., *Zbl. Bakt., I. Abt. Orig.*, 21 (1897) 769.

OGATA, N., *Zbl. Bakt., I. Abt. Orig.*, 163 (1955) 171.

POLLITZER, R., *Bull. Wld Hlth Org.*, 4 (1951) 475; 6 (1952) 381.

POLLOCK, J. S. and MACKENZIE, *Trans. roy. Soc. trop. Med. Hyg.*, 41 (1948) 647.

RIJCKMAN, R. E. *et al.*, *J. Econ. Entomol.*, 46 (1953) 598; 47 (1954) 604.

SEMENOVA, E. L. *et al.*, *Ž. Mikrobiol. (Mosk.)*, 28 (1957) 428.

SPIVACK, M. C. and A. KAILER, *J. Immunol.*, 80 (1958) 441.

SWELLENGREBEL, N. H., *Docum. Med. geogr. trop. (Amst.)*, 5 (1953) 151.

5

J. ZIDON

Tularaemia

The disease nowadays called tularaemia has been known under various names for many years. In the U.S.A. it has been called Pahvant valley plague, deer-fly fever or rabbit fever, in Japan yato-byo or Ohara's disease and in Norway Olaus Wormius, in his book *Historia Naturalis,* described it as early as 1653, as lemming fever. It may safely be assumed that the disease reported in Japan by Homma (1837), affecting wild rabbits and humans alike, and the "plague" prevailing in the Astrakhan district during the Turko-Russian War in 1877 were outbreaks of tularaemia.

McCoy and Chapin demonstrated the aetiologic agent of a plague-like disease of ground squirrels which prevailed in Tulare County, California, between 1908 and 1911 and named the organism *Bacterium tularense.* Further research led to the discovery of the same microorganism in man, two years after it had been found in rodents.

Francis, to whom we owe the name tularaemia, conducted, with his co-workers at the Washington Public Health Bureau, extensive investigations into the nature of the disease. Present knowledge of the bacteriological and clinical aspects of the infection are largely derived from achievements of these workers.

Tularaemia has since been reported from and investigated in all the states of North America (with the exclusion of Vermont), and also in several Asiatic, European and North African countries.

Thus, the disease was recognized in Japan by Ohara, in 1924; he postulated that hares constitute the source of infection in 86.5% of all cases. As a result of its high incidence in the U.S.S.R., research on tularaemia, initiated in that country in 1926, led to the establishment of anti-tularaemia stations in most of that country's provinces. In Norway,

:ularaemia was recognized in 1929 by Thiotta and two years later by Olin n Sweden. In these countries, the main reservoir of the causative agent is n lemmings.

For additional information on the discovery of the disease in other :ountries, see Table X.

Pasteurella tularensis * is a strictly aerobic, non-motile, non-spore-'orming, gram-negative, extremely polymorphic microorganism, which :akes the form of either coccus, bacillus or filament. It is a facultative ntra-cellular parasite and does not grow on ordinary media.

A species, *P. novicida* (Larson, 1955), closely resembling *P. tularensis,* has been isolated 'rom the Ogden Bay waters in Utah (U.S.A.). It is pathogenic to rodents, but is not known to infect man.

Pasteurella tularensis is not endowed with high resistance to elevated :emperatures, exposure to sunrays or bactericidal chemicals. It is readily destroyed by such common germicides as lysol and cresol. At 56–58° the organism is killed within 10 minutes and, when it is exposed to direct sunshine at 29°, after 3 hours. It possesses, on the other hand, a high viability, not only *in vitro* (*P. tularensis* survived in cultures at 10° for 22 years), but also under different and variable conditions in nature. Thus the organism remained alive in humid soil for 30 days, in water for 90 days and in wheat grain for 133 days. The bacterium may maintain its virulence inside the body of the tick *Ornithodoros turicata* up to 764 days. This high viability accounts for the continuity of the disease in nature and affects its epizootiology and epidemiology.

In *lagomorphs* and *rodents* the disease may appear as an acute or sub-acute bacteraemia or in a chronic form. The course of the naturally acquired disease in wild animals can be observed only rarely. The affected hare moves about slowly, sometimes leaping in a strange fashion, becomes unwary of his natural enemies, such as cats and dogs, and is easily caught by man. Full clinical symptoms have been recorded after experimental inoculation of hares by the intracutaneous route (Skrodzki, 1954). In addition to the signs described above, lack of appetite, weakness, rise of body temperature to 40–42° were observed. At the site of injection ulcers and abscesses developed and the regional lymph glands became

---

* Synonyms: *Bacterium tularense* (McCoy and Chapin, 1912), *Brucella tularensis* (Foshay and Wilson, 1931), *Francisella tularensis* (Olsufiev and Emelianova, 1959).

TABLE X

TULARAEMIA CASES IN MAN REPORTED IN VARIOUS COUNTRIES IN THE YEARS 1924–1957

Country	Years	Number of cases	Source of recorded data
Africa			
Tunesia	1933	?	Anderson
America			
Canada	1930–50	79	Olsufiev *
	1951–57	45	W.H.O.**
Mexico	1944	?	Tovar
U.S.A.	1924–50	23308	Olson *et al.*
	1951–57	3758	W.H.O.**
Venezuela	1948–50	17	Olsufiev *
	1951–57	44	W.H.O.†
Asia			
Japan	1924–57	720	Ohara, Muto
Turkey	1936–53	700	Bilal
Europe			
Austria	1935–50	500	Schaffer
	1951–57	248	W.H.O.**
Belgium	1949–57	52	Nelis
Czechoslovakia	1936–52	585	Drbohlav *et al.*
Finland	1939	?	Siewers
France	1946–50	294	Thiery
	1951–57	140	W.H.O.**
Germany	1943–47	152	Jusatz
(Fed. & Dem. Rep.)	1948–56	405	Lenz
Greece	1939	?	Lorando *et al.*
Italy	1931	"few cases"	Bardella *et al.*
Netherlands	1953	7	Hemmes
Norway	1929–31	50	Thiotta
Poland	1950–55	390	Wysocka
Rumania	1948–49	820	Olsufiev *
Sweden	1931–50	650	Olin
	1951–57	418	W.H.O.**
U.S.S.R.	1926–42	73300	Jusatz ††
Yugoslavia	1952–56	45	Falisevac

* From data quoted by this author.
** Epidemiological and Vital Statistics Reports.
† Reported area including 55.6% of the total population.
†† Comprising a fraction of the total number of cases.

enlarged. All inoculated animals died in 8–14 days. Post-mortem findings resembled those of plague and pseudotuberculosis. The swollen lymphatic glands frequently contained caseous and softened foci, the 3–4 times enlarged spleen showed grayish-white spots and dots. Usually the liver, adrenals and bone marrow also contained a large number of granulomatous foci; they were less numerous in the lung and in the kidneys (Fig. 11).

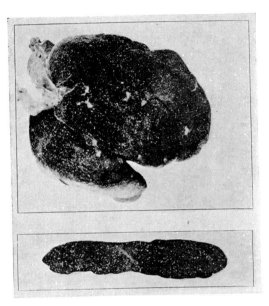

Fig. 11.   Liver and spleen of rabbit succumbed from tularaemia.
(Photo: Dr. E. Francis, Washington, D.C.)

In very sensitive animals, such as the water rat, in the beginning the disease takes the course of haemorrhagic septicaemia acompanied by haemorrhage in the spleen and lymphatic nodes, swelling and degeneration of the parenchymatous organs and a tendency to proliferation. Sometimes only swelling of the spleen or central deterioration of lymphatic nodules accompanied by fistules is found.

Of all domestic animals among which tularaemia is relatively widespread, *sheep* are the most frequently involved, constituting at times a source of infection for man. Epizootics in sheep have been recorded in Alberta, Canada, in 1942 and in neighbouring districts in the U.S.A (Montana, 1928, 1934 and Idaho, 1928, 1949, 1952) as well as in the U.S.S.R. (northern Caucasus in 1940 and Transcaucasus in 1954).

In most instances *wood ticks* act as vectors of the disease, by attacking flocks on pastures in springtime. Lambs and yearlings are chiefly affected as compared to mature sheep (Jellison).

In these animals the earliest symptoms of illness are prostration and loss of weight; the sheep strays from the flock, its movements become heavy and stiff, and sometimes it lies down and begins to roll to-and-fro. The regional lymph nodes of the head and neck become swollen at the sites of concentration of ticks. Rise of body temperature, increase of respiration rate, nasal discharge and coughing are present in conjunction, in the advanced stage, with diarrhoea. Respiration becomes laborious and is accompanied by grinding of teeth. In severe cases weakness progresses to the point of complete exhaustion, death occurring within a few hours. In most cases, whenever the infesting ticks are removed before exhaustion sets in, uneventful recovery ensues.

Post-mortem examination reveals specific changes in the swollen prescapular and mesenteric lymph nodes; small abscesses, caseous foci or necrotic areas can also be noted. Hepatitis is frequent; changes in the spleen and liver are characterized by subcapsular white foci and small yellowish necrotic areas, whereas in the lungs atalectatic areas may be found. The kidneys are little, if at all, involved. This is also true of the heart and skeletal muscles. In most cases, *P. tularensis* may be recovered from the spleen and liver.

In *goats* which have died of tularaemia, similar changes may be at hand. This animal is, however, rarely affected by the illness.

Natural infection occurs in *swine,* as in sheep, as a result of tick bites; ingestion of infected rodents may be another mode of infection. Young swine are chiefly affected. Clinically, swine show inappetency, general weakness and rise of body temperature accompanied by profuse sweating, coughing and swelling of the lymphatic nodes. On necropsy, characteristic changes are found in the lymphatic glands in conjunction with splenomegaly and occasional inflammation of the lungs.

The disease in *cattle* is commoner than is sometimes thought. Apart from several isolated cases in California and Montana (U.S.A.) in 1938, Sinai and Uzunov, in the U.S.S.R., found positive serotitres in 12 (2.2%)

 out of 543 examined cows in areas where foci of tularaemia had been discovered. Similar results were obtained by Skrodzki and co-workers, after examining 354 cows of the "tularaemia area" of Szcezcin (Poland) in 953, of which 2.5% showed positive serum reactions.

Cattle are infected by: (1) infected ticks, especially ticks of the genus *xodes*, (2) the bites of insects (mosquitoes or bloodsucking flies), (3) grazing on contaminated pastures or ingestion of water from sources polluted by the excretions of diseased rodents.

Like most young mammals, calves are particularly susceptible to tularaemia. The commonest clinical symptoms observed include rise of temperature with coughing and diarrhoea, followed by progressive weakness, exhaustion and death.

In *horses*, the modes of infection are much the same as those of cattle, but susceptibility to the disease is lower. The onset is marked by a rise of temperature usually to over 41°, oedema, stiffness of limbs and dyspnoea. There is swelling of the lymph nodes in the region of the neck and prescapular area. In pregnant mares in contaminated areas, a considerable number of abortions can be ascribed to tularaemia. In a district of the U.S.S.R., out of 103 abortions of mares, only 8 could be definitely traced to *Salmonella abortus equi*, while in the remaining instances there was unmistakable evidence indicating that these were due to tularaemie (Isakow). Post-mortem examinations reveal numerous infected areas with focal necrosis in the lung. Involvement of the heart is mostly characterized by dilatation. Swelling of the spleen, liver and kidneys, which are dotted with small necrotic foci, are observed (Claus).

The *cat* may be included among domestic animals which show a relatively high susceptibility to tularaemia. As a carnivore, primarily preying on various rodents, it is understandable that it was chosen by early investigators as an object for studying the modes of spread of tularaemia. Thus, Francis in 1924 and Green and Wade in 1928, investigated the disease in experimentally infected cats. It remained for Collins to report the first cases of naturally infected cats in 1933. Tularaemia infection in cats has also been reported from Austria and Turkey. In 1940, during epizootics occurring in the Caucasus (U.S.S.R.), there was high morbidity and mortality among the feline population. The clinical picture in cats includes such features as loss of weight, progressive debility and swelling of regional lymphatic glands of the neck and head. On necropsy, enlarged submaxillary, cervical and mesenteric lymph nodes, with coagulative or caseous necrotic foci, are noted, whereas in the lung the alveoli are filled with coagulated cells and fibrin. The septa of the lung appear necrotic. In the compressed and atrophic liver, multiple nodule containing necrotic cells with fibrin are observed. Some major veins are partly or totally obstructed by necrotic cellular thrombi. In the swollen spleen, small nodules with caseous centre or areas of confluent necrosis are encountered (Francis). In most instances the causative agent could be recovered by animal inoculation of material from the liver and spleen.

Although resistance to the disease in *dogs* seems to be higher than it is in cats, numerous cases of natural infection of dogs have been recorded in Austria (David), U.S.A. (Calhoun, Kunkel) and in the U.S.S.R. (Dorofejew). Most of the dogs were hunting-dogs and dogs on sheep-breeding ranches. The clinical picture often showed suppurative abscesses or ulcers of the skin, swelling of lymphatic glands and sometimes paralysis of hind legs. On necropsy, swollen lymph nodes with widespread necrotic foci are revealed; the lungs appear inflamed, with a muco-purulent exudate. Contrary to what is found in most other susceptible mammals, the spleen, liver and kidneys of dogs are little, if at all, involved. The aetiological agent may be isolated from the blood or abscesses, but rarely from the liver or spleen.

Among *wild fowl,* and particularly among birds of prey that feed on cadavers, tularaemia is not an uncommon occurrence. When one considers that some ectoparasites, such as ticks *(Dermacentor andersoni* and *Ixodes ricinus),* mosquitoes *(Culex pipiens, Aedes aegypti),* fleas *(Cerato-pyllus),* affect rodents and birds alike, it is natural that under certain conditions, birds should become both vectors and reservoirs of the causative agent.

Among *domesticated birds,* the chicken, is resistant to the infection, but is not entirely immune to it (Francis, Tumanski). This is apparently also true of pigeons and turkeys, whereas wild birds such as quail, the different species of grouse, gulls and other birds, seem to be more susceptible.

The pathological findings in naturally infected birds are scarce and may be altogether inapparent, although the aetiological agent may be demonstrated by inoculation of guinea pigs with material taken from the liver and spleen of the birds.

American and Soviet publications (Nowikow *et al.*) remark on the relative susceptibility of frogs *(Rana esculenta, Rana catesbeiana)* to tularaemia; an epizootic among these animals was correlated with a prevailing illness of rodents in the environment. The occurrence of tularaemia among crabs and snails has been reported from Armenia.

The disease in *man* takes a varied course determined not only by his resistance, the virulence of the bacterium and the density of infection, but also by the portal of entry.

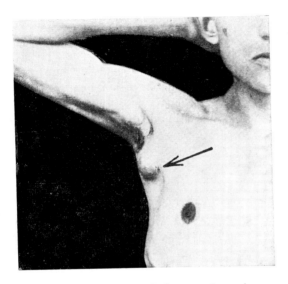

Fig. 12. Axillar bubo in human tularaemia.
(Photo: Dr. E. Francis, Washington, D.C.)

Tularaemia is classified into five principal clinical types, according to its specific clinical manifestations: (1) ulceroglandular, (2) glandular, (3) oculoglandular (4) typhoidal and (5) pulmonary.

The onset is similar in all 5 types and does not differ much from the initial stage of any other acute infectious disease. It is sudden and dramatic, after an incubation period of 1 to 10 days (in most instances 3 to 4 days) and is associated with chills, general weakness, inappetence, muscular and lumbar pain as well as articular pain in the limbs, headache and vomiting. Flushing of the face and conjunctivitis are sometimes pronounced. The tongue is coated and dry.

During the first few days the body temperature rises to 38–39°, and is mostly of the remittent or undulant type. In many cases there is a brief remission of fever after 3 days with subjective improvement, only to be followed by a renewed bout of fever lasting for 2 to 3 weeks, which gradually subsides afterwards. Convalescence is slow and protracted.

The blood picture exhibits no characteristic changes and only seldom is moderate leucocytosis observed. The blood sedimentation rate is somewhat accelerated.

The most common form seen in man (85%) is the *ulceroglandular type,* which begins with a primary lesion. Usually the lesion follows a scratch of cut occurring chiefly on the fingers that have been in contact with blood or excretions from infected animals. About 24 hours after manifestation of the first clinical symptoms, a painful papule develops at the site of infection, with ensuing swelling of the regional lymph nodes, even though no lymphangitis develops between the papule and the bubo. The bubo is formed as a result of penetration of the microorganisms into the lymph node and their multiplication there, and the node may attain the size of a hen's egg (Fig. 12). Simultaneously, the primary lesion, the papule, spreads out into painful edges and heals slowly. In about 50% of all cases, the bubo may become suppurative and, in others, ulcerative, with slow healing and cicatrization. Sclerotization is not rare, the gland remaining tense and painful for many months.

In the *glandular type* no primary lesion is present, although in all other respects the clinical picture is reminiscent of the ulceroglandular type with formation of one or, rarely, several buboes. This variety of tularaemia is particularly common in Japan.

The *oculoglandular type,* which is usually unilateral, evolves after penetration of the causative agent into the conjunctiva by spattering of blood or excreta of the infected animal into the eye, or by wiping the eye with contaminated hands. At the site of the primary lesion an ulcerated papule is formed with widely differing ensuing local reactions, such as conjunctivitis and swelling of the preauricular, submaxillary or cervical lymphatic glands. The clinical picture suggests that of Parinaud's conjunctivitis. The incidence of this type appears to be higher in Turkey, as compared with other tularaemia endemic countries.

The most serious clinical manifestations are associated with the *typhoidal type* of the disease, which is a generalized process with no apparent involvement of the lymphatic glands. This form, the incidence of which is estimated at about 10%, is chiefly prevalent among laboratory workers and it is doubtful whether there is any laboratory engaged in tularaemia research, which can boast that tularaemia has not occurred among its workers. In the severe forms of this type of infection, fever may persist unabated for 4 to 6 weeks and it is followed by slow subsidence of the temperature with profuse sweating. Severe signs of a generalized toxic state, mental clouding, delirium and vomiting are not uncommon. The spleen, which is considerably increased in size from the third day of onset of the disease, is painful; the liver is enlarged as well.

Encephalitis or *meningitis,* rarely occurring in tularaemia, are serious complications. In the typhoidal type, pleuropulmonary involvement is characterized by bronchitis, and sometimes also by pneumonia. The infection may, when it extends to the pleura, cause pleurisy.

The *pulmonary type,* tularaemic pneumonia, is frequently encountered in the U.S.S.R. as a primary disease. Agricultural workers engaged in threshing and handling straw contaminated with mouse excreta, may inhale dust bearing the causative agent, whence the clinical picture of an atypical pneumonia emerges with roentgenological findings in one or both lungs.

Cases of tularaemia associated with a rash resembling erythema nodosum have been reported.

In addition to the just mentioned types *rhinoglandular* and *tonsilloglandular forms* have been described.

Until the advent of antibiotic therapy, the mortality rate during outbreaks in the U.S.A. fluctuated between 5 and 7%, as compared to 1 to 2% for Europe and Asia.

Pathological findings on necropsy bear strong resemblance to post-mortem findings in rodents. Tularaemic lesions in the form of small abscesses may be found on the skin and in the lymphatic and endothelial systems. Necrotic areas are also present in the liver and spleen.

Isolated, necrotic foci of the lungs may be found, with occasional lobar involvement. The myocardium and pericardium are less often involved.

Diagnosis of the ulceroglandular and oculoglandular types offers no difficulties, particularly when a history of contact with tularaemia-carrying rodents or lagomorphs can be evoked, or when the individual has been bitten by flies or ticks in an endemic region. In doubtful cases, an early diagnosis can be obtained with Foshay's intradermal test, which yields positive reactions after the third or fourth day of illness.

The serum agglutination test is a laboratory procedure universally employed for the diagnosis of tularaemia, although the blood sometimes exhibits specific antibodies only from the tenth day after onset of illness or even later. An agglutination titre of 1:80 indicates infection, but the ultimate evidence of tularaemia will be a rise of the agglutination titre. At its peak in the fourth or fifth week of illness it may attain 1:5000. Cross-agglutination with *Brucella* is likely to occur; in this event the titre for the specific organism will, in most cases, be higher.

Other noteworthy diagnostic laboratory procedures are: (1) the culture method, by means of which blood, material from lesions, sputum or pleural fluid taken during the first fortnight of illness, are cultivated upon a blood–dextrose–cysteine–agar medium; (2) animal inoculation with such materials injected into guinea pigs or mice. In spite of the reliability of both procedures, their practical application is limited, because of the time-consuming and complicated techniques involved.

The diversity of clinical manifestations calls for differentiation of tularaemia from a series of other diseases. Thus the typhoidal type may be confused with typhoid fever, influenza, brucellosis, septicaemia, malaria and pulmonary tuberculosis. Anthrax, syphilis, lymphogranuloma venereum and sporotrichosis can be confounded with the ulceroglandular type of tularaemia. The glandular type may be mistaken for lymphadenitis, plague, infectious mononucleosis, parotitis, lymphoma and leucaemia; the oculoglandular type, for conjunctivitis of other aetiology or blepharitis ulcerosa; the pulmonary type for atypical pneumonia.

Tularaemia is a specific infectious disease of rodents and lagomorphs, which are, in enzootic regions, the chief reservoirs of the causative microorganism. In rare instances domestic animals (sheep, cats) and birds (pheasants, quail) may be also considered as sources of human infection. This is also true of blood-sucking arthropods, which are the main vectors of the microorganism.

In American, Soviet and Japanese literature on the subject, some 60 different species of animals are listed as natural hosts of *P. tularensis*. In the U.S.A. *Leporidae* (the cotton tail rabbit, *Silvilagus floridanus;* the snowshoe hare, *Lepus bairdii;* and jack rabbits) constitute the reservoir of about 90% of tularaemia cases. In the U.S.S.R., *Muridae* (the water rat, *Arvicola amphibius;* the common vole, *Microtus arvalis* and the house mouse, *Mus musculus*) play a similar role. For additional natural host animals of *P. tularensis* in other countries, see Table XI.

Tularaemia prevails in most countries of the northern hemisphere. As in other zoonoses with a wild animal reservoir, the propagation of the disease is influenced by a large variety of factors which form part of their biocenosis.

There is everywhere clear evidence of a causal relationship between the rapid increase in numbers and density of rodent populations and epizootics followed by epidemic-like spread among humans. This is best illustrated by the cyclical mass infestation (approximately every 9 to 11 years) of mice which invade fields and settlements; it was observed in Southern U.S.S.R. in 1941–42, 1932–33, 1922–23 and earlier.

The modes of infection and transmission are many and varied. Thus, Francis recorded some 20 ways of infection, of which the most frequent are:

(1) Contact, while hunting, dressing game or bathing in rivers contaminated with infected animals or their excreta. It should be mentioned that the organism can penetrate the apparently unbroken skin. (2) Alimentary infection by ingestion of undercooked meat of an infected animal, or drinking of water polluted by cadavers or excreta from such animals. (3) Bites from infected blood-sucking arthropods, carnivores or rodents. (4) Inhalation of dust while threshing polluted wheat or gathering hay in which infected rodents have nested. (5) Laboratory infection.

As in domestic animals, man may be infected *in utero*. American and Soviet authors reported isolated cases of diaplacental transmission from the infected mother to the foetus, terminating, in a single instance, in foetal death during the eighth month of gestation (Foshay, 1950). In another case, a live infant was delivered, with a titre of 1:2000 for *P. tularensis* which gradually declined until in the third postnatal month it became negative (Ovasapyan, 1956).

Since the disease is rarely transmitted from man to man, there is no practical value in isolating affected individuals, nor is it epidemiologically necessary to disinfect their dwellings.

Regarding transmission from animal to animal (homo- and heterologous infections), as well as from animal to man, apart from bites and abrasions which may be the commonest way of infection, the blood-sucking arthropods play an important role as vectors. 70 different types of arthropods have been listed as being capable, under favourable conditions, of transmitting the causative agent of tularaemia (Table XI). Epidemiologically, ticks form the most important group of these arthropods. In some ticks, up to 10 billion microorganisms of tularaemia have been found. It is also noteworthy that the adult female tick may pass the infection transovarially to the next generation and that the ectoparasite will serve as vector during all the stages of metamorphosis of the tick, from the

TABLE XI

DISTRIBUTION OF TULARAEMIA IN VARIOUS COUNTRIES

Natural reservoirs, hosts and vectors of *P. tularensis*

Countries	Main animal hosts (reservoirs)	Other natural hosts	Vectors
Africa			
Tunisia	Rabbit		
America			
Canada	Hare, Meadow mouse, Rabbit	*Mammals:* Beaver, Polecat, Squirrel *Birds:* Franklin gull	
Mexico	Hare	Wood rat	
U.S.A.	Snowshoe hare, Cottontail rabbit, Jack rabbit	*Mammals:* Badger, Beaver, Cat (domestic and wild), Cattle, Chipmunk, Coyote, Deer, Dog (domestic and prairie dog), Ferret, Fox (gray, red and silver), Goat, Gopher, Hog, Horse, Marmot, Mink, Mouse (deer, field, meadow and pocket), Opossum, Polecat, Porcupine, Raccoon, Rat (house, kangaroo,	*Ticks: Amblyomma americanum, Dermacentor andersoni, D. occidentalis, D. parumpertus, D. variabilis, Haemophysalis cinnabarina, H. leporis palustris, Hyalomma cincumbarina, Ixodes californicus, I. dentatus, I. ricinus, I. pacificus, Ornithodoros parkeri, O. turicata*

Countries	Main animal hosts (reservoirs)	Other natural hosts	Vectors
		musk, wild and wood), Sheep, Shrew, Skunk (spotted and striped), Squirrel (ground and tree), Weasel *Birds:* Mallard duck, Grouse (columbian, ruffed, sharptailed), Franklin gull, Chicken hawk, Hen (domestic, sage), Horned owl, Pheasant, Pigeon, Quail *Amphibia:* Bull frog *Reptilia:* Bull snake	*Fleas: Cediopsylla inaequalis, Diamanus montanus, Malareus telchinum, Xenopsylla cheopis* *Flies: Chrysops discalis, Stomoxys calcitrans* *Mosquitoes: Aedes aegypti, A. cinereus, A. excrucians, Culex tarsalis* *Lice: Haemodipsus ventricosus, Neohaematopinus laeviusculus, Polyplax serratus*
Asia Japan	Rabbit	*Mammals:* Black bear, Marmot *Birds:* Hen, Pheasant	
Turkey	Hare, Rabbit, Harvest mouse	*Mammals:* Cat, House mouse *Amphibia:* Frog	*Ticks: Ornithodoros lahorensis*
Europe Austria	Hare, Field mouse, Rabbit	*Mammals:* Cat, Dog, Rat (musk, water) *Birds:* Crow	

Table XI (cont.)

Countries	Main animal hosts (reservoirs)	Other natural hosts	Vectors
Belgium	Hare, Rabbit	Field mouse	
Czechoslovakia	Hare, Field mouse, Rabbit	Cat, Ferret, Rat (musk, water)	Mosquitoes
Finland	Hare(?)		
France	Hare, Rabbit	Mammals: Wild boar, Dog, Fox, Hog, Field mouse, Sheep, Squirrel Birds: Hen	Ticks: Dermacentor marginatus, D. pictus, Ixodes ricinus Fleas: Haemodipsus lyriocephalus
Germany	Hare, Rabbit	Rat	Ticks
Greece	Hare		
Hungary	Hare, Rabbit	Mouse, Rat, Squirrel	
Italy	Hare		

Countries	Main animal hosts (reservoirs)	Other natural hosts	Vectors
The Netherlands	Hare		
Norway	Hare, Lemming		
Poland	Beaver, Hare, Rabbit	Wild boar, Hog. Mouse (field, harvest, house)	*Ticks: Ixodes ricinus, I. persulcatus Flies: Chrysops discalis, Stomoxys calcitrans Mosquitoes: Aedes theobaldia, Anopheles claviger, A. maculipennis, Culex pipiens, Mansonia richardii*
Rumania	Hamster, Field mouse		
Sweden	Hare, Lemming	Mouse, Rat, Squirrel	*Fleas: Megalobothris rectangulatus* (lemming flea) *Mosquitoes: Aedes aegypti, A. cinereus, A. vexans, Theobaldia incidens*
U.S.S.R.	Field mouse, House mouse, Water-rat	*Mammals:* Beaver, Camel, Cat, Cattle, Chipmunk, Dog, Hamster, Hare, Hedgehog, Horse, Jerboa, Mole, Mouse (harvest, meadow), Rabbit, Rat (house, musk, wood),	*Ticks: Dermacentor marginatus, D. pictus, D. silvarum, Haemophysalis cinnabarina, H. otophila, Hyalomma marginatum, H. plumbeum, Hystionyssus isabellinus, H. musculi*

Table XI (cont.)

Countries	Main animal hosts (reservoirs)	Other natural hosts	Vectors
		Spotted skunk, Squirrel (tree, ground), Shrew, Weasel *Birds:* Crow, Hen *Amphibia:* Toad *Reptilia:* Snail *Crustaceae:* Crab	*Ixodes apronophorus, I. laguri, I. persulcatus, I. ricinus, Laelaps echidinus, L. pachypus, Ornithodoros lahorensis, Rhipicephalus rossicus* *Fleas: Ceratophyllus acutus, C. orientalis, C. walkeri; Ctenocephalus canis, Ct. assimilis, Ct. pollex, Neopsylla setosa* *Flies: Chrysops discalis, Chr. pelictus, Chr. relictus, Chr. punctifer, Chrysozona pluvialis, Colicoides pulicaris, Limnephilus stigma, Stomoxys calcitrans* *Mosquitoes: Aedes caspius, A. cinereus, A. excrucians, A. flavescens, A. vexans, Culex apicalis; Mansonia richardii* *Lice: Hopopleura acanthopus*
Yugoslavia	Hare		

larva to the adult. As a rule the disease is transmitted by the bites of the ticks, but infection may also occur by crushing the tick on the skin.

The ticks which are the principal transmitters of the infection to rabbits, domestic animals and man in the U.S.A. are: in the Western States, the wood tick *(Dermacentor variabilis)* which, like the Lone Star tick *(Amblyomma americanum)* acts as both host and vector; the tick responsible for rabbit-to-rabbit infection is *Haemophysalis leporis palustris*, but the rabbit flea *(Cedopsylla inaequalis)* and the rabbit louse *(Haemodipsus ventricosus)* are just as commonly vectors. Although the human body louse *(Pediculus humanus)* is under experimental conditions susceptible to infection with tularaemia, its epidemiological significance as vector of the bacterium is negligible (Price, 1956).

In the U.S.S.R., the chief vectors are ectoparasites of the different species of Muridae and these also pass the infection to domesticated animals. This applies to *Dermacentor marginatus* (Southern Russia) and the meadow tick, *Dermacentor pictus* (Central U.S.S.R.), two species which also act as vectors for tularaemia in France.

In the districts of Arkhangelsk (Northern U.S.S.R.) and Alma Ata (Kazakhstan) in the South, the prevailing tick is *Ixodes apronophorus* and this is here the principal vector.

In addition to these and other ticks, *Ixodes persulcatus* and *Ixodes ricinus* are also transmitters of tularaemia (the latter two in Poland as well).

The Russian water-rat louse *(Hoplopleura sp.)* and waterrat flea *(Ceratophyllus walkeri)* also, like the ectoparasites of rabbits in the U.S.A., maintain and disseminate tularaemia.

Blood-sucking *Diptera*, especially *Tabanidae* and *Culicidae*, are responsible in no small way for causing tularaemia; these insects may mechanically infect animals and man after they have sucked the blood of infected rodents. The annual outbreaks of the disease in Utah (U.S.A.) are, in fact, caused by mechanical infection of this kind by the deer fly.

The stable fly, *Stomoxys calcitrans*, may also be, to a lesser extent, a mechanical vector, in both the U.S.A. and the U.S.S.R.

Mosquitoes *(Aedes cinereus* and *Aedes excrucians)* are vectors of tularaemia in both the New and Old World, but the cosmopolitan house fly, *Musca domestica*, probably transmits the disease only under experimental conditions. The same is true for the bedbug, *Cimex lectularius*, the epidemiological significance of which in the transmission of the infection is negligible. Research workers, however, succeeded in transmitting tularaemia from mouse to mouse by means of this ectoparasite, although human infection as a result of contact with faeces from bedbugs is very rare.

When the largest zone of the spread of infection is demarcated, it is apparent that the distribution of tularaemia is restricted to the northern hemisphere, a fact which suggests that in this area ecological factors prevail which may influence the propagation of the disease (Table XI).

In Eurasia, from Japan in the east to France in the West, and from Norway in the North to Turkey in the South, the chief endemic regions are:

References p. 94

(a) Along the waterways and lakes where climatic and soil conditions favour the multiplication and migration of rodents, particularly of the water rat, the field mouse and the hare. In the U.S.S.R. for instance, the basins of the Lena in the north-east, the Volga in the centre and Dniepr in the south-west, and the lake district in Kazakhstan, have all been theatres of epizootics of tularaemia, followed by epidemics in the twenties and early thirties. The same pattern was repeated in Germany, along the Oder (1949–50) and the Main (1951–52) and, in Austria, along the Danube and its affluents, the March and the Raab rivers (1936–37).

(b) The steppes or wastelands with a characteristic continental climate, where the average annual rainfall is less than 750–1000 mm (Jusatz) and where the flora and soil structure favour the survival of rodents. These conditions are encountered in the Kirghiz and Kalmuck steppes (U.S.S.R.), in Thrace (Turkey), in Moravia (Czechoslovakia) and in the districts of Doubs and the Côte d'Or in the East of France, where the *Muridae* and *Leporidae* constitute the main reservoir of the infection.

In the parts of the North American countries (U.S.A., Canada and Mexico), in which tularaemia is endemic, the climatic conditions and vegetation are, however, very different and in these areas the vectors are of primary importance. The most important of these are ticks and deer flies, which are most active during the summer. Thus, from March to June, there is an increase in the incidence of tularaemia in the western states, caused by the wood tick *(Dermacentor andersoni);* between July and September the increased incidence is attributed to deer flies. In the southern states the seasonal peak occurs between February and October and is ascribed to the activity of the dog tick *(Dermacentor variabilis)*. When jack rabbits are hunted from April to October, and when in the eastern states cotton-tail rabbits are hunted from November to December, the risk of human infection is increased.

This seasonal incidence of tularaemia has also been reported by Soviet workers (Washkow, Pronin). Thus in extensive territories of the U.S.S.R. (Siberia, the Urals, Altay, Astrakhan and northern European Russia), where the chief reservoir of the disease is the water rat, outbreaks occur in the spring and summer. Wherever the field mouse is the main reservoir of the organism (Central and Western Russia), the rise of incidence occurs during the threshing and wheatgathering season (autumn and winter). In the southern part of the U.S.S.R., however, where the house mouse is the source for tularaemia, outbreaks occur in the winter and spring.

From the modes of spread of tularaemia, *i.e.* by direct contact with infected animals, their excreta, or products, or with objects in their environment polluted by these animals (water, grain, foodstuffs), as well as by different vectors (ticks, flies, mosquitoes), it may be inferred that the infection is always derived directly or indirectly from a particular species of rodent. This inference indicates the measures that must be taken to avert the greater part of these infections. The most radical measure would be the extermination of all infected animals. Because in endemic regions only partial eradication can be contemplated, measures to control the infection should be directed towards preventing the transmission of the infection from animal to man. This may be accomplished by: (a) providing the population of infected areas with adequate information about the modes of spread of the disease and the hazards inherent in handling animals known to harbour the infection; (b) advocating the use of rubber gloves during the skinning of animals and the dressing of furs, cautions against smoking and eating during such work and the recommendation that the hands should be thoroughly cleaned when this work has been done; (c) enforcing strict rodent control in grain and foodstuff stores; advising that game should be well cooked for consumption; (d) warning against drinking and bathing in water suspected of being polluted; (e) extensive use of rodenticides, insecticides and acaricides with a view to preventing arthropod infestation of animals. Because the extermination of each type of arthropod requires specific methods and materials, their proper selection according to local conditions is of primary importance; (f) enacting veterinary public health regulations designed to protect rodent-hunting animals such as foxes, hawks, buzzards, and prohibiting the importation of rabbits, hares and sheep from infected countries, in order to prevent introduction of the infection into a nonendemic area.

In endemic countries, research workers have been endeavouring for years to develop a vaccine which will effectively reduce the incidence of tularaemia in exposed persons, such as hunters, farmers, butchers, and laboratory workers. Results have, so far, not been satisfactory. Thus, Francis, Foshay and Kadull in the U.S.A., and Khatenever, Sinai and Verenikova in the U.S.S.R., did not succeed in preparing a useful heat- or chemically killed vaccine. Their vaccines either conferred insufficient immunity, or they provoked side-reactions (Saslaw et al., 1961).

In 1941–42, Gaisky and Elbert developed a living attenuated vaccine, which was improved by the Scientific Research Institute of Epidemiology and Hygiene (NIIEG); it was later applied in a large-scale vaccination scheme at the anti-tularaemia stations throughout the U.S.S.R. Soviet literature claims that immunity was obtained in 97% of all vaccinated persons (Olsufiev). The W.H.O. Experts Committee on Zoonoses, in their August–1958 session, mentioned the beneficial results obtained with this living vaccine in the U.S.S.R.

References p. 94

Therapy of tularaemia has undergone various stages of development.
For decades treatment was purely symptomatic. The endeavours of
Francis and Foshay in the U.S.A. and of Khatenever and Volferts in the
U.S.S.R., brought only partial success with the introduction of specific
serotherapy. Furthermore, chemotherapy with the sulfacompounds did
not meet expectations. With the advent of antibiotics, penicillin was tried,
but without success. In 1944, however, Heilmann took the first step towards
discovery of effective treatment when he obtained in experimental
tularaemia favourable results with streptomycin. Equal results were
obtained when tetracycline and chloramphenicol were used. Thus an
effective means was found for the treatment of the disease, particularly
when it is applied in the first week after its onset.

In conjunction with general antibacterial therapy, topical treatment of
primary lesions and buboes with wet saline dressings is advocated. In the
oculoglandular type of disease, the antibiotics just named should be
supplemented with instillation of homatropin into the affected eyes, which
must be protected by dark sunglasses. In severe cases with allergic
reaction to tularense-protein, application of corticosteroids should be
considered.

REFERENCES

BIEGELEISEN, J. Z. and M. D. MOODY, J. Bact., 79 (1960) 155.
BURROGHS, A. L., R. HOLDENFRIED, D. S. LONGANECKER and K. F. MEYER, J. Infect. Dis., 76 (1945) 115.
FRANCIS, E., Publ. Hlth Rep. (Wash.), 36 (1921) 1731.
HEILMANN, F. R., Proc. Mayo Clin., 19 (1944) 553.
HEMMES, G. D., Ned. T. Geneesk., 97 (1953) 990.
JELLISON, W. L. and G. M. KOHLS, Publ. Hlth Monogr., 10 (1955) 28.
JUSATZ, H. L., Z. Hyg. Infekt.-Kr., 134 (1952) 350.
KADULL, P. J. and J. H. V. METRE, Ann. Internal Med., 70 (1959) 621.
LARSON, C. L., W. L. JELLISON and W. WICKT, Publ. Hlth Rep. (Wash.), 70 (1955) 253.
McCoy, G. W. and C. W. CHAPIN, Publ. Hlth Bull. (Wash.), 53 (1912) 18.
McKEEVER, S., J. H. SCHUBERT, M. D. MOODY, G. W. GORMAN and J. F. CHAPMAN, J. infect. Dis., 103 (1958) 120.
OLSUFIEV, N. G., Vestn. Akad. med. Nauk, 11 (1958) 63, Ž. Mikrobiol. (Mosk.), 9 (1956) 13.
PARNAS, J., T. ROZOWSKI and F. WYSOCKA, Tularemia, Warszawa, 1957, 332 pp.
SASLAW, S., H. T. EIGELSBACH et al., Arch. Int. Med., 107 (1961) 702.
SYLTCHENKO, V. S., Ž. Mikrobiol. (Mosk.), 10 (1957) 35.
TRAUB, A., J. MAGER and N. GROSSOWICZ, J. Bact., 70 (1955) 270.
WORLD HEALTH ORGANIZATION, Epidem. vital Statist. Rep., 11 (1958) No. 9; 12 (1959) No. 11.
WYSOCKA, F., Ann. Univ. M. Curie-Sklodowska, 10 (1956) 229.

6

J. VAN DER HOEDEN

Brucellosis

Brucellosis is an infectious disease of animals of world-wide distribution; it particularly affects herbivores and swine, which are the main sources of human infection.

The first clinical report on the disease in man is ascribed to Hippocrates, as early as the 5th century a.D. In later times, diseases resembling brucellosis have time and again been reported in the Mediterranean area, their designation being usually based on their analogy to other well-known maladies, according to the most characteristic symptoms or the locality in which they prevailed.*

During the Crimean War, the disease was differentiated as a special one, distinct from other febrile ailments in the area (Marstan, 1863).

The discovery of the aetiologic agent of Mediterranean fever is due to David Bruce (1886), who found numerous small microorganisms in the spleen of soldiers who had died of the disease in Malta. Shortly afterwards he cultivated the same organism from the blood and spleens of patients suffering from the infection, and named it *Micrococcus melitensis*. This organism was specifically agglutinated in the blood serum of the patients (Wright, 1896). Full light was thrown on the epidemiology of the disease by the research of the British Royal Commission on Mediterranean Fever under Bruce's direction (1904). The natural history of Malta fever has been gradually revealed since Zammit (1905) found a strikingly high concentration of agglutinin for the *melitensis*-organism in the blood of numerous apparently healthy Maltese goats.

---

* Some of the historical names, partly still used are: pseudotyphus, intermittent typhoid fever, febris typho-malariae, fièvre sudorale, undulant fever, bovine contagious-, infectious- or enzootic abortion, Bang's disease, melitococcia, Mediterranean (gastric remittent) fever, Gibraltar-Rock fever, Cyprus fever, Malta fever, Neapolitan fever.

Further investigations revealed that the sera of about half of the 20,000 caprines on the island agglutinated the organism and that approximately 10% of the animals excreted viable *micrococci* in their milk or urine. It soon became evident that milk from these goats was a potential source of human infection. This assumption became a certainty when, in 1906, after the military authorities on Malta had prohibited the consumption of goat's milk by all military and navy personnel, the disease disappeared among the British forces stationed there, whereas among the civilian population, to whom the military ordinances did not apply, Malta fever continued to take its toll (Table XII).

TABLE XII

NUMBER OF CASES OF MEDITERRANEAN FEVER IN THE ARMY, NAVY AND CIVILIAN POPULATION
ON MALTA
(After Eyre)

Year	Army	Navy	Civilians *
Average 1900–1905	310	355	618
1906	145	163	822
1907	12	9	714

* The following figures representing the yearly incidence in the civilian population over the period of 1950–54 have been reported: 1950: 1668, 1951: 1226, 1952: 1100, 1953: 850 and 1954: 1096.

For at least two centuries, cattle breeders have been aware of the periodic recurrence of multiple cases of bovine abortion. In the late seventies of the nineteenth century, the contagious character of these abortions was established by Franck (1876) and others, who succeeded in inducing the disease by introducing the vaginal secretion or placental tissue of aborting cows into the vagina of pregnant cattle.

In 1885, countless *micrococci* were observed by Nocard in smears taken from the uteri and foetuses of cases of bovine abortion. Organisms which had the same appearance were isolated in pure culture by Bang and Stribolt (1897), who gave them the name *Bacterium abortus infectiosi*. Injection of these organisms into pregnant cows resulted in abortion.

It was, however, not until 1918 that the close morphological, cultural and antigenic resemblance of the "micrococcus" of Bruce and the "bacterium" of Bang was demonstrated by Alice Evans. Since 1920, both microorganisms have been designated by the generic name *Brucella* (Meyer and Shaw).

The pathogenicity of *Br. abortus* to man was first suggested by Bevan (1922), who observed in Rhodesia several cases of a disease which resembled Malta fever in persons working on farms on which cattle suffered from contagious abortion; no goats were present. Brucellae were isolated from one of these patients, a man employed as a butcher.

Some 4 to 5 years later, several "Bang-infections" in human beings were reported almost simultaneously from North America, Germany, Denmark and Holland.

A strain which Traum had isolated from American pigs in 1914, showed differences from *Br. melitensis* and *Br. abortus*. The first culture which was supposed to be *Br. abortus,* isolated from a human being in the U.S.A. (Keefer, 1924), proved later to be identical with *Br. suis* of Traum.

Thomsen (1929) cultivated from pigs in Denmark, brucellae which in some respects differed from the American strain of porcine origin. Afterwards, the Danish variety was found also in hares.

Another variety of *Brucella, Br. ovis,* has been isolated by Buddle and Boyes in Australia (1953) from sheep with genital lesions. Some bacteriologists still regard the incorporation of this microorganism in the genus *Brucella* as tentative.

All brucellae are tiny, more or less coccoid, nonmotile, nonsporulating, gram-negative, aërobic bacteria which form, on solid media, colonies which have a characteristic appearance. Differentiation of the various species * of the genus *Brucella* is based upon rather subtle laboratory methods which were, for the greater part, first described by Huddleson in 1928.

On artificial media, *Brucella* tends to a rapid dissociation from "smooth" to "rough" growth, with a change in its ability to agglutinate. This interferes with the serological differentiation of such strains. *Br. ovis* is only known in the rough state and cannot, therefore, be satisfactorily classified on the basis of its antigenic structure.

No difference can be noticed between the three main species of *Brucella* by simple agglutination tests. A practical method of distinguishing between *Br. melitensis* and *Br. abortus* or *Br. suis* is based on the finding of Wilson and Miles (1932) that, although the two antigens present in all three species are similar, their proportion differs. For differentiation, monospecific agglutinating sera are used which are prepared in rabbits by injection of either a *melitensis* or *abortus* strain and thereafter partially absorbed with the heterogenous *brucella* species. Smooth strains of *Br. melitensis* are agglutinated by the monospecific *melitensis* serum alone, *Br. abortus* and *Br. suis* by the monospecific

---

* In the literature, the terms types and varieties have been arbitrarily used in the classification of *Brucella*.

abortus serum. Unlike *Br. melitensis,* which develops under ordinary atmospheric conditions, *Br. suis, Br. abortus* and *Br. ovis* require a higher concentration of carbon dioxide (optimal 10%) for their initial growth. Production of hydrogen sulfide by *Br. melitensis, Br. ovis* and the Danish porcine strain is absent or low; *Br. abortus* produces only a moderate amount of H_2S during 2 to 3 days, *Br. suis* (Traum) a considerable amount for 4 to 5 days. Other means of classification are based upon inhibition of growth on culture media containing various aniline dyes, and on the production of urease.

This rather complex system permits differentiation between most of the *Brucella* strains recovered from goats, cattle and pigs (species: *melitensis, abortus* and *suis* respectively). Several strains, however, exhibit an intermediate position. In certain regions these varieties are even more frequently encountered than the "classical" species are.

Renoux *et al.* (1955) investigated 230 strains from various sources, all of which behaved biochemically as *Br. melitensis* does. Serological examination revealed that only 51 of these strains reacted like *Br. melitensis,* while the other 179 reacted like *Br. abortus* (A/M variety). Similar strains have been found many times in Tunisia, India, Indonesia, Israel, Southern Russia, Switzerland and Poland. The reverse (*i.e.* serological reactions like those of melitensis, biochemical reactions like those of abortus; M/A variety) has been demonstrated in strains of cattle in Great Britain and Israel.

Brucellae are rather resistant to various environmental conditions. They have remained alive in bovine foetuses for as long as 182 days after abortion, and in the afterbirth for 147 days. Bosworth (1934) recorded survival of the organisms in manure for two months, Kurdaz and Morse (1954) for even 385 days at 8°.

Simple desiccation kills brucellae in 3 to 5 days; their resistance to direct sunlight and to the action of most of the common disinfectants is rather weak. In tap water, the organisms remain viable for 10 to 120 days at 25°, in bovine urine up to 4 days. They are readily destroyed by ordinary pasteurization.

Under normal conditions, *goats* are affected only by the melitensis species of *Brucella.* The animals reach the peak of susceptibility during their first gestation.

In feeding experiments of goats, the incubation time varied from 3 to 4 weeks, but evidence exists that sometimes illness appears much later after infection.

The microorganisms enter the body through the mucous membranes of the eye, mouth or vagina, or by way of abrasions or wounds of the skin. Milking seems to favour penetration of brucellae into the skin of the teats.

At the onset of the disease, the microorganisms circulate in the blood and a brief febrile period may be noticed. Usually, however, no clinical signs are observed. Occasionally the animals are dull, their coat is rough, they lose weight and have slight diarrhoea. Sometimes chronic bronchitis develops, which causes a frequent short, hacking cough. Most of the affected goats recover quickly, the agglutinin titre of their blood often declining rapidly to a non-significant level. Nevertheless, bacteraemia may continue, as well as excretion of the organisms in the milk.

When mastitis develops, the course is usually mild and spontaneous recovery follows rapidly. More exceptionally the secretion of the mammary gland is altered to a clear, watery fluid containing clot. Generally, the milk yield is not appreciably reduced. Up to 60% of the infected milking goats excrete brucellae in the milk. For 4 to 6 weeks after kidding considerable numbers are usually present, but later their number gradually diminishes. Apparently healthy goats sometimes continue to excrete brucellae until their next pregnancy. In these cases, the secretion of them may proceed uninterruptedly during two consecutive lactation periods.

The organisms are also discharged in the urine and vaginal secretions and this may go on for a period of up to 5 months. Although discharge from the vulva is often initiated shortly before abortion and proceeds thereafter, sometimes brucellae are also excreted at the termination of an uneventful pregnancy, after normal delivery or this may even happen in virgin goats (Renoux, 1959).

The most characteristic symptom of caprine brucellosis is abortion. In herds primarily infected, 50 to 90% of the pregnant goats may abort, but in herds repeatedly infected, abortion usually occurs in no more than 10 to 20%. Contrary to earlier opinion, Renoux (1955) contended that young-born, apparently healthy kids from affected mother-goats are often infected. This observation is important from an epidemiological point of view.

Exceptionally, bucks suffer from brucellar orchitis.

Spontaneous recovery ensues in the majority of goats with only few remaining chronic carriers.

Unlike *Br. abortus, Br. melitensis* prevails only in restricted regions of the world. It has spread to territories formerly free from it by importation of goats or sheep suffering from latent infection. Apart from the classical endemic foci in the countries of the Mediterranean basin, *melitensis* infection of goats has been reported from the Asiatic Arab countries, the Southern regions of the U.S.S.R., South Africa, China, South America (in the western section of Argentina there are 5 to 80 % of goats affected), and the U.S.A. (in the western and south western States of Colorado, Arizona and New Mexico).

For a long time, *melitensis* infection of goats was unknown in European regions above the 43rd degree of northern latitude. Since 1932, it has extended to northern France, in 1948 it penetrated into Switzerland, in 1950 into southern Germany.

The incidence of caprine brucellosis is to a large extent determined by local conditions. Whereas in France, Malta-fever in goats is mostly rural in its occurrence, in Tunisia the disease is practically restricted to town-bred caprines.

Sheep show greater resistance to brucellae than do goats; most infections in this animal are caused by *Br. melitensis,* only few by *Br. abortus.* Huddleson, in 1943, found two strains of the latter species among 48 of ovine origin in France.

Usually the course in sheep is subclinical. The syndrome in ewes is similar to that of goats. Excretion of the organisms in the milk rarely continues for longer than 1 to 2 months. Brucellae usually disappear from the vaginal secretions within a month following abortion; they are very rarely found in urine.

Ovine brucellosis has a tendency to self-limitation; unlike goats, sheep rid all their tissues rather rapidly of the organism. Non-pregnant sheep, in particular, quickly recover from the infection. In France, Russia and some other European countries, brucellosis of ovines is more widely distributed than brucellosis of caprines. This may be related to the habit of communal pasturing of the sheep of several owners during a large part of the year, with the result that infected and susceptible animals are mingled in a small area for a protracted period.

After World War II, several heavily infected Italian flocks of sheep were driven into the region of Trieste, where they pastured with Yugoslavian herds. In 1947 this resulted in serious outbreaks of brucellosis–melitensis among the population of Fiume. The opposite took place in south-western Germany, where before 1950 *Br. abortus* had been the only cause of human and animal brucellosis, except for a few localized outbreaks of brucellosis *suis* in pigs. Large herds of sheep had been pastured during war time in the areas of northern France (Alsace-Lorraine) endemically infected with *Br. melitensis* and, on the return of these animals to the Pfaltz region (which serves as winter pasture for sheep flocks of S.W. Germany), about half of 20,000 of them proved to be infected with *Br. melitensis.* The infection spread to Hesse, Württemberg and the right bank of the Rhine and also involved cattle and man. Wundt (1959) recorded

39 human infections, of which 23 could be traced to sheep and 5 to cattle excreting *Br. melitensis.*

In addition to the countries just mentioned, ovine brucellosis has been reported from Switzerland, Hungary, East and Southwest Africa and Mongolia. In southern districts of U.S.S.R. brucellosis is wide spread in sheep. In the U.S.A. it is a problem of minor importance; only 2% of ewes slaughtered during 1939 reacted with rather low agglutinin titres to *Brucella.*

The A/M variant of *Brucella* was encountered in 77% of the small ruminants in Tunisia (Renoux, 1952). A similar intermediate strain was recovered in sheep of the Crimea (Matweew, 1937).

A special place in brucellosis of sheep is taken by the genital disorders (epididymitis, orchitis, abortion) caused by *Br. melitensis, var. ovis,* first observed in Australia and New Zealand (Buddle and Boyes; Simmons and Hall, 1953). The organism has been isolated from ovine foetuses, foetal membranes, vaginal secretion, the regional lymph nodes, the colostrum and the semen. It has also been found in sheep in California and in a ram with epididymitis in Czechoslovakia.

As a rule the only symptom observed in brucella-infected *cows* is abortion, but even this sign is often lacking and in such cases, as well as in non-pregnant cows, the infection often remains clinically inapparent. Thorough examination not uncommonly reveals shortly after infection a slight rise of temperature which takes a wavy course.

The incubation period is subject to considerable variation; variations of from 1 week to 7 months have been recorded.

In general, the period between infection and expulsion of the foetus is inversely proportional to the age of the foetus at the time of penetration of the microorganisms into the bovine body. Brucellae entering the mucosae of the digestive tract are carried to the regional lymph nodes. When they survive, they are carried through the thoracic duct to the bloodstream. The initial bacteriaemic stage is usually brief, but in a certain number of animals it persists intermittently for a long period. By way of the blood stream the organisms may settle in various lymphatic nodes, spleen, bone marrow and liver. Localization in the pregnant uterus provokes purulent, necrotic inflammation of the uterine wall and foetal membranes, which severs the chorion from the maternal cotyledons, and causes expulsion of the foetus. After abortion, the uterus promptly recovers and the microorganisms disappear from the organ within a few weeks to a month. Frequently the foetal membranes, which contain enormous numbers of brucellae, remain attached for a prolonged period (*retentio secundinarum*).

Not only are cattle herds stricken by brucellosis subject to multiple abortions, but decreased fertility is an added liability, and this not infrequently leads to total sterility in individual animals.

The milk yield of infected cows often remains below normal level during the year of abortion. Even when infected animals are delivered of healthy full-term calves, an average decrease of nearly one quarter of the normal milk production may ensue. Brucellae can be excreted in the milk of cows which do not show agglutinins in their bloodserum. Close investigation may reveal slight focal, nonpurulent interstitial proliferations in the udder tissue without a manifest mastitis developing. Superficial examination of the milk does not reveal abnormal changes.

In most instances, brucellae appear in the milk from 1 to 7 days after abortion, occasionally later. The organisms are discharged intermittently, their number varying from day to day. This may continue for a long period of time (Cotton, in 1913, recorded secretion of *Br. abortus* during more than 6 years; Renoux, in 1953, established excretion of *Br. melitensis* for longer than 3 years).

The persistence of brucellae in the mammary gland and its regional lymph nodes is of considerable pathogenic importance. Starting from these latent foci the organisms occasionally reach the bloodstream via the lymph ducts and are deposited in internal organs. In this fashion, reinfection of the sensitive uterus can readily be provoked in any ensuing pregnancy.

About 20% of infected cows are liable to have a second abortion and sometimes a third follows. The first one most often occurs in about the sixth month or pregnancy. Subsequent abortions usually happen at later stages of gestation.

Rather exceptional symptoms of bovine brucellosis are arthritis and tendovaginitis with particular involvement of the femoro-tibial joint.

Schaal in Germany (1957) recovered *Br. abortus* from 65% of the kidneys of slaughter-cows which gave positive serotests for *Brucella*.

Br. abortus has been frequently isolated from the serous contents of knee boils (bursitis precarpalis, carpal hygroma) of cows, the fluid also containing high antibody concentration (Fig. 13).

Full-term calves from infected cows are usually free of brucellae. Whenever the organisms are present, however, they are soon eliminated from the digestive tract by excretion in the faeces.

BRUCELLOSIS 103

Enormous numbers of brucellae are discharged in the uterine excretions and afterbirth. Calves born healthy may be covered with countless brucellae without giving rise to infection.

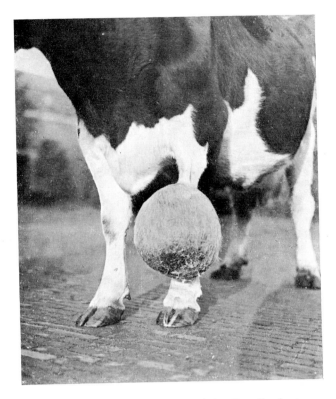

Fig. 13. Bursitis precarpalis containing *Brucella abortus*.
(Photo: Department of Veterinary Surgery, State University, Utrecht)

The natural resistance of calves during the first 3 to 5 months of life gradually declines with approaching sexual maturity.

The lesions caused by *Br. abortus* in the bull may be serious. They are chiefly localized in the genital organs (orchitis, periorchitis, epididymitis, ampullitis and vesiculitis seminalis), these organs displaying necrotic or purulent foci accompanied by chronic indurative inflammation. The considerably enlarged testicles remain swollen for several months when, due to retraction of the fibrous wall surrounding the necrotic tissue, the swelling gradually subsides. In other cases the orchitis has a marked tendency to purulent liquefaction, the necrotic testicle finally hanging in a pus-filled cavity surrounded by the much thickened fibrous tunica vaginalis (Jepsen and Jörgensen, 1938). In spite of the presence of viable brucellae in the sperm, transmission of infection by copulation or artificial insemination with such semen is very rare; when it does occur, it seldom causes abortion (Bendixen and Blom, 1947).

In herds in which cows have not previously been infected, brucellosis usually makes swift inroads. If no new cattle are added to the stock, the enzootic loses its serious aspect, the infection remaining latent for several consecutive years. As a rule, abortion occurs more frequently in large herds than in those comprising 20 or less head of cattle.

Brucellae usually enter the bovine body through the lymphatic tissue of the throat, the conjunctival and enteric mucosae, or the soft parts of the skin, especially above the hoof.

Some investigators attach special epizootiological importance to the role of water and contaminated dust. In a considerable number of cases it was suggested that the infection had passed from udder to udder by the act of milking, particularly when milking machines had been used, slight abrasions of the teats being the portals of entry.

The susceptibility of the bovine organism to brucellar infection tends to increase with progress of pregnancy. As in tuberculosis, dairy cattle are usually more often affected than the meat-yielding races are.

Bovine brucellosis caused by the *abortus* species has occurred in nearly every country. Stableforth (1950) claimed an infection rate of 10 to 30% in most European and South American regions. Herd infection in Great Britain amounted to 10–15%. Serological evidence of brucellosis was established in 25% of the dairy herds of northern Scotland (1954–1956). In West Germany an overall infection rate of 20% was estimated (Götze, 1954), but significant differences of incidence (0.3 to 62%) were recorded in various localities. In the different provinces of the Netherlands, herd infection varied between 36 and 82% in 1956 with an infection rate in individual adult cows of between 5 and 10%.

Thanks to systematic veterinary control, there has been, in recent years, a steep decline of bovine brucellosis in several countries. The number of infected herds in Sweden (which in 1945 still amounted to 16,000) has now been reduced to nil. Although, according to the results of serotests, the incidence of bovine brucellosis in the U.S.A. has decreased from an average of 14% in 1935 to less than 5% in 1952, herd infection rates have remained at about 20%.

The original conception that cattle are affected only by *Br. abortus* had already been questioned in publications of the British Commission on Mediterranean Fever (Shaw, 1906). However, as long as the methods of differentiation between the various *Brucella* species had not been satisfactorily standardized, no reliable conclusion on the prevailing types could be made.

In 1920, human *melitensis* infections of bovine origin were found in southern France. Since 1930, various foci of brucellosis *melitensis* in bovines have been established in the northern regions of that country. These were related to commercial transfer of contaminated sheep from Algiers to Lorraine. The disease did not appear in goats (Taylor *et al.*, 1932).

Recent investigations have confirmed the presence of *Br. melitensis* in the bovines of several European countries, *e.g.*, S.W. Germany, Czechoslovakia, Poland, Switzerland, the Soviet States and Turkey. Out of 16 *Brucella* strains isolated from Turkish cows, 11 showed similarity with the *melitensis* type and only 5 with *Br. abortus*. In the U.S.A., *melitensis* infection of cattle is very rarely observed, but, since 1940, several cases of this infection have been revealed in British cattle. In a report of the Animal Health Services of England for the 3 years prior to 1956, 27 cattle herds were recorded in which *Br. melitensis* infection was established and from an additional 17, intermediate M/A strains had been isolated. In most cases all cultures from milk and foeti in a herd were of the same type, although mixed infections have also been observed. Similar experiences have been reported from the northern regions of Germany (Sleswick-Holstein) since 1956. The origin of these strains, which were isolated from milk, placentas and aborted foetuses, remained unknown. It is noteworthy that neither in England nor in N. Germany have *melitensis* infections of cattle been transmitted to in man or other animals. Contrary to this, Moldavskaya *et al.* (1960) reported in the U.S.S.R. a severe epidemic outbreak of brucellosis which involved 68 persons who had drunk milk of cows which had been in contact with infected sheep; typical *Br. melitensis* were isolated from the blood of these patients and the cows' milk.

The most reliable method of diagnosing brucellosis is by isolation of the organisms from blood, milk, foeti, placenta or pus. The procedure of choice for mass examination, however, is the agglutination test with blood-serum or milk, carried out with standardized antigens. The reliability of this method is, however, not absolute.

Sometimes no agglutinins are found in cattle for several months after infection, the antibodies only appearing after abortion has taken place. For this reason, the result of a single serum test may be misleading. In some cases the titres of milk whey, semen or uterine secretion reach higher levels than those of blood sera of the same animals. This might indicate local antibody production. According to Kerr *et al.* (1958) the vaginal mucus test is always positive within 3 weeks after abortion when brucellae are found in the foetus; consequently this test could take the place of bacteriological investigation of the foetal stomach contents.

Cross-agglutination has been noticed with tularaemia. Particularly in these cases the author's "tropin test" (1940) may offer most reliable diagnostic information.

Milk containing *Brucella* antibodies, mixed in tubes with diphenyl-tetrazolium-chloride-stained *Brucella* culture, shows a purple-red disk of cream after 1 hour incubation at 37°.

For field use, an immediately readable test can be performed by mixing on a glass plate drops of the whole blood or milk with stained concentrated brucella suspension. A method applied all over the world for screening purposes is the Abortus Bang Ring Test (A.B.R.).

After rapid demonstration of herd infection by means of the A.B.R. test, examination of blood sera will identify the individual affected cows.

Zaki (1948) recorded a rather marked susceptibility of *camels* to *Br. abortus*, 14 % of the female camels slaughtered in Cairo reacting to the agglutination test with titres ranging between 25 and 1,600.

Global distribution of *porcine brucellosis* is far less extensive than bovine brucellosis and its local incidence is usually much more restricted.

The first porcine *melitensis* infections in the U.S.A. were recorded in 1943. McCollough (1951) isolated 10 strains of *Br. abortus*, 11 of *Br. melitensis* and 14 of *Br. suis* from 5,000 submaxillary lymph glands of slaughtered hogs. *Br. suis* in North America is chiefly confined to the midwestern states. During the 6 years prior to 1958, 501,160 swine in 57,666 herds were tested, of which 5.3 % reacted. Weeter (1923) established brucella agglutinins in 14.7 % of sows and 5.3 % of boars slaughtered in Chicago. During the period between 1938 and 1949, an average 41.6 % of 994 swine herds and 11.8 % of 19,937 individual pigs examined in Illinois, revealed significant agglutinin titres for *Brucella* (Cameron, 1957).

For correct evaluation of these figures one should bear in mind that the decline or even total disappearance of *Brucella* agglutinins from the blood does not preclude the continued presence of *Br. suis* in the tissues and its excretion in the urine.

The disease is frequently encountered in the porcine population of the Latin American countries, especially in Argentina and Brazil. Narcis (1925, 1928) observed serious annually recurring outbreaks among swine in Hungary, caused by *Br. abortus* as well as by *Br. suis*.

Numerous enzootics have been recorded from the U.S.S.R. (particularly from the hog-raising Baltic areas and White Russia), Switzerland, Italy, France, Portugal, Roumania and Germany. In most of these countries *Br. suis* predominates over the other two species. Also in Upper Egypt it was found responsible for the disease in pigs (Zaki, 1948).

Russian workers claim that hogs are infected when they are fed on skimmed milk from plants which produce sheep cheese, by eating aborted foetuses and manure in the vicinity of sheep pens and blood or tissues from slaughter offal.

All the pregnant sows in Malta, which had been fed on unpasteurized goat's milk aborted and *Br. melitensis* was recovered from their foeti (Huddleson, 1938).

Of special interest are three enzootics of porcine brucellosis which occurred in Denmark (Thomsen) during 1929–1932, 1940 and 1951, and were caused by Thomsen's variety, which differs from *Br. suis* Traum.

Swine are affected more than cattle, by serious local purulent and necrotic brucellar inflammations. Multiple abscesses are found in the spleen and other organs, and these often show a tendency to calcification. The *suis*-species of *Brucella* is most frequently localized in the genital tract, and it provokes abortion, still-births and infertility (metritis). The testes may become enormously enlarged (orchitis, epididymitis, vesiculitis seminalis, prostatitis). This is often associated with spondylitis, arthritis, lameness and paralysis.

In swine the course of the disease is usually chronic and abortion occurs at various stages of pregnancy. In five herds comprising more than 5,100 pigs, about 50% showed positive *brucella*-serotests and 8% arthritis; one-third of the sows were unproductive, one-tenth aborted and one-third of the boars had orchitis (Makkawejski *et al.,* 1933).

Contrary to what is usual in young calves, kids and lambs, weanlings and suckling-pigs possess a high degree of susceptibility to *Brucella* infection.

The boar often plays a much more important part in the spread of porcine brucellosis than the bull plays in the spread of bovine *Brucella* infection. The semen of infected boars usually contains huge numbers of *Brucella* organisms. Sudden outbreaks of brucellosis often occur after the introduction of a newly bought boar or breed gilt into the piggery.

Besides transmission of infection from boar to sow and *vice versa,* the portals of entry into the pig may also be the conjunctival mucosae, skin and upper digestive tract. As in other domestic animals, the organism is present in vaginal discharge, the placenta, foetal membranes, in aborted foetuses and in sow's milk. Spread of infection among the omnivorous swine is promoted by the swallowing of tissues delivered by abortion.

Because of the differences in breeding systems in pure bred swine herds which raise brood stock for commercial purposes, brucellosis generally persists for a prolonged time, whereas the infection is rather rapidly eliminated from pork-producing herds (Cameron, 1957).

The clinical manifestations of brucellosis in *horses* differ in several respects from those of other animals. This may account for the late discovery of equine brucellosis.

At the end of the first world war, Fontaine and Lütje (1919) recorded a remarkably great number of horses in the German army, which suffered from a suppurative inflammatory process of the neck and withers and showed positive complement-fixation tests with *Br. abortus* antigen. 9 years afterwards, similar experiences were observed in France by Rinjard and Hilger who isolated the micro-organism from two cases of fistulous withers.

In 1930 the author investigated several horses in the Netherlands upon which the following data were recorded (Table XIII).

TABLE XIII

	Number of horses serologically examined	Significant serotitres established	Number of horses culturally examined	Br. abortus isolated
Horses suffering from:				
fistulous withers	36	36	33	24
poll-evil and/or neckboil	17	16	10	5
bursitis presternalis	8	3		
tarsitis	1	1	1	1
Total	62	56	44	30
Clinically healthy horses	560	8		

Positive seroreactions were also revealed in cases of lameness due to tendovaginitis, arthritis (especially coxitis and tarsitis), bursitis podotrochlearis and osteomyelitis. In most cases, the disease started with protracted intermittent fever (38.5–40°), laziness and general weakness, although the animals remained in good bodily condition and their appetite was not impaired. This situation often persisted for 2 or more months. Sometimes multiple lesions of different localization appeared simultaneously or one shortly after the other.

The main portal of entry of the organism is most probably the digestive tract. Experimental oral infection of horses was seen followed by high concentration of antibodies, as well as by circulation of brucellae in the blood.

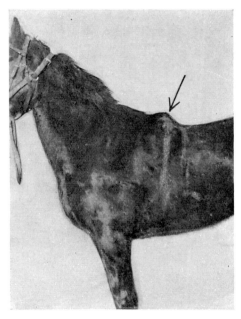

Fig. 14. Fistulous withers caused by *Brucella abortus* in a horse.
(Photo: Department of Veterinary Surgery, State University, Utrecht)

Characteristic of equine brucellosis is the localization of pathological foci in pre-existent subcutaneous or subligamentous bursae of the poll, neck, withers (Fig. 14) and presternal area (Fig. 15), as well as of the synovial sacs of joints and tendons. The inner wall of the bursae is inflamed and altered by strongly proliferating granulative tissue, profuse amounts of exudate being produced. Voluminous hygromas are formed, which contain sero-fibrinous fluid in which coagulates and necrotic material of the adjacent tendinous and osseous tissues are suspended.

References p. 131–132

In most cases the sacs finally drain themselves through one or more
fistulae which penetrate the skin.

Roderick *et al.* (1948) isolated *brucella* strains from 65 out of 80 cases of poll evil and
fistulous withers and found *Actinomyces bovis* as well as *Br. abortus* or *Br. suis*. Experimental infection of the supra-spinous bursa of horses with either of these microorganisms by itself did not have pathogenic effects. A combined injection of brucella
and actinomyces, however, provoked pathological lesions similar to those observed in
cases of spontaneous infection.

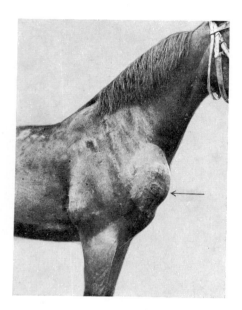

Fig. 15.   Presternal hygroma caused by *Brucella abortus* in a horse.
(Photo: Department of Veterinary Surgery, State University, Utrecht)

Exceptionally, *Brucella* infection is observed in other equine species.

It may safely be assumed that many more *dogs* are infected by *Brucella*
than can be inferred from the scanty records in the literature. This is
probably due to the rarity of pathological reaction in dogs, so that
investigations of them have not been made.

In Malta (Kennedy and Eyre, 1914), 4 out of 162 dogs gave serological
indication of *Brucella* infection and *Br. melitensis* was isolated from one of
the reacting animals. Experimental infection of dogs with this *Brucella*

species did not reveal pathological effects, although the microorganism was recovered from their blood, urine and milk (Eyre).

Very few cases of abortion in dogs have been connected with *Br. abortus* infection. The author (1932), examining 442 blood sera of dogs chosen at random in Holland, found significant agglutinin titres for *Brucella* in 16.3% and complement-fixing antibodies in 10.2% of them.

Experimental infection of puppies 6 to 8 weeks old, by instilling *Br. abortus* culture into the mouth or conjunctival sac, or by rubbing it into the scarified skin, produced high antibody titres; but neither fever nor any other signs of disease were noticed over an extended period of observation. Contact between infected and non-infected dogs in a narrow room brought about transmission of brucellae within 8 days. As early as 3 days and as late as 105 days after exposure, *Brucella* organisms were recovered from the spleen, liver and mesenterial lymph nodes of the dogs, after 32 days from the blood and up to 42 days from the bone marrow. These data explain how young dogs may easily acquire long lasting *Br. abortus* infection, which is clinically inapparent.

In Denmark, Thomsen (1932) demonstrated the presence of *Brucella* antibodies in the blood only of dogs living on farms, but not in dogs from Copenhagen. A similar experience was established on American farms. Out of 102 clinically healthy shepherds' dogs in Germany, 32 showed positive serotests for *Brucella* and *Br. melitensis* were isolated from 15 out of 25 of these animals, especially from the pharyngeal tissues. Most of these dogs had been in contact with infected sheep (Ostertag and Mayer, 1958).

Rementsova *c.s.* (1956) isolated in Russia brucellae from 4 out of 10 dogs (2 *abortus* and 2 *melitensis* species).

Veterinary literature contains a limited number of clinical observations of spontaneous *Brucella* infections in canines. The symptoms recorded comprise listlessness, fever, loss of weight, abortion (*Br. abortus* isolated from bitch and foeti), metritis, chronic vaginal discharge, orchitis (*Br. suis* recovered from pus of testicular abscess), epididymitis (*Br. abortus* isolated) and lameness.

Because the kidneys of dogs are very rarely affected, it is not likely that urine plays an important part in the conveyance of brucellosis to man or other animals.

As dogs appear to be attracted by material, pelled from aborting cows, they may spread *Brucella* infection about by dragging such material to other farms.

In recent years, brucellosis has been rather frequently observed in wild fauna.

Since 1930, infection has been spreading among *buffaloes* (bisons) in the

Montana Range of the U.S.A. (44% of steers, 62% of cows and 70% of bulls serologically reacting and *Br. abortus* isolated from a case of orchitis). A lower rate of infection has been recorded in *elks* (Katz, 1941), *chamois, deer* and *roes* (Burgisser, 1954), *moose* and *polecat*.

Available data on spontaneous *Brucella* infection in *rodents* are meager.

Investigation of 34 *grey rats* trapped on three Russian farms on which infectious abortion prevailed among bovines, revealed the presence of *Br. abortus* in the spleens and livers of 11 and in the blood of 2 of the rats (Karkadinovsky, 1936). Occasionally, brucellae have also been isolated from the organs of rats in England, France and the U.S.A. Rats are infected by ingestion of contaminated food and the brucellae are excreted in urine and faeces (Bosworth, 1937).

In Tunisia, *Br. melitensis* has been recovered from *Mus musculus;* in the U.S.S.R. *Br. abortus* was isolated from the *common vole (Microtus arvalis)*, the *Siberian marmot, gerbils, gophers, gerboas* and *hamsters*.

Leporine brucellosis was recorded for the first time by Witte (1941), who noticed in Germany a partly paralysed hare with multiple subcutaneous abscesses and isolated *Br. abortus* from these lesions. Similar findings were obtained by Roux and Bouvier (1946) when they examined two hares in Switzerland which had purulent lesions of the internal organs.

In 1949, Burgisser established *Brucella* infection in about 10% of the hares in Switzerland. The strain which he isolated differed from the three main species. It was considered to be an atypical *suis*-type, adapted to hares, and a special name, *Br. leporis,* was suggested for it. *Br. melitensis* infections of hares have been reported from France (Jacotot and Vallée, 1951) and from the U.S.S.R. (Rementsova, 1959), whereas in Czechoslovakia leporine infection was caused by *Br. abortus* (Niznansky *et al.,* 1952).

In 1951, brucellosis of hares was recognized in Denmark. During the hunting season of 1954–55, 16 strains were isolated from hares which showed similarity with the Danish variety of *Br. suis*. Significant differences existed in the incidence of infection in various regions of the country. Among 1941 hares from three localities, 82 (4.2%) infected animals were found, whereas 38.7% of 150 hares in a small area in another part of the country exhibited significant serotitres for *Brucella* (Christiansen and Thomsen, 1956).

In Denmark, the importance of brucellosis of hares is reflected in the incidence of the infection among hogs, for which hares seem to be the main source. This has been substantiated by the high susceptibility of swine to experimental infection with brucellae of leporine origin. In Poland, Hay (1960) found a positive serum reaction in 207 out of 911 hares, and the Thomsen variety of *Br. suis* was isolated from some of these animals. In the northwest of Hungary, hares were found to be affected in the proportion of 2 to 23% (Kardeván *et al.*, 1961), the disease being chronic; it was caused by the Danish type of *Br. suis*.

Brucellosis is a serious disease in hares. The extensive lesions are characterized by suppuration and necrosis with the production of creamy or viscid caseous pus. Roundish nodules of different sizes with soft contents, as well as abscesses, are found in various organs. The uterus may accumulate a large quantity of pus. The spleen is more often involved than are the liver, kidneys or lungs. Proliferative necro-purulent orchitis and epididymitis are frequently observed. The lymph nodes often contain yellowish-green caseating foci.

Spontaneous melitensis infection was reported in *chickens* in Italy as early as 1907. Fiorentini noticed fever, inappetency, loss of feathers and emaciation. The microorganism was isolated from the spleen.

A highly fatal outbreak of melitensis infection among fowl was described in France by Dubois (1910). As well as the signs just mentioned, dullness, stiffness, drooping wings and diarrhoea were observed.

In the U.S.A., *Br. abortus* was isolated from the spleen and kidneys of chickens spontaneously infected (Huddleson and Emmel, 1928) and *Br. suis* was recovered from fowl in the State of New York (Gilman and Brunett, 1930.)

Pigeons, turkeys, ducks, pheasants and *geese* exhibited susceptibility to experimental infection after they were fed or inoculated with the three main species of *Brucella*. Turkeys often succumb to the disease.

Experimental *Brucella* infection in chickens provoked general weakness, paleness of the comb and wattles, a brittle pale liver with numerous necrotic foci, degenerative processes in the ovaries, decreased egg production and signs of paralysis. Agglutinins appeared within 7–10 days after exposure and disappeared within a month. The chickens usually succumbed in from 18 to 96 days after infection. It must, however, be mentioned that other investigators were unable to reproduce such marked lesions.

Infection among poultry is probably transmitted by their droppings. No conclusive evidence exists as yet which might enable us to evaluate the role of chickens in the propagation of brucellosis among mammals.

References p. 131–132

Some investigators have postulated that ectoparasites play a role in the epidemiology of brucellosis in man and animals.

Horrocks and Kennedy (1906) recovered *Br. melitensis* from 3 *Culex* and 2 *Aedes* out of 896 mosquitoes caught in a hospital in Malta in which patients suffering from Mediterranean fever were interned.

In *Aedes* and *Stomoxys, Br. melitensis* remained viable for 4 to 5 days following an infective meal, and the organisms were excreted in their faeces (Lustig and Vernoni, 1928). *Houseflies (Musca domestica)* contaminated by *Br. melitensis* remained carriers for from 2 to 7 days (Negro, 1927).

Wellmann (1950–51) successfully transmitted *Br. melitensis, Br. suis* and *Br. abortus* to guinea pigs, goats, cows and swine by means of biting flies *(Stomoxys* and *Tabanids)* which had previously infected themselves on bovine foetal tissue or artificially contaminated milk. *Br. abortus* could be transmitted to cattle by non-biting *Musca domestica*.

In Mexico, Tovar (1947) recovered *Br. abortus* from ticks of cattle *(Boophilus annulatus)* and *Br. melitensis* from bedbugs *(Cimex lectularius)*. He also demonstrated infection of ticks, bugs and fleas in experiments with the three main species of *Brucella*, most easily, with *Br. suis*. The two arthropods first mentioned still eliminated brucellae in their faeces 3 months after the infective meal. They transmitted the infection to healthy test animals by consecutive feeding on them. The brucellae passed on from the adult ticks via their eggs to the larvae.

Natural *melitensis* infection of *Ornithodoros, Rhipicephalus* and *Hyalomma* was found in Russia. In *O. lahorensis* of sheep, *Br. melitensis* remained viable for 27 months and the organism was excreted in the coxal fluid. On the other hand, examination of several thousands of ticks collected from cattle, goats and sheep in enzootic areas of the U.S.S.R. showed negative results (Rementsova, 1956).

In the light of this, it should not be overlooked that brucellae can be maintained for a considerable time in the body of ectoparasitic arthropods, although their epizootiological and epidemiological role does not appear to be very important in itself.

The great extension of the *Brucella* reservoir in nature has been elucidated by Pavlovski (1957), who stated that, in the U.S.S.R., 30 kinds of wild vertebrates (including mammals, birds, reptiles, amphibians and even fish), as well as 14 kinds of ticks, and 4 kinds of insects, have been found either to be spontaneous *Brucella* carriers or to be capable of contracting *Brucella* infection under experimental conditions.

Most of the morbid manifestations of animal brucellosis are also observed in *human beings*. In man, however, the disease is much more polymorphic. Its most characteristic features are prolonged intermittent bacteraemia and recurring bouts of fever. Human brucellosis differs from the disease in ruminants and swine in that the reproductive organs are seldom involved, nor is gestation interfered with. Although a few human cases of uterine infection by *Br. melitensis* and *Br. abortus* have been recorded, miscarriages do not form part of the picture usually seen.

In man the average incubation period is about 14 days. In the first stage after infection no characteristic symptoms are noticed. The disease usually develops gradually, but sometimes the onset is sudden.

A sensation of general discomfort, weariness and weakness are the earliest common complaints. They are followed by fever, now and then accompanied by chills. More or less pathognomonic is profuse nocturnal sweating, headache and pains in different parts of the body, especially in the legs, large joints and the lumbar regions, irritability, depression and insomnia. Laryngitis and bronchial catarrh may cause painful coughing. Persistent constipation often alternates with diarrhoea.

In many cases the body temperature runs a characteristic course. The daily fluctuations are of the intermittent type, with high levels in the evenings and subfebrile temperature earlier in the day. After 1 to 3 weeks, an apyrexial interval of a few days follows, and then a second period of intermittent fever sets in. These alternating stages of high temperatures interrupted by afebrile intervals are several times repeated and usually they show decreasing length and height of the successive waves (febris undulans, see Fig. 16a-b). Cases have been recorded of fever lasting for as long as 2 or more years.

The blood picture indicates a progressive secondary anaemia, accompanied by a relative lymphocytosis, monocytosis and sometimes leucocytosis; the eosinophil count remains normal.

The tissues most affected are those associated with the reticuloendothelial system (liver, spleen, bone marrow, lymph nodes, etc.). The intracellular localization of the micro-organisms gives rise to rather characteristic, but non-specific, tissue reactions (hyperplasia of the cells of the R.E.S.; epitheloid cell granulomata comparable with those seen in tuberculosis, syphilis and sarcoidosis), and suppurative or destructive lesions.

The repeated circulation of brucellae in the blood may lead to various metastases resulting in phlebitis, subacute endocarditis, lung infiltration, nephritis, cholecystitis and pericholecystitis, spondylitis, encephalitis, meningitis, orchitis, epididymitis and suppurative processes in various tissues. The spleen and liver are soft and swollen, the latter becoming firmer when the duration of the disease is prolonged (hepato-splenomegaly). Neuralgic conditions of the peripheral and central nervous system often develop. Neuritis is frequently localized in the coxal region. The clinical

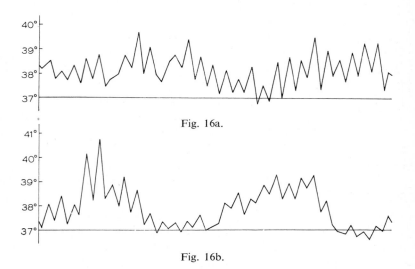

Fig. 16a.

Fig. 16b.

Fig. 16.   Temperature curves of two persons suffering from brucellosis (undulant fever).

picture is not seldom dominated by extreme depression, attacks of delirium, excitability or apathy and amnesia.

In extensive clinical surveys of brucellosis in Minnesota, Spink recorded the following percentage incidence of symptoms:

fever	97.9	coughing	30
weakness	91.5	hepatomegaly	20.6
profuse sweating	76.5	visual disturbances	11.6
chills	75.5	diarrhoea	9.6
generalized aches	69	cardial affections	7.5
headache	63.8	genito-urinary disturbances	7.4
nervousness	52	neuralgia	5.3
lymphadenopathy	45.7	spondylitis	± 4
joint pain	43.6	erythematous skin eruption	3.3
splenomegaly	40.5	orchitis	2.1
depression	40		

In veterinary obstetricians, in addition to an allergic reaction of the skin which is due to hypersensitivity to the bovine or placental proteins, a specific "erythema brucellum" occurs, which is an expression of dermal *Brucella* allergy or *Brucella* infection. The lesion appears on the hand and arm soon after assisting at delivery of an infected foetus (Fig. 17) as a rash

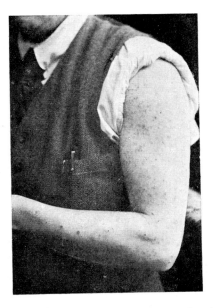

Fig. 17. Erythema brucellum in a veterinary practitioner after delivery of an aborted foetus. (By courtesy of Dr. A. Thomsen, Copenhagen)

of papules and pustules which quickly undergo necrosis. These skin lesions tend to recur on nearly every occasion when a similar task is performed. Sometimes it forces the veterinarian to give up practising this branch of his profession.

Uncomplicated brucellosis often assumes an ambulatory course with quick recovery. In a considerable number of cases, however, the disease develops more severe symptoms, or complications set in, especially when elderly persons are affected or when hygienic conditions are unfavourable.

The average duration of the disease ranges between 2 or 3 months. Spink, in Minnesota, found that complete recovery occurred in about 80% of the patients within a year. Signorelli (1941) recorded in Italy a mortality of 5% of cases, partial recovery in 10% and return to full health in 85%.

Mortality in the U.S.S.R. was estimated at 3 to 5%. The "Vital Statistics" of the W.H.O. give the following percentages of deaths from brucellosis: in Malta 0.6, in the U.S.A. 0.9, in France 1.1, in Greece 0.13, in Denmark and Italy 1.3, in Portugal 1.6, in Holland 1.7, in West Germany 2, in Switzerland 2.7 and in Mexico 12.3.

Exceptionally, human brucellosis takes, from its first onset, a malignant course. In such cases the body temperature remains constantly high, the tongue is thickly coated; pulmonary congestion, diffuse bronchial ronchi and profuse diarrhoea are conspicuous symptoms. The pulse soon becomes weak. Vomiting, incontinence, cardial weakness and coma are prodromes of early death (febris undulans acutissima).

Since Alice Evans, in 1934, called attention to prolonged conditions of ill health with no detectable cause, and their probable relation to hidden *Brucella* infection, the problem of "chronic brucellosis" has been of foremost medical interest. Except for patients from whom brucellae are recovered, this diagnosis carries a great deal of risk. Only in a negligible proportion of suspect cases can a history of a previous acute febrile phase, compatible with brucellosis, be evoked. Usually in these cases, antibodies against brucella are not present in significant amounts, the organism does not circulate in the blood, and even physical signs of illness are often lacking. There are constant complaints of muscular weakness and extreme weariness. Neuro-psychiatric conditions are in the foreground. They involve chronic pachy- and leptomeningitis, neurasthenia, psychoneurosis, hypochondriasis and anxiety. Spink and Magoffin (1950) assume that in emotionally unstable persons *Brucella* infection may tend to accentuate and intensify the already existing psychoneurotic disposition.

Local lesions are frequently found in the long bones and joints (suppurative arthritis mostly of the knee and hip). Spondylitis and osteomyelitis especially occur in the vertebral column, with destruction and granulation of adjacent tissues.

Rheumatic conditions (periarticular, articular, pelvo-rachitic, osteitic affections) have frequently been ascribed to *Brucella* infection ("rhumatisme mélitococcique", Mériel *et al.,* 1960).

Serious complications are due to cardiovascular localization of the infection, the formation of vegetations and ulceration, chronic hepatosplenomegaly, and sometimes suppurative processes of the genital organs (epididymitis, orchitis, tubo-ovarial abscesses, etc.), ocular involvement (optic neuritis and atrophy, corneal ulcer, iridocyclitis) and other lesions.

In the period between 1947 and 1954 Zammit examined in Malta 115 patients with brucellar spondylitis. The localization in 62 of them was as follows: 37 lumbar, 16 dorsal, 4 dorsal and lumbar and 5 cervical.

McVay *et al.* (1950) cultivated from 250 specimens of chronically affected human tissues 6 strains, *viz.* 2 *Br. melitensis* and 2 *Br. abortus* from prostates and 2 *Br. melitensis* from Fallopian tubes. None of the 6 patients reacted in the serum test with *Brucella*, 2 showed a positive intradermal reaction. In all of them there was a history of farm life, contact with cattle and consumption of raw milk.

As a rule infection by *Br. melitensis* causes more serious and more manifold complications than those caused by the other brucella species. Patients suffering from Mediterranean fever feel and look very ill. Soon there is utter weakness and exhaustion and marked weight loss. Peripheral neuritis inflicts acute pain. Psychiatric and neurological disturbances, spondylitis, orchitis and epididymitis occur more frequently than they do in brucellosis caused by the *abortus* or *suis* species.

On the other hand it cannot be overlooked that strains of *Brucella*, which are classified by laboratory methods as belonging to the same species, may exhibit a degree of pathogenicity widely divergent from what is usually observed. Several examples can be given. The "*melitensis* strains" encountered in Great Britain and Northern Germany were not virulent to human beings. Nearly all *Br. abortus* strains which the author isolated from horses in the Netherlands were markedly less pathogenic to guinea-pigs than those recovered from cattle.

As a rule the pathogenicity of *Br. suis* is, on the average, between that of *Br. melitensis* and *Br. abortus,* being characterized by a strong tendency to cause suppurative lesions in man and pigs alike. Whereas in Denmark no case of human infection caused by the local variety of *Br. suis* is on record, in Roumania this strain provoked infection in more than 10% of the pig-breeders exposed to it (Pop *et al.,* 1958).

In contrast to what occurs with *Br. melitensis,* only a minor number of the persons infected by *Br. abortus* develop symptoms of illness. Gould and Huddleson (1937) estimated the infection-rate of brucellosis in the North-American population at 10%, but they concluded that no more than 1% of the persons reacting serologically would be likely to show clinical evidence of illness.

Only very exceptionally do several persons in a contaminated environment or in one family suffer at the same time from brucellosis caused by *Br. abortus.* It has been postulated that certain additional factors must

prevail in order to enable this species to injure human health; in other
words, it only becomes pathogenic to man when the biological balance
between host and potential parasite is disturbed by such factors. This may
happen as a result of weakened local or general resistance of the host,
brought about by extreme fatigue, intercurrent illness, trauma, wounds and

TABLE XIV

AVERAGE YEARLY INCIDENCE OF BRUCELLOSIS

(1951–1956)

Country	Population (approximately)	Average number of cases registered	Average number per 100,000 inhabitants
Italy	46,600,000	8,437	181.7
Malta	300,000	515	171.7
Greece	7,600,000	662	87.1
Mexico	26,300,000	1,040	39.5
France	42,200,000	926	21.9
U.S.A.	154,800,000	2,046	13.2
Portugal	8,600,000	376	4.4
Switzerland	4,800,000	175	3.6
Denmark	4,300,000	53	1.2
West Germany	48,100,000	376	0.8
Netherlands	10,300,000	52	0.5
Egypt	20,700,000	81	0.4

other damages. The requirement of these stress factors offers a plausible
explanation for the numerous failures in experimentally inducing oral
infection in volunteers with milk contaminated with *Br. abortus*.

Invasion through the abraded skin and the conjunctiva seems to cause
infection in man more readily than along the gastro-intestinal route.

Evaluation of the actual incidence of human *Brucella*-infections is
hampered by the protean character of the symptoms and the frequency of
non-specific courses of the disease, especially in subclinical and chronic
cases. This difficulty applies particularly to *Br. abortus*. Official reports
record only data on patients with clinically evident illness, whereas the
other cases remain unidentified and are therefore not notified.

For some countries the annual case-incidences are recorded in
Table XIV which was derived from the Vital Statistics of the World
Health Organization (1958) over the 6-year period of 1951–1956.

It should be borne in mind that there were great differences between the various methods used for the collection of these data, so that the accuracy of the figures given above also varies greatly. However, it may be safely concluded that the prevalence of human brucellosis varies considerably in different countries.

Reliable estimates of the actual incidence, elicited figures a great deal higher. Thus it has been stated that in France about 9,000, in the U.S.A. 40,000–100,000 (Kaplan, 1950) and in the U.S.S.R. (Smirnov, 1956) three to four million persons were infected by *Brucella* annually.

The incidence of human brucellosis in any region depends primarily on the spread and density of the infection among livestock and on the closeness of contacts between man and animals or their excreta. This accounts for the epidemiological importance connected with certain occupations (Fig. 18).

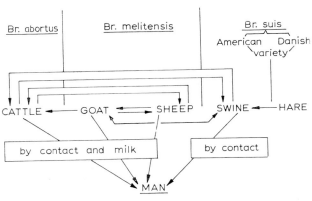

Fig. 18.   Routes of natural infection with *Brucella abortus*, *-melitensis* and *-suis*.

Control measures in animals have a beneficial effect on the incidence of the disease in man.

In the U.S.A. the number of notified cases declined from about 6,000 in 1946 to 3,139 in 1951 and 1,300 in 1956. Wholesale vaccination of livestock in the U.S.S.R., starting in 1955, achieved a decrease of approximately 50% of cases among human beings. Between the years 1951 and 1956 the human incidence of brucellosis diminished in France from 1,104 to 715 cases, in Denmark from 153 to 11, in the Netherlands from 64 to 37. Between 1939 and 1957 it fell in Sweden from 114 to nil and in Finland between 1938 and 1952 from 28 to nil. Contrary to this, propitious local conditions in other countries gave rise to increased incidence in man. In Argentina 1,825 cases of brucellosis were notified in 1951 and 3,398 in 1956; and in Greece 189 and 618 cases respectively were recorded in these same years. The role of ecological factors is illustrated in Algeria where the urban-kept goats were most heavily infected and consequently *febris melitensis* became a malady almost exclusively of European town dwellers.

In the South-Eastern districts of France the disease occurs especially among the rural population. In Argentina, the species of *Brucella* are distributed in a similar manner among human beings and domestic animals, *i.e. Br. melitensis* occurs in the western regions, while *Br. abortus* and *Br. suis* are predominant in the eastern part of the country.

The distribution of *Br. melitensis* and *Br. abortus* differs among the various population groups in Kenya, the former particularly occurring in natives, the latter among Europeans (Manson-Bahr, 1956).

Whatever the species of the causative agent may be, brucellosis appears more frequently in males than in females. This higher incidence in males is apparently connected with their greater exposure to occupational contacts, because wherever the infection is due to the consumption of milk or dairy products, both sexes are about equally affected.

Most cases of brucellosis are noticed in people belonging to the age group 20 to 40 or 50 years, a fact which may likewise be explained by their greater occupational exposure.

Humans, like calves, kids and lambs, show high resistance to *Brucella* infection during the early years of life. This is to be regarded as being a specific function of the youthful organism which is lost with advancing age. Brucellosis, especially when it is caused by the *abortus* species, is seldom encountered in individuals below the age of 15 years and it is extremely rare in children under 5 years. Spink (1937–1954) found that less than 3% of the brucellosis patients in the State of Minnesota were under 12 years; Hemmes (1950) recorded the infection in 7% of the patients in Holland below the age of 15.

According to the author's experience (1934) a woman suffering from acute brucellosis Bang may give birth to a healthy child which can be nursed for several months with the heavily contaminated mother's milk without showing any pathological effect and without even producing specific antibodies. The low incidence of brucellosis during the early years of life is patently in contrast with other milk borne infectious diseases. Another opinion has been expressed by certain observers, who explained the rarity of brucellosis in infants and children by the failure of physicians to diagnose the disease which – in this age-group – most frequently appears in a subclinical, mild or chronic form (Harris, 1951).

Comparatively high rates of attack are encountered among the intensively exposed workers in the veterinary profession. Steele (1953) recorded 250 per 100,000 veterinarians affected, as compared with 45 per

100,000 among farm workers in the U.S.A. High incidence of infection in these groups is also expressed by serological and allergic reactivity, which increases with the duration of employment in contaminated environments.

In the years 1930–1932, about 94% of the Danish veterinarians practising for more than 1 year showed positive *Brucella*-serotests, whereas no agglutinins could be established in the blood of students at the Veterinary College in Copenhagen (Thomsen). Antibodies against *Brucella* were established among various professions in Poland (Szmuness and Parnas, 1960) as follows: 47.94% in veterinarians and zootechnicians, 16.48% in individual farmers, 12.71% in workers in collective farms, 2.36% in employees of the meat industry and 0.84% in laboratory personnel. In 1949, an average of 25.6% of the American veterinarians gave serological evidence of *Brucella* infection.

The appearance of erythema brucellum was recorded in 171 out of 796 Danish veterinarians, in 186 out of 449 Dutch and in 86 out of 166 Swiss veterinary surgeons.

A much smaller number of veterinarians are affected by the general disease. Out of 449 engaged in rural practice in Holland, 15 reported that they had actually suffered from the disease and another 8, that they presumably had. Among 651 veterinarians in Prussia 55 (8.4%) evoked a history of brucellosis, and in Poland one third of the sero- logically reacting veterinarians reported the disease. Out of 329 veterinary surgeons in Southern Italy, 67 (20.4%) had contracted a clinical form of brucellosis and 121 (36.8%) suffered from exanthema brucellum. Of all these cases, 74% were associated with manual removal of placentae of cows and 15% with other obstetrical interventions. In 89%, cattle were the source of infection as compared with 8% infected from goats (Battelli, 1959).

Brucella infection not seldom occurs by accidental pricking or scratching with a needle mounted on a syringe filled with live vaccine, or by wounds inflicted by a glass-splinter from an ampule containing the vaccine. Splashing or spraying of vaccine into the eyes of the vaccinator has also been mentioned as cause of infection.

Strain B19 of *Br. abortus,* which is used for preparation of the bovine vaccine, has practically lost its pathogenicity for cattle. In several cases accidental penetration of the vaccine into the skin of a veterinarian caused marked local painful swelling within the following 1/4–3 hours. Shortly afterwards a systemic reaction sometimes developed (chills, fever, sweats, headache, myalgia, arthralgia and other signs of acute brucellosis). Antibodies were produced up to high titres and it was possible to recover strain-19 organisms repeatedly from the blood. This rapid pathogenic action seems to warrant the view that workers in the veterinary profession are sensitized to *Brucella* as a result of their frequent exposure to these organisms. Furthermore, it seems that although strain B19 has lost its pathogenicity for bovines, it has not lost it for man.

References p. 131–132

Ranking next to the heavy exposure of veterinary surgeons, is the exposure of employees in meat-packing plants, slaughter-houses and establishments for the destruction of animal carcasses. Repeated and often massive and close exposure to this large reservoir of infection results in high incidence among meat processors, butchers, delivery men and other workers in the plants.

The incidence of brucellosis per 100,000 persons employed in miscellaneous occupations in the U.S.A., recorded by Jordan (1948), amounted to 562 for veterinarians, 276 for slaughter-house workers, 59 for farmers and only 4 for individuals not coming into contact with farm animals. The infection generally develops after penetration of the micro-organisms through small abrasions or wounds of the skin. Most seriously affected in meat packing plants are the "beefkillers", but brucellosis also prevails among persons not concerned with the actual handling of carcasses or animal products. This indicates that contamination is possible everywhere on the premises of such plants. Intensive exposure to *Brucella* infection is an especially potential menace to handlers of pork, because the organisms are more widely distributed throughout the tissues of swine than they are in those of cattle.

In the period between 1937 to 1954, 134 out of 244 cases of brucellosis observed in the Minnesota University Clinics, occurred among packing-plant personnel, and 51 strains of *Br. abortus*, 11 of *Br. suis* and only 1 of *Br. melitensis* were isolated from them.

On the basis of serological investigation, evidence of *Brucella* infection among butchers amounted, in Hungary to 22.6%, in the Netherlands to 14.3, in England and the U.S.A. to 13.7 and in Argentina to 10.8%. In a regional animal destructor plant in Holland (1953) 34 out of 74 employees showed significant agglutinin titres as compared with 4 out of 70 workers in dairies. In the southern districts of the U.S.S.R., where *melitensis* infection prevails enzootically, 37.2% of the brucellosis cases occurred in sheep breeders (Drankin, 1955), and 17 to 25% of the *Br. abortus* infections occurring in the country were recorded from cattle ranch workers.

In the pig-breeding districts of the U.S.A., the frequent infection of man with the *suis* species is reflected in the overall incidences. According to Borts (1954, quoted by Stableforth and Galloway, 1959) among 362 strains isolated from human beings in Iowa, 207 were *Br. suis*, 140 *Br. abortus* and 15 *Br. melitensis*. Damon (1944) recovered 69 *suis*-strains among 91 isolates from clinical cases of brucellosis in Alabama. The risk of infection to workers in the American meat industry is reflected by the finding that at least 1.25% of the carcasses of slaughtered cattle and 1.15–3.5% of swine carcasses were contaminated with one or more of the three *Brucella* species (Sadler, 1960).

Exposure of dairy men and livestock producers employed in heavily infected farms is not restricted to direct contact of the bare abraded skin of their hands and arms with aborted foetuses, foetal membranes or allantoic fluid, but is connected with contaminated dust entering the mucous membranes of the respiratory tract and the eyes as well. Milking of cows, goats or sheep excreting *Brucella* may represent another way of infection in farm workers.

It is often difficult to evaluate the role of either contact or consumption in the rural population which may be contaminated along both routes of infection. Various statistics have estimated that 10–25% of cases of human brucellosis are associated with the consumption of fresh milk, non-fermented cheese or ice-cream.

Unheated milk or dairy products containing *Br. melitensis* or *Br. suis* (the latter proceeding from cattle) are much more dangerous than are the foodstuffs which harbour *Br. abortus*. However, Dalrymple–Champneys (1953) recorded that about 69% of 1,134 brucellosis patients in Great Britain probably acquired *Br. Bang* infection from drinking non-pasteurized milk or cream. Brucellae are largely concentrated in the cream-layer of milk. Vershilova and Pavlov suggested that nearly half the cases of human brucellosis in the U.S.S.R. are due to alimentary infection. Steele stated, in 1957, that 16% of all *Brucella* infections in the United States were even then due to the consumption of milk. In 79% of human infections the source was traced back to cattle, in 19% to swine and in less than 1% to sheep.

Brucellosis has practically disappeared from the large towns where pasteurization of milk is compulsory. The few cases occurring in Copenhagen since 1942 have been ascribed to ingestion of "childrens milk", the only unpasteurized dairy product available in that city.

In fresh milk, at body temperature, brucellae perish within a few hours; at 8° they survive for about 2 days.

Infection experiments have proved that large numbers of *Brucella* are necessary to cause human infection by ingestion.

The viability of brucellae in cheese depends on the methods of processing applied. The low pH reached in the manufacture of butter and the adverse influence of the undissociated lactic acid molecule render this product harmless. It is assumed that in hard fermented cheeses the organisms are destroyed within 3 months. Aged-ripened cheese does not represent any hazard. On the other hand, in Israel, in brynza-cheese prepared from fresh goat's milk, *Br. melitensis* remained viable for up to 8 weeks.

Br. suis has been cultivated from stored meat and the viscera and lymph nodes of infected pigs, more than a month after killing of the animals. Viable *Brucella* organisms were recovered from cured and commercially pickled hams of naturally infected swine after 21 days of refrigeration.

There is, however, no evidence to show that the consumption of such food actually caused infection in human beings. The process of smoking kills *Brucella* present in pork.

Records on the prevalence of *Br. abortus* in meat and organs of slaughter cattle are rather contradictory.

Leresche *et al.* (1957), in Switzerland, isolated brucellae from the meat of 3 and from the blood of 2 out of 9 cows which had recently aborted. However, brucellae could not be revealed in the muscles of 62 cows with chronic brucellosis. Other investigators obtained similar negative results.

From these facts it can be elicited that no great pathogenic significance must be attached to the eating of meat from animals infected with *Brucella*.

Interhuman transmission of brucellosis is very rare, and even doubtful. Cases of mechanical transmission as a result of blood transfusion are on record. The donors may be subclinically infected, but nevertheless have brucellae circulating in their blood (Wood, 1955). In the Minnesota-Hospitals low *Brucella* agglutinin titres were established by Spink in 18.57% of the bloodsamples collected for the blood-bank (1.66% showing a titre of 1:160 or higher). In human whole-blood, refrigerated at 4°, the three species of *Brucella* remained viable for 6 months. However, in view of the small number of organisms present in stored blood, it can be expected that infection of the receiver will be most exceptional.

The relatively high incidence of laboratory infections is mainly due to the extreme virulence of *Br. melitensis* and *Br. suis* in artificial culture. These strains are, in fact, among the most dangerous microorganisms handled in the laboratory.

Up to 1940, Meyer and Eddie reviewed 74 cases of brucellosis which had occurred in 17 American laboratories. 21 of 34 strains isolated from the patients were of the *melitensis* species, 12 were *Br. suis* and only 1 *Br. abortus*. In a survey of laboratory-acquired infections, based upon data from a questionaire submitted to approximately 5,000 laboratories, Sulkin and Pike (1951) concluded that the hazard of infection with brucellae is far greater than that with all other infective agents.

In 60% of the 224 recorded cases, the species of *Brucella* involved was known, and, in contrast to the data mentioned by Meyer and Eddie, nearly even numbers of *Br. melitensis, Br. suis* and *Br. abortus* were listed.

A high incidence of *melitensis* infection is reported among laboratory personnel in the centres of brucellosis-research in Tunis and Montpellier. Handling of cultures or infected test-animals, inhalation of dust, sucking of a bacterial suspension and droplet spraying from a pipette, are among the recorded causes of infection. In the U.S.A., accidental contamination of the general water supply in a laboratory has been mentioned as the source of numerous infections among the personnel.

Brucellosis, particularly when it is provoked by the *melitensis* species, may represent a public health problem of primary importance. Besides this, substantial economic losses are sustained and considerable reduction in the production of valuable human foodstuffs is caused by the *abortus* species. Most heavily affected are the meat and dairy industries.

There is loss of manpower as a result of reduced working capacity due to physical and mental suffering, protracted convalescence or chronic course of disease.

According to the Bureau of Economics of the U.S.A. Department of Agriculture, in Michigan State, 222,804,000 pounds of market milk were lost as a result of bovine brucellosis in 1945, which is equivalent to an amount as large as that consumed annually by 557,000 persons. As a result of brucellosis, an expected production of 800 million pounds of cows' milk a year were not produced in the State of New York (Fagan, 1949). In addition to these huge losses sustained by the dairy industry, vast damage is inflicted on the meat producers. The estimated annual loss of veal in Michigan amounted in 1945 to 1,299,200 pounds.

The following figures based upon officially recorded incidences may give an impression of the total annual economic damage in different countries: in the U.S.A. originally 100 million dollars (1947), which has been reduced to an estimated 40 million dollars in 1957; in France (1953) 37 milliard old Fr. frcs.; in Argentina 172 million pesos; in Germany (1946) 200 to 250 million R.Mk.; in the Netherlands (1956) 45 million H.fl.; in Switzerland (1945) 20 million Sw.frcs. In the U.S.S.R. the number of infected animals has been estimated in the millions and the losses are accordingly extraordinarily high.

The enormous economic losses and the serious hazard to human health demanded enforcement of energetic measures, which should aim at total elimination of sources from which the infection primarily originates, namely enzootic brucellosis in livestock.

A successful campaign would require adaptation of the control measures to locally prevailing conditions. To be taken into account are: the size of the herds, their infection rate, housing and hygienic conditions, the distance between, and contact with, neighbouring herds, the economic situation and educational status of the livestock owners and several others factors.

Full cooperation of the owners is most desirable. First, it is necessary to establish which herds in a presumably infected area contain animals which react to the milk-ring-test (A.B.R., see page 106). The next step should be general screening by agglutination tests performed with the bloodsera of individual cows in the "positive" herds.

The main measures of control in a brucellosis eradication program are: serological testing, elimination of the reacting animals from a herd and vaccination of the remainder. In addition to this, the hygienic conditions on the farm should be improved, and contamination from the outside prevented. This includes restriction of movement of the cattle and preliminary testing of animals before they are permitted to join the herd. Very important are the separation of cows shortly before parturition, disposal of aborted foetuses and afterbirths, disinfection of the animals and their quarters, and segregation of the cows until secretion from the uterus has stopped (at least for 10 days post partum). Rats should be exterminated. In regions where the small ruminants and swine are also affected, prevention of interspecies transmission is necessary.

A most beneficial method in the control of bovine brucellosis is vaccination at an early age. The vaccine, consisting of a live suspension of an attenuated strain of Br. abortus ("Buck 19"), has found worldwide application. In cattle it does not produce disease, but it is still capable of inducing a high grade resistance against Brucella infection.

The vaccine is injected subcutaneously, intradermally or sometimes intracaudally. Administration of this vaccine offers many important advantages. Strain B19 is remarkably stable; after passage through cows its properties remain unchanged. It does not settle in the uterus or mammary glands of vaccinated non-pregnant animals and pregnant cows excrete the organism only during about a week's time after parturition. The resistance induced by one subcutaneous or intradermal injection in calves lasts for a long time (at least 7 years as has been claimed), a fact which makes revaccinating practically unnecessary. Vaccination at the age of 6–8 months does not provoke lastion presence of agglutinins in the blood, but when older animals are vaccinated the antibodies tend to persist for an indefinite time, so that it becomes difficult to differentiate between vaccinated and naturally infected animals. According to Andersen (1961) and others, unspecific reactions can be excluded when carrying out the tests at a temperature of 50–55°.

The most effective procedure would be the eradication of all reacting animals, as is done for control of bovine tuberculosis. For reasons of economy, however, such a radical method can only be applied to herds with a low incidence of infection. In these herds, the "reactors" are slaughtered or removed from the farm. Because virulent Brucella organisms may be excreted in the milk of serologically nonreacting cattle and in the urine of swine showing negative serum tests, segregation of reactors alone may be inadequate. Gradual replacement of the older cattle by the new healthy generation supports control measures.

The following are examples of different systems of Brucella control and their results in various countries under varying local conditions.

In 1938, a campaign against bovine brucellosis was launched in Finland, where the initial infection rate was 3.4% of herds. The radical control program then initiated yielded very satisfactory results. In 1956, infectious abortion was completely wiped out among Finnish livestock and consequently brucellosis was also banished from the population of the country. In Norway, energetic nation-wide measures were undertaken in 1934, with financial aid from the Government. Without milk-testing and vaccination, the disease has been practically eliminated within a period of 10 years.

The wide-spread infection among the dense cattle population of Denmark required unabated activity. With the full support of the Cooperative Dairies and a large sub-vention from the State, a collective campaign-program was set up. In the fiscal year 1954–1955, 700,179 blood samples were examined, as well as 683,835 milk samples and 32,406 placentas. The original infection-rate of 25% of the herds in 1944 had declined to less than 5% towards 1957.

In the Swiss canton of Zürich some 15% of the cattle herds were infected in 1951, in 1957 the figure was only about 1%. In Yugoslavia the percentage of cows reacting to Brucella was 4.1 in 1951, and 1 in 1956; in the U.S.S.R. the corresponding percentage was estimated at almost 8 in 1932, 3 in 1940 and 1.5 in 1953.

In the U.S.A. the first organized efforts to combat bovine infectious abortion were made in 1934, when a Cooperative State-Federal-Brucellosis-Eradication-Program was instituted on an areal basis. Great improvement was achieved when, in 1941, vaccina-tion with strain-19 was added to the program. Since 1947, a uniform nation-wide campaign has been carried out, which is flexible enough to cope with the different herd- and regional conditions. In the 2 decades following 1934, approximately 127 million heads of cattle in 11 million herds have been blood-tested. The number of infected herds fell in this period from 38–14.2% and that of the infected animals from 10–2.6%. Between 1941 and 1955 more than 21 million calves were vaccinated and during the following 3 years, 20.9 million. In 1958 the infection rate of all bovines throughout the U.S.A. had fallen to 1.6%, while 15 States and Puerto Rico were certified as having been completely free from brucellosis for a period of at least 1 year.

This favourable condition in the bovines is clearly reflected in the gradual decrease of notified incidences of human brucellosis (4,991 cases in 1948 as compared with 802 cases in 1958).

Comparatively little has been accomplished in several countries in the systematic eradication of brucellosis among sheep, goats and swine. Because Brucella infection tends to be self-limiting in sheep, serotesting and segregation or slaughtering of the reacting animals are often sufficient to attain satisfactory control. Reacting goats should be slaughtered. In the U.S.A. simple control-measures have reduced the original infection rate of 7.8% of goats to 1.3% between 1944 and 1947.

Vaccination of swine proved of little or no avail, and until recently it was accepted that it did not confer adequate immunity on the small ruminant animals either. Russian experiences of the last years seem, how-ever, to be very favourable. In addition to the B19 vaccine various other products have been used in several countries. (Attenuated strains of Br. abortus, -suis or -melitensis, prepared for example, by addition of formalin and aluminium hydroxide or glycerin, or by combination of a formalinized *(ana-)* culture of *Br. melitensis* and a live avirulent *Br. abortus* strain). Most of these vaccines have not been tested beyond the stage of field-trial, so that a final evaluation of their practical value cannot yet be made. Workers in several countries have, however, reported promising results with a vaccine introduced by Elberg in California (1957) which is prepared from an attenuated living *Brucella melitensis* strain, not dependent on streptomycin, derived from a culture, dependent on streptomycin.

Education of the public is a valuable aid in the fight against human brucellosis.

People whose occupations expose them to *Brucella* infection should take care to protect themselves. Wounds and abrasions on the hands or arms should be cleansed and covered before the individual attends to parturition or abortion in ruminant animals. Veterinarians who must explore the bovine vagina and uterus should wear long-sleeved rubber gloves or they should at least cover the skin of the hands and arms with a thick layer of ointment. Employees in meat-packing plants and slaughter-houses must wash and disinfect their hands when their work is finished. Every cut or scratch incurred during work must be thoroughly treated at once.

Alimentary infection can be effectively prevented by the compulsory sterilization or pasteurization of milk destined for direct consumption or for dairy production.

In some countries in which many persons are heavily exposed to *Brucella* infection, vaccination of these individuals is performed. Some experts recommend vaccination with strain B19, but others contest the usefulness of this strain. Very remarkable results were obtained with B19-vaccine in the U.S.S.R. In 1947–51 in a trial involving 5,000 people an index of effectiveness of 1 :24 was recorded. Since 1952 human vaccination with the live attenuated American B19 strain (designated in the Moscow Institute: BAJ/19), or with another locally isolated *Br. abortus* strain (M) has been officially adopted. During the following 4 years more than 2 million persons received preventive vaccination. By comparing the morbidity rates of vaccinated and non-vaccinated groups of exposed persons under similar conditions, it has been claimed that the efficacy of this procedure has been definitely proved.

Treatment must be initiated as soon as the diagnosis has been made.

The brucellae settle chiefly inside the cells and in this position they are fairly well protected against noxious influences and drugs. Before the discovery of antibiotics, no specific medical treatment was known. Penicillin is not effective and it has been found that the administration of one single antibiotic is of little avail. Great advances have been made by the combined application of broad-spectrum antibiotics, supported by sulfonamides, vitamin-B-complex and small doses of cortisone. Protection of human beings against brucellae is imperative so long as brucellosis prevails among animals. The aim of both public health authorities and veterinarians is therefore the total eradication of brucellosis from the whole animal world.

REFERENCES

ANDERSEN, F. M., *Nord. Vet.-Med.*, 13 (1961) 289.
BATTELLI, C., *Vet. ital.*, 10 (1959) 799.
BENDIXEN, H. C. and E. BLOM, *Månedsskr. Dyrlæg.*, 59 (1947) 61.
BUDDLE, M. B. and B. W. BOYES, *Aust. vet. J.*, 29 (1953) 145.
BURGISSER, H., *Schweiz. Arch. Tierheilk.*, 91 (1949) 273; 96 (1954) 521.
CAMERON, H. S., *Advanc. vet. Sci.*, 3 (1957) 275.
CHRISTIANSEN, M. and A. THOMSEN, *Nord. Vet.-Med.*, 8 (1956) 841.
DALRYMPLE–CHAMPNEYS, W., *Brucella infection and undulant fever*, London, 1960, 196 pp.
DAMON, S. R., J. H. SCRUGGS and E. B. PARKER, *J. Amer. vet. med. Ass.*, 117 (1950) 39.
EVANS, A. C., *J. Amer. med. Ass.*, 103 (1934) 665; *Amer. J. publ. Hlth*, 37 (1947) 139.
GRUMBACH, A., in GRUMBACH and KIKUTH, *Die Infektionskrankheiten des Menschen*, II, Stuttgart, 1958, p. 862.
HARRIS, H. J., *Brucellosis*, New York, 1950, 617 pp.
HOEDEN, J. V. D., *Z. Infekt.-Kr. Haustiere*, 42 (1932) 1; *T. Diergeneesk.*, 59 (1932) 1383; 1446; *Antonie v. Leeuwenhoek*, 7 (1941) 211.
HUDDLESON, I. F., *Brucellosis in man and animals*, New York, 1943, 379 pp.
JACOTOT, H. and A. VALLÉE, *Ann. Inst. Pasteur*, 80 (1951) 99; 214.
Joint F.A.O./Wrld Hlth Org., *Expert Comm. on Brucellosis Rep.*, I, 1951; II, 1953; III, 1958.
KARKADINOVSKY, *C. R. Soc. Biol. (Paris)*, 121 (1936) 1611.
KATZ, J. S., *J. Amer. vet. med. Ass.*, 99 (1941) 24.
KERR, W. R., J. K. L. PEARSON and J. E. F. RANKIN, *Vet. Rec.*, 70 (1958) 503.
MÉRIEL, P., R. RUFFIÉ and A. FOURNIE, *Gaz. Hôp (Paris)*, 132 (1960) 7.
MOLDAVSKAYA, A. A., A. A. LIFSHITS, M. K. YANCHENKO, J. J. POLYAKOV and V. S. URALEVA, *Ž. Mikrobiol. (Mosk).*, 9 (1960) 113.
REMENTSOVA, M. M., *Veterinariya*, 36 (1959) 11.
RENOUX, G., *Ann. Inst. Pasteur*, 83 (1952) 814; *Advanc. Control Zoonoses*, F.A.O. Agric. Studies, No. 25 (1953) 61; *Arch. Inst. Pasteur Tunis*, 32 (1955) 51; *Advanc. vet. Sci.*, 3 (1957) 242.
RENOUX, G. and L. W. MAHAFFEY, *Ann. Inst. Pasteur*, 88 (1955) 528.
SADLER, W. W., *Amer. J. Publ. Hlth*, 50 (1960) 504.

SCHAAF, A. V. D. and M. ROSA, *Ned.-Ind. Bl. Diergeneesk.*, 52 (1940) 1.
SIMMINS, G. C. and W. T. K. HALL, *Amer. vet. J.*, 29 (1953) 33.
SZMUNESS, W. and J. PARNAS, *Arch. Inst. Pasteur Tunis,* 37 (1960) 457.
SPINK, H. W., *The nature of Brucellosis,* Minneapolis, 1956, 464 pp.
TAYLOR, R. M. and R. H. HAZEMANN, *Rev. Hyg. Méd. soc.,* 54 (1932) 481.
THOMSEN, A., *Månedsskr. Dyrlæger,* 43 (1931) 46; *Rev. gén. Méd. Vét.,* 41 (1932) 597;
　　Brucella infection in swine, Copenhagen, 1934, p. 253; *Advanc. vet. Sci.,* 3 (1957) 198.
TOVAR, R. M., *Amer. J. vet. Res.,* 8 (1947) 138.
WELLMANN, G., *Zbl. Bakt., I. Abt. Orig.,* 156 (1950) 414.
WOOD, E. E., *Brit. med. J.,* I (1955) 27.
WUNDT, W., *Arch. Hyg. (Berl.),* 143 (1959) 145.
ZAKI, J., *J. comp. Path.,* 58 (1948) 145.

A. CLARENBURG

Salmonelloses

Salmonelloses are infectious diseases caused by one of the many types of bacteria included in the genus *Salmonella*. Since the clinical symptoms are not characteristic of the disease, ultimate diagnosis depends on bacteriological examination.

The following definition of *Salmonella* has been adopted by the Salmonella Subcommittee of the Nomenclature Committee of the International Association of Microbiologists:

"A large genus of serologically related, gram-negative and non-sporing bacilli; 0.4 to 0.6 × 1 to 3 microns in usual dimensions but occasionally forming short filaments; showing, with certain exceptions, a motile peritrichous phase in which they normally occur; in fact adhering to the pattern of *S. typhi* in staining properties and morphology. Rarely fermenting lactose or sucrose, liquefying gelatin or producing indol, they regularly attack glucose with, but occasionally without, gas production. All the known species are pathogenic for man, animals, or both" (Edwards and Ewing, 1957).

The members of the genus *Salmonella* are characterized by their antigenic structure. Classification is based on distinction between O (somatic) antigens and H (flagellar) antigens. So far, more than 50 O antigens and an equal number of H antigens of actual importance from the point of view of diagnosis have been identified.

A particular antigen is the Vi (virulence) antigen which, unlike the other O antigens, is thermolabile; it only occurs in a few species of Salmonella *(S. typhi* and *S. paratyphi C).*

Particular antigenic combinations provide the basis for the Kauffmann–White scheme, in which the O antigens form the basis for the classification of the genus into 27 groups. These groups are divided in individual types (species) according to the H antigens present (Kauffmann, 1941 and 1954; Edwards and Ewing, 1957). This classification into groups and types is founded on agglutination tests with sera obtained by injection of the respective O and H antigens into rabbits. So far, more than 700 serologically different *Salmonella* types have been identified, although several other combinations (about 3,000) are theoretically conceivable (Kauffmann, 1956). The future will show how many of these occur in nature.

Several serotypes can be subdivided into varieties which may be of special importance from an epidemiological point of view. This subdivision is based on particular biochemical characteristics. As examples may be cited 2 biochemical varieties of *S. enteritidis, i.e., S. enteritidis* var. *danysz* and *S. enteritidis* var. *essen.* Of these varieties, the former occurs in rats, the latter mainly in ducks. Recently, Kallings and Laurell (1957) have subdivided *S. typhimurium* into 20 different biochemical varieties.

The bacteriophage typing method may be used to make a further subdivision of certain *Salmonella* types into "bacteriophage" subtypes (Craigie and Felix, 1947). This method is mainly employed in the case of *S. typhi, S. paratyphi B* and *S. typhimurium* and it has been found very useful in epidemiological studies.

In salmonelloses, as in tuberculosis, an important question is whether the types are either constant units or are capable of changing into one another. In considering this problem, it should be borne in mind that the requirements of bacteriological differentiation are less strict than those usually necessary in biological arrangements. A classification into types of bacteria is fully justified when it is useful in clinical and epidemiological studies and when the characteristics adopted as distinctive criteria are retained under natural conditions. In this sense, the *Salmonella*-types may undoubtedly be regarded as constant units.

Salmonelloses are extremely common in the animal world. As a rule, young, and especially newborn animals show a particular degree of susceptibility, as a result of which clinically perceptible infections are liable to occur. These infections may become widespread and may be associated with a high death rate. The animals become less susceptible as they grow older, so that salmonellae are not infrequently present as commensals in the intestines of adult animals. When the local or general resistance of such hosts is lowered, the organisms may be able to enter the internal environment and so cause infection. The lowering of resistance may be due to various causes, such as irrational diet, physical factors, fatigue, disease, injury, hard labour, abortion and agonal exhaustion. In various animals, virus infection is not infrequently followed by salmonelloses. This is observed in conditions such as swine fever and foot-and-mouth disease.

The change from commensalism to parasitism has frequently given rise to incorrect conclusions, when the secondary infections with *Salmonella* have been mistaken for the primary cause. A number of classic instances of mistakes of this type have been reported in the literature. In the United States, Salmon and Smith (1885) were the first to detect the bacterium of paratyphoid fever in pigs affected with swine fever, mistaking this bacterium for the causative organism of the disease "*Bact. cholerae suis*". Swine fever was subsequently found to be due to a filterable virus, *S. cholerae suis*, which is common in apparently healthy pigs and is a secondary cause of intestinal disease in a number of pigs affected with swine fever.

During an epidemic of psittacosis in parrots and human subjects in Paris, Nocard (1892) isolated a *Salmonella* strain which for a long time was termed *Bact. psittacosis* and was believed to be the cause of psittacosis, until the disease was found to be due to a filterable virus. Nocard's bacillus (identical with *S. typhimurium*) occasionally gives rise to secondary complications in these cases.

Sanarelli believed that yellow fever is also due to this *Salmonella* type ("*Bact. icteroides*").

Salmonellosis may give rise to a wide variety of clinical syndromes and the following conditions may be differentiated:

(1) Primary salmonelloses, diseases which are primarily and solely due to salmonellae and may be naturally transmitted to the homologous animal species. It is known that these salmonellae occur in animals such as horses, cattle, sheep, pigs, poultry, furred animals and rodents. The causative organisms are particularly pathogenic to the animal in question and they produce a fairly characteristic clinical picture.

(2) Secondary salmonelloses, following other diseases or accidents. This group includes, among other conditions, *Salmonella* infections in animals slaughtered in emergency. They are caused by a wide variety of *Salmonella* types.

(3) Chronic carriers. These are usually animals which have recovered clinically from a primary salmonellosis. They are particularly observed among adult bovines suffering from enteritis due to *S. dublin*.

(4) Temporary carriers are clinically normal animals which are excreting salmonellae for brief periods only. This condition mainly occurs among pigs, poultry, dogs, cats and insects. In recent years, vectors have also frequently been identified among reptiles (tortoises, lizards, snakes).

(5) Latent infections are often found in the mesenteric lymph nodes of various slaughter animals, above all pigs. Sometimes they are also identified in the internal organs, especially the liver.

Infections by salmonellae are common in *cattle*. They occur all over the world and are usually due to *S. dublin*, sometimes to *S. typhimurium*; bovine infections caused by other serotypes are exceptional. The lesions in young animals differ markedly from those observed in adult cattle.

Clinical symptoms in the calf usually appear towards the end of the first week of life. In addition to acute signs of septicaemia, enteritis (white scours in calves) and pneumonia are the chief symptoms. When they are left untreated, a large number of animals will die within a few days or weeks. In cases running a less rapid course, inflammation of the joints (osteomyelitis) frequently occurs (Fig. 19 A. B). On many farms, the disease in calves reappears every year.

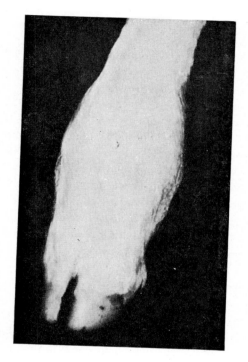

Fig. 19 A.

Hind leg of a calf with osteomyelitis after oral infection with *Salmonella dublin*. (Photo: J. Frik; courtesy Prof. A. van der Schaaf, Institute for Veterinary Bacteriology, State University, Utrecht)

In adult cattle, salmonellosis is usually characterized by a sudden onset marked by high temperature and profuse diarrhoea, the faeces often being mixed with mucus, fibrin membranes and/or blood. In these cases, the disease often terminates fatally within 24 hours. In other cases the

enteric symptoms are less severe and the animal may recover spontaneously. Abortion is common, the calf being born from 2 to 4 months
before term. Salmonellae may be isolated from the foetuses. In some
cases more or less serious mastitis occurs.

Unlike salmonellosis in calves, the disease in adult cattle is usually
confined to a few animals only of a herd.

After recovery from the disease, adult cattle almost always continue to
excrete the pathogen in the faeces; this is exceptional in the calf. Not

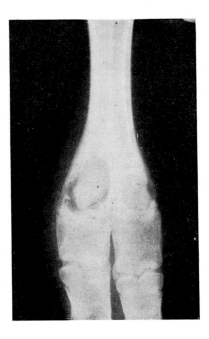

Fig. 19 B.

Röntgen-photo of the same leg as in Fig. 19A. In the epiphysical line of both me-
tacarpal bones a focus with demarcated sequester is visible. (Photo: Clinic for
Veterinary Surgery, State University, Utrecht; courtesy Prof. A. van der Schaaf)

seldom adult cattle are found to be carriers, although they have never
shown symptoms of the disease (Sjollema, 1959). In a recent statement
British authors estimated that the proportion of carriers among apparently healthy cows is 1 %. In the Netherlands, a study of 1,600 normal

slaughter cattle showed that 0.5% were infected (Kampelmacher, 1956). On the whole, salmonellosis is relatively uncommon in small ruminants. In the U.S.A. the disease frequently caused serious losses among *sheep* and it affected lambs especially. Newsom and Cross (1924, 1930 and 1935) reported three outbreaks of "paratyphoid dysentery" in lambs, the first of which involved 30,000 animals, with a death rate of 6.2%. The causative *Salmonella* type was always *S. typhimurium.* In each instance a long railroad journey and insufficient feeding predisposed the lambs to the disease.

An outbreak of enzootic gastro-enteritis in Überruhr (Germany) in 1919 was notorious for its severe effects on human subjects (meat poisoning in over 1,000 individuals). Of a flock of 300 sheep, 160 died or were subjected to forced slaughter. Crowding of the animals during transportation and in the pens was a predisposing factor.

Infection with *S. typhimurium* in sheep is characterized by an acute gastro-intestinal disease accompanied by diarrhoea and high temperature. As a rule, the animals die within from 1 to 3 days, at any rate within 1 or 2 weeks.

"Infectious abortion" of sheep is an entirely distinct form of salmonellosis. This septicaemic disease is caused by *S. abortus ovis.* Changes in the foetus and foetal membranes result in abortion. Of 81 cases of abortion in sheep, Weikl (1957) found that 49 were due to salmonellae.

De Jong (1915) observed a severe outbreak of salmonellosis among 50 Saanen *goats* in the Netherlands; 44 died shortly after infection, most of the animals showing symptoms of acute septicaemia and severe diarrhoea, while in others the disease ran a slower course, the symptoms being enteritis, fibrinous peritonitis and pneumonic lesions.

Caprine infections with *Salmonella* were subsequently observed in Germany and England. Gibson (1957) recently described an outbreak of infection by *S. dublin* in goats, which was contracted from dairy cattle.

Healthy solipeds not infrequently harbour salmonellae, particularly *S. typhimurium* and *S. dublin,* in their intestinal tract. These latent infections may give rise to overt disease when the resistance of the host is seriously impaired, especially during tiring transport, or in cases of colic, or following severe injuries. Salmonellosis usually runs a very grave course in *horses.* The clinical picture, which bears a marked resemblance to that of human typhoid fever, is characterized by a rapid onset, symptoms of septicaemia, high temperature, a relatively slow pulse and, particularly at a later stage, profuse diarrhoea. In some cases the animals die as early as within from 24 to 36 hours after onset. Recovery is rare.

An entirely different disease is infectious abortion in mares, a primary salmonellosis caused by *S. abortus equi*. This species of *Salmonella*, first identified by Smith and Kilborne in 1893, has a particular affinity for the reproductive organs (uterus, testes). The disease is wide-spread in several countries. Infection of the animals occurs by the oral route; in exceptional cases, however, it is transmitted during coitus. Because stallions sometimes develop a testicular form of infection, the semen may continue to be infective for a considerable period (Jansen, 1946).

This highly infectious disease is septicaemic in character. Abortion may appear at any stage of pregnancy, though as a rule it occurs during the period from the sixth to ninth month. It is due to exudative inflammation of the foetal membranes and infection of the foetus. If the foal is live-born, it will very likely be infected and develop septicaemia or polyarthritis.

Several investigators observed latent infection in equines of all ages and both sexes. Under certain predisposing conditions, the infection may become apparent in these carriers. Besides abortion, *S. abortus equi* may also cause local inflammatory lesions (fistulous withers, orchitis, abscesses, tendinitis).

Salmonellosis is one of the most important infectious diseases of *pigs*. An acute and a chronic form are differentiated.

Acute salmonellosis occurs in young animals up to about the sixth month of life and is usually caused by *S. cholerae suis*. But normal pigs may also be infected with this organism, particularly in the intestinal canal. As a result of factors which lower resistance, and especially when the animals are infected with the virus of swine fever, or with the bacterium of swine erysipelas, the commensal salmonellae may enter the tissues and blood stream, with the result that clinical symptoms of salmonellosis appear. These are: fever, vomiting, diarrhoea and bluish-red discolouration of various areas of the skin. Often death occurs within a few days, although the disease may also take a chronic course.

Chronic salmonellosis affects adult pigs and is relatively rare. It has been recorded from Germany and Hungary and is caused by *S. typhi suis*. The main symptom is a foetid form of diarrhoea which usually terminates fatally within a few weeks.

In addition to the above forms of porcine salmonellosis, latent infections due to various types of *Salmonella* are common in pigs. Together

References p. 160–161

with poultry, swine are assumed to be the chief animal reservoir of salmonellae. Buxton (1957) reported the proportion of infected pigs in various countries as ranging from 2.5 to 16.7%. In the vast majority of cases the mesenteric lymph nodes are infected, and much less frequently the portal lymph glands and interior organs, such as the spleen and liver. Recent studies have shown that not infrequently the faeces are also infected. The incidence of latent *Salmonella* infections shows an upward trend. Kampelmacher and Guinée (1960) who examined 2,100 clinically normal pigs, found that 25% of the animals were infected with salmonellae (mesenteric lymph nodes and faeces in 13%, portal lymph nodes in 3%). Contaminated feeding-stuffs of animal origin seem to be an important factor in the creation of latent infections.

Dogs and *cats* are susceptible to infection by salmonellae. Symptoms of acute gastro-enteritis (vomiting, diarrhoea) occur, particularly in young animals, and these symptoms are soon followed by death. Intermittent diarrhoea is observed in mild cases. In adult carriers clinical symptoms are frequently absent. Various investigators have stressed the fact that distemper acts as a predisposing factor in the pathogenesis of canine salmonellosis.

Infection of these carnivores is due to contact with infected dogs, cats and human subjects, but particularly to ingestion of contaminated food. Van der Schaaf (1960) observed infection by *S. typhimurium* two days after the ingestion of contaminated sausages which had given rise to clinical symptoms in a number of elderly persons.

As regards the food of dog and cat, infection mainly derives from contaminated meat, eggs (rejected chandled eggs!) and egg products. Galton *et al.* (1955) isolated salmonellae from a high proportion of American dog meals.

In view of the risk of transmission of *Salmonella* infection to human subjects, extensive investigations have been carried out, particularly in recent years, in dogs and, to a smaller extent, in cats. These studies showed that such infections are common in dogs, especially those in kennels. Galton *et al.* (1952) found 53 different types of salmonellae by examination of 2,252 samples of infected dog faeces. On the whole, *typhimurium* is the most common type. In the Netherlands (National Salmonella Centre), eleven different serotypes were identified; these cases included *S. dublin* in 19, and *S. typhimurium* in 16.

The incidence of infection varies markedly with the feeding habits. It is usually rather low in European countries. In Great Britain, for instance, Cruickshank and Smith (1949) isolated salmonellae from the faeces in 1 % of the normal dogs examined. In the U.S.A. this proportion is much higher. Thus Wolff *et al.* (1948) observed *Salmonella* carriers in 18 % of the dogs in Michigan.

Infection by *Salmonella* is also frequently observed in cats, the proportion rising up to 12%. Over 20 different types of *Salmonella* have been identified from cats, mainly *S. typhimurium*. The author found 4 serotypes in the Netherlands, including *S. typhimurium* in 5 cases, and *S. dublin* in 3. Infections by *S. typhimurium* are frequently attributed to the catching of infected wild mice.

Watt and De Capito (1950) examined rectal swabs from a large number of pet dogs and cats exposed to known human infections which occurred in the home of their owners These studies showed that of 1,156 dogs 3.4%, and of 625 cats, 3.0% were carriers of *Salmonella*.

In *poultry* salmonelloses are common and widespread in many countries. Increasing interest is being taken in these infections, especially in view of their role as possible sources of human disease. They are mainly known to occur in fowls, ducks, pigeons, geese and turkeys. Apart from commercial poultry, infection with *Salmonella* is also observed in canaries, pheasants and other wild birds.

Salmonelloses are particularly common in young fowls a few days to several weeks old. The death rate in chicks varies from a few to almost 100%. Chickens which survive the disease usually continue excretion of salmonellae in the faeces for some weeks and they may do so throughout life.

Adult poultry, on the other hand, are much more resistant and usually do not show any symptoms of disease. From the point of view of food-hygiene it is of special importance that the infection is in adult birds localized in the ovary, so that the eggs may become infected with salmonellea from the inside (yolk !). Moreover, normal animals clinically infected may continue to discharge salmonellea in the faeces for a considerable period, so that the eggs are contaminated externally.

Salmonelloses in poultry may be due to a wide variety of *Salmonella* types. Among the best known are *S. pullorum* and *S. gallinarum*, which are serologically identical and are grouped together in the Kauffmann–White Scheme under the name of *S. gallinarum pullorum*.

Extensive studies have been made in the United States, particularly by Edwards, Bruner and Moran (1948). These investigators examined 6,387 cultures isolated from poultry, mainly young turkeys and fowls, and identified no fewer than 60 different types of *Salmonella* which, with a few exceptions, are found in human subjects as well. Their conclusion was that, in the U.S.A., poultry are the main reservoir of *Salmonella*.

Buxton (1957) recorded the following numbers of various *Salmonella* types isolated from poultry: in fowls 78, in turkeys 62, in ducks 31, in pheasants 10, in pigeons 8, in geese 7, in partridges 4, in canaries 3, in quail 3, in budgerigars 3, in guinea fowl 4, and in sea birds 3.

Unlike *S. gallinarum* and *S. pullorum,* the other types of *Salmonella* show little if any host-specificity. Consequently, the latter may constitute a greater danger to public health.

The most common and earliest known salmonelloses in fowls are fowl typhoid and pullorum disease which are caused by *S. gallinarum* and *S. pullorum,* respectively. Fowl typhoid is commonest in adult birds, whereas pullorum disease occurs mainly in chicks. The two diseases may cause serious losses on poultry farms. Infection may be congenital (latent infection of chickens hatched by hens or in the incubator), or by ingestion, or it is air-borne (in the incubator).

The symptoms of pullorum disease are dullness, loss of appetite, laboured breathing, greenish or whitish diarrhoea, obstruction of the cloaca by incrusted faeces and emaciation.

Fowl typhoid is chiefly marked by dullness, blue combs and diarrhoea.

In recent years, salmonelloses caused by serotypes other than *S. pullorum* and *S. gallinarum* have been increasingly observed. *S. typhimurium* heads the list, and is followed by *S. thompson* and *S. niloese. S. bareilly* was found to be an important pathogenic organism in chickens as well (Clarenburg and Roepke, 1952). The clinical symptoms in chickens are similar to those of pullorum disease. Adult birds usually do not show any symptoms, although they may excrete salmonellae in the faeces.

In *turkeys,* next to *S. typhimurium,* the most important causes of the disease are *S. pullorum* and *S. gallinarum.* The mode of spread of these is similar to that in fowls. Infection by *Salmonella* is common in *ducks* and *geese,* particularly in the former. It has been studied in detail in view of the high incidence of human food poisoning resulting from the use of contaminated duck's eggs. A large number of serotypes were found, *S. typhimurium* and *S. enteritidis* var. *essen* being the most important pathogens. In addition, *S. anatum* and *S. saint paul* have been frequently isolated.

In view of the ubiquity of *S. typhimurium* in various hosts, the fact that the rhamnose-negative type is usually found in ducks, but not in several other animals, may be important from the point of view of epidemiology.

In addition to the intestines, infection also is fairly often localized in the ovaries, resulting in the laying of germinally infected eggs and congenital infection of the chicks.

Clinical symptoms mainly appear in young chickens. Adverse conditions (*e.g.*, a long journey in narrow space) are decisive factors in outbreaks of salmonellosis. Adult birds usually do not show any clinical symptoms, although egg production is frequently decreased.

As early as 1895 Moore described a disease due to *Salmonella* in *pigeons* in the U.S.A. Salmonelloses are very common in these birds and are among their most dreaded diseases. They usually are due to *S. typhimurium*, from which organism Kauffmann (1934) and Edwards (1935) showed that the 0.5 antigen is absent.

Pigeons, a few weeks old, are particularly liable to die after a brief period of disease with diarrhoea as its main symptom. In the older birds the infection usually runs a chronic course. The most marked signs are emaciation and drooping wings, the latter being due to inflammation of the joints. Apparently normal animals may excrete salmonellae in the faeces. The infection, like that of ducks, is localized in the intestines or ovaries and rarely in the testes.

There are probably no birds which are not occasionally affected by salmonellosis. The disease has been frequently recorded as the cause of death of *partridges, canaries, parrots, parrakeets, sparrows* and other birds. Urbain (1938) reported an epizootic due to salmonellae in white *swans, wild ducks* and African *pelicans* swimming together in a pond, most of them dying within from 2 to 3 days after infection.

Salmonelloses are frequently observed in *gulls*. Besides other serotypes, *S. typhimurium* is usually isolated in these cases. A large number of deaths occur in the young birds.

Salmonelloses are common in rodents, particularly in *rats* and *mice* but also, though to a smaller extent, in *rabbits, hares, guinea-pigs* and related species. They may cause tremendous losses among rats and mice; in some cases laboratory animal breeding establishments are rapidly depopulated by the disease. The chief clinical symptom is diarrhoea; the animals die from systemic septicaemia within 24 or more hours. Infectious abortion and endometritis may occur in rabbits.

A large number of types of *Salmonella* have been identified in rodents. The main types are *S. typhimurium* and *S. enteritidis,* particularly var. *danysz*. In several cases *S. bovis morbificans* was isolated from mice.

Rats and mice excreting salmonellae were frequently found to be capable of transmitting the disease to man and animals; their faeces may continue to be infective for several months.

The extent to which carriers of *Salmonella* occur among rats and mice has been investigated in various countries. The incidence varied markedly (from 0–14%). A relatively large proportion of rats caught in the neighbourhood of docks and slaughter-houses were found to be infected.

Salmonelloses may become widespread and cause serious losses on breeding-farms of *furred animals*. They are particularly common in foxes and mink. The young animals are highly susceptible to acute infections which terminate fatally. The chief symptoms are diarrhoea (haemorrhagic in some cases), loss of appetite and emaciation. Mortality may be high. The more chronic disease is mainly characterized by intermittent diarrhoea, emaciation and a harsh coat.

Various serotypes are usually transmitted by meat, when this forms a considerable part of the diet.

In America, Green and Schillinger (1929) observed an outbreak of infection in silver-foxes, in which the death rate among young animals was up to 60%. Extensive investigations have been especially carried out in the Scandinavian countries, where it was found that the percentage of infection in foxes varied from 8–20. In Sweden, 335 carcasses of silver-foxes were examined by Thal *et al.* (1957), who isolated *S. dublin* in 13 cases, *S. cholera suis* in 6 cases, *S. typhimurium* in 3 cases, *S. newport* in 3 cases and *S. derby* in 1 case. These investigators found about 1% of the mink to be infected with *Salmonella*. In the Netherlands, de Blieck and Jansen (1935) isolated *S. dublin* only from silver-foxes, this type also being present in the fleas living as parasites on the sick animals. This probably indicates the epidemiological role of these arthropods.

Epizootics of salmonellosis in wild animals are undoubtedly not confined to rodents.

It has been found that *monkeys* are highly susceptible to infection with *Salmonella;* Jansen (1938) recorded *S. typhimurium* as the cause of gastro-enteritis and diphtheric and ulcerative enteritis from which the 15 monkeys belonging to a single owner died. The rhamnose-negative variety of this strain of *Salmonella* was identical with that which is common in ducks and the monkeys had in fact been regularly eating raw duck's eggs.

In recent years, 29 cultures of *Salmonella* from monkeys have been studied in the Netherlands (National Salmonella Centre). 8 different serotypes were observed, including *S. typhimurium* in 14 cases and *S. stanley* in 6.

Urbain and Guillot (1933) found that *Salmonella* was the cause of a fatal form of septicaemia in the *elephant*.

Jansen (1937) isolated *S. dublin* from two *raccoons* living on a fox-farm and *S. typhimurium* from a *civet-cat*.

During an outbreak of endemic enteritis in the buildings of a zoological garden housing *beasts of prey*, Van der Hoeden (1946) isolated *S. typhimurium* from two tigers, a lion and a few of the smaller wild carnivores. In this instance, the disease might have been imported by mice or rats.

Apart from mammals, salmonellae are also found in various lower animals, such as *reptiles* and *arthropods*.

In recent years, the author observed infections in the following reptiles: in *tortoises* in 5 cases (3 different serotypes, including *S. newport* in 3 cases), in *snakes* in 18 cases (9 serotypes including *S. enteritidis* in 4 and *S. carreau* in 3 cases) and in *lizards* in 14 cases (14 serotypes including *S. give* in 4., *S. typhimurium* in 3 and *S. urbana* in 3 cases). These animals are usually symptomless carriers capable of transmitting the infection to man and other mammals.

Various *insects* (flies, fleas, cockroaches), as well as *ticks*, may be infected with salmonellae by contact with infected animals. The author isolated *S. bredeney* from ticks.

Human salmonellosis is a common disease in many countries. In recent years, considerable interest has been taken in its constantly increasing incidence. In most instances, this increase is not caused by the salmonellae occurring autochthonously in man *(S. typhi, S. paratyphi A, B* and *C)* but by various other types, many of which had been seldom if ever observed previously. This is illustrated in Table XV, which gives data supplied by the Chief Medical Inspectorate of the Netherlands Public Health Service.

The number of *Salmonella* serotypes occurring in human subjects in the Netherlands showed a constant increase from 10 in 1949 to 67 in 1959. The total number of serotypes identified during this period amounted 92. Of these, *S. typhimurium* was the commonest, being present in about 70% of the cases notified.

Similar findings were obtained in several other countries. Dauer (1959) in the U.S.A. recorded: "During the past decade, while typhoid fever has been reported less frequently and has caused fewer deaths from year to year, other *Salmonella*-infections have shown the opposite trend. In 1950 twice as many cases and deaths from typhoid fever were recorded as for other *Salmonella* infections. In 1957, however, there were 5 times more cases of the latter than of typhoid fever, and the number of deaths was also in excess of those for typhoid fever".

TABLE XV

CASES OF INFECTION WITH *S. typhi*, *S. paratyphi B* AND OTHER SALMONELLAE NOTIFIED IN THE NETHERLANDS DURING THE PERIOD FROM 1953–1959

Year	S. typhi	S. paratyphi B	Other salmonellae
1953	161	309	360
1954	79	622	563
1955	100	313	1,009
1956	87	219	825
1957	87	317	1,537
1958	77	277	3,204
1959	62	301	6,670

It is generally agreed that all types of *Salmonella* may cause disease, although the degree of pathogenicity varies with the type. There are types which are adapted to man *(e.g., S. typhi, S. paratyphi A, B and C)*, and other types adapted to particular species of animals *(e.g., S. gallinarum pullorum* in poultry) to the extent that they will only exceptionally cause clinical symptoms in other species.

On the whole, it can be stated that, with the exception of the types of *Salmonella* specifically pathogenic to man, a large number of salmonellae are necessary to produce clinically perceptible lesions. It is often found, for instance, that ingestion of recently contaminated food does not cause any symptoms, whereas the use of this food after it has been stored for a period of a few hours or longer, will do so. This is in accordance with the findings reported by McCullough and Eisele (1951), whose experimental infection of volunteers with various types of salmonellae showed that from hundreds of thousands to millions of these organisms are necessary to produce illness.

The incubation period partly depends upon the number of bacteria that have entered the body. In cases of food posioning, the symptoms usually appear within about 12 hours, but this period may be longer or shorter, according to the density of the pathogenic organisms in the contaminated food. In one case alarming symptoms were observed as early as within 2 hours; it was found that the offending food (brawn) contained millions of *S. typhimurium* organisms per gram of food.

In addition to the number of bacteria, the resistance of the subject plays a part in the appearance or absence of symptoms. Individuals affected with another disease, or suffering from traumata, seem to be more susceptible to infection. This also is true of young children and elderly persons, as well as of patients after gastrectomy (Hemmes, 1952).

Infection by salmonellae may result in the appearance of a wide variety of clinical manifestations. The following 4 main forms are differentiated:

(1) The typhoid form is chiefly marked by persistent, severe systemic symptoms (bearing a resemblance to those observed in typhoid fever, though usually running a milder course), a prolonged incubation period (about 10 days), contact infections between men and the appearance of chronic *Salmonella* carriers. It is usually due to types of *Salmonella* occurring autochthonously in humans. There are, however, several exceptions to this rule. Salmonellae of animal origin may cause systemic infections which produce a clinical picture bearing a marked resemblance to the classical symptoms of typhoid fever. In the case of these salmonellae, infections transmitted from one human subject to another and prolonged excretion of bacteria have been observed as well.

(2) The gastro–enteritic form is mainly characterized by a shorter incubation period (about 12 hours), symptoms which persist for a shorter period, the infrequent occurrence of contact infections and the fact that salmonellae are usually discharged for brief periods only (a few weeks at the maximum). As a rule, this form is due to salmonellae of animal origin. Here too there are several exceptions; *S. paratyphi B,* for instance, may give rise to a gastro–enteritic syndrome as well. Unlike the typhoid form, in several countries the incidence of the gastro–enteritic form is increasing.

(3) Localized infections appear in the form of abscesses, empyema, arthritis, meningitis, osteomyelitis, orchitis and cholecystitis, due to various types of *Salmonella.*

(4) Temporary or chronic excretion of salmonellae in subjects who have not shown any clinical symptoms is caused by types particularly adapted to man, and also by those which are commoner in animals. These carriers, especially when they handle food stuffs, become a potential source of transmission of salmonelloses.

Apparently normal carriers, and especially clinically sick animals excreting large numbers of salmonellae, present a grave risk of infection from one animal to another, contaminated food and drinking-water being among the most important vehicles of the agent. The infection may be transmitted to animals of the same species as well as to others. A case in point is that of a fatal infection due to *S. anatum* transmitted from ducks which were clinically normal carriers to a cow.

In addition, food-stuffs of animal origin, such as meat–bone meal, meat-meal, bone-meal, fish-meal, etc., constitute important sources of infection. In view of their high protein or calcium and phosphorus content, large quantities of these products are fed to pigs and poultry. Recent studies in various countries showed that, in a considerable proportion of cases, these food-stuffs are contaminated with a wide variety of types of *Salmonella*.

During the past 5 years in the author's laboratory a total number of 75 different serotypes were identified in imported food-stuffs of animal origin. Animals thus infected may, without showing any symptoms, discharge, for longer or shorter periods, the salmonellae that have entered their bodies and so may infect other animals and indirectly man.

Danish authors sounded an early warning against the risk of this kind of infection in live-stock and man. Wöldike Nielsen (1954) defined this risk as follows: "It is as if a delayed action bomb had been introduced into the country".

In recent years, attention has also been drawn to vegetable food-stuffs. Extensive investigations led Hauge and Bøvre (1958) to the conclusion that "the imported vegetable protein concentrates constitute an important source of *Salmonella* infections in domestic animals".

Waste-water represents another hazard to farm animals. Recently investigations were carried out on the risk of contamination by waste-water from slaughterhouses. Schaal (1959) reported that, quantitatively as well as qualitatively, this water should be regarded as an extremely important reservoir of salmonellae; 70% of the water samples were found to be contaminated by 17 different types of *Salmonella*.

All salmonelloses in animals constitute a potential source of direct infection of man. This is mainly due to close contact with animal carriers, particularly when the latter show clinical symptoms. These animals often excrete large numbers of salmonellae and these salmonellae may have acquired increased virulence.

Although a rather limited number of cases of human infection due to direct contacts with mammalian animals have been reported so far, the possibility of infection from this source must be taken into account. Animals should therefore be included in epidemiological investigations of human salmonellosis of unknown origin. It should, however, be borne in mind that, conversely, infection in animals may originate from man.

Literature provides several instances of direct infection by contact with poultry. In the U.S.A., salmonelloses caused by turkeys have often been observed. Clarenburg *et al.* (1952) frequently observed human infections with *S. bareilly* due to the handling of infected one-day-old chicks. Lockett (1959) reported an outbreak of salmonellosis caused by *S. typhimurium* in a family, the infection having been probably contracted from ailing "day-old" cockerels.

Occasional infections have been known to occur by contact with other species of farm animals. Brunner (1946), for instance, reported infection of a veterinary surgeon in Japan, after manual vaginal investigation of an aborting horse infected with *S. abortus equi*. Four furuncles appeared on the arm of the man, *S. abortus equi* being isolated from the pus of the lesions.

Several cases of human infection have been reported, in which salmonellae had been transmitted from dogs or cats. In the Netherlands, a number of infections due to contact with infected tortoises were observed in children.

Various food-stuffs may give rise to *Salmonella* infection in their consumers. The more suitable the medium provided by the contaminated food, the more rapidly the salmonellae will develop when it is stored or transported at a favourable temperature. Meat, milk, eggs and their products are among the chief food-stuffs producing food poisoning in man.

Several observations suggest that animal food-stuffs are important factors in the increased incidence of infections due to the so-called rare types of *Salmonella*, not only in animals, but also in man.

In Western Germany an epidemic form of enteritis following the use of "Braunschweiger Wurst" (Brunswick sausage) prepared from pork was observed in 1955, the number of patients being from 1,500–2,000 and 3 deaths occurring in elderly subjects. The causative organism was found to be *S. blockley,* a type of *Salmonella* previously unknown in Germany. Shortly before, the same type had been isolated from imported fish-meal used in feeding pigs (Handloser, 1956). In Israel, Hirsch and Sapiro-Hirsch (1959) observed an outbreak of food poisoning caused by *S. hadar* and *S. infantis* following a festive dinner in a collective settlement. The infection had been transmitted by chopped chicken-liver. The fowls were infected by the contaminated bone-meal fed to them.

Several investigators identified in man rare types of *Salmonella*, which had been previously isolated from meat and bone-meal or fish-meal. Writing on the subject, Newell *et al.* (1959) stated: "In Northern Ireland the first isolations of *S. orion, S. infantis* and *S. schwarzengrund* were made from human cases in 1959 after it had been confirmed that these types were being imported and were causing animal infections".

To gain a proper understanding of the mechanism of "meat poisoning", a differentiation should be made between *intravital* and *post-mortem contamination* of the meat. In intravital infections, the tissues of the slaughtered animal harbour the causative organism. In post-mortem contamination, which occurs after the animal has been slaughtered, the organisms originate from elsewhere.

Primary salmonelloses in slaughter animals constitute an extremely important source of intravital infection. They are very common in cattle, both in adult animals and calves. The fact that a considerable proportion of carriers are found among adult cattle is highly significant. These animals not only harbour the salmonellae in their intestines, but also in other organs and the muscles, particularly in the liver and gall-bladder. Because symptoms are usually not observed on inspection of the living animals, and because anatomical lesions are frequently absent after slaughter, there is a risk of the meat being released for consumption without examination for the presence of *Salmonella*. The number of salmonellae in the organs, and particularly in the muscles of the animals, may be very small. When, however, meat-products are prepared, or the meat itself is stored under adverse conditions (*e.g.*, at moderately high temperatures), the number of the salmonellae may increase considerably.

In addition to primary salmonelloses, secondary salmonelloses are also important in meat-poisoning, particularly in cases of forced slaughter, or following accidents.

A third form of intravital contamination is latent infection of the organs; this has been particularly observed in pigs during recent years. These latent infections are a nightmare to veterinary meat-inspectors, because they are not detectable at routine examination.

Human carriers also play an important role in meat-poisoning. In addition, attention should be paid to contamination of the meat by rodents (mice and rats), or insects (flies), and particularly by the tools used in handling and preparing meat and meat-products, *e.g.*, chopping-blocks and mincing-machines. The author frequently isolated salmonellae from scrapings of these objects.

As instances of contamination by rodents may be mentioned an outbreak of food-poisoning involving over 100 individuals following consumption of sausages prepared from liver, soiled by rats excreting *S. enteritidis* var. *danysz* (Clarenburg, 1953), and an explosive outbreak due to *S. typhimurium* after eating smoked beef contaminated by mice.

Special attention should be paid to preparations used for the eradication of mice and rats, which consist of suspensions of live cultures of *S. typhimurium* and *S. enteritidis* var. *danysz* ("ratin") respectively. The view that the ratin strain is pathogenic only to rodents and is not dangerous to man is definitely incorrect, as is shown by various cases of human infection with it.

Both chronic and temporary animal carriers are highly important in producing post-mortal infections. Studies on slaughtered pigs in the United States have shown that the skin, as well as the interior organs and muscles are frequently infected by the faeces and the contents of the intestine. As a result, salmonellae are found in a considerable proportion of meat-products (Galton *et al.*, 1954). A recent report on the subject was published by investigators in Northern Ireland (Newell *et al.*, 1959). Studies on the infection of pigs during slaughter are also in progress in the National Institute of Public Health in the Netherlands. From the results so far obtained, it could be concluded that infected pigs brought to the slaughter-house frequently cause the spread of salmonellae to pigs initially free from infection; this occurs during stabling and in the subsequent process of slaughter, especially in depilating machines.

In the vast majority of cases meat-poisoning is caused by meat-products. This is not surprising, because the salmonellae show a marked increase during the process of manufacture and storage. Meat-poisoning mainly occurs during the warm summer months.

Food-poisoning may also originate from meat and organs of infected poultry. This is particularly true in countries where the meat is used without sufficient heating. In Germany, for instance, several cases of food-poisoning occurred after the consumption of smoked breast of goose.

In the U.S.A., there have been numerous reports incriminating poultry or poultry-products in outbreaks of the disease in man (Galton and Arnstein, 1959). Wide-spread outbreaks were due to *S. blockley* in commercially prepared chicken salad and to *S. typhimurium* in cold sliced turkey.

Chronic carriers of *S. dublin*, and occasionally of *S. typhimurium*, are fairly common among cattle. As a rule, these animals are clinically healthy and have a normal milk yield. They discharge, however, enormous numbers of salmonellae in the faeces, so that contamination of the milk is bound to occur from the outside. Its consumption may result in human infections which sometimes run a fatal course (Clarenburg and Ten Bokkel Huinink, 1948). In the United Kingdom, about 600 children developed infection due to *S. dublin* in 1952, mainly within from 24–30 hours after drinking unpasteurised milk supplied to 12 schools. A cow which had recently calved was found to be excreting *S. dublin* in the milk and faeces (Report, 1954).

Infrequently, a form of bovine mastitis due to *S. dublin* occurs, which occasionally causes wide-spread disease among the population. Bovine infections with *S. paratyphi B* transmitted by human carriers are not seldom observed. The infected cows usually develop enteritis. The milk of these animals may cause severe epidemics of paratyphoid fever. An epidemic of this type involving 52 individuals was described by Dijkstra and Van der Hoeden (1929). *S. paratyphi B,* phage type Dundee, was isolated from the faeces and samples of milk of a number of cows by Clarenburg and Kampelmacher (1958) and also from the faeces of 6 children who had fallen ill following consumption of milk of these animals.

Human carriers of *S. paratyphi B* not infrequently contaminate milk; dairy products (ice-cream, butter and fresh cheese) made from it are serious hazards to their consumers.

As has previously been pointed out, a wide variety of *Salmonella* types are very common among poultry. Infection of the eggs may actually take place in the ovary or oviduct, *i.e.,* internally, or externally in the cloaca, or through the faeces in the laying-nests. Experiments have shown that salmonellae may penetrate the shell of the egg and infect the contents. The possibility of penetration is governed to a large extent by the degree of humidity of the environment, and the presence or absence of the protecting cuticle on the egg-shell.

As a rule, infected fresh eggs contain only very few salmonellae, so that their consumption carries comparatively little risk. An entirely different problem, however, prevails when these eggs are used in the preparation of food which is not heated to a temperature sufficient to kill the salmonellae. If these foods are stored under environmental conditions favourable to the multiplication of the pathogens, there will be considerable danger of food-poisoning.

As regards the hazard to human health, marked differences exist between the various kinds of eggs, as is shown by the following findings.

Large numbers of hen's eggs have been examined for the presence of salmonellae by various research workers. With the exception of *S. pullorum*, which is frequently isolated, other types of *Salmonella* are rarely observed.

Bernstein (1952) examined 2,184 British hen's eggs and 1,464 eggs from other countries and did not find a single one of them to be infected. Similar results were obtained in Sweden and Norway. Watts and Mander (1953) found no salmonellae in 3,312 Australian hen's eggs, with the exception of *S. pullorum*. In the Netherlands, Clarenburg *et al.* (1952) examined the contents of more than 800 hen's eggs obtained from farms infected with *S. bareilly*. They did not discover a single egg infected with *Salmonella*.

Salmonellae are chiefly present on the shells. The incidence of contamination mainly depends on the cleanliness and quality of the shells. Goresline (1946) isolated salmonellae from the shells in 1% of clean, undamaged eggs, compared with 5% in the case of soiled and washed soiled eggs. Cantor and McFarlane (1948) examined 2,132 samples of scrapings from egg shells and found 0.6% to be contaminated. The consumption of shell-eggs hardly ever gives rise to *Salmonella* infection of man. However, several outbreaks of human salmonellosis due to the use of food prepared from hen's eggs are reported in the literature. The causative type of salmonella was usually *S. typhimurium*.

Möller (1955) reported food-poisoning in 10 individuals, the poisoning being due to a potato salad prepared from hen's eggs several days before it was actually consumed; *S. typhimurium* was isolated from the eggs. An outbreak of food-poisoning reported by Jellard (1956), which involved no fewer than 56 individuals, was due to the consumption of a cold egg custard pudding, which had been cooked only lightly and allowed to cool slowly during a summer night. Broomhead and Mann (1959) reported an outbreak of food-poisoning due to *S. thompson*. The source of infection was a whip prepared from raw eggs. Watt (1945) described an infection among a ship's crew resulting from the mixing of hen's eggs infected with *S. montevideo*, in mayonnaise and salad.

Up to about 15 years ago, *S. pullorum* was almost universally regarded as being non-pathogenic to man. Since then, however, several human infections with this type have been recorded, more or less certainly attributed to the consumption of contaminated eggs. A paper by Mitchell *et al.* (1946) describes the first reported, large-scale epidemic of human gastroenteritis associated with *S. pullorum*. Of 423 individuals affected, 172 had to be admitted to hospital. It was found that a rice-pudding containing eggs was the source of the infection.

Unlike hen's eggs, duck's eggs have frequently been the cause of food poisoning. The chief risk consists in the use of duck's eggs in the manufacture of food in which the salmonellae can multiply. Cases of food-poisoning were observed after eating minced meat, pudding, cakes, mayonnaise, ice-cream, currant bread and liver sausage, for the preparation of which duck's eggs had been used.

S. typhimurium and *S. enteritidis* var. *essen* are the most common cause of these outbreaks. In exceptional cases other types such as *S. saint paul* were found.

The considerable risk involved in the use of duck's eggs may be explained by the high incidence of the "classic" types of *Salmonella* in ducks.

In 1936, the author examined 7,000 eggs obtained from large duck farms. About 2% were found to be internally infected with salmonellae, both *S. enteritidis* var. *essen* and *S. typhimurium* being isolated. Gernez-Rieux *et al.* (1949) recovered *S. typhimurium* from 6.5% of eggs sold in the main Paris market.

The percentage of eggs stated to be infected by the Salmonella Subcommittee of the Public Health Laboratory Service in Great Britain (1954) was much lower; examination of a total number of 13,562 duck's eggs showed only 0.15% infection. *S. typhimurium* was the type mainly isolated, *S. pullorum* and *S. enteritidis* being isolated in a few instances only.

It has been found that the eggs of turkeys and geese also harbour salmonellae. Yamamoto *et al.* (1952) reported on human infection due to *S. typhimurium* caused by the consumption of goose eggs. Of the 9 persons infected, 1 died. The *Salmonella* type found in these patients was also present in the geese.

When conditions favour the multiplication of salmonellae, pigeon eggs may also cause food-poisoning. This was clearly established in an outbreak occurring in a military unit after consumption of pudding prepared from the eggs of pigeons carrying *S. typhimurium*. 20 soldiers were simultaneously affected. *S. typhimurium* was isolated from the contents of 6 out of 200 eggs of the infected birds (Clarenburg and Dornickx, 1932).

Eggs of wild birds have also been found to be infected with salmonellae. Lerche (1938) isolated *S. typhimurium* from the eggs of sea-gulls.

Egg products are frequently contaminated with a wide variety of types of *Salmonella*.

A report published by the Medical Research Council of the United Kingdom in 1947 described the examination of 7,584 samples of spray-dried eggs from the U.S.A., Canada and the Argentine. The average proportion of infection was found to be 9.9%, involving 33 serotypes. As a rule, only very small numbers of salmonellae were found, never more than 30 per gram. Soloway *et al.* (1947) isolated salmonellae from 35% of 5,198 samples of dried eggs obtained from 100 dehydration plants in the U.S.A.; 52 different serotypes were identified. On the other hand an extensive investigation of British egg products revealed a much lower rate of infection (Report, 1955): of a total number of 1,649 samples of untreated or chilled liquid hen's eggs, 9 (0.5%) were found to be infected; of 65 samples of liquid duck's eggs, 2 (3.1%) harboured salmonellae. In Germany, before the adoption of protective measures in 1957, examination of 82,594 samples from various countries showed that 5,301 (6.4%) were contaminated; of 50,154 samples examined after these measures had been adopted, 580 (1.1%) were found to be infected (Bischoff, 1959). Emmenegger (1959) reported that, of a total number of 353 samples of egg-products imported into Switzerland, 42 (11.9%) were contaminated. Several investigators found that Chinese egg-products were infected with different types of *Salmonella,* including *S. paratyphi B,* in a considerable proportion of cases.

During the period from 1952–1958, a total of 3,091 batches of various sorts of egg-products partly prepared from hen's eggs, and partly from duck's eggs, were examined by the author in the Netherlands. They comprised imported products as well as those intended for export. The results obtained in these studies are summarized in Tables XVI and XVII.

TABLE XVI

EGG PRODUCTS EXAMINED FOR SALMONELLAE DURING THE PERIOD FROM 1952–1958 IN THE NETHERLANDS

	Hen's egg products		Duck's egg products	
	Number of batches examined	Number found to be positive for salmonellae	Number of batches examined	Number found to be positive for salmonellae
Dried white (crystals)	371	57	19	3
Dried white (spray-dried)	56	6	13	1
Dried yolk	43	5	24	0
Dried whole egg	377	7	103	6
Frozen white	533	11	20	5
Frozen yolk	288	14	30	2
Frozen whole egg	522	13	36	12
Liquid yolk	470	17	156	54
Total	2690	130 (4.8%)	401	83 (20.8%)

TABLE XVII

TYPES OF *Salmonella* ISOLATED FROM HEN'S AND DUCK'S EGG PRODUCTS IN THE
NETHERLANDS DURING THE PERIOD FROM 1952–1958

Type of Salmonella	Hen's egg-products	Duck's egg-products
S. amager	1	—
S. anatum	7	2
S. bareilly	54	8
S. bredeney	1	—
S. chicago	3	—
S. dublin	1	1
S. enteritidis	5	28
S. gaminara	—	1
S. irumu	2	—
S. montevideo	6	—
S. ness-ziona	1	—
S. newington	3	—
S. newport	1	—
S. niloese	5	—
S. oranienburg	1	—
S. thompson	11	—
S. thompson var. berlin	8	—
S. typhimurium	19	43
S. virchow	1	—

From these Tables it can be concluded that infected egg-products may constitute a latent threat to public health.

There was, during the second world war, a marked increase in the number of cases of food-poisoning in the United Kingdom. A report by the Medical Research Council (1947) presents a detailed review of the outbreaks of food-poisoning and other forms of *Salmonella* infection resulting from the use of American egg-powder. In addition, 24 new species of *Salmonella* were identified in man during the period from 1942 to 1944. "Of these new species, the 6 commonest, in order, were *oranienburg, montevideo, meleagridis, anatum, tennessee* and *bareilly,* the same 6, in fact, as headed the list of *Salmonella* strains isolated from dried eggs".

Attention has been drawn to the hazards involved in the storage of reconstituted dried eggs before these are cooked. This risk is apparent, for instance, from a report by Zeman (1949), who described an outbreak of infection with *S. tennessee,* which involved 45 subjects who had used scrambled eggs prepared from American egg powder.

Not only egg powder, but also other egg products (albumen, frozen egg) have caused several outbreaks of food-poisoning. Kwantes (1952) reported a case involving 203 individuals, following consumption of cream pastries prepared from duck egg albumen contaminated with *S. typhimurium*.

A number of infections with *S. paratyphi B* were traced to egg products. Newell *et al.* (1955) reported 2 outbreaks of paratyphoid fever due to the consumption of cakes filled with synthetic cream, which had apparently been contaminated with *S. paratyphi B* from Chinese frozen whole eggs.

Salmonelloses do not, so far as is known, occur in fish. *Salmonella* infections have, however, been frequently transmitted by the eating of fish, particularly by smoked or steamed fish, the pathogen originating from human carriers. In the Netherlands, an outbreak of infection with *S. paratyphi B* was caused by eating smoked eel. The living eels were stored overnight in containers filled with harbour water into which the faeces of patients with type-B paratyphoid fever drained. Salted herring contaminated by a carrier has also given rise to outbreaks of salmonellosis. A case in point is an epidemic of typhoid fever caused by this food in Amsterdam in 1946.

Salmonellae do not normally occur in plants. Vegetables, however, may be contaminated by man or animals and may then transmit infection to humans. A widespread outbreak of typhoid fever and infection with *S. senftenberg* was caused by desiccated coco-nut in Australia (Wilson and Mackenzie, 1955). Galbraith *et al.* (1960), examining 851 samples of this product imported into the United Kingdom from Ceylon, found that 76 of them (9 %) were contaminated with salmonellae; 18 different serotypes were identified.

Measures designed to prevent salmonelloses in large domestic animals should be directed mainly towards improving the sanitary conditions in stables and sheds and avoiding contact with faeces. In doing this, systematic elimination of chronic carriers is an important factor.

Attention should be paid to food and drinking-water. Waste-water should be rendered innocuous on the spot.

For the protection of cattle, it is essential to take into account, not only infection transmitted from one animal to another, but also infection derived from human carriers.

On poultry farms, the houses, floors, incubators and artificial breeders should be cleaned and disinfected at regular intervals. Other measures to be considered are the detection and elimination of infected animals and the disinfection of the incubators and the shells of hatching eggs.

The results obtained from the agglutination test have been very useful in controlling *pullorum* disease; in other salmonelloses this procedure is far less satisfactory.

Hatching eggs are disinfected in the incubator by formaldehyde fumes which kill the salmonellae on the egg-shells and do not have any adverse effects on the results of hatching (Clarenburg and Romijn, 1954). This method is compulsory in the Netherlands. It is, however, not effective against infection of the contents of the eggs before.

Measures against the risk of infection by foodstuffs of animal origin should be adopted in the places in which these foodstuffs are prepared, packed and transported. When these measures are inadequate from the point of view of public health, decontamination of imported foodstuffs may be necessary. In Denmark, this procedure was made compulsory for all batches imported as from 1954; in the German Federal Republic the foodstuffs have been, since 1958, examined for salmonellae before importation. As the salmonellae are present only in small numbers and their distribution in the foodstuffs is irregular, failure to detect bacteria does not provide reliable evidence of their absence. For this reason decontamination of consignments of suspected origin is to be preferred.

Inspection of slaughter animals, before as well as after slaughter, is essential for the prevention of infection due to meat from animals infected during life. Examination for the presence of salmonellae is particularly indicated in cases of forced slaughter. When salmonellae are isolated from the meat or organs, the animal must be declared unfit for consumption.

This inspection does not permit the identification of chronic carriers (cattle) and animals with latent infection of organs (pigs). In order to reduce to a minimum, the risk from apparently normal carriers control of salmonellosis in live-stock is essential, compulsory notification being among the most important measures. To control latent infections, their origin in animals should be traced and eliminated (animal foodstuffs).

Strict hygienic measures should be exercised both in slaughter-houses and in butcher's shops, as well as during cold storage and transport of meat and meat products to prevent postmortal infections. The issue of sanitary regulations should be preceded by expert education of the employees.

Pasteurization is the most effective measure to prevent infection by milk. When it is desired to market uncooked milk, dairy-cattle, rinsing-water and employees should be rigidly supervised.

It is hardly necessary to stress the fact that the trade in duck's eggs should be governed by strict regulations. In the Netherlands, these regulations are laid down in a Royal

Decree (1953), the main points of which may be summarized as follows: The eggs must be stamped with the words "duck's egg, boil for 10 minutes"; duck's eggs may not be supplied to an establishment in which food or beverages are processed, *e.g.*, bakeries, restaurants, etc. Exemption certificates are only granted to establishments manufacturing rusks, because the temperature to which these products are heated during baking ensures that any *Salmonella* initially present will be killed. These regulations do not apply, however, to eggs that have been pasteurized in the shell in an establishment holding the necessary licence. These eggs must be stamped: "Duck's egg, pasteurized". The measures governing duck's eggs should also be applied to goose eggs.

All egg-products, should undergo a form of preliminary treatment designed to reduce risk of infection to a minimum (pasteurization or other methods).

As regards infections due to handling, a high standard of hygiene in the preparation of food is essential. Employees should be trained in the habit of washing their hands with soap and hot water after using toilet facilities, and before starting work, and they should get into the habit of keeping their nails closely cut. Carriers, if any, should be eliminated.

Rats and mice must be exterminated in food factories, kitchens and store-rooms. It will be advisable to ensure that the premises are rat-proof. The use of bacterial preparations as rat and mouse exterminators should be prohibited.

Multiplication of *Salmonella* is best prevented by storage of the foodstuffs at temperatures below 10°. In addition, it is essential that foodstuffs heated during processing are consecutively cooled as rapidly as possible.

The sensitivity of the various types of *Salmonella* to antibiotics and chemotherapeutic agents *in vitro* follows a fixed pattern marked by only slight individual variations. They are usually sensitive to streptomycin, chloramphenicol, the tetracyclines (oxytetracycline, chlortetracycline, tetracycline), polymyxin, kanamycin, furazolidone (furoxone) and the sulphonamides.

Of the agents effective *in vitro*, only chloramphenicol is of importance in treatment, particularly in salmonellosis characterized by typhoid manifestations. Unlike most other drugs, chloramphenicol is capable of reaching the bacteria in therapeutically active concentrations in almost every part of the body. In addition to chloramphenicol, the tetracyclines are also used in salmonelloses in which the bacteria do not penetrate beyond the intestine. Sulphonamides as well as streptomycin are usually not effective in salmonellosis.

References p. 160–161

Treatment of salmonellosis with chloramphenicol will result in recovery in the majority of cases, although the disease may recur, probably because this antibiotic has a bacteriostatic rather than a bactericidal action. If there is a recurrence, the patient may ultimately become a carrier. Administration of antibiotics may occasionally result in bacterial resistance. The tetracyclines are more likely to induce this phenomenon than is chloramphenicol.

In view of the ubiquity of *Salmonella* in nature it is likely that eradication of salmonelloses will remain utopian for the present. The possibility, however, exists that the chain of infections may be broken in several places.

Any approach to the many outstanding problems requires detailed epidemiological studies. It is likely that these will be most successful when veterinary surgeons and physicians cooperate to carry them out. It is gratifying that the view is gradually gaining ground that health services should be reorganized for this purpose.

REFERENCES

BUXTON, A., *Salmonellosis in Animals*, Commonwealth Agricultural Bureau, Bucks, 1957, 209 pp.
BISCHOFF, J., *Berl. Münch. tierärztl. Wschr.*, 72 (1959) 129.
CLARENBURG, A. and C. G. J. DORNICKX, *Ned. T. Geneesk.*, 76 (1932) 1579; *Z. Hyg.*, 114 (1933) 31.
CLARENBURG, A., G. D. HEMMES and W. WAGENVOORT, *Antonie v. Leeuwenhoek*, 8 (1952) 171.
CRAIGIE, J. and A. FELIX, *Lancet*, 252 (1947) 824.
DAUER, C. C., *Publ. Hlth Rep. (Wash.)*, 74 (1959) 940.
DIJKSTRA, O. H. and J. V. D. HOEDEN, *Ned. T. Geneesk.*, 73 (1929) 1458.
EDWARDS, P. R. and W. H. EWING, *Identification of Enterobacteriaceae*, Minneapolis, Minn, 1957, 179 pp.
GALBRAITH, N. S., B. C. HOBBS, M. E. SMITH and A. J. H. TOMLINSON, *Monthly Bull. Minist. Hlth Lab. Serv.*, 19 (1960) 99.
GALTON, M. M., W. D. LOWERY and A. V. HARDY, *J. infect. Dis.*, 95 (1954) 236.
GALTON, M. M., M. HARLESS and A. V. HARDY, *J. Amer. vet. med. Ass.*, 126 (1955) 57.
GALTON, M. M. and P. ARNSTEIN, *Poultry diseases in public health*, U.S. Dept. Health, Education and Welfare; P.H.S. Comm. Disease Center, Atlanta, Ga., 1959.
HANDLOSER, M., *Arch. Hyg. (Berl.)*, 140 (1956) 569.
HAUGE, S. and K. BÖVRE, *Nord. Vet.-Med.*, 10 (1958) 255.
HIRSCH, W. and R. SAPIRO-HIRSCH, *Harefuah*, 54 (1958) 57.
JANSEN, J., *T. Diergeneesk.*, 71 (1946) 160.
JELLARD, C. H., *Monthly Bull. Minist. Hlth Lab. Serv.*, 15 (1956) 34.
KALLINGS, L. O. and A. B. LAURELL, *Acta path. microbiol. scand.*, 40 (1957) 328.

KAUFFMANN, F., *Die Bakteriologie der Salmonella-Gruppe,* Kopenhagen, 1941, *Enterobacteriaceae,* Kopenhagen, 1954, 382 pp.

KWANTES, W., *Monthly Bull. Minist. Hlth, Lab. Serv.,* 11 (1952) 239.

McCULLOUGH, N. B. and C. W. EISELE, *J. infect. Dis.,* 88 (1951) 278; 89 (1952) 209; 259.

MITCHELL, R. B., F. C. GARLOCK and R. H. BROH-KAHN, *J. infect. Dis.,* 79 (1946) 57.

MÖLLER, A., *Zbl. Bakt. I. Abt. Orig.,* 164 (1955) 535.

Monthly Bull. Minist. Hlth Lab. Serv., 13 (1954 a) 12; 13 (1954 b) 38; 14 (1955) 65.

NEWELL, K. W., *Bull. Wld Hlth Org.,* 21 (1959) 279.

NEWELL, K. W., R. McCLARIN, C. R. MURDOCK, W. N. MacDONALD and H. L. HUTCHINSON, *J. Hyg. (London),* 57 (1959) 92.

NEWSOM, J. E. and F. CROSS, *J. Amer. vet. med. Ass.,* 66 (1924) 289; 76 (1930) 91; 86 (1935) 534.

SCHAAL, E., *Berl. Münch. tierärztl. Wschr.,* 72 (1959) 66.

SJOLLEMA, P., *T. Diergeneesk.,* 84 (1959) 1047.

Spec. Rep. Ser. med. Res. Counc. (Lond.), No. 260 (1947).

THAL, E., L. RUTQVIST and H. HOLMQVIST, *Nord. Vet.-Med.,* 9 (1957) 822.

WILSON, M. M. and E. F. MACKENZIE, *J. appl. Bact.,* 18 (1955) 510.

WÖLDIKE NIELSEN, F., *Bull. Off. int. Épiz.,* 42 (1954) 746.

ZEMAN, W., *Dtsch. med. Wschr.,* 74 (1949) 121.

J. VAN DER HOEDEN

Erysipeloid

(swine erysipelas, rouget du porc, Rotlauf der Schweine)

In 1878, R. Koch discovered a microorganism which he believed to be the cause of a septicaemic disease of mice *(Bac. muriseptica,* Flügge, 1886). Four years later, Pasteur and Thuillier isolated, during an outbreak of swine erysipelas ("rouget") in France, a similar organism from hogs, and soon afterwards (1885–86), Loeffler in Germany, described in detail the same bacterium, recovered from the skin of a pig which had died from "Schweinerotlauf".

The causative agent of erysipeloid in human beings was recorded in 1909 by Rosenbach as an organism indistinguishable from the above bacteria isolated from mice and swine.

At the present time, these three strains of different origins are considered to be culturally and serologically identical, representing one single genus, denominated *Erysipelothrix.* By this conception, *B. muriseptica, E. rhusiopathiae (= E. porci)* and *E. erysipeloides* are simply synonyms.

Together with the genera *Listeria* and *Corynebacterium, Erysipelothrix* belongs to the family of *Corynebacteriaceae.* On the basis of priority, the type species should be called *E. insidiosa,* Trevisan, 1885 (Bergey's Manual, 1957, VII).

Erysipelothrix is a thin, non-motile, grampositive rod. In the animal body it may show some morphological resemblance to *Actinomyces.* An important cultural criterion in identifying *E. insidiosa* is its growth in gelatin stab-culture with delicate lateral filamentous side-growth from the line of inoculation, so that the culture has the appearance of a tube-brush.

Despite the absence of capsules and spores, the resistance of *Erysipelo-*

thrix to adverse physical and other antagonistic influences is much greater than that of most bacteria.

Several scientific workers consider that the organism is a saprophyt which can become parasitic in the animal body.

In addition to its presence in diseased and apparently healthy animals, the erysipelas bacterium is widely disseminated in the outer world, particularly where decaying nitrogenous substances of animal or vegetable origin are present. *E. insidiosa* is also to be found in sewage water and soil, and evidence exists that it proliferates in these media, particularly in humid, sandy soil, which is rich in lime and humus.

It has been shown that the organism retains its viability in decomposing material for 4 months, in sewage for 2 weeks (but in tap water for only 4 to 5 days) and in buried carcasses for several months (up to 280 days).

Drying, especially in cool and dark places, and the various methods used for the preservation of meat, such as pickling and salting, delay the natural death of *E. insidiosa*. It survived in salted and salpeter-treated hams for 30 days; in concentrated brine for 26 days and in the stomach contents of normal swine, at pH 4.3, for at least 3 hours.

Although it is fairly resistant to freezing, the bacterium's susceptibility to elevated temperatures is rather high. It is destroyed at 44° in 4 days and at 52° in 15 minutes.

Virulence usually diminishes rapidly in artificial culture media as well as in the bodies of test-animals. Passage through pigeons, however, generally raises its virulence.

The drastic change of virulence observed under laboratory conditions suggests that natural factors connected with climate and soil play a significant part in the epizootiology of erysipelas in swine. It is an established fact that it is very difficult or even impossible to reproduce the disease by introduction of a culture of *E. rhusiopathiae* (syn. *E. insidiosa)* into susceptible swine. This has led to the assumption that the organism requires, after it has left the animal body, a sojourn in the outer environment in order to render it capable of causing disease.

The ubiquitous distribution of the swine erysipelas bacterium in nature and its ability to change easily from a saprophytic to a parasitic state and *vice versa,* are important factors influencing the natural spread of the disease. It has often been contended that, in the absence of certain stress factors, the organism cannot become pathogenic in the animal body. Favorable influences may increase the virulence of *Erysipelothrix* already present in the body of apparently healthy animals. Moreover, weakening of local or general resistance of the carriers (by other diseases, infestation with helminths, poor feeding, inadequate management, adverse climatic conditions, etc.) may help the saprophytic microorganism to penetrate into the tissues. These factors may explain, to a certain extent, the capricious epizootiological course of swine erysipelas in different places and at various times.

The periods between successive outbreaks of the disease may differ widely. General experience has shown that after one infection of a herd, reappearance of the disease in later years is to be expected.

It has been found that *E. insidiosa* remains viable in the soil for approximately 21 days. For this reason permanent contamination of the soil can be achieved only by repeated pollution by the faeces or urine of animal-carriers. Transfer of apparently healthy swine from chronically infected piggeries to healthy herds has often introduced erysipelas into regions previously free from the disease.

The infection is wide-spread in different animal species and over various continents of the world.

Mortality is mostly confined to *swine,* although turkeys may also be severely affected. Other domestic and wild mammals and birds are prone to the disease, or appear to be clinically undetected carriers of the bacterium. These animals, too, contribute to the spread of infection through their faeces and urine.

Occasional infections occur in sheep, horses, cattle, dogs, cats and farm-bred mink.

Wild and laboratory mice, rats and voles have been found infected with *E. insidiosa,* and the mortality among them is sometimes high (Drake and Hall, 1947). Outbreaks among these rodents are favoured by adverse conditions, such as those prevailing during mass-migration or over-crowding.

In the steppes of the Transbaikalian regions of the U.S.S.R., Timofeeva *et al.* (1959) recovered *E. insidiosa* from the blood, sputum and bubos of two hunters and from the organs of 87 out of 43,166 rodents, mostly tarbagans, as well as from fleas on these animals. Olsuf'ev *et al.* (1959) found the same organism, together with *Listeria mono-cytogenes,* in several water-voles and isolated them also from the streams in which these animals lived.

Although the role of *mice* and *rats* in the conservation and distribution of swine-erysipelas is not often mentioned in the literature, its importance should not be underestimated.

Because white mice and pigeons are highly susceptible to the organism, they are usually selected as test animals for research on erysipelas of swine.

Large numbers of virulent *E. insidiosa* are frequently present in the surface layer of the slime of fishes, especially on mackerel, but the organism does not appear to be pathogenic to these animals. Apparently, the slime is a favourable medium for further saprophytic development.

It is generally assumed that *Erysipelothrix* thrives well on contaminated carcasses and in refuse thrown into the water.

The question whether blood-sucking arthropods contribute to the spread of erysipelas has been widely explored. Wellmann (1949, 1950, 1955), successfully transmitted *E. insidiosa* from infected mice and pigeons by a single bite of *Aedes* sp., *Anopheles* sp., *Stomoxys* and *Chrysozona*. The insect's role was merely mechanical, the arthropods remaining vectors for 1 to 4 days after the contaminative feed. The stable fly, *Stomoxys calcitrans*, produced erysipelas in swine after it had fed on a mixture of swine-blood and a culture of *Erysipelothrix*.

It is noteworthy that the organism has been isolated from mosquitoes collected in a piggery in which swine were suffering from erysipelas. The insects are infected by sucking blood during the septicaemic stage of the disease or by feeding on contaminated excretions or filth.

Although it is difficult to produce the disease experimentally by feeding or injection of a culture of *E. insidiosa,* swine frequently show marked susceptibility when they are exposed to this organism in their natural biotope.

Wherever hogs are raised in large numbers, erysipelas used to be a rather common disease. It was differentiated from hog cholera about a century ago. For many years erysipelas was one of the most serious diseases of swine in Europe. In the New World its significance was not recognized earlier than in the twenties of this century. Since then, swine erysipelas has become a major hazard to animal husbandry in the U.S.A., particularly in the Mid-Western states (S. Dakota, Nebraska, Iowa).

The losses due to swine erysipelas in the U.S.A. have been estimated at 24 million dollars yearly (U.S.A. Yearbook of Agriculture, 1956).

In certain parts of Europe and North America, recurrence of the enzootic has been noticed every 4 to 5 years. It has been suggested that this periodicity of the disease is due either to fluctuations in the strength of the naturally acquired immunity of the swine population in a contaminated area, or to periodic changes of virulence of the causative organism, or even to variations in local stress factors.

Most outbreaks occur during the hot months of the year, although they may be observed at any time. Animals between the age of 3 to 10 months are particularly affected. Pigs below the age of 3 months and old hogs show a fairly strong resistance. The immunity of sucklings is probably due to protective antibodies in the sow's colostrum and milk; in the older animals, it may be a result of antibody formation by repeated natural exposures to the infection. In certain races and breeds of pigs, extraordinarily strong resistance against infection has been observed.

Portals of entry of the infection can be the mucosa of the digestive tract or the skin.

In swine-erysipelas, three distinct syndromes are distinguished.

(1) The *acute septicaemic form*, which is a very serious disease. In European countries it has been known for many years; in the U.S.A. its increasing importance has been recognized since 1930.

The micro-organism circulates in the blood during the acute attack and is excreted in the faeces and urine.

In a susceptible herd outbreaks have a sudden onset, and many animals are simultaneously affected. Signs of septicaemia are evident. The spleen and several lymph nodes are enlarged and reddened. Acute inflammation and minor haemorrhages, and sometimes ulcerative lesions, are found in the mucous membranes of the stomach and small intestines; cloudy swelling of the kidneys is usually observed. The animals lie prone on the floor and look very ill. Pulmonary oedema and swelling of the snout cause difficulty in breathing. On the second or third day of the disease, an erythematous eruption occurs in the form of irregularly shaped patches, particularly localised on the ears, snout, thorax and abdomen, the inner sides of the thighs, groins and perianal region. Originally pink, these patches turn bright or dark red and eventually purple. By confluence of the patches, irregular designs appear over large parts of the skin. Sometimes these lesions are succeeded by an eruption of petechiae. In many cases, necrosis of the affected areas occurs, particularly in the skin on the back, ears and tail. Eventually, the dark skin cicatrizes or sequestrates.

A considerable number of hogs may succumb overnight or within a week's time. Other animals recover or suffer from a chronic form of the disease, remaining backward in growth, unthrifty and crippled. After survival from the acute or subacute form of the disease, infection of the joints may develop into a chronic arthritic condition.

The mortality rate of the septicaemic attack varies in different outbreaks, sometimes reaching 80% or more of the herd.

(2) The *urticarial form* of swine erysipelas usually takes a mild course. It is characterized by sharply circumscribed quadrangular or rhomboidal,

slightly oedematous blotches on the skin ("diamond skin disease"; Fig. 20). When the eruption appears, the initial constitutional symptoms rapidly improve. The size of the geometric lesions varies from 1 to 10 cm in diameter. They are principally localized on the abdomen. The changes of colour of the urticaria resemble those of the erythema in the septicaemic form. In the regressive stage desquamation usually starts at the periphery of the lesion, and ends with the formation of brownish crusts.

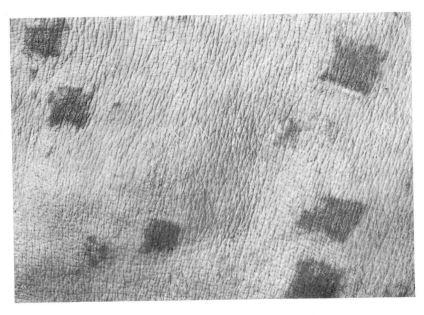

Fig. 20.   Diamond skin ("urticaria") in *erysipelas suis*.
(Photo: Institute for Veterinary Pathology, State University, Utrecht)

Mild attacks subside within a fortnight. When local lesions become confluent, covering large areas, dry gangrenous sloughing may cause loss of these parts of the skin, and of the ears and tail. The urticarial form of swine erysipelas is seldom fatal.

(3) Survival from a septicaemic attack may be followed by the *chronic form*. It is known that chronic erysipelas of swine may also start independently and may assume this form from the beginning. It is characterized by proliferative polyarthritis with pannus formation and vegetative bacterial endocarditis.

References p. 174

Lesions of the joints are not only characteristic of the chronic form of the disease; they are also associated with the septicaemic and urticarial syndromes. In the U.S.A. nearly 80% of all the arthritic lesions of swine from several slaughterhouses revealed *E. insidiosa,* and in Canada (1958) the organisms were isolated from 63.5% of the joints of lamed hogs with arthritis. In many pigs in which "rheumatism" is diagnosed, the chronic arthritis did result from *E. rhusiopathiae* infection. Although both the bony and soft parts of the joints are affected, no suppuration will occur. The joints mainly involved are the knee, hip, carpus and tarsus. Lameness and stiffness, followed by stunted growth of the animals, render breeding uneconomic. It has been assumed that allergic sensitization is an aetiological factor in the development of arthritis in porcine erysipelas. The anaphylactic response which is often observed after vaccination with *Erysipelothrix* is suggestive in this respect.

Cardiac trouble is often observed after acute symptoms of septicaemia have subsided. In a large piggery in Germany, a sudden outbreak of endocarditis from which *E. insidiosa* was isolated, was observed by Hupka (1957). No preliminary signs of infection had been noticed. In this instance it was assumed that the circulating organisms settled on the heart valves as a result of the steady intake of the bacteria to which the pigs were exposed while they lay on an infected dung-heap.

Vegetative endocarditis especially affects the mitral valves, which are eroded and covered with a gradually growing deposite of fibrin (Fig. 21). Heart function and blood-circulation are often seriously impaired, sometimes causing sudden death. Healed endocardial lesions have been established at slaughter in more than 10% of apparently normal hogs and in some instances the erysipelas bacterium has been recovered from the vegetations.

In advanced cases of chronic erysipelas of swine, changes of the adrenal glands and fibrosis of the kidney tissue have been found.

In chronically infected pigs, the microorganisms are concentrated in the lymphoid tissues of the tonsils and intestines.

In Germany (1925, 1927) about 50% of swine were found to be carriers without giving clinical indication of infection. Out of 220 slaughter pigs examined at random (in 1954), 88 harbored *E. insidiosa* in the tonsils or ileocoecal valves. *Erysipelothrix* was isolated from 82% of the tonsils of 275 non-selected hogs in Poland (in 1956) whereas in Yugoslavia (in 1956) the organism was identified in only 6.15% of 1007 pigs. Rowsell (1958), in the U.S.A., recovered the largest numbers of infected tonsils from the higher age groups among the animals: almost none were found in swine aged 4 to 5 months, while 36% were positive at the age of 6 to 8 months, and 50% at 1 to 1½ years of age. In Roumania (1956) the swine-erysipelas bacterium was isolated from 9 out of 240 tonsils of apparently healthy slaughter cattle.

In 1913, Poels in Holland first isolated *E. insidiosa* from *lambs* suffering from joint ill. 6 years later, in Denmark, a similar outbreak occurred in *sheep*, which was complicated by haemorrhagic enteritis with enlarged mesenteric glands. Enzootics of a septicaemic form in lambs have also been recorded in Germany (1923) and the U. K. (Harbour and Kershan, 1949).

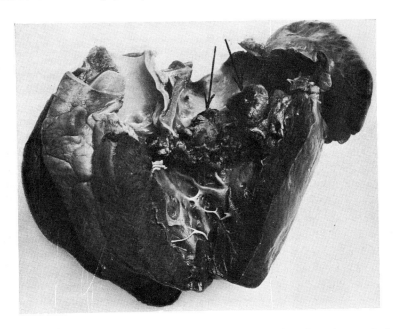

Fig. 21.   Chronic endocarditis verrucosa of the mitral valves in swine erysipelas.
(Photo: Institute for Veterinary Pathology, State University, Utrecht)

In New-Zealand, since 1948, many cases of *E. insidiosa* infection have been observed among *sheep* and these were due to the common use of antiparasitic dips contaminated by soil (McLean, 1948). The animals developed fever, lameness and sometimes arthritis and skin lesions comparable to those found in human erysipeloid. Similar outbreaks have been recorded in Uruguay (since 1949) and in England (Kent, 1949). In the latter country, the disease appeared 2 to 5 days after the sheep had been dipped in a DDT–Gammexane mixture. Fatal septicaemia occurred in newly weaned lambs.

Since the turn of the century, *E. insidiosa* has been increasingly established as the cause of disease in *domestic turkeys, ducks, pheasants, peacocks, pigeons,* and *chickens* as well as in different species of *wild birds (e.g. quail)*. The birds most severely affected are turkeys, although great damage can also be caused to ducks and chickens. Turkeys have shown even stronger resistance than swine to experimental infection by laboratory strains of *E. insidiosa*. Thus, environmental conditions and stress factors seem to carry decisive weight in the development of the infection among these birds. The virulence of the organism was increased by interavian passage. The first major outbreak among turkeys in the U.S.A. was observed in 1934 (Beaudette and Hudson, 1936).

E. insidiosa infection of chickens was unknown in New Jersey prior to 1951, but has been twice observed in that region in 1952–53, simultaneously with outbreaks in 22 flocks of turkeys. Between the years 1942 and 1951, the annual economic loss to the turkey- and duck-breeding industry in the U.S.A. has been estimated at nearly two million dollars. In 1956–57 the disease was frequently encountered among pheasants and ducks in France, mostly in the acute septicaemic form. Even before the outbreak becomes obvious and without prodromal signs, some birds in a flock may suddenly die. In other instances there is at first general weakness and listlessness, followed by a purplish-red swelling of parts of the head and neck. A pathognomonic symptom is the haematoma-like swelling of the caruncle, comparable with that of the ears in man and swine. Thick mucal excretions fill the nasal cavity. Lameness is caused by arthritis, which most often involves the tibio-metatarsal joints. At post-mortem examination, small haemorrhages are found in the muscles and pericardium, as well as a dark, swollen, friable liver and spleen and congested kidneys. The death rate fluctuates between 2 and 40% of the affected birds.

Most of the infections in *man* are the result of skin injuries, but exceptionally they may also be produced by penetration of the agent through the digestive tract.

In human beings and swine alike, *E. insidiosa* may adopt three clinical forms of disease, *i.e.,* a benign localized dermal affection, a septicaemic syndrome including vegetative endocarditis, and a severe dermal generalization of long duration.

Acute erysipeloid in human beings (Rosenbach, 1884), had been earlier described by Morrant Baker (1873) under the name of *erythema serpens*. It appears 1 to 4 days after penetration of the organism into the skin, and begins with itching, tingling or burning pain at the site of the infection. The skin lesion consists of sharply defined purplish-red, slightly elevated tense patches, which progress slowly from the periphery as the center gradually heals. The erythematous eruption, which is mostly localized at

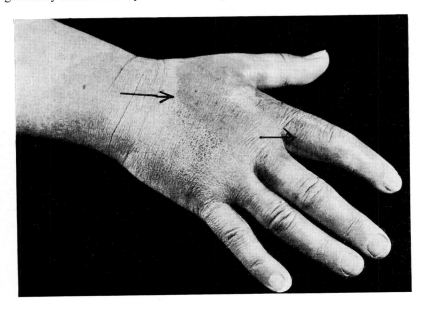

Fig. 22.   Erysipeloid (Rosenbach) due to injury by fish bone.
(Photo: Department of Dermatology, Medical Faculty, State University, Utrecht;
by courtesy of Prof. L. H. Jansen)

the thumb or fore-finger, extends to other parts of the hand, but seldom progresses beyond the wrist. Suppuration does not occur (Fig. 22). Lymphangitis and arthralgia occasionally develop. The joint-pain and stiffness of the affected fingers may persist for a long time. Usually general symptoms of disease are lacking or very slight. Spontaneous remission is followed by total recovery within 1 to 6 weeks. In some cases the cutaneous eruption progresses by uninterrupted spreading from the edges, which remain sharply defined, to give rise to a diffuse pink to purplish-red generalized erythema. The parts affected earlier gradually return to normal without marked desquamation. In addition to this creeping spread of the erythema, new patches may suddenly appear on distant parts of the body, or relapses occur after an asymptomatic remission. *E. insidiosa* can be isolated from the affected skin, but not from the blood.

Subjective constitutional complaints and polyarthritis have been recorded in the course of this form of chronic erysipeloid. Infections lasting for more than a year have been observed.

Apart from the presence of cutaneous lesions, a septicaemic form of erysipeloid may develop. It is sometimes accompanied by a generalized skin rash of purple or bluish-red spots, comparable to those observed in the septicaemic form of hog erysipelas. In the course of the disease, characteristic painful purplish-red swellings of the ears resembling haematomata are not unusual. They tend to become necrotic and to amputate spontaneously, as the similar affections of the ears of swine and the caruncles of turkeys also do. Anaemia and leucopenia with monocytosis are rather pathognomonic of the septicaemic syndrome of human erysipeloid.

As in the septicaemic form of erysipelas in swine, in man endocarditis of the aortic and mitral valves occur in addition to skin eruption and joint involvement. In these exceptional cases the organism can be easily isolated from the blood and endocardial vegetations. Other complications have also been recorded, such as lymphangitis, lymphadenitis, meningitis, neuritis optica, delirium and bone-necrosis.

Most cases of erysipeloid are occupationally contracted by persons engaged in handling of meat, slaughter products, manure, fish or crustaceans (veterinarians, butchers, meat-inspectors, fishermen, sewer workers, cooks, workers in skin and bone processing factories, laboratory personnel, etc.). In several instances it was found that the entire environment in the fish industry was heavily contaminated with *Erysipelothrix* organisms.

85 out of 115 cases of erysipeloid among 2300 patients attending the Septic-hand Clinic at Charing Cross Hospital, London, were directly attributable to an animal source, and 7 to organic plant matter (King 1946).

In a survey of 100 cases, Klauder (1938) recorded 74 butchers and fishmongers. Out of 500 other cases of erysipeloid, 260 were employees in meat-packing plants (Nelson, 1955). An "epidemic" affected about 200 men handling fish from the Dniepr and Bug in Russia (Stefansky and Grunfeld, 1930). Approximately half of the workers in button factories in the U.S.A., especially those who sawed or polished wet cow- or hog bones, presented a history of previous attacks, which had often recurred several times on the same hand (McGinnes and Spindle, 1934).

In an inquiry among Dutch veterinarians in 1938, 231 out of 534 of them reported that they had suffered from the disease. In 88 % of these cases, erysipeloid was contracted, while vaccinating swine with virulent *E. insidiosa* suspensions, by means of a prick of the needle or a wound from a glass-splinter of the ampule. 53 of the veterinarians had a single recurrence of the disease, 12 had 2 recurrences, 2 had 3 and 18 had 4 or more. The significance of this accidental mode of infection should not be overlooked, especially in view of the comparatively small number of cases among veterinarians in Denmark (only 43 out of 796), where vaccination with a living culture was not applied in practice.

The recurrence of attacks in the same persons exposed to occupational infection demonstrates the weakness, or lack, of persistant immunity in human beings. It may also indicate allergic sensitization to the erysipeloid organism.

In view of the prevalence of *E. insidiosa* as a saprophyte both in the environment and inside the animal body, it is obvious that eradication of swine erysipelas, once it has become established in an area, is hardly possible. Only limitation of its incidence can be expected.

It has been shown that repeated cleaning and disinfection of the hog pens will reduce the number of infected swine. Newly purchased pigs should, if possible, be isolated for at least a month before they are added to a clean herd.

Injection of erysipelas-immune serum has little or no therapeutic value, except for treatment at the acute stage of disease. Its use is only advisable in cases which progress rapidly and when arthritic involvement appears.

Pasteur's vaccine (1883) consisted of living bacteria the virulence of which had been reduced by passage through rabbits. Lorenz (1893) introduced simultaneous injection of virulent bacteria and potent immune serum. Both methods run the risk that the vaccine itself may cause the disease ("Impfrotlauf"), or may spread the infection by the establishment of clinically healthy carriers and may endanger the vaccinator.

More widely adopted at present are Traub's bacterin of killed micro-organisms of high immunising capacity adsorbed on to aluminium hydroxide, and vaccines prepared from selected non-virulent strains (Staub, Wiidik). Different authors claim that postvaccinal immunity lasts from 3–12 months. It is obvious that varying local conditions will influence the validity of vaccination procedures. Even when dead vaccines have been employed cases of illness, or of death soon after the injection, have been described (Saxer, 1954: 26 ill, 11 dead out of 596 pigs vaccinated in Switzerland). This has been explained as a result of a lowering of tissue resistance against "saprophytic" *Erysipelothrix* already present in the body.

In the treatment of pigs, turkeys and other birds, administration of large doses of penicillin, terramycin and erythromycin has been recommended as providing satisfactory results. Sulfonamides are useless.

Protection of human beings includes disinfection and covering of scratches and wounds on the hands of persons exposed to infection. Under certain conditions, the wearing of rubber gloves by fish- and meat-handlers and kitchen-personnel is to be recommended.

REFERENCES

BAUDETTE, F. R. and C. B. HUDSON, *J. Amer. vet. med. Ass.*, 88 (1936) 475.
CROUGUE, O., *Bull. Acad. vét. Fr.*, 9 (1936) 438.
DRAKE, C. H. and E. R. HALL, *Amer. J. publ. Hlth*, 37 (1947) 846.
HARBOUR, H. E. and G. F. KERSHAW, *Vet. Rec.*, 61 (1949) 37.
HETTCHE, H. O., *Arch. Hyg. (Berl.)*, 119 (1938) 178.
HOEDEN, J. v. D., *T. Diergeneesk.*, 66 (1939) 219.
HUPKA, E., *Dtsch. tierärztl. Wschr.*, 64 (1957).
KING, P. F., *Lancet*, ii (1946) 196.
KLAUDER, J. V., *Ann. N.Y. Acad. Sci.*, 48 (1947) 535; *J. Amer. med. Ass.*, 111 (1938) 1345.
MCGINNES, G. F. and F. SPINDLE, *Amer. J. publ. Hlth*, 24 (1934) 32.
MCNUTT, S. H., *Vet. Sci.*, 1 (1953) 304.
NELSON, E., *Rocky Mtn. med. J.*, 52 (1955) 40.
OLSUF'EV, N. G., V. G. PETROV and K. N. SHYGINA, *Ž. Mikrobiol. (Mosk.)*, 30 (1959) 112.
ROOTS, E., *XV Internat. Vet. Congr.* I, 1 (1953) 44.
SAXER, E., *Schweiz. Arch. Tierheilk.*, 96 (1954) 151.
STEFANSKY, W. K. and A. A. GRÜNFELD, *Zbl. Bakt., I. Abt., Orig.*, 117 (1930) 376.
TIMOFEEVA, L. A. and V. I. GOLOVACHEVA, *Ž. Mikrobiol. (Mosk.)*, 30 (1959) 106.
WELLMANN, G. C., *Zbl. Bakt. I. Abt., Orig.*, 155 (1950) 109; 162 (1955) 265.

9

J. DONKER-VOET

Listeriosis

Listeriosis was first described in 1926, when the causative organism was isolated by Murray, Webb and Swann, during an epizootic among laboratory rabbits and guinea pigs in Cambridge. Because the disease in these animals was characterized by an increase in the number of monocytes, these authors gave the organism the name *Bacterium monocytogenes*.

One year later, Pirie remarked on a similar disease in a South African gerbil *(Tatera lobengulae)*. In honour of Lister, and because the organism produces liver lesions, Pirie named the organism *Listerella hepatolytica,* a name which was later changed to *Listeria monocytogenes* (see Bergey's *Manual of Determinative Bacteriology,* 7th edn.).

L. monocytogenes is a member of the family *Corynebacteriaceae*. It is a small, grampositive rod with rounded ends. Although it may at times be difficult to isolate the organism, it grows, once it has been cultivated, freely on most of the culture media commonly employed. Acid, but no gas, is produced from different sugars; esculin is hydrolyzed in 24 hours. Grown at room temperature the organisms show a rather peculiar tumbling motility. On horse-blood medium there is a small zone of β-haemolysis around the slightly raised colonies. The organism is catalase-positive and grows best under aerobic conditions. Rough variants are often non-pathogenic, but they produce monocytosis when they are inoculated into laboratory animals.

L. monocytogenes was first recognized as a possible cause of disease in man by Nyfeldt (1929) in Denmark. He isolated the organism from the blood of persons suffering from infectious mononucleosis (glandular fever). Stanley (1949) found significant agglutinin titres for *L. monocytogenes,* together with agglutinins for red blood cells of sheep (the Paul–Bunnell reaction which is indicative of glandular fever), in 7 out of 20 cases of the disease. Although the illness had already been described by Pfeiffer as early as 1889, its cause is still obscure. All attempts to establish a causative relationship between Pfeiffer's disease and the *Listeria* organism have as yet failed. It may be that the name "glandular fever" and its symptoms cover more than one entity, one of which might result from infection by *Listeria.*

References p. 183

Gill (1931) recovered *Listeria* from sheep in New Zealand. Since then it has been shown that *L. monocytogenes* can attack a wide range of animal species, including cattle, sheep, goats, pigs, horses, dogs, cats, rabbits, guinea pigs, rats, mice, chinchillas, mink, chickens, turkeys and canaries. Seeliger (1958) listed all the susceptible animal species and the countries in which listeric infections have been observed. Gray recorded the isolation of *L. monocytogenes* from 11 different species of domestic and wild birds. The only animal that resists even heavy experimental infection is the racing pigeon, but this bird sometimes remains a carrier for a long period of time.

Listeriosis has been reported from all parts of the world, usually in sporadic cases.

The disease is seldom diagnosed in its early stages, chiefly because ignorance of its aetiology and the great variability of the symptoms easily lead to confusion with other diseases. A tentative diagnosis can be based upon clinical signs, post-mortem lesions and serological tests. The most dependable method, however, is isolation and identification of the causative organism.

This has been most successfully achieved by macerating aseptically a portion of the tissue to be investigated, and plating the resulting suspension on to tryptose agar directly and after refrigeration at 4° for several weeks. The fact that *L. monocytogenes* is often intra-cellular may partly explain the need for tissue maceration.

Isolation of the organism may be facilitated by inoculation of the tissue material into rabbits or mice. It may be advantageous to inoculate embryonating chicken eggs rather than to use dead media.

Two distinctive characteristics of *L. monocytogenes* can be used as aids in identifying suspected cultures. Instillation of *L. monocytogenes* into the conjunctival sac of rabbits or guinea pigs evokes a specific conjunctivitis and subsequent keratitis. In pregnant animals it may produce abortion. If a sublethal dose of the organism is injected intra-venously into rabbits, there is a striking increase in the number of monocytes in the peripheral blood. Under certain conditions this may reach 30 to 50% or more.

The most important contribution to the antigenic characterization of *L. monocytogenes* has been made by Paterson (1939, 1940), who demonstrated the presence of both H- and O-antigens and distinguished 4 serotypes. There seems to be little correlation between the antigenic type and the kind of host species, or its geographical origin. Seeliger (1953) as well as the author (1957) subdivided Paterson's types, but it is most probable that in addition to the serotypes which are at present known other types exist as yet unknown.

In general, serotests are of only limited value in the diagnosis of listeriosis. The sera of a relatively high percentage of human beings and animals with no history of exposure to the disease contain agglutinins for the organism. The antibody response of both man and animals to infection is quite variable. Often there is only a low production of antibodies, even in natural listeric infections (Hood, 1957) and their specificity may be questionable. Investigations by Seeliger (1958) and Flamm (1958) showed that certain strains of *Staphylococcus aureus, enterococci*, haemolytic *streptococci* and *Corynebacteriae* gave serological cross-reactions with one or more serotypes of *L. monocytogenes*. For this reason great caution should be exercised in interpreting the serological results. They may, however, have diagnostic significance if a series of consecutive tests show a rise in titre during the development of the disease.

The incubation period of natural infections is not exactly known. After experimental infection of large animals it is at least 7 days, but it may be prolonged to a month or more. It appears that some animals harbour *Listeria* for long periods of time before infection becomes manifest. Symptoms of disease may differ considerably in the various host species.

Listeriosis is often associated with meningo-encephalitis, septicaemia, abortion, stillbirth or neonatal death. In ruminants, the disease is most commonly characterized by a localized encephalitis, while in monogastric

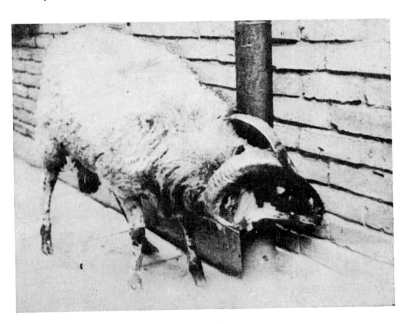

Fig. 23 A.

Dutch sheep suffering from the encephalo-myelitic form of listeriosis, 2 days before death. (Photo: Prof. A. van der Schaaf; Institute for Veterinary Bacteriology, State University, Utrecht)

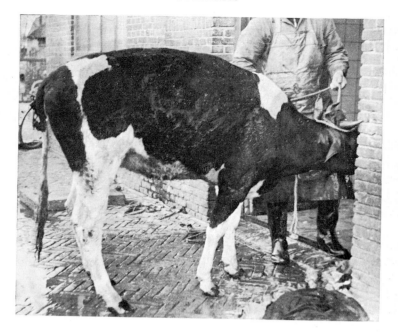

Fig. 23 B.
Heifer with meningo-encephalitis caused by *Listeria*. The head, especially the horn, is
pressed against the wall; the right ear hangs down.
(Photo: Provincial Animal Health Service in Friesland. Courtesy: Prof. A. van der Schaaf)

animals there is usually a septicaemia with focal hepatic necrosis.
Conjunctivitis and a granulomatous condition have been occasionally
recognized in man.

In *ruminants* with listeric encephalitis, mortality is very high. Only a few
of the animals showing definite symptoms of disease will recover. In
sheep and goats the disease is highly acute and death may occur within a
few hours after the appearance of the first signs. In cattle the course is less
acute; some animals recover spontaneously.

Symptoms in sheep, goats and cows are similar and vary only in
severity. At the onset, the infected animal segregates from the rest of the
herd. It appears depressed and indifferent to its surroundings. Incoordination and sometimes torticollis may ensue. Often local paralysis of the
facial and throat muscles interferes with swallowing and results in marked
salivation and drooping of one or both ears. The animal may appear to be

blind. In the early stages it tends to lean against stationary objects (Fig. 23A, B). If the animal walks, it often moves in a circle. This circling movement is always in the same direction and has given rise to the name "circling disease" (Gill, 1931). In the terminal stage the animal falls down and cannot get up without assistance.

The lesions in the central nervous system are characterized by peri-vascular infiltration, "cuffing" with lymphocytes and necrosis. Less constant lesions are focal and perivascular oedema, haemorrhages and degenerative changes in the nerve cells and tracts. The most marked changes occur in the medulla oblongata.

Although it is, as a rule, difficult to recover *Listeria* from the living animal, it is relatively easy to isolate the organism from the medulla oblongata of animals which have died from the disease.

In *swine* the most common form of listeriosis appears to be a septic-aemia with focal hepatic necrosis. Affected pigs may also show signs of encephalitis. Hale (1959) recorded diarrhoea, weakness and stiffness as the most characteristic clinical signs in piglets. The frequent isolation of *L. monocytogenes* from pigs which had obviously died from some other cause, suggests that this animal may be a carrier which may play a part in the transmission of listeric infections.

In wild and domestic *rodents Listeria* infections are usually septicaemic. Infected pregnant animals often abort. The blood usually shows large numbers of mononuclear cells, mainly monocytes. In general the principal lesion is a focal hepatic necrosis and the bacterium can be isolated from the affected liver.

In *fowls* also listeriosis is most commonly manifested by septicaemia. *L. monocytogenes* can be recovered from most of the viscera, particularly the liver and spleen. Usually the most conspicuous lesions are: extended areas of myocardial degeneration, pericarditis and an increased amount of pericardial fluid. In some instances the heart shows greyish-white foci of necrosis. Occasionally birds show symptoms of localized central nervous disorder, and *L. monocytogenes* can be isolated from the brain.

Perinatal listeriosis in animals is similar to that seen in man (see below). Numerous abortions have been observed in cattle, sheep, horses, swine, chinchillas and rabbits. In Holland, 1 % of all abortions in cattle are due to this organism. Perhaps the most important form of the disease in *man* is abortion and/or perinatal death. Although the foetus or new-born infant may be heavily infected with *L. monocytogenes,* the mother is usually not ill. In some instances she may initially show clinical evidence of mild indisposition, which is, with few exceptions, followed by complete recovery. This is in contrast with other forms of listeriosis which, until the advent of antibiotics, showed very high mortality.

From observations of subsequent pregnancies it appears that there is no great danger of infection for the next child. Newborns may be infected prenatal through the placenta or amniotic fluid, or intrapartum in the birth canal. The source of infection usually remains obscure.

The course of the disease in the newborn is always severe and is especially so when it is not suspected or recognized before parturition. Birth is usually premature and the child is either stillborn or survives for only a few days. Long lasting brain damage is a common sequel in infants surviving *Listeria* infection.

Potel (1950–51), who observed in East Germany a large number of perinatal cases of listeriosis, called the disease "granulomatosis infantiseptica". This name is based on the presence of focal necrosis especially in the liver, and sometimes in other viscera. It is thought that necrosis in the liver develops in the hepatic cells surrounding the Kupffer's cells which have ingested large numbers of organisms. The foci enlarge and often become infiltrated with neutrophils or mononuclear cells.

Usually *L. monocytogenes* can be isolated without difficulty from the foetal liver, blood, stomach contents, meconium and foetal membranes. In order to institute therapy as quickly as possible, the meconium should be examined in all suspected cases. When listeriosis is suspected in pregnant women, urine removed with a catheter should be bacteriologically investigated. It is also essential to watch the antibody level of the blood during the course of the disease.

In man, *L. monocytogenes* also affects the central nervous system; meningitis and encephalitis are similar to those seen in other diseases.

There is often an increase of the monocytes and decrease in the sugar level of the spinal fluid. These changes may be used for differential diagnosis. *L. monocytogenes* can be directly observed in gram-stained smears or it can often be cultivated from the cerebro-spinal fluid. The course of the disease is determined by the location of the infection within the central nervous system.

In listeric septicaemia there is high temperature, but there are no typical symptoms which indicate its aetiology. In these cases the correct diagnosis can only be made by blood culture. In cases of chronic septicaemia, protracted disorders of the central nervous system and habitual abortion in women, listeriosis should be considered.

The oculo–glandular form of listeriosis is rare. In the few cases reported in man there was unilateral chemosis of the conjunctiva with swelling of the preauricular, and sometimes also of the cervical and submaxillary, glands. Skin lesions on the hands and arms have been observed in veterinarians who had treated aborting cows. The same type of *L. monocytogenes* was isolated from their arms and from the foetuses.

Although it is well established that *L. monocytogenes* can attack a wide range of animal species, very little is known about its epizootiology. A main reservoir in nature has never been established. The wide host range suggests the occurrence of symptomless carriers, and that predisposing factors and stress promote the chance of infection. This supposition is made likely by the occasional recovery of *L. monocytogenes* from either apparently normal people and animals, or from those which have died from other causes. The difficulty in producing the disease experimentally also suggests that factors still unrecognized contribute to infection under natural conditions.

The source and route of human infection are as yet undetermined. No direct evidence exists that the disease is transmitted by immediate contact with animals. It is most likely that infection of newborn infants takes place in the maternal genito-urinary tract.

It has been suggested that farm workers and veterinarians may become infected, not only by direct contact with sick animals or apparently healthy carriers, but also by handling aborted foetuses or by removing foetal membranes from otherwise normal animals.

The meat of animals slaughtered during the period of listeric bacteriaemia may also be a source of infection.

The possibility that poultry plays a part in human listeriosis has been put forward by Felsenfeld (1951), who reported listeric conjunctivitis in workers employed in poultry processing plants. Gray (1958) stated that, although eggs laid by infected birds will not necessarily contain the organism, the shells may be contaminated by the faeces.

Consumption of raw infected milk has also been considered a potential danger to man. In a few instances, *Listeria* infection in man has been associated with mastitis in cows. Although this does not appear to be a common event, it might represent a definite health hazard to anyone, especially pregnant women, who drink raw milk from such an animal. It appears that in all cases of generalized listeric infection of lactating animals the microorganisms may be shed through the milk.

Hyslop and Osborn (1959) isolated *L. monocytogenes* from 8 lactating milk cows, 2 of which excreted the organism in their milk. *Listeria* were shed during a period of several months. In this way milk from cows with mild subacute listeric mastitis can reach the public. Since *L. monocytogenes* is able to multiply at relatively low temperatures, the addition of infected milk could result in contamination of a large amount of milk otherwise safe for consumption. *L. monocytogenes* possesses a greater heat tolerance than most other pathogenic microorganisms. Bearns and Girard (1958) showed, that if the viable cell count exceeded 5×10^4 per ml, *L. monocytogenes* might survive pasteurization.

Gill (1931) suggested that the sheep-nasal-fly, *Oestrus ovis*, can transmit ovine listeriosis. *Dermanyssus gallinae* may play a part in its transmission among poultry and canaries. The organism has been isolated from ticks found on infected cattle.

Osebold *et al.* (1957), in a study of the role of wild fauna in the epizootiology of listeriosis in ruminants, recovered the micro-organism from a striped skunk, found on a pasture grazed by infected sheep. The amount of direct contact between infected wild animals and domestic livestock and/or pasture contamination may constitute the greatest potential hazard. The ingestion of the carcasses of dead animals by carnivorous animals or birds constitutes another probable mode of spread of the infection.

It has often been suggested that there may be a link between silage feeding and listeric infection in ruminants. Recently Gray (1960) reported the isolation of *L. monocytogenes* from mice fed with silage thought to have been responsible for listeric abortion in cattle. Although the significance of this observation cannot be fully evaluated at present, it does lend support to the above suggestion.

Contaminated food or dirt is probably the most important source of infection.

Sanitary measures are of the greatest importance in preventing listeric infection.

The present widespread use of poultry foods containing antibiotics may be an effective prophylactic measure against listeric infection in these animals.

Active immunization against *L. monocytogenes* would be valuable on premises on which outbreaks of listeriosis occur in successive years. Such attempts have, however, led to controversial results. At present there is no effective vaccine or bacterin available. It has, moreover, not been possible to confer passive immunity on mice with sheep- and rabbit-antiserum.

In listeric infection of man, treatment with a combination of sulfonamides and antibiotics, especially tetracyclines, has often proved successful, provided that it has been promptly initiated.

Among animals, the brain may already have been irreversibly damaged before any symptoms of the disease have been noticed. Although the therapeutic agent may reach the brain quickly, the animal seldom survives. Gray and Moore (1953) reported moderate success with tetracyclines in the treatment of cattle, but no recovery in sheep.

It is imperative that treatment should be initiated as early as possible and that a sufficiently high dose should be maintained over a relatively long period.

Although the disease is usually sporadic, it must be emphasized that listeriosis in animals constitutes a potential public health hazard. This should be stressed to bacteriologists, physicians and veterinarians.

REFERENCES

BEARNS, R. E. and K. F. GIRARD, *Canad. J. Microbiol.*, 4 (1958) 55.
GRAY, M. L., *Zbl. Bakt. I. Abt. Orig.*, 169 (1957) 373; *Avian Diseases*, 2 (1958) 296; *J. Amer. vet. med. Ass.*, 136 (1960) 205.
HOOD, M., *Amer. J. clin. Path.*, 28 (1957) 18.
HYSLOP, N. ST. and A. D. OSBORNE, *Vet. Rec.*, 71 (1959) 1082.
MCBRIDE, M. E. and K. F. GIRARD, *J. Lab. Clin. Med.*, 55 (1960) 153.
MURRAY, E. G. D., *Canad. med. Ass. J.*, 72 (1955) 99.
OSEBOLD, J. W., G. SHULTZ, and E. W. JAMESON, *J. Amer. vet. med. Ass.*, 130 (1957) 471.
POTEL, J., *Wissenschaftl. Z. Martin Luther Univ., Math. Nat.*, Halle-Wittenberg, 6 (1957) 311.
ROOTS, E. and D. STRAUCH, *Zbl. Vet.-Med.*, Beiheft 1 (1958).
SEELIGER, H. P. R., *Listeriose*, II, Leipzig, 1958, 194 pp.

10

A. VAN DER SCHAAF

Malleus

(English: glanders; French: morve; German: Rotz)

Since the horse lost its importance as a transporter of man and goods, glanders has become a disease of no practical significance in Europe. It was especially a hazard under the unfavourable circumstances of wars, during which a sharp rise of the number of glanderous horses formerly occurred. Nowadays, in countries where motorcars and motorised army vehicles are scarce, the incidence of malleus may still be significant.

In some parts of Asia the veterinary services have not been able to eradicate this usually chronic contagious disease from horses, mules and asses.

Natural infection is characterized by the formation of nodules in the skin and internal organs, especially the lungs, and swelling of the lymph glands. Breakdown of these nodules causes the appearance of ulcers on the mucous membranes and skin.

Although other animals, such as carnivora and man can be occasionally infected and may even die of the disease, its cause, *Actinobacillus mallei,* will become extinct when the sanitation of equines has reached a satisfactory high level, as it has in western Europe and North America.

As early as in the fifth and fourth century A.D. malleus was mentioned by Vegetius and Apsyrtus as a malignant disease of horses.

In the seventeenth and eighteenth century it was considered, like plague and smallpox, to be an infectious disease of man, and already in 1784 strict regulations were decreed in France to prevent the propagation of the disease, especially among army horses. De Solleysel should be mentioned as the *auctor intellectualis* of these regulations, notwithstanding that La Fosse, the famous veterinary surgeon of the French court, considered that the disease was a local non-infectious ailment (1749). The Danish veterinarian Viborg (1797) demonstrated the identity of "glanders" and "farcy", its cutaneous form.

Similarly, in Germany, Greve declared in 1818 that "Rotz" and "Hautwurm" are of the same nature and are actually identical.

In spite of these observations Dupuy, of the "Ecole Vétérinaire d'Alfort", declared again on the grounds of negative results from experimental infections, that it was doubtful whether glanders and farcy were contagious. As a consequence of this change of view, the enforcement of the usual regulations slackened and thus it happened that in the second half of the nineteenth century the disease again became widespread in the whole of France. When, finally, the Veterinary School of Lyon gave definite proof of the infectiousness and similarity of glanders and farcy, the eradication measures were resumed.

Since then, in the Western countries, the number of glanderous horses constantly declined until the first world war, when unfavourable conditions again caused a flare-up of the disease. Whereas in the first half of 1914, for instance, not a single case was reported among the civil and army horses in Germany, from August of that year until the end of the war in 1918, the Military Veterinary Service condemned 15,776 clinically or latently infected animals; these contaminations mainly originated from captured Russian horses. Almost everywhere on the European continent a tendency to increased incidence of glanders was observed. In the French Army, during the First World War, 58,843 animals were affected, of which 294 died from generalised malleus, while 20,585 had to be destroyed. In geographically isolated Great Britain, however, wartime did not bring about an increase of the disease: in 1910, 1014 cases had been diagnosed; in 1915, 85; in 1920, 22 and in 1925 only 2. In neutral Netherlands a few malleus cases were observed, the largest outbreak appearing in 1925 in Rotterdam, due to the importation from eastern countries of infected horses, which gave negative mallein tests.

After the publication of Löffler and Schütz's (1882) exhaustive study of the causative organism of glanders, only a few fundamental facts remained to be added. These investigators demonstrated the rods in closed lesions of the lungs and obtained a pure culture on Löffler's blood-serum medium, with which healthy horses could be infected. They also established the marked pathogenicity of *A. mallei* to guinea pigs and mice and described the peculiar swelling of the scrotum in the infected animals. Some years later Strauss gave a detailed account of the characteristic phenomenon which appears after intraperitoneal injection of a suspension of the organisms into male guinea pigs. In some cases considerable time may elapse before the typical manifestation is observed, although when a pure culture is used the scrotal swelling may appear within 3 or 5 days.

A. mallei (formerly called *Bacillus-, Pfeifferella-, Malleomyces-* and lately also *Loefflerella mallei*) is a slender, straight or slightly curved bacterium with rounded ends, 2 to 5 micra long and 0.5 micron broad. In materials from glanderous lesions the rods often stain irregularly and, although they are not acid-fast and do not take the Gram-stain, they bear some morphologic resemblance to tubercle bacteria. The characteristic bead-like appearance in older cultures is caused by partial degeneration of the organisms. As a rule, these "rough" forms are less virulent than the recently isolated "smooth" cultures.

A. mallei can be easily stained with ordinary aniline dyes, Löffler's alkaline methylene-blue giving the clearest picture. In histological sections demonstration of the bacteria is much more difficult.

Cultivation from closed abscesses in the lungs or in a lymph node can be carried out on ordinary media. The direct isolation of the organism from ulcerated skin lesions or muco-purulent exudate from the nostrils rarely succeeds. In chronic cases it is particularly hard to establish the aetiology of the disease by bacteriological means. The most suitable media for cultivation are glycerin–agar, glycerin–serum–agar and glycerinated potatoes.

Overgrowth of contaminating organisms, such as *Escherichia coli,* cocci and sarcina, inhibits the appearance of the small transparent blueish-grey colonies of *A. mallei.* When incubation is prolonged for a few days, the colonies become whitish, yellowish or even slightly brownish in colour; finally their consistency turns slimy. On glycerinated potato the growth resembles drops of honey and is more pigmented than it is on an agar-medium.

A. mallei is very sensitive to light, heat and desiccation. It is difficult to keep it alive on agar media. On glycerinated potato-slants in closed tubes it will survive in darkness at room-temperature for at least a month. The virulence of the strains to be used for mallein production can be maintained by injecting guinea pigs intraperitoneally every 2 months.

A. mallei is pathogenic to equines (horse, mule, ass), camels and felines. Wild felines in particular such as lions, tigers and leopards, can easily be infected. The incidence in these carnivores depends on their feeding on the meat and internal organs from glanderous horses.

It is possible to infect guinea pigs, laboratory- and field-mice and cats experimentally. Dogs and rabbits are more resistant. Whereas cattle and sheep are only slightly susceptible, goats are more sensitive. Horses are readily infected with their food or drinking water. Marxer (1915) was able to cause the disease in horses by subcutaneous inoculation of 1/250,000 loopful of virulent culture.

Lobel *et al.* (1941) observed a strain of *A. mallei* isolated from a native horse in Indonesia which had a high degree of virulence, although in that country glanders usually takes a chronic course and is not dangerous. The disease which occurs rather frequently in horses in Java has never been observed in lions and tigers in the local zoological gardens there.

It is often possible to recognise chronic malleus by diagnostic tests before clinical symptoms become manifest and before the animals are spreading the organisms.

In 1896 McFadyean found specific agglutinins in infected horses at titres of 1:1000 or higher. Other investigators concluded that only titres above 1:640 were of diagnostic significance. The complement fixation and conglutinating complement-absorption tests are free from this drawback of the agglutination test and are now commonly applied; the antigen used in these tests consists of an extract of glanders bacteria cultivated on glycerol–agar. Non-specific reactions are very rare. In Indonesia misleading results have mainly been found in West-Java and Celebes, where pseudo-malleus (melioidosis) prevails both in man and animals (Van der Schaaf, 1940). The conglutinating complement-absorption test is the most sensitive; it allows the detection of antibodies in chronically infected man and animals for a long period of time.

The mallein skin and ophthalmic tests are very reliable in the detection of infected horses. Mallein can be prepared by growing *A. mallei* in a thin layer of glycerol broth for 4 weeks. For the ophthalmic test it is concentrated by evaporation of the water by heating the culture to a temperature of 80°. The tested horses must remain under constant supervision for a period of 48 hours.

Much easier and more specific is the intrapalpebral test, which is carried out by injecting 0.1 ml of the concentrated mallein into the skin of the lower eye-lid. The development of oedema, mucopurulent exudate in the corner of the eye and acute inflammatory changes of the conjunctiva are signs of a positive reaction. A drawback of the intrapalpebral test is that it causes, in a certain percentage of the horses, an increase of agglutinating and complement fixing antibodies, the increase being maintained during a maximum period of 30 days (Kelser and Hardenberg, 1920).

The intradermal test has also been applied for diagnostic purposes in man. The mallein then has to be diluted 1:10.000 (Miller *et al.*).

The "Strauss-reaction" is still generally used for diagnostic purposes. It should however be taken into consideration that not only *A. mallei*, but also *Pseudomonas pseudomallei* and *Ps. aeruginosa* can produce a similar purulent periorchitis a few days after injection.

A. mallei has a specific affinity for the lungs and mucous membranes of the nose, larynx and trachea. Furthermore, abscesses can be found in the lymph nodes, liver, spleen and subcutaneous lymph vessels. The cutaneous form (Fig. 24), which formerly was called *farcy,* can be caused by wound infection or appears as a sequel of generalisation of lung lesions. In *horses* the infection usually takes a chronic course, but sometimes they die in 3 to 4 weeks. In such acute cases the animals run high temperatures of an undulant type. Some days after infection the mucous membrane of the nose becomes hyperaemic with the formation of small nodules and very soon also of ulcers, upon which the slimy exudate of the nostrils becomes more purulent and sometimes blood stained. The respiration rate is more frequent than usual and, if there are also lesions in the bronchi, trachea

References p. 193

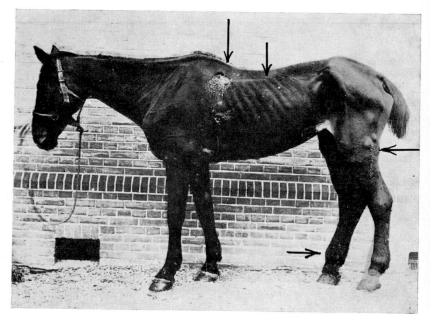

Fig. 24.   Subacute malleus in a horse.
(Photo: Department of Veterinary Bacteriology, State University, Utrecht)

and larynx, a suppressed cough frequently occurs. In the meantime the submaxillary lymph nodes, unilateral or on both sides, can show considerable swelling, but they never burst as in strangles.

In very chronic cases the typical "icefern scars" appear on the inter-

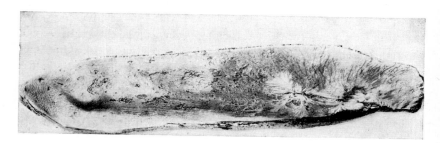

Fig. 25.   "Ice fern scars" on the internasal septum of a horse with chronic malleus.
(Photo: Institute for Veterinary Pathology, State University, Utrecht)

nasal septum or in the trachea, and are often combined with fresh ulcers on other places (Fig. 25).

The hidden form of glanders is very common in horses. This form can be diagnosed only by allergic and sero-tests. In the Austrian army, in 1915, squadrons equipped with only allergically and sero-logically positive horses were formed. Wintersberger had the opportunity to observe these horses over a considerable period of time and was thus able to make many bacteriological and histological examinations. Of 64 *post mortem* examinations of horses of such a "Rotzstaffel", which had all shown positive allergic reactions and complement-fixation tests, only 23 were considered histologically positive and 6 dubious. Had those horses been kept under more favourable circumstances, the percentage of cured cases would undoubtedly have been much higher.

Notwithstanding the very low incidence of malleus in *mules* and *asses*, the disease is generally far more acute in these animals as compared with horses. They often die in a few weeks from severe pneumonia and generalised pyaemic conditions.

Among wild animals kept in captivity, considerable losses were observed during and after the first world war. Reiff (1919) mentions that the circus of Sarrasani in Dresden lost 14 *tigers* and 12 *lions* from malleus. In Hagenbeck's menagerie in Hamburg 12 *lions*, 8 *tigers*, 10 *polar bears*, 1 *Malayan bear*, 1 *leopard* and 1 *jackal* died from glanders. The disease was also observed in *hyaenas*, but these animals were more resistant and recovered.

The symptoms mentioned in these wild animals were dullness, painfulness of the pads, conjunctivitis and mucous discharge, often streaked with blood from the nose. The animals sniffled as though they had difficulty in breathing through the nose. Abscesses or ulcers on the skin of the paws or the head were regularly observed. The ulcers did not show any tendency to heal and the lymphatics leading from them were thickened cords. At *post mortem* examination a penetrating smell of the brown-reddish fluid from the nose was most evident. The mucous membranes of the nasal cavities were intensely eroded. The lungs showed acute broncho-pneumonia, but the abdominal organs were not affected.

Glanders of *man*, is an occupational disease which affects persons having close contact with glanderous equines or carcasses of such animals (coachmen, cavalrymen, veterinarians, butchers).

References p. 193

Rainard, of the École Vétérinaire in Lyon, reported in 1842 on malleus infection of himself and 11 veterinary students, of whom 8 died of the acute form of the disease, while 3 were chronically ill for a considerable time.

During the first world war some cases were observed amongst the military forces. Lührs described an accidental, acute infection of a veterinary surgeon. A young healthy officer scratched himself in the left forefinger at the autopsy of a glanderous horse. He disinfected the small wound, but nevertheless, 2 days later, he did not feel well and was feverish. The finger was somewhat swollen, and from a small vesicle around the scratch wound he could press a drop of pus. The regional axillary lymph node was painful. The following day he felt better, but from the seventh to the tenth day his temperature rose every day to 39°, dropping to normal in the evening. On the 20th day after infection the nose started to swell and during the following days the skin showed erythematous swelling, spreading to the right cheek and the right eye. Abscesses were formed, which burst, giving rise to malignant ulcers, and causing pronounced deformation of the face. Several days later the nose became blue and covered with haemorrhagic vesicles and this was followed by gangrene and complicated by lung lesions. The diagnosis was confirmed by a positive complement-fixation test 5 days before death.

The risk of laboratory infections with A. mallei has been clearly demonstrated in a publication by Roelofs (1929). He described the lethal disease in a laboratory technician from the Amsterdam slaughterhouse. The young man had handled cultures of the glanders bacterium isolated from the lungs of a naturally infected horse. About 5 days after contamination, perhaps of conjunctival origin, the man fell ill with high fever, headache and nausea. 2 bluish coloured tumours developed on his left leg and the left eyelids were red and swollen. The swelling then extended to the left half of his nose with the formation of a pustule containing a haemorrhagic purulent exudate (Fig. 26). Afterwards the septum nasi and the left nosewing necrotised and pneumonia became obvious. Blood culture gave a pure growth of A. mallei.

The virulence of strains of A. mallei is subject to changes. Relatively low virulence has been claimed for several strains of Asiatic origin. This may perhaps explain why, in spite of the rather high frequency of glanders among horses in the Indonesian archipelago, no proven cases of infection have been reported in veterinarians or their attendants in these regions for the last 50 years.

Neither have human infections been noticed among the numerous personnel of the Veterinary Institute in Bogor (Buitenzorg, Java), where, ever since its foundation in 1910, large amounts of concentrated mallein have been prepared yearly. Several infected horses and test animals have been constantly at hand and the precautions taken for protection of the workers were rather elementary.

The papers of Murase et al. (1952) on equine glanders in Manchuria support the belief that in that part of East-Asia also the virulence of the malleus bacterium for human beings is slight. Contrary to this, the

incurable cases of malleus in man published by Sabolotny (1926) in
Russia, and those earlier recorded by Breithor (1919) and Lührs (1920)
among German army personnel, demonstrated a high mortality rate of
the disease in Europe. Robins had already shown as early as 1906 that, in
Canada, man rarely recovers from glanders. Of 43 grooms, 18 coachmen,

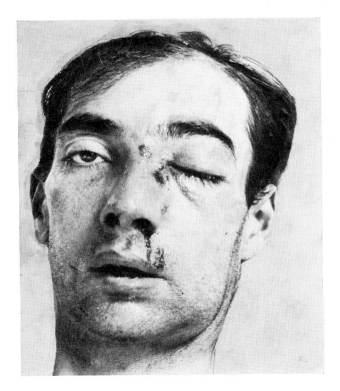

Fig. 26.   Acute malleus of a slaughter-house employee.
(By courtesy of Dr. D. Herderschêe, Amsterdam)

17 veterinarians, 5 surgeons and 73 other people, 147 (94%) died during
the acute or chronic stage of the disease.

Only a few serious cases in man have been reported from South Asia.
Gaiger, of the Indian Civil Veterinary Department, contracted the infection from an Arab pony in 1911 and, after he had been treated surgically several times during two years, he was cured, but lost an arm. Hunter

(1920) described a fatal case in a veterinary officer employed in laboratory work in Naini Tal in the North of India. In 1919, von Brunn summarized 394 cases of glanders in man; 110 were reported from Germany, 58 from Russia, 23 from North America, 109 from Cuba, 2 from Belgium, 7 from Rumania and 1 from Switzerland. Since the first world war the frequency of the infection in horses in the Western hemisphere has declined to practically nil, human glanders being restricted now to accidental contaminations of laboratory workers engaged in the production of mallein and antigens for serological tests*.

Acute glanders of man and animals was formerly incurable. In the more chronic phase, many humans and even horses suffered acute exacerbations, dying after the disease had run a course of over half a year.

After the introduction of sulfa-drugs and antibiotics as therapeutic agents in glanders the prognosis has changed from unfavourable to favourable.

Miller *et al.* (1948) showed that sulfathiazole and streptothricin are bacteriostatic to *A. mallei.* They have been recommended as drugs for topical and systemic treatment. The therapeutic effect of streptothricin is limited because of its toxicity. According to the experiments of Miller *et al.,* sulfadiazine is very active in guinea pigs with acute infections. Howe and Miller used it successfully in 6 rather benign cases of glanders occurring in laboratory staff.

The three severely ill patients recorded by Tezok (1958), regained health after treatment with tetracyclines, streptomycin and penicillin. Similar good results were reported by Ansari and Minou (1951) in Iran with sulfadiazine. Favourable effects are also recorded in horses after oral application of sulfadiazine and sulfamezathine, but in most countries treatment of animals is not allowed because of the risk of recidival spread.

In 1899 Nocard had already observed that glanderous horses could recover, but after disappearance of the bacteria from the body the recovered animals were as susceptible as the controls. The immunizing capacity of dead and living attenuated bacilli has been investigated many times, generally with negative results. Experiences with vaccines based on various principles have not yielded satisfactory results.

---

* In 1963, Rubin *et al.* speculated that *P. pseudomalleus* (see next chapter) might have been the aetiologic agent of many of the past cases of diagnosed "glanders" in man and animals.

Control of the disease in horses by hygienic procedures alone offers no difficulty in countries which dispose of a modern and comprehensive veterinary service. Because of the reliability of allergic and serological tests in bringing to light clinical and hidden infections, the disease can be promptly eradicated by slaughtering all affected animals. This method, if it is legally enforced, will soon turn the glanderous horse into an oddity. The low resistance of the glanders bacteria against certain conditions in nature and to disinfectants is to be looked upon as one of the reasons for the beneficial results of the usual control measures.

Nevertheless, both of the following contradictory opinions of Bory and Panisset respectively seem to be valid for this disease at the present time: "Glanders is a disease of the past", and "The question has lost none of its actuality".

REFERENCES

Ansari, M. and M. Minou, *Ann. Inst. Pasteur*, 81 (1951) 98.
Breithor, *Berl. tierärztl. Wschr.*, 35 (1919) 35.
Howe, C. and R. Miller, *Ann. intern. Med.*, 26 (1947) 93.
Hunter, T., *Vet. J.*, 77 (1920) 156.
Lührs, Z. *Veterinärk.*, 32 (1920) 133; *Mh. prakt. Tierheilk.*, 30 (1920) 359.
Mc Fadyean, J., *J. comp. Path.*, 17 (1904) 295.
Mc Gilvray, C. D., *J. Amer. vet. med. Ass.*, 55 (1919) 627; 104 (1944) 255.
Murase, N., A. Juraki, J. Tien and F. Shimzu, *Jap. J. vet. Sci.*, 14 (1952) 157.
Murase, N., A. Juraki, J. Tien, F. Shimzu and H. Ashirawi, *Jap. J. vet. Sci.*, 14 (1952) 175.
Nocard, M., *Bull. Soc. Sci. méd. vét.*, 48 (1894) 225 and 367; 53 (1899) 502.
Overbeek, A. A., *T. Diergeneesk.*, 52 (1925) 808.
Rainard, J. *Méd. Lyon*, (1842) 333.
Reiff, J., *Dissertation*, Mainz, 1919.
Robins, G. D., *Stud. Roy. Victoria Hosp., Montreal*, 2 (1906) 1.
Roelofs, J. W., *Ned. T. Geneesk.*, 73 (1929) 3272.
Rubin, H. L., A. D. Alexander and R. H. Yager, *Military Med.*, 128 (1963) 538.
Schaaf, A. v. d., *Jaarverslag Burgel. Veeartsenijk. Dienst in Ned.-Indië*, (1940) 90.
Solleysel, De, *Le parfait maréchal qui enseigne à connoistre la beauté, la bonté et les défauts des chevaux*, 1691.
Stableforth, A. W. and I. A. Galloway, *Infectious diseases of animals*, 1 (1959) 296.
Strauss, I., *Arch. exp. Vet.-Med.*, 1 (1889) 460.
Tezok, F., *VII. Internat. Congr. Microbiol., Abstr.*, 1958, p. 344.

11

A. VAN DER SCHAAF

Melioidosis

(Pseudo-malleus, Whitmore's disease)

Melioidosis is an acute, subacute or chronic septic or pyaemic infection which has, in man, some similarity to glanders. Most probably the disease originated from south-east Asia. In the chronic form the lungs, joints and kidneys are often affected, and sometimes abscesses are localized in the skin or subcutaneous tissues only.

In animals, natural infection usually takes a chronic course, the malignant character being less pronounced. Unlike glanders, melioidosis is, particularly in horses, rarely a serious disease.

Pseudomonas (Malleomyces) pseudomallei (Bacillus whitmori) was first recognized as the causative agent of a malleus-like disease in undernourished people by Whitmore and Krishnawami (1912). Of the 38 cases described, 31 patients were morphine-addicts, and the infections were probably caused by injection with a contaminated needle. The patients, all of them males, often had cutaneous and subcutaneous abscesses, but Whitmore's bacterium could be isolated from only 1 case.

Fletcher, in 1913, studied an outbreak of a septicaemic disease among laboratory animals, conveyed through contaminated food, in which the causative organism was identified. A few years later, Stanton and Hennessy, in the Governmental Laboratories of the Federated Malay States, demonstrated the same organism at post mortem examination of lesions in patients who had recovered from an initial attack of a disease resembling asiatic cholera; they suffered from a pyaemic condition and had lesions in the lungs and other viscera, which resembled those of tuberculosis. They also described clinical cases with cutaneous vesicles containing pus, from which the pseudoglanders bacterium could be cultivated. Later on, the same investigators were able to isolate the organism from blood, sputum and urine. Identical lesions could be reproduced in laboratory animals, monkeys, sheep and goats.

Fletcher (1919) compared the micro-organism isolated by Stanton and Hennessy with the organisms he had found and could not indicate any differences. Stanton and Fletcher further established the identity of *B. pseudomallei* of Whitmore with the micro-organisms they had isolated and proposed to call the disease melioidosis, according to the word *melis* given to a glanders-like condition already described in early times by Greek physicians.

Several publications on the disease in south-east Asia appeared thereafter.

According to the seventh edition of Bergey's Manual the name *Pseudomonas pseudomallei* should be given to Whitmore's bacillus instead of *Malleomyces pseudomallei*.

The organism has 1 to 4 polar flagella, produces a yellow pigment which can be extracted by a weak solution of hydrochloric acid, and slowly liquefies gelatine and bloodserum; all these properties are closer to those of *Pseudomonadaceae* than to those of the *Brucellaceae*. The bacterium of pseudoglanders is gram-negative, aerobic, motile and has, especially in animal- or human tissue or exudate, a safety-pin like form, whereby it could be mistaken for *Pasteurella pestis* or *P. pseudotuberculosis*.

Its growth in artificial media is typical. On glycerine–agar and glycerine–potato it forms flat, smooth, greyish-white colonies with a metallic luster. After several days most of the colonies become rough, wrinkled and lace-like. The odour of the culture is typical and reminds one of the urine of mice. In broth, the growth is turbid and forms a supernatant pellicle which might suggest that there is a contamination with *Alcaligenes faecalis* or *B. laterospores*.

An extensive description of the first clinically recognized case in a native farmer in Java was given by De Moor, Soekarnen and Van de Walle (1932). Several years later, the author and Rosa (1938) identified as *M. pseudomallei* a glanders-bacterium-like organism isolated in the same district (Bantam) from a *horse* suffering from subacute purulent pneumonia. They found that a considerable number of horses in West Java had specific complement-fixing antibodies for this micro-organism in their bloodserum without showing any clinical symptom suggestive of glanders. Davie and Wells (1952) observed 3 similar cases in race horses in Malay. The diagnosis was made only after sudden death occurring 4 to 6 weeks after the animals had raced for the last time. It was shown that gross lung lesions had developed within a short period.

The first case of melioidosis in *cattle* was diagnosed *post mortem* by Nicolls in Ceylon (1927). The only lesion found was a splenic abscess.

In Australia (Cottew, 1955) the disease has been more frequently recognized in *sheep* and *goats*. During the first observed outbreak in 1949, about 2 % of a herd of 4,000 sheep died, many animals showing staggering gait and inability to continue walking after they had been driven (Cottew *et al.,* 1952). The organism often caused not only suppurative arthritis, but also purulent meningo-encephalitis. In Queensland enzootic outbreaks have been recorded in goats as well. Olds and Lewis examined 6 herds comprising 385 goats. Out of 66 destroyed animals, all of which agglutinated *P. pseudomallei* and/or reacted in the allergic test, 27 exhibited typical lesions. In only 3 of the goats the fatal disease was more or less acute, while the others had chronic abscesses in the lymph nodes, lungs or joints and one showed lesions of the udder with excretion of the organisms in the apparently normal milk.

Melioidosis has also been demonstrated in *pigs*. The first recorded isolation of *P. pseudomallei* from a hog was described in 1936 by Girard from Tannarif, Madagascar. All he found was an abscess in a submaxillary lymphnode. It was suggested that pigs can be healthy spreaders of the melioidosis organisms. Lewis and Olds, in 1953, demonstrated lesions in a pig living with infected goats and sheep on an Australian farm. Enzootic outbreaks in hogs only have been observed in Vietnam by Nguyen-Ba-Luong (1956).

Melioidosis in man and animals has seldom been reported from the Western Hemisphere. The cases on record are of American soldiers who had returned from the Pacific area (Guam); 2 single autochthonous cases are known of persons who had never left the U.S.A.

An enzootic outbreak of melioidosis in sheep, goats and pigs on Aruba (Netherland Antilles), recorded by Sutmöller, Kraneveld and Van der Schaaf (1957) probably originated from an imported ram (Clara Nigg, personal communication).

Melioidosis is limited in its distribution to certain tropical and subtropical regions. Its incidence is highest amongst man and animals in south-east Asia. Most reports emanate from Burma, Thailand, Malaya, Indochina and Vietnam. In Indonesia the infection has rarely been diagnosed in man and only once, *post mortem,* in a horse. Australian publications mention cases in ruminants and in one pig, while human infections have not been recorded. From Africa there are only a few communications about the disease in man and only one on melioidosis in animals (a pig in Madagascar).

The assumption that in cool climates Whitmore's bacterium loses its virulence is supported by the observation that freeze-dried cultures are often much less virulent for guinea pigs than are original cultures kept in a milk medium at room temperature for several months.

Doubt has been expressed whether the disease is a true zoonosis, because it has not been possible so far to demonstrate immediate transmission of animal melioidosis to man. In several cases, the infection seems to be connected with polluted pond-water, mud or paddy-fields.

Investigations by Leclerc and Sureau on the presence of two specific anti-*P. pseudomallei* bacteriophages in North-Vietnam showed that 30 out of 152 samples from stagnant pond-water contained a specific phage. This significant percentage of positive findings suggests that pond-water is much more often contaminated than might have been expected from the small number of positive cultures.

Abrasions of the skin and wounds are often the portal of entry of the agent.

It has been suggested that the alimentary tract is another route of infection. Spraying of vegetables with polluted water and contamination of foodstuffs by the urine of infected rodents *(Rattus diardi* and *Mus griseiventer)* are possible means of spread of the infection. Moreover, since milk is a suitable medium for the preservation of *M. pseudomallei,* it may, together with soft cheese, be a vehicle for transmitting the organisms from infected animals to man.

Goats and sheep which sometimes develop lesions of the udder after septicaemic infection, shed the microbes in their milk (Cottew). Other excretions also, such as the nasal discharge, urine and bronchial exudate, may contain numerous organisms. Abscesses in lymph nodes resembling those of pseudotuberculosis may break through the skin and thus may contaminate paddocks and barns.

In *human beings,* skin-affections often take a chronic course with periodic flare-ups. Abscesses and ulcers in the intestinal wall result in faecal contamination of water. Biting insects such as the fleas of rats and man and also mosquitoes and stable flies, can easily transmit the organism from sick to healthy animals in a shed. Morphine-addicts with open skin lesions not only contaminate their bedding, but may also be the source of the infection of bloodsucking and non-biting arthropod parasites.

Blanc and Balthazard have shown that *Xenopsylla cheopis* and *Aëdes aegypti* readily become infected by sucking blood from diseased laboratory animals. The organisms multiply in the digestive tracts of these insects and survive for a considerable time in their faeces.

Natural infections of man are not very frequently diagnosed and are not epidemic. General weakness, exhaustion, avitaminosis and other stress factors have been mentioned as influences which diminish resistance. Most human infections, however, result from the contamination of wounds under unhygienic conditions. Accidents and injuries often promote the development of the disease.

As in brucellosis, tularaemia and malleus, laboratory infections occur in persons working with *P. pseudomallei*. Phung Van Dan mentioned 3 cases of melioidosis amongst members of the staff of the Pasteur Institute in Saigon. In 1 person the infection originated from a small wound of the forefinger, accidentally caused by manipulating a broken pipette loaded with a suspension of *P. pseudomallei*. In the other 2 cases the infection was attributed to inhalation or oral contamination. In 2 patients the organism was isolated from an axillary lymph node and from the bronchial exudate respectively and in the third case, the diagnosis could only be made by serological methods. According to Rubin *et al.* (1963), by 1932, 83 buman cases with a mortality rate of 80 to 95 percent had been reported. After World War II, both severe and chronic cases of melioidosis were recognized in the U. S. A., France, India and Guam. Most were soldiers or veterans who had served in S. E. Asia (Fournier *et al.*, 1958).

The pathogenicity for man and different kinds of animals is approximately equal.

In man, according to De Moor *et al.* (1932), 3 different syndromes can be distinguished. These are:

(1) The peracute septicaemic condition which is usually characterized by high fever, diarrhoea, chest-pain and collapse, symptoms which would also indicate cholera, plague or tropical malaria. A correct diagnosis can eventually be made by cultivating the organism from the blood.

(2) The subacute pyaemic form of the disease may be confused with typhoid fever, miliary tuberculosis and endocarditis. Abscesses are often formed in various organs, including the lungs, kidneys, joints and testes. In these cases, diagnosis can be made by cultivating the organism from the pus.

(3) The chronic local inflammation resembles, in some respects, lues, tuberculosis or chronic osteomyelitis. Cutaneous and subcutaneous abscesses are not very painful and general health is usually not much

impaired. Puncture of the lesions for diagnostic purposes is advocated. In animals the disease is very seldom diagnosed during life. The pathogenic effect of artificial infection depends mainly on the portal of entry and the number of the bacteria. Guinea pigs and rabbits are very susceptible and can be readily infected by conjunctival contamination or through scarifications of the skin. The pathological changes resemble those of pseudotuberculosis rodentium.

After intraperitoneal injection of a small number of virulent organisms, male guinea pigs show a Strauss reaction (see page 187).

Experimental infections always take a chronic course, with abscesses in different organs and lymph-nodes. As in the spontaneous disease, artificial infection often provokes polyarthritis and lameness. Goats and sheep can be infected orally with melioidosis-pus or culture of *P. pseudomallei*. Pigs are easily infected subcutaneously.

According to the author's observation the organisms can still be cultivated from abscesses in lymph-nodes, lungs and spleen after several months. Horses are very resistant, although they become sensitized against melioidin and sometimes more or less against mallein as well.

The clinical symptoms of spontaneous melioidosis are so polymorphic that laboratory methods are essential for diagnosis during life.

Body excretions, with the exception of pus obtained by puncture from abscesses, are usually heavily contaminated with saprophytic organisms and this makes direct isolation of the causative agent very difficult.

Not all guinea pigs are uniformly susceptible. Hamsters and ferrets, on the other hand, are regularly killed by the introduction of a small number of *P. pseudomallei*. Loss of virulence of a culture markedly hampers the biological test (Miller *et al.*, 1948).

Serological tests are, therefore, usually indispensable. The agglutination reaction is often not sufficiently reliable. Most cultures exhibit a tendency to grow in a rough form and this fact makes them unsuitable for agglutination. Nigg *et al.* (1956) proved that the virulence of some strains can be enhanced and the R (rough) variant be changed into an agglutinable S (smooth) variant by serial passage through white mice.

According to a communication from Lapeysonnie, 4% of human sera give false positive reactions, especially those of persons affected by salmonellosis or rickettsiosis. The haemagglutination test of Middlebrook-Dubos is more sensitive, but even with this technique there still remain 3% of non-specific results.

The most reliable serological method is the complement-fixation reaction. In the author's experiments with goats, sheep, pigs and horses, no non-specific reactions were observed.

The antigen is prepared according to the same principles as those recommended for the complement-fixation test in glanders. False positive results with melioidosis antigen have been noticed only in horses and men suffering from malleus. The simultaneous test with both titrated antigens has proved useful for the differentiation of malleus from pseudomalleus in horses. In cases of glanders the serum-titres are higher with the malleus antigen; in the usually benign melioidosis infection of horses, the Whitmore-antigen provides a higher titre (personal observation by the author).

Australian investigators found that the allergic test with melioidin (concentrated broth or culture on synthetic medium) is very useful for diagnostic purpose in sheep. Reactions following intracutaneous injection of 0.1 ml of melioidin into the caudal fold or the lower eyelid were observed on the third or fourth day. Mallein provokes a much weaker reaction in sheep or horses infected with melioidosis. On the other hand, in glanderous horses the reverse is seen.

Sulphonamides and various antibiotics have been tried for the treatment of human melioidosis. It was found that early treatment with sulfadiazine had a favourable effect (Miller *et al.,* 1948). *In vitro,* all cultures of *P. pseudomallei* are sensitive to chloromycetin. Thus application of this antibiotic in combination with sulfamezathine or sulfadiazine, both in massive doses, is probably the treatment of choice for the arrest of the subacute, usually malignant course of the infection in man.

Prevention of the disease in man and animals is a complex matter.

Delbove and Reynes (1942) state that there was, in most cases of human melioidosis, a history of lowered resistance due to shock, malnutrition, chronic intoxication or another chronic disease. In south-east Asia, white people are more sensitive than natives are.

In regions where the infection is endemic, every person with serious wounds, who has been in contact with stagnant water or the mud of ponds, canals or ricefields, should be treated prophylactically with the drugs mentioned above. Pollution of vegetables and fruit by the urine of rodents should be prevented. Infected sheep or goats must be slaughtered. Methods of eradication based on serological and allergic tests in infected herds have sometimes been successful.

Heat-killed and formalinized cultures have occasionally been used as vaccines, but the results are doubtful. Stanton and Fletcher (1932) found that rabbits and guinea pigs could not be immunized by inoculation with the heat-killed bacteria. The chronic course and frequent recurrence of the disease suggest that infected human beings do not develop immunity.

The incidence of melioidosis in human beings and animals seems to be higher than the meager data recorded in the medical and veterinary literature suggest. Further study is needed of its transmission, direct or indirect, from animals to man.

REFERENCES

BLANC, G. and M. BALTHAZARD, *Arch. Inst. Pasteur Maroc.*, 3 (1947) 574.

BRYGOO, E. R. and C. RICHARD, *Ann. Inst. Pasteur*, 83 (1953) 822.

COTTEW, G. S., A. K. SUTHERLAND and J. F. MEEHAND, *Aust. vet. J.*, 23 (1952) 113.

COTTEW, G. S., *Aust. vet. J.*, 31 (1955) 155.

DAVIE, J. and C. W. WELLS, *Brit. vet. J.*, 108 (1952) 161.

FOURNIER, J. and L. CHAMBON, *La Mélioidosis*, Paris, 1958, pp. 106.

LAPEYSONNIE, L., *Ann. Inst. Pasteur*, 95 (1958) 334.

LECLERC, H. and P. SUREAU, *Bull. Soc. Path. exot.*, 49 (1956) 874.

LEWIS, F. A. and R. J. OLDS, *Aust. vet. J.*, 28 (1952) 145.

MILLER, W. R., L. PANNEL, L. VRAUTZ, W. A. TANNER and T. ROSEBURRY, *J. Bact.*, 55 (1948) 127.

MIRICK, G. S., H. M. ZIMMERMAN, G. D. MANER and A. A. HUMPHRY, *J. Amer. med. Ass.*, 130 (1946) 1063.

MOOR, C. E. DE, SOEKARNEN, and N. V. D. WALLE, *Geneesk. T. Ned. Indië*, 72 (1932) 1618.

NGUYEN-BA-LUONG, *Bull. Soc. Path. exot.*, 49 (1956) 25.

NIGG, C., J. RUICK, E. SCOTT and K. NOBLE, *J. Bact.*, 71 (1956) 530.

OLDS, R. J. and F. A. LEWIS, *Austr. vet. J.*, 30 (1954) 253; 31 (1955) 273.

PATON, J. P. J., C. R. PECK and A. V. D. SCHAAF, *Brit. med. J.*, 1 (1947) 336.

PHUNG VAN DAN, *Thèse*, Lyon, 31 (1957).

RUBIN, H. L., A. D. ALEXANDER and R. H. YAGER, *Milit. Med.*, 128 (1963) 538.

SCHAAF, A. V. D and M. ROZA, *Ann. Rep. Indonesia*, (1938) 92.

STANTON, A. T. and W. FLETCHER, *J. Hyg.*, 23 (1925) 347.

SUTMÖLLER, P., F. C. KRANEVELD and A. V. D. SCHAAF, *J. Amer. vet. med. Ass.*, 130 (1957) 415.

12

J. VAN DER HOEDEN

Anthrax

(Splenic fever, charbon (bactéridien), fièvre charbonneuse,
Milzbrand, malignant carbuncle, pustula maligna, wool sorter's disease)

Anthrax is a disease known from early history. Investigation of its cause was the first of the studies of pathogenic micro-organisms ever made and from this study much of the fundamental knowledge of microbiology has been derived.

There are, in ancient Hindu, Hebrew, Indian, Greek, Roman and Arabic literature, numerous descriptions of diseases which are suggestive of anthrax. If these suggestions are right, the incidence of anthrax in ancient times was very high and represented a serious hazard to human and animal health. Several communications indicated the occurrence of epizootics over vast geographical regions, causing tremendous ravage. Tens of thousands of human beings, and still larger numbers of animals, perished.

At the turn of the 17th century, a considerable number of cattle were destroyed by a plague which seems to have been anthrax, some 60,000 people dying from the same disease. In the middle of the 18th century, anthrax apparently killed off from 25–50 % of the sheep in Europe. A hundred years later, the disease still prevailed panzootically throughout the European continent. In France, nearly half of all the cattle and sheep succumbed, with the result that animal industry was almost ruined.

French publications of the 18th and early 19th century contain interesting records of the frequent occurrence of "charbon malin" (Chabert, 1780). Fournier described the "malignant pustule" in man in 1767, and in 1788 Andreevskii recorded the "Siberian ulcer" in the Ural province of Russia.

In 1823, Barthélémy proved the infectious character of anthrax by inoculating healthy animals with the blood of sheep which had died of the disease. Rayer and Davaine (1850) discovered sticks and filaments in the blood and organs of affected sheep. 5 years later, Pollender published a complete description of these bodies, which he compared with vibrios. Delafond (1860) established their living nature and diagnostic value, and laid the foundations of further classical research.

In 1863–64, Devaine recorded the important fact that anthrax could be transmitted to various species of animals only if the "bactéridies" were present in the injected material. The demonstration of similar rods in the malignant pustules of man strongly suggested that the aetiology of this disease was the same as that of anthrax in animals. It was these investigations which gave rise for the first time to the idea that there is a causal relation between microorganisms and infectious diseases.

Scientific confirmation of Davaine's thesis was provided by R. Koch's researches in 1876–77, when he grew in pure culture the bacillus with which anthrax could be produced. He also detected the formation of the highly resistent spores within the anthrax bacillus. Pasteur (1881), applying the method of multiplication *in vitro*, finally produced the first prophylactic vaccine ever made with attenuated bacteria.

Bacillus anthracis is a large, non-motile, aerobic, gram-positive, capsulated and sporulating organism. The ovoid spores appear only in the presence of oxygen.

On a solid medium the colonies have a characteristic groundglass-like appearance. At low magnifications they grow as long, convoluted, parallel chains of bacilli, which have a polar arrangement, so that the chains give a picture of wavy locks of hair, the "medusa's head". In gelatine stab-cultures, the growth resembles an inverted fir tree.

The spores, unlike the bacilli, are little sensitive to high or low temperatures, chemical disinfectants, drying or sunlight. In water at 120°, anthrax spores are destroyed within 5–15 minutes; in flowing steam at 100°, in 2 minutes; in dry heat at 120° only after about 1 hour. In the soil and in buried carcasses spores may survive for several years or decades. They are not destroyed in hides, which have been dried and salted in the usual way. Disinfectants in the usual dilutions fail to kill anthrax spores within several days. The vegetative form is killed at 60° within a few minutes and, in the unopened carcass, in which, owing to the absence of oxygen, no spores are produced, these forms soon die, chiefly because the putrifying organisms are antagonistic to them.

The resistence of the spores to heat is used to isolate *B. anthracis* from contaminated materials (carcasses, soil, hides, etc.). For the demonstration of anthrax bacilli, a suspension of the sample is heated at 80° for 10 minutes and then spread over an agar medium, or inoculated into a guinea pig, which will, if anthrax spores are present in the inoculum, die after 1 to 7 days, and will show at autopsy the characteristic picture of anthrax.

A method commonly applied for the detection of anthrax infection is the thermoprecipitin-test of Ascoli. A suspension of the material is heated at 100° and filtered. The clear fluid is placed over an immune serum (prepared in the donkey or horse by immunisation against *B. cereus (anthracoides)*, which is antigenically related to *B. anthracis*). If anthrax infection is present, a whitish disk of precipitate appears at the level of contact of the two fluids.

References p. 222–223

Anthrax still has a wide global distribution and affects a large range of animal species. In several countries in which no systematic control is enacted, the disease remained a major hazard to livestock. Extensive destruction of stock still occasionally occurs, *e.g.* in Siberia ("boil plague"), and other parts of Asia, in Southern Europe and Northern Africa and in some Latin American countries.

In certain areas, the soil is so heavily contaminated with anthrax spores that the disease is enzootic and endemic ("anthrax regions", "champs maudits", in France, Germany, Russia, Central-, South- and Minor Asia, Japan, Australia, South Africa, South America, Mexico, etc.). Epizootics, reported from Australia, claimed 200,000–300,000 victims among sheep. In Russia more than 43,000 cattle were lost from anthrax during the first months of 1914. In Lousiana, where the occurrence of anthrax in livestock can be traced back to the days of the French colonization, 2,000 farm animals perished from anthrax even in 1946.

Among domestic animals, *cattle, sheep* and *goats* are mainly affected. All herbivores are highly susceptible, whereas carnivores and omnivores are less affected. No mammal, however, possesses absolute natural immunity. Birds have often been considered refractory to natural infection, although by heavy exposure to spores and under adverse environmental conditions, they can contract the disease. Outbreaks in chickens have been reported.

Anthrax is relatively rare in adult *dogs,* but puppies are fairly susceptible. *Cats, rats* and several other small rodents showed little resistance to artificial infection.

In some localities (Texas and England) anthrax occurs among *wild deer,* and in countries where *camels* and *elephants* are domesticated, the disease is not uncommon among these animals. *Ostriches* (in Madagascar) and various mammals in zoological gardens, circuses *(lions, bears)* and on fur farms *(foxes, minks)* have been recorded as dying from anthrax contracted through ingestion of infected food. Sometimes spontaneous anthrax has also been observed in wild rodents *(gerbils).* Cold-blooded animals are not affected.

It seems that among various races and breeds of a given animal species resistance to anthrax may differ significantly. Thus, Algerian sheep and albino rats have been noted for their relatively low susceptibility.

The incidence of anthrax in domesticated animals often varies considerably from country to country (Table XVIII). This may be related to differences in the manner in which they are kept and fed.

TABLE XVIII

INCIDENCE OF ANTHRAX IN DOMESTIC ANIMALS

Country	Period	Total number of cases recorded	Cattle	Horses	Pigs	Sheep and goats	Other animals
Gr. Britain	1914–37	annually 400–700					
	1937	743 *	820	13	30	1	15
	1952	1215	729		479		7
Belgium	1930–45	3585	3321	114	122	28	
France	1926–39	2786					
Germany	1931–35	2948 *					
	1935	977	728	28	83	138	
Netherlands	1931–34	1164					
	1953–56	201					
Denmark	1934–38	240					
Poland	1935–38	2926 *					
Rumania	1935	7940	3383	523	71	3963	
Turkey	1928–39	3477 *					
Palestine	1942–47	405	151	24		228	1 **
U.S.A.	1945–54	3447 *					

* = outbreaks.
** = camel.

In several Mediterranean and Near Eastern countries, as well as in Australia and South America, small ruminants are the main victims of anthrax. Delpy and Kaweh reported that 1 million of the 15 million sheep in Iran had died from the disease during 1945.

Infections in equines are rather common in Japan and the Balkans. In the U.S.A. the loss of animals as a result of anthrax-infection amounted to 4,003 in 1946, 1,645 in 1948 (120 outbreaks in 14 States), 2,753 in 1951 (483 outbreaks in 25 states) and only 247 in 1956. During 10 years, between 1945–1955, the total losses amounted to 17,604 heads of livestock in 39 States.

If no measures of control are applied, the total number of anthrax cases in the animals of a given country usually remains fairly stable. Enforcement of prophylactic measures has markedly decreased the incidence of anthrax in several countries, or has even practically eradicated it. However, the risk of its reappearance in a "cleaned" area is constant when raw materials of animal origin, animal food stuffs and fertilizers continue to enter the country from heavily contaminated regions of the globe.

Every live or dead animal infected with *B. anthracis* is a potential hazard to *man*. The incidence of anthrax in humans parallels that found among the animals. Because animal products intended for industrial use are transported to remote parts of the world, the spread of the disease in the human population does not depend only on the density of the indigenous reservoir of infection, but is also correlated with the introduction of foreign materials contaminated with anthrax spores. In some countries fluctuations in the frequency of human infections are due to a greater extent to the incidence of anthrax among livestock of countries from which raw animal materials are imported than from its incidence in animals of the given country itself.

According to statistics supplied by the World Health Organization, the total number of annually reported cases of human anthrax in the world amounts to approximately 9,000. It is, however, thought that this figure underestimates the actual situation and it has been reasonably concluded that the world incidence in recent years fluctuated between 20,000 and 100,000 cases per annum (Glassman, 1958). The considerable improvements achieved in countries in which anthrax is systematically combated, show that, at the present time, the number of infections is out of proportion both to the total population of these countries and also to the number of agricultural and industrial workers in them. This can be elicited from data collected by the W.H.O. in its Epidemiological and Vital Statistics Reports (1958), (Table XIX).

Although the skin has been considered to be the tissue most susceptible to anthrax infection (Besredka), the principal portal of entrance of the anthrax bacillus into animals other than man is the digestive tract. Man, on the other hand, usually acquires his primary infection through minor wounds, abrasions or scratches of the skin. In animals the spores find their way unharmed through the animal stomach to the intestines, where they germinate. After they have gained access to the internal tissues, rapid multiplication occurs, and this is, most probably, further aided by the antiphagocytic property of the capsule which envelops the bacillus. Whenever the natural defenses of the body are sufficiently high, the animal soon overcomes the infection and recovery follows. If, however, bacteria

TABLE XIX

INCIDENCE OF HUMAN ANTHRAX DURING THE SIX-YEAR PERIOD 1951–1956

Reported from	Number of cases
Portugal	6,932
Spain	5,912
Italy	5,027
Yugoslavia	4,835
Kenya	4,178
Tanganyika	3,166
Ruanda-Urundi	1,967
Argentine	1,760
Chili	1,736
Iraq	1,333
Greece	828
Germany	104
Norway	4
Denmark	0

succeed in avoiding phagocytosis and the bactericidal action of the host animal, they invade the blood stream, but are mainly confined to the capillary system of the internal organs. Shortly before death, massive invasion of the general circulation occurs *(septicaemia ante mortem* of herbivores).

The duration of the incubation period in animals depends on the susceptibility of the host, the portal of entry, the number of spores and the virulence of the bacillus. In sheep it can be as short as 1 day; in cows and horses about 3 days (in less severe cases up to 6 or 10 days); in hogs about a week.

The course of the disease may be peracute, acute, subacute or chronic.

The *peracute (apoplectic) form* is commonest in ruminants, especially in sheep at the beginning of an enzootic, and it is also characteristic of anthrax in mink. The onset is sudden and a fatal fulminant infection follows, with the result that in many cases the animals are found dead without any prodromal evidence of disease having been noticed.

In other cases, sudden tremor, heavy convulsions, pounding heart beat and marked dyspnoea precede death only by a few minutes. Sometimes the process lasts from 1 to 2 hours. Often no definite changes are found at post-mortem examination, excepting those which indicate death by suffocation, bloody liquid flowing from the natural body openings, or incomplete rigor mortis and unclotted blood.

In birds an apoplectic form of anthrax has been noticed, with bloody excrements, spasms and cyanosis from which the animals soon succumb.

The *acute or subacute disease* is seen in the majority of cases. It starts with a rapidly rising temperature, a short stage of restlessness and excitement, followed by staggering gait, trembling, spasms, convulsions and a condition of heavy depression. Horses often limp, and, when they suffer from intestinal anthrax, are subject to severe attacks of colic. In cows gastric phenomena are accentuated. Pregnant animals abort. The milk secretion falls markedly or stops altogether. Subcutaneous oedema appears on several parts of the body, especially in horses, in which oedema is particularly found on the neck, the lower abdomen, the perineal region and external genitalia. In pigs, massive swellings have a jelly-like consistency and are mostly found around the head, particularly the throat and glottis, where they interfere with swallowing and breathing. Oedema of the glottis often causes death by suffocation. Considerable swelling of the tongue (glossanthrax) occurs in cows and swine. A dark bloody discharge flows from the nostrils, mouth, anus and vulva of ruminants and equines. *B. anthracis* can be recovered from the reddish coloured urine and faeces, as well as from the saliva.

In the *subacute form* of the disease carbuncles develop, which are at first usually located near the shoulder, neck and head. At the out set circumscribed and firm, they soon become diffuse and smooth. In cases of *glossanthrax* these lesions are often found in the tongue and mucosa of the mouth, where they soon ulcerate. Anthrax in dogs is particularly confined to the head, throat, tongue and intestines, showing ulcerating carbuncle-like swellings on the lips, tongue and toe-pads. Lesions of the intestines are predominant. Sometimes typical anthrax carbuncles are observed on the comb, tongue and legs of chickens.

The duration of fatal anthrax in cattle is usually from 10–36 hours, sometimes up to 2 days, rarely 5 days. In horses, the course of the disease is somewhat slower.

Topley, Wilson and Miles, excluding very mild and latent infections, claimed a mortality rate of untreated anthrax in animals, of 75–100%.

Rapid decomposition sets in in the carcasses of anthrax victims. Rigor mortis is incomplete. The blood is very dark and unclotted, with a tarry or muddy appearance. Much bloody effusion is present in the body-cavities. All internal organs are congested, and show several haemorrhagic spots. The spleen may be 3 to 5 times its normal size, the pulp being soft, dark and greasy, the surface wrinkled and the organ easily torn. The sub-cutaneous and sub-serous tissues, intestines and lymphatic glands show oedema and multiple haemorrhages.

The *chronic form* of anthrax is most frequently encountered in pigs and usually it starts in the tonsils. Exceptionally this infection develops a fatal septicaemia; but as a rule, it remains circumscribed to the places at which the bacilli entered and brings about a serohaemorrhagic or necrotic pharyngitis with regional and mesenteric lymphadenitis. This localized chronic form of porcine anthrax may appear to be so mild that it remains entirely unnoticed throughout life, and will be diagnosed only by chance at meat inspection of apparently healthy slaughter animals. Similar ob-servations have been recorded from "normal cows" showing hypertrophic lymphatic glands as the only visible lesions ("charbon bactéridien cryptique" of Provost and Trouette, 1957). In the spleen of obviously healthy horses, small metastatic anthrax carbuncles are casually detected.

It is claimed that these apparently normal carriers of *B. anthracis* are sometimes excreting the organism in their faeces, so that they represent an epizootiological hazard.

As compared to its primary importance in animals, alimentary infection in man is of little significance. Among 106 cases of anthrax in Germany (1923) and 405 in France (1910–1920), only 3 intestinal infections were reported in either statistics. In the U.S.A., alimentary anthrax has not been recorded. In places where the meat of slaughtered or dead animals affected with anthrax is eaten, it is only very exceptionally followed by intestinal infection.

According to Boquien (1950), the French department of Morbihan was the site of an anthrax epizootic in cattle. The meat of 3 of the animals was consumed by several persons but no intestinal infection ensued, though 14 of them, who had handled the animals and prepared the meat, suffered from multiple anthrax pustules and 1 died from meningitis.

In 1958, cutaneous anthrax accounted for more than 95% of all reported anthrax cases in the North American population.

Between 1919 and 1943, Smyth established the primary affection in the skin of 629 out of 640 human beings suffering from anthrax (98,3%). Among the small number of remaining cases, pulmonary, intestinal and meningeal localizations dominated the clinical picture. In the U.S.S.R. (1957) about 90% of cases in rural regions and 80% of those in industrial centres were of the cutaneous type.

Development of the malignant pustule starts after an incubation period of

References p. 222–223

2 or 3 days. At the point of infection a central vesicle appears, which is surrounded by an indurated, red area. This vesicle rapidly increases in size and the originally serous fluid becomes bloody. The infiltrated area then becomes tensely oedematous and several small blisters are formed at its edges. At the same time the central vesicle desiccates. As a result of coagulation-necrosis, a blue-blackish eschar develops and this soon turns into dark-brown or black ("charbon") (Fig. 27). The slough widens in

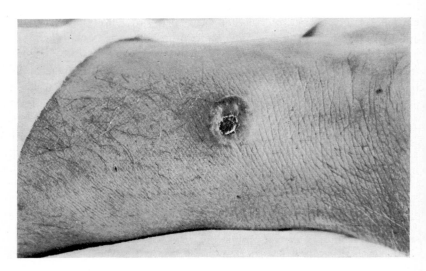

Fig. 27.   Malignant pustule *(anthrax)* on the wrist of a butcher.

surface area as well as in depth. The carbuncle itself is almost painless and in this respect differs from the regional lymphangitis and lymphadenitis which may be painful. At this stage, fever reaches a high degree and general malaise and prostration have developed.

The subsequent course depends greatly on the virulence of the bacilli and the site of the pustule.

With or without medical treatment, regression of the dermal affection may lead to recovery; but when this does not occur and, if the infection spreads into the lymphatics and the bloodstream, fatal bacteraemia may ensue. On the other hand, it is not rare that the development of the anthrax pustule deviates from the classical course just described. In these cases, it is difficult to distinguish skin anthrax from ordinary pustules or boils caused by other microorganisms, although the absence of pus and the black eschar are rather typical features of anthrax aetiology.

Because the malignant pustule develops at the site of the penetration of the bacilli into the skin, it is evident that the pustules are practically restricted to those parts of the skin that are unprotected (Table XX).

TABLE XX

LOCATION OF THE MALIGNANT PUSTULE IN MAN
(in percentage)

	Data collected by		
	Wolff and Heimann (1951) * *in the U.S.A.*	*Legge (1934)* ** *in England*	*Shliakhov (1957)* † *in the U.S.S.R.*
Arms	36	20.4	28
Legs	3	1.9	2.8
Hand	9	⎱ 44.6	
Face	23	⎰	⎱ 50.6
Head	11		⎰
Neck	14	31.2	14.5
Trunk	3	1.9	1.6
Shoulder	1		
Other sites			2.5

* 2,447 cases over the period 1919–1949.
** 937 cases.
† "several hundreds of cases".

Primary infection of the lungs or intestines and the entry of anthrax bacilli circulating in the blood into the very susceptible brain and meningeal tissues occurs in only 5% of the total number of human infections. Infection of the lungs, brain or meninges is serious. The lungs are invaded when dust particles laden with anthrax spores are inhaled. This form (wool sorter's disease) usually starts with a sudden, steeply rising body temperature and runs a swift, fatal course. It appears as an atypical pneumonia followed by signs of cardiac failure. Sometimes, the upper respiratory tract is also involved and empyema develops. The lungs, as a portal of entry, may also play a purely mechanical role when dry spores in particles, one or more micra in diameter, enter the alveoli and are carried through the lymphatic glands and the efferent lymph ducts to the blood stream, and thus initiate generalized anthrax (Ross, 1957).

The digestive tract is the most unlikely route of anthrax infection in human beings. Intestinal anthrax shows the clinical picture of haemorrhagic enteritis (bloody faeces), and multiple carbuncles are usually located in the mucosae of a limited part of the small intestines and the coecum.

In several countries the mortality rate of human anthrax has significantly decreased within the last two decades, partly as a result of earlier recognition of the aetiology of the infection and more efficient modern treatment. It should, however, be borne in mind that changes in recording techniques may also have influenced the statistical data.

The fatality rates of anthrax for the period 1919–1938 in the U.S.A. in general, and for the State of Louisiana in particular, amounted respectively to 22 and 30%; in the last 5 years of that period, the figures were 16 and 22% respectively. Anthrax mortality in North America decreased from approximately 20% in 1910–1920 to about 8% in the period 1939–1943 and to almost nil in the last few years.

Whereas the average percentage of fatal cases of external anthrax in Great Britain amounted to 19.6 in the years 1905–1909, it was only 2.3 during the period 1950–1954; the average percentages of deaths over the same periods were 19 and 1.2 respectively.

Holtzmann (1935) established an average fatality rate of 9.3% of anthrax cases occurring in the tannery industry in Germany, during the years 1929–1932, as compared to 12% among workers suffering from anthrax in the same industry, during the same period in the U.S.A.

Recurrent anthrax infection in one and the same individual has been reported. In Louisiana, where biting flies play an important part in the transmission of the disease, repeated infections within a year have been observed (Haren, 1947). Shliakhov recorded a case in Russia with attacks occurring 8, 15 and 30 years respectively after the initial infection.

The primary source of anthrax infection is always traceable to the animal world. Direct inter-human transmission is extremely rare.

Although carnivores are, as a rule, infected by eating parts of dead or slaughtered animals, and man is generally infected through contact with infected animals or their products, herbivores are usually indirectly contaminated by means of soil, water, food and objects polluted by the excretions, blood or tissues of animals which have died of anthrax.

The degree of multiplication of *B. anthracis* in nature outside the animal body has not been ascertained. Russian investigators, however, claim that spores may develop in soil rich in organic material, when the humidity, temperature and pH are favourable. The vegetative form is capable of sporulating and sporulation may repeat itself several times. In any event, once the soil has been contaminated, the extraordinarily resistant anthrax spores will stay in it for many years as a source of infection of all animals grazing on these fields or eating the crops grown on the contaminated soil.

In several Western countries, differences have been noticed in the seasonal incidence of anthrax among both cattle and sheep and the farmers who tend these animals. Until the beginning of the century, most anthrax cases occurred during the summer season on pasture ground, especially on marshy lands with a loose soil structure. In the Southern hemisphere (Australia) 70–80% of the total annual anthrax cases occur in the period between December and March.

The increased use of foodstuffs imported from countries in which anthrax is enzootic caused a shifting of the highest incidence of infections to the winter season, when the animals are fed in barns. Fertilizers containing products of animal origin (bone meal, bone dust) imported from enzootic parts of the world have also introduced new infections and have created anthrax reservoirs in previously uninfected regions.

During an unusually virulent outbreak of anthrax among animals in England in 1952, the sources of infection were traceable 1,001 times to imported foodstuffs, 42 times to contaminated fertilizers and 38 times to both. 20 cases were connected with the waste of tanneries and 21 occurred on premises known as "anthrax farms".

Many cases of anthrax recorded in the Midwestern states of the U.S.A. during 1951–52 were connected with imported bone meal. In contrast to the formerly sporadic cases in the State of Ohio, which affected only one or two farms of a certain region, the most severe outbreak on record, which occurred in 1952, affected all the counties in this State. The epizootiological spread was ascribed to the distribution of imported raw bone meal, which was mixed with local foodstuffs, the anthrax spores having been demonstrated in the foreign material.

The considerable reduction of the incidence of anthrax in several European countries during the first world war has been explained as a result of the interruption in the importation of artificial foodstuffs, fertilizers and raw animal materials for industrial uses from countries where anthrax used to prevail enzootically. In Germany, for example, as a result of the blockade, a tenfold decrease was recorded between 1914 and 1919, while immediately after the reinstatement of foreign commercial relations, an increase in the incidence became noticeable.

The rise of the incidence of human anthrax in the U.S.A. during the second world war has been causally related to the sharp increase of war demands for textiles and leather wares.

In many countries the incidence of anthrax among sheep and goats is highest by the end of the summer season. This seasonal increase has been attributed to the scarcity of edible green food available, which forces the animals to close grazing and furrowing of the earth with their noses. When the water-holes in the fields are partially dried up, the contaminated mud is easily stirred to the surface. It has often been pointed out that heavy rains and flooding, followed by dry summer weather, create optimal conditions for the occurrence of outbreaks in areas known to be contaminated.

Ploughing of infected land brings to the surface anthrax spores derived from buried carcasses, with the result that the risk of infection among grazing livestock is increased.

The spread of anthrax can be furthered by dogs, wild carrion feeders and birds of prey, which carry off parts of cadavers lying about in the fields; these carrion feeders subsequently excrete anthrax spores in their faeces, often without developing the disease themselves.

In certain regions an important epidemiological role is played by biting insects. In these areas the incidence of anthrax in animals and agricultural workers is, as a rule, highest during the season when these flies are abundant.

Kraneveld (1939) established in Indonesia that, after the biting flies suck infected blood, the anthrax organisms adhere for some time to the probosces of the flies, the spores being discharged in the faeces of these vectors for the remainder of their lives.

It has also been shown that the blood-sucking flies (the pupiparous fly; *Hippobosca,* especially in South Africa), the stable fly *(Stomoxys calcitrans)* and mosquitoes, and also some flies which do not suck blood, such as the house fly *(Musca domestica)* and the blowflies *(Calliphora vomitoria)* may transmit anthrax mechanically. The anthrax bacilli, however, do not seem to develop within the bodies of these insects.

Heeren (1947) pointed out the great importance of biting flies in the epidemiology of anthrax in Louisiana. He quoted 8 human cases of the disease recorded as early as 1830 (1 occurring after consuming meat from a sick cow, another in a man who had skinned an anthrax carcass, and 6 in persons who had been bitten by insects). In recent times, several infections were traced to *Tabanidae* (grey biting flies and gad flies) and pupiparous flies *(Lipoptena)* which attack a wide range of host species.

Outbreaks of cutaneous anthrax in cattle and buffaloes in the dense forest areas of India, ascribed to transmission by blood sucking flies, have been recorded by Mohiyddeen and Krishna Rao (1958). According to Russian statistics 2% of all animal infections were attributable to the bites of stable or horse flies and other biting insects (Shliakhov, 1957).

In animals bitten by contaminated flies the disease runs a course which characteristically contrasts with that due to alimentary infection. The lesions in insect-borne anthrax of animals are located in and under the skin at the site of the insect bite and develop nodules and carbuncles comparable to the malignant pustules seen in man.

The risk of contracting the disease by the intake of milk from anthrax animals is negligible. The bacilli do not appear in the milk until shortly before the death of infected cattle, when the secretion of milk has already greatly decreased or has stopped altogether, the milk being visibly abnormal (yellowish, bloody).

Intestinal anthrax resulting from consumption of contaminated meat is not infrequently observed in carnivores kept at zoological gardens or on fur farms, most often when the meat of animals slaughtered in emergency without regard to the rules of food inspection, has been distributed. Huge losses have been attributed to this mode of infection, especially on mink farms in the U.S.A. and in France (Verge *et al.*, in 1952, recorded a fatal epizootic of anthrax envolving 600 mink).

The intestinal tract of human beings offers rather strong resistance to anthrax infection. Even in under-developed countries where meat inspection is not enforced, and among native populations who are used to eating their dead animals, intestinal anthrax rarely occurs.

During a serious epizootic in Haiti, however, in 1943, Steele recorded many human cases of anthrax of the intestinal type, which were attributed to the consumption of the flesh of dying animals.

Although the bacilli are rapidly destroyed by the gastric juice, they may enter through minor wounds of the upper digestive tract. Their spores, however, can pass unharmed through the stomach and infect the intestines.

By and large, human anthrax is connected with occupational exposure to sick or dead animals or their excretions and products. Formerly the incidence of anthrax in human beings was almost directly proportional to that found in local livestock. The people most often affected were farmers, herdsmen, shepherds, butchers, skinners, tanners and veterinarians. An inquiry into occupational infections made among 975 veterinary surgeons in Prussia by Jopke (1934) revealed 28 cases of anthrax (23 malignant pustules, 4 septicaemia, 1 pulmonary anthrax). Thomson (1937) recorded 26 instances among 796 Danish veterinarians. The author (1938) collected 10 among 532 veterinary surgeons in the Netherlands.

It is understandable that the favourable results of control-measures in farm-animals have also contributed to the decrease in the incidence of the infection in individuals employed in agricultural occupations. In several countries this change, together with the increasing importation of raw animal materials from heavily contaminated foreign regions, has shifted the rate of incidence of the disease from the agricultural to the industrial sector. In the U.S.A. an average of 80% of human anthrax cases are now industrial in nature.

Table XXI records the sources of notified cases among industrial workers in Great Britain.

TABLE XXI

SOURCES OF HUMAN ANTHRAX IN INDUSTRY IN GREAT BRITAIN

| | Number of cases * | |
Source of infection	Period 1913–1924 (12 years)	Period 1933–1952 (20 years) according to Brennan, 1953
Wool	414 (59) ⎫ 471 (72)	159 (11) ⎫ 185 (14)
Horse hair	57 (13) ⎬	26 (3) ⎬
Hides and skins	208 (20)	236 (20)
Other industries	32 (7)	58 (12)
Stevedores	32 (10)	
Total	743 (109)	479 (46)

* Between brackets: number of deaths.

During the 5-year period between 1939 and 1943, Smyth and Higgins (1945) collected data concerning 408 cases of anthrax in the U.S.A. 20% of these persons had supposedly been infected by handling hides and skins, 60% by industrial contact with wool and hair, 16% by direct agricultural exposure to sick animals and contaminated soil, and 4% from other sources.

Table XXII is based on the statistics of Wolff and Heimann concerning anthrax in the U.S.A. over the period 1919–1949:

TABLE XXII

INCIDENCE OF HUMAN ANTHRAX IN DIFFERENT OCCUPATIONS IN THE U.S.A. OVER VARIOUS PERIODS

Source of infection	Period 1919–1928	Period 1929–1938	Period 1939–1949	Total: period 1919–1949
Industrial				
Hair and wool	131 ⎱ 369	139 ⎱ 316	479 ⎱ 585	749 ⎱ 1270
Skins and hides	238 ⎰	177 ⎰	106 ⎰	512 ⎰
Agricultural	71	162	97	330
Other sources	85	63	19	167
Unknown source	404	213	63	680
Total	929	754	764	2447
Percentage of industrial infections *	70	58	83	72

* Cases of unknown origin have been dispensed with in the calculation.

In most industrial areas a large increase in human anthrax cases occurred in textile mills, less so, in brush making factories. Recently, Brachman and Fekety (1958) pointed out the favourable effect of the substitution of natural raw materials by synthetic fibers. This applies to a lesser extent to goat's hair and consequently most infections in textile workers are now associated with this material. Coarse wool used in the manufacture of carpets seems to have more bearing on human anthrax than fine wool intended for textile products.

Among anthrax cases in American hair-workers, the source of infection could be traced 84 times to goats, compared with 5 times to horses and 1 to cows, camels and pigs, respectively. Most of the infected raw products were imported from Pakistan, Iraq, Iran or India.

The early stages of the industrial process are the most hazardous to the textile worker. The dust associated with the operation of the vacuum picking machine (in which the fibers are separated and impurities removed) is most dangerous, as are also carding and combing procedures.

In 3 textile mills, during 15 years, an average of 4.4% of cases were recorded as having originated during picking and carding processes, while 4% were attributed to combing, 3 to drawing, 2.2 to spinning, 0.2 to weaving and 0.8 to the finishing stage of the production (Brachman and Fekety).

The heavy rate of exposure to the anthrax spores in certain textile industries has been clearly demonstrated by the investigation of Carr and Rew (1957), who recovered *B. anthracis* from swabs of the nose and pharynx of 14 out of 101 healthy labourers, taken $1\frac{1}{2}$ to $4\frac{1}{2}$ hours after they had finished employment in goat-hair processing mills.

Even in 1960, Abbrink *et al.* reported 3 fatal cases of disseminated anthrax infection and 4 non-fatal cases of cutaneous anthrax in mill workers in Manchester during a period of 10 weeks.

Several cases are known of workmen carrying the infection home on their work-clothes and thus conveying anthrax to members of their families. Nor can be denied that there is a certain amount of risk in living in the neighbourhood of plants which process raw animal material.

In addition to the occupational infections in tanneries and factories which process wool, hair and bristles, the finished product can also be a source of infection. Sporadic cases of anthrax have been attributed to the use of woollen and fur clothing, as well as to contact with prepared skins and carpets.

The role of the bone industry in the epidemiology of the disease should not be overlooked. Large cargoes of raw bones are continuously imported for the production of bone meal, which is used as fertilizer, or of charcoal used in sugar refining, or in the manufacture of glue, gelatine and buttons. The frequency of contamination of these bones has been demonstrated by Davies and Harvey (1955), who isolated anthrax bacilli from 5 out of 41 cargoes from India, Pakistan and Argentina. The very fine bone dust of the crushing mills is easily conveyed to the respiratory tracts of the workers.

Epidemiologically, shaving brushes are especially instrumental in causing the disease. During and after the first world war, many cases of malignant pustules, connected with the use of brushes originating from China, Japan or Siberia, were observed in America, England and Holland. In the U.S.A. Army, 149 cases with 22 ensuing death were recorded, and in New-York City, 32 cases have been notified between 1919 and 1923. It should be borne in mind that the sporebearing brush may remain hazardous for many years, minor cuts or abrasions offering to the pathogenic organism an excellent portal of entry.

The nature of the exposure to the infection definitely determines the site of the anthrax lesions. In butchers, skinners, veterinarians, pathologists and bacteriologists the hands or arms are mainly involved; stevedores carrying hides and skins usually develop lesions on the back or the neck; most cases of pulmonary anthrax occur among workers in wool, hair and bone meal factories. Skin anthrax, caused by the use of a contaminated shaving brush, is confined to the face.

Prevention of infection in animals requires enforcement of strict measures regarding contaminated pastures, artificial fertilizers and foodstuffs. Protection of man demands that attention be given to sick or dead animals and their products.

In modern, well developed countries, the decrease in incidence of anthrax in domestic animals is achieved by: (1) adequate provision of laboratory facilities for prompt diagnosis, (2) immediate reporting of suspect cases to veterinary and health authorities, (3) prohibition of skinning and opening of anthrax carcasses, (4) covering the carcass with kerosene or crude oil to keep flies, dogs and prey animals away until the carcass is disposed of, (5) complete incineration or deep burial of the carcass under quick-lime, (6) burning of all manure in the environment of the animal and thorough disinfection and prevention of access to the place in which it has been lying, (7) removal of apparently healthy animals of a herd in which anthrax has occurred, to other pasture grounds, (8) quarantining of the carefully examined herd for at least the 2 weeks following the last case of anthrax, (9) vaccination every 10 to 12 months of all livestock in a potentially contaminated environment. The last mentioned procedure has proved to be highly successful in the protection of domestic animals, particularly in "anthrax districts".

When Pasteur's original method of double vaccination with attenuated culture was used, it soon became evident that, in spite of the beneficial effect of the vaccine, a certain number of animals succumbed as a result of infection by the vaccine itself. Less hazardous was the method of simultaneous inoculation with a culture and a potent immune serum (Sobernheim, 1902; Eichhorn, 1925), and administration of vaccines composed of the spores of a strain which had lost its virulence.

Two products of the latter type have found world wide application to several millions of animals every year. In 1934, Mazzucchi introduced "carbozoo", which is composed of a virulent anthrax culture suspended in 2 % saponin; the saponin produces in the host a local gelatinous oedema which prevents the rapid dissemination of the bacilli. The other product is Sterne's anthrax spore vaccine (1939), prepared from a non-capsulating avirulent variant of *B. anthracis,* the spores of which are suspended in 50 % glycerol saline solution. This latter vaccine gives results as good as those obtained with carbozoo, and causes less local reaction. In the U.S.S.R. extensive use is made of an aluminium hydroxide vaccine. Because the immunity produced by these protective inoculations does not last for more than 9 to 12 months, the vaccination must be repeated every year, preferably in advance of the "anthrax season".

Subcutaneous or intradermal vaccination of all livestock in epizootic areas has checked the disease in many parts of the world in which in the past, animal industry functioned precariously or not efficiently enough.

Prolonged employment of workers in factories which process animal material does not ensure significant immunity. Brachman and Fekety (1958) recorded an annual infection rate of 1.8 per 100 workers who had been employed for a period of up to 4 years in goat-hair plants, and a rate of 1.2 among those employed for 17 to 20 years.

Under certain circumstances immunization has been considered for the protection of those individuals who are most heavily exposed to contaminated materials. In the U.K., the U.S.A. and U.S.S.R. promising results have been obtained by the vaccination of industrial workers (*e.g.* with alum-precipitated anthrax antigen). Recently, Wright's alum-treated vaccine prepared from a noncapsulated, nonproteolytic mutant of *B. anthracis* was clinically and epidemiologically evaluated in the U.S.A. (Brachman *et al.*, 1962). The results of this investigation are highly suggestive of its usefulness in the protection of occupationally exposed population groups.

Protective measures in these occupational institutions are mainly based on improvement of the hygienic conditions of the plant and disinfection of raw materials. At the turn of the century, pulmonary anthrax was more frequently observed in these industries than anthrax of the skin. This situation has since reversed itself, especially so in bone crushing plants, where the problem of fine dust has to be dealt with by supplying proper exhaust and ventilation devices. All waste must be burned or autoclaved. Properly constructed floors and walls must be regularly cleaned and disinfected. Flies must be destroyed. In order to avoid contamination of the environment of the plants, wastes must be made harmless by disinfection with liquid chlorinated compounds before they are discharged. The use of special protective working clothes, shoes, caps, gloves and masks, must be enforced. The clothing must be disinfected by steam under pressure and should remain on the premises. Before the workers change into street-clothes, they should take a shower and thoroughly wash their hands.

Wounds and abrasions of the skin require adequate disinfection and dressing. Constant medical supervision of personnel is a prime requisite.

Experience has proved that consular certifications of the animal by-products, which state that these products come from supposedly anthrax-free areas, are not always reliable. This implies that raw materials imported for industrial uses must be sterilized before they are allowed to reach the factories. Although it would be better to have this done at the shipping port, it must, for practical reasons, be done in the country that receives these raw materials.

When a method of disinfection of the animal materials is selected, it is necessary to bear in mind the extraordinarily high resistance of anthrax spores and the eventual damage to the product itself causing depreciation of its economic value.

In Great Britain, since 1921, a satisfactory system has been enforced in the hair and wool industry. At the central sterilization station of wool and hair in Liverpool, these products undergo preliminary treatment with a sodium carbonate solution and soap at 40°, followed by exposure to a 2 % formaldehyde solution, and by rinsing and rapid drying at 120°.

In view of the high operation costs of this system, cheaper though less safe methods of disinfection have been adopted in several other countries. Such compromises, however, arise from economic considerations rather than from concern for human welfare. Steaming under pressure is a useful method for the disinfection of hair and bristles, provided that the steam circulates freely between small bundles of the raw materials. For the sterilization of wool and hides, this procedure is less satisfactory. Destruction of anthrax spores in wool in the raw state can, however, be achieved by the dyeing process.

The disinfection of hides and skins without causing depreciation of their industrial value is rather difficult and costly. In Great Britain solutions of bichloride of mercury and formic acid are used (Seymour–Jones method); in the U.S.A., milk of lime (for goat skins) and bichloride (for cattle hides), whereas in the U.S.S.R. sodium bisulfite, together with sodium chloride and hydrochloric acid are employed (Boyarshinov).

The importation of bones, bone meal and flour, horn and meat meal, or of hooves and hoof meal requires an official certificate which states that adequate sterilization of these materials has been carried out in plants approved by the Government.

Treatment of anthrax pustules formerly consisted of excision, cauterisation, the application of iodine and the injection of phenol into the local lesions. Significant progress was achieved by the introduction of specific anthrax immune serum, which brought about reduction of the mortality to less than one-tenth of its original rate. This treatment, however, had several drawbacks, among which was the fact that the repeated injection of huge doses of a foreign serum often caused serious allergic reactions. In 1926, treatment with neoarsphenamine was recommended (Pijper). This chemical, either by itself or combined with serum injections, was a great improvement on the former treatment (Eurich). Sulfonamides (*e.g.* sulfathiazole) have been successfully applied since 1942.

A dramatic turning-point was the introduction of penicillin for the treatment of human infections (Murphy *et al.*, 1944) and those of animals (Sugg, 1948). When penicillin and broad-spectrum antibiotics (*e.g.* chlortetracycline) were used, the original mortality rate of 10 to 20% in the U.S.A. was reduced to almost zero.

During 7 years, White (1956) had treated over 500 cases of cutaneous anthrax in the African population of Kenya with procain penicillin in oil, with only 3 deaths.

The fight against anthrax in man and animals has taken a marked turn, for the better in extensive parts of the world. These successes, however, should not lead to relaxation of the enacted measures of control.

The ubiquity of the bacillus, its great tenacity and high pathogenicity to many mammals, together with the ease with which it is transmitted when it is hidden, as it may be, in materials and products of animal origin, over large distances, necessitate the constant vigilance of medical and veterinary authorities and practitioners, to whom the prevention of the scourge is entrusted.

REFERENCES

ABBRINK, W. S., S. M. BROOKS, R. E. BIRON and M. KOPEL, *Amer. J. Path.*, 36 (1960) 457.
BOQUIEN, I., *Bull. Acad. Nat. Méd. (Paris)*, 134 (1950) 585.
BRACHMAN, P. S. and F. R. FEKETY, *Ann. N.Y. Acad. Sci.*, 70 (1958) 574.
BRACHMAN, P. S., H. GOLD, S. A. PLOTKIN, F. R. FEKETY, M. WERRIN and N. R. INGRAHAM, *Amer. J. publ. Hlth*, 52 (1962) 632.
BRENNAN, A. D. J., *Vet. Rec.*, 65 (1953) 255.
CARR, E. A. and R. R. REW, *J. Infect. Dis.*, 100 (1957) 169.
DARLOW, H. M., F. C. BELTON and D. W. HENDERSON, *Lancet*, II (1956) 476.
DAVIES, D. G. and R. W. S. HARVEY, *Lancet*, ii (1955) 86.
DELPY, L. P. and KAWEH, *Arch. Inst. d'Hessarek*, 2 (1946) 3.
Epidem. Vit. Statist. Rep., 11 (1958) 476.
GLASSMAN, H. N., *Publ. Hlth Rep. (Wash.)*, 73 (1958) 22.
GOOD, G. M., *J. Amer. vet. med. Ass.*, 129 (1956) 470.
GREEN, D. M. and W. M. JAMIESON, *Lancet*, II (1958) 151; 153.
GRUMBACH, A., in GRUMBACH and KIKUTH, *Die Infektionskrankheiten des Menschen und ihre Erreger*, II, Stuttgart, 1958, p. 943.
Joint W.H.O.–F.A.O. *Expert Group on Zoonoses, Rep.* 1 (1951) 47 pp.; *Rep.* 2 (1959) 83 pp.
KLEMM, D. M. and W. R. KLEMM, *J. Amer. vet. med. Ass.*, 135 (1959) 458.
LAMB R., *Lancet*, II (1958) 151.
MINETT, F. C., *Bull. Office internat. Epizot.*, 37 (1952) 238.
Rep. Comm. Inquiry on Anthrax, Ministry Labour, London, 1959, 222 pp.

Ross, J. M., *J. Path. Bact.*, 73 (1957) 485.

Shliakhov, E. N., *Ž. Mikrobiol. (Mosk.)*, 28 (1957) 748.

Smyth, H. F. and W. D. Higgins, *Amer. J. publ. Hlth*, 35 (1945) 850.

Steele, J. D. and R. J. Helvig, *Publ. Hlth Rep. (Wash.)*, 68 (1953) 616.

Stein, C. D., *Ann. N.Y. Acad. Sci.*, 48 (1947) 507; *Vet. Med.*, 50 (1955) 579.

Verge, J., P. Goret, L. Joubert, L. Gauchy and M. Fuerxer, *Bull. Acad. nat. Méd. (Paris)*, 136 (1952) 53.

Wolff, A. H. and H. Heimann, *Amer. J. Hyg.*, 53 (1951) 80.

Wundt, W., *Arch. Hyg. (Berl.)*, 143 (1959) 145.

13

J. VAN DER HOEDEN

Necrobacillosis

The bacterial genus *Sphaerophorus* (family: *Bacteroidaceae)* includes anaerobic gram-negative, non-sporulating rods of extreme pleomorphism, which may be fusiform, or coccoid, or filaments 80 to 100 micra long. In culture these organisms produce a characteristic foul odor. The genus contains more than one serological type.

The protean appearance of the bacteria has resulted in much confusion in differentiating various strains, more than a dozen names having given in literature to closely related or identical organisms *(Sphaerophorus necrophorus, S. Persoon, Sphaerophorus-, Bacillus-* or *Bacteroides funduliformis, Bac. pyogenes anaerobius, Streptothrix-* or *Actinomyces cuniculi, A. necrophorus, Bac. funduliformis,* etc.). Dack *et al.* (1938) stated that no distinction exists between *S. funduliformis* isolated from man and *S. necrophorus* from animals; he considered that these two names are synonyms of a single species. In Bergey's Manual of Determinative Bacteriology (1957) this organism has been classified in the genus *Sphaerophorus,* under the name *S. necrophorus* or *Necrobacterium necrophorum.* In experimental infection some strains are pathogenic to rabbits, guinea pigs and mice, but not to white rats.

Necrobacterium is a frequent inhabitant of the mucous membranes of healthy humans and animals and has an inherent capability to cause serious and often lethal septic or pyaemic diseases.

Wild and domestic animals are subject to sporadic or epizootic necrobacillosis. Among the many diseases caused, the following may be mentioned: ulcerative necrotic stomatitis of calves ("calf diphtheria"), lambs, pigs, rabbits (labial necrosis) and several wild animals; necrotic angina, panaritium and abscesses of dogs; "foot-rot" (panaritium) of cattle and sheep; gangrenous dermatitis and fistulae of the hooves of horses and mules; multiple abscesses and embolic necrosis of the lungs, liver, udder and heart-muscle of cattle, lambs and swine; gangrenous foci in the vagina and uterus of cows appearing post partum; navel-ill of young-borne calves and still other ailments. Early therapeutic measures are indicated in order to avoid high mortality rate.

On the other hand, a high incidence of encapsulated necrotic foci is observed in apparently healthy slaughter animals. In English slaughter houses such lesions were found in about 50 % of the animals slaughtered. According to Beveridge (1937), in the U.S.A. 2–10 % of bovine livers were condemned at meat inspection because of the presence in them of abscesses and in 80 % of these abscesses *N. necrophorum* was the only micro-organism found.

It is generally assumed that, as happens with other pyogenic organisms, commensalism may be converted into parasitism when necrobacilli present on the exterior of the body invade the tissues, as may happen, for example, when local resistance has been weakened by trauma, bacterial infection or other favourable circumstances. The potential pathogenicity of this usually saprophytic organism may be demonstrated in man, after tonsillectomy, parturition or intestinal surgery.

Symbiosis with other, especially aerobic micro-organisms, or penetration of a foreign body, may promote the pathogenic action of the anaerobic *Necrobacterium*. As in human Plaut-Vincent's angina, the accessory organism in many instances is a spirochaete.

It is often difficult to ascertain whether epizootic spread of necrobacillosis is due to animal-to-animal infection, or to environmental factors which promote the entrance of the bacterium into the internal tissues.

In New-Zealand the annual economic loss from foot-rot in sheep has been estimated at one million pounds Sterling (Ensor, 1957). Although as a rule only 1 or 2 animals in a herd are affected with calf diphtheria, in the U.S.A. an incidence of up to 70 % has been occasionally recorded. During a 6-month period of World War I, Kelser observed more than 4,000 cases of gangrenous dermatitis with 212 deaths among American army horses.

According to Alston, 269 *human* cases of necrobacillosis had been recorded in the literature until 1955 (94 in Germany, 87 in the U.S.A., 31 in France, 10 in Great Britain, 24 in Hungary, 15 in Holland, 6 in French Indo-China and 2 in Scandinavia). The ages of 21 patients reported by this author from Great Britain fluctuated between 5 and 65 years. 13 of them died between 6 days to 7 weeks after the onset of the disease. Recovery required 1 to 17 weeks.

In a Memphis (Tennesee) hospital, McVay and Sprunt (1952) observed 35 cases of necrobacillosis in the course of 5 years. 2˙ of these persons were seriously ill and 11 died. The incubation period varied greatly.˙ cultures of necrobacteria were isolated and also a mixed flora of 2 to 4 different orga ms.

Four clinical forms of necrobacillosis have been differentiated in *human beings*. Benign lesions are caused by direct infection of the skin and sub-cutaneous tissues. In this group no deaths have been recorded.

The other three forms have a triad of symptoms in common, *viz.* (a) sudden rise of temper. ure to high levels, accompanied with violent cold shivers and abundan perspiration, (b) embolic lung infarcts and (c) arthralgia or arthritis. Concurrent abscesses and empyema are not uncommon. Purulent-necrotic lesions may be localized in various organs. A serious septicaemia may follow tonsillitis or a peritonsillar abscess (post-anginous necrobacillosis); this occurs most frequently in young persons. Prolonged circulation of the bacteria may lead to the formation of embolic foci and infarcts of the lung, which often suppurate and pro-duce abscesses.

The intestinal form, which usually affects older persons, takes a very serious course and has a grave prognosis. It is characterized by repeated vomiting, diarrhoea and severe abdominal pain. Sometimes the lungs are also involved and show infarcts. The genital form usually appears about a week after abortion or parturition and is frequently associated with peritonitis; the mortality may be high.

It is most probable that only the group of direct skin or wound infections first mentioned are in fact true zoonoses. The majority of cases in the three other syndrome groups seem to be the result of auto-infection, *i.e.* these syndromes appear when the bacteria in a pre-existing latent focus become pathogenic.

Transmission of infection from animals to man is brought about by bites or other injuries of the skin. The following examples may be quoted from the literature.

Schmorl, as early as 1891, described necrobacillosis in two laboratory workers who were accidentally infected when they were handling experimentally infected rabbits.

A veterinary surgeon in the Netherlands wounded his arm when he was exploring the mouth of a cow suffering from suppurative retropharyngeal lymphadenitis (van Wering, 1923). 3 weeks later local abscesses, lymphangitis and lymphadenitis developed with high fever and general malaise. The abscesses turned into coalescing ulcers which spread over the forearm. *N. necrophorum* was isolated from the lesions. Recovery followed prolonged therapy.

Stemen and Shaw (cited by van Gelder, 1930) reported very painful voluminous ulcerations on the hand and forearm, accom⸱ ⸱nied by general symptoms, occurring in a government meat-inspector, 5 days after ⸱⸱ had wounded himself while excising a necrotic ulcer on the lip of a sheep. Reco⸱ ⸱y began after 3 weeks. *N. necrophorum* was recovered in pure culture.

Alston (1955) quoted two accidental infections by *N. necrophorum*. A veterinarian acquired a skin lesion with central necrosis, lymphangitis and lymphadenitis on the forearm, 3 days after manual removal of a cow's placenta. Another person had been bitten by an infected cow 3 weeks before the onset of small abscesses at the site of the wound. A week later regional lymphangitis and ax⸱ ⸱ary lymphadenitis developed; *N. necrophorum* was isolated from these lesions.

In the treatment of necrobacillosis, aureomycin has been found the most effective antibiotic.

There is ample reason to believe that the significance of necrobacillosis in human pathology is insufficiently recognized. This particularly concerns cases of lung infarcts, empyema, liver abscesses and infections of the urinary tract. However, the relationship of most of these cases with necrobacillosis in animals can hardly be substantiated.

It is clear, in the light of all these facts, that necrobacterial infection deserves more attention from clinicians and bacteriologists.

REFERENCES

ALSTON, J. M., *Brit. Med. J.,* (1955/II) 1524.

BEEUWKES, H., J. B. M. VISMANS and A. H. SMEETS, *Ned. T. Geneesk.,* 95 (1951) 1143.

BEVERIDGE, W., *Necrobacillosis, Infectious Diseases of Animals,* II, in STABLEFORTH and GALLOWAY, Eds., London, 1959, 397 pp.

DACK, G. M., L. R. DRAGSTEDT, R. JOHNSON and N. B. McCULLOUGH, *J. infect. Dis.,* 62 (1938) 169.

ENSOR, C. R., *N.Z. J. Agr.,* 94 (1957) 218.

GELDER, R. I. v., *Derm. Z.,* 58 (1930) 368.

McVAY, L. V. and D. H. SPRUNT, *Ann. intern. Med.,* 36 (1952) 56.

SHAW, F. W., *Zbl. Bakt. I. Abt. Orig.* 129 (1933) 132.

14

J. VAN DER HOEDEN

Vibriosis

Although *Brucella*, *Leptospira* and *Trichomonas* are frequent causes of abortion, *Vibrio* is also important in its aetiology.

In 1909–1913 McFadyean and Stockman, working in England, demonstrated the aetiological relationship between abortion in sheep and cows and a spirillum- or vibrio-like organism found in the uterine exudate of these animals. The disease was reproduced by experimental infection of pregnant ewes and cows with a culture of the organism isolated from aborted ovine foetuses. Theobald Smith recovered in 1918 the same agent *(Vibrio fetus)* from aborted cattle foetuses in America.

Vibriosis has been recorded in *cattle* and *sheep* in all continents of the globe. In some countries *V. fetus* is the most frequent cause of bovine abortion. Thus, Levi *et al.* isolated from the foetuses of aborted cattle in Israel, during the period 1948–1951, 203 strains of *V. fetus,* only 70 of *Brucella abortus* and 61 of *Corynebacterium pyogenes.*

In 1949, Stegenga and Terpstra, in Holland, established that *V. fetus* is the main factor in enzootic or infectious sterility in cattle. This disease, the aetiology of which had hitherto been obscure, represented a serious hazard to the cattle industry in their country, with an estimated annual loss of 40–60 million guilders from reduced breeding efficiency.

In Belgium, Willems (1957) suggested causative relationship between a vibrio which he isolated from young *pigs* and the acute enteritis from which the animals suffered.

Trueblood and Post (1959) recovered the same vibrio from aborted foetuses in a herd of *antelopes* in America among which fertility had considerably declined.

Vibrio fetus in tissues and in the initial culture appears as small, slender, comma- or S-shaped, gram-negative rods which, when artificial cultivation of them is continued, tend to grow into longer spirilla-like elements. The organism can only successfully be cultured in an atmosphere of increased concentration of carbon dioxide, the culture medium requiring the addition of blood or other animal fluids. Growth is slow and delicate. *V. fetus* is microaërophilic and actively motile. It does not ferment carbohydrates and does not produce indol. Its resistance to unfavourable environmental conditions is rather low. The antigenic composition of most strains of bovine origin differs partly from that of strains isolated from sheep.

After natural infection of *cows,* the vibrio settles in the reproductive organs, where it induces a mild subacute or subchronic vaginitis and sometimes endometritis and salpingitis, which prevent conception. Young sexually mature heifers are the most susceptible to infection.

The least serious consequence of vibrio infection is a delayed, irregular oestrus cycle. Most often failure to conceive ensues. Early death and expulsion of the young embryo usually remains unnoticed, so that the number of obvious cases of infertility is increased. *Vibrio fetus* also causes necrotic foci and oedema in the foetal membranes.

Abortion of ewes and cows occurs when the foetus dies at a later stage of gestation, this being due to placentitis and obstruction of the foetal circulation. The placenta is often retained for an extended period of time.

Vibriosis in cattle is primarily a veneral disease transmitted when an infected bull mates with a susceptible cow, or as the result of artificial insemination with contaminated sperm. The reverse process, *i.e.,* transmission from infected cows to a bull, is also known to occur. Once a bull is infected, he usually continues to carry the vibrio in the prepuce for an indefinite period of time without showing any clinical sign of illness and the semen is not altered in appearance or inseminating quality. The presence of *V. fetus* in the testicular secretion classifies the bull as a poor breeder, a fact which is evidenced by the fact that frequently repeated services by these bulls are necessary before the cows conceive.

Vibrio fetus is excreted in large numbers by infected cows in the uterine exudate and the placenta. In the aborted foetuses the vibrio is concentrated in the stomach and, in sheep particularly, in necrotic foci in the liver.

Small test animals are refractory to infection, with the exception of pregnant guinea pigs and hamsters, which often abort, revealing at postmortem examination haemorrhages, oedema and necrosis. Atrophic testicles have been observed in infected hamsters.

Ewes are most susceptible during pregnancy, especially when this is advanced. This accounts for the high rate of abortion or premature lambing in this animal. In the U.S.A., incidences of 50–70% of the sheep in an infected flock have been reported. The uterine wall, placenta and subcutaneous tissue of the sheep foetus are oedematous and blood-stained fluid is found in the foetal body-cavities.

It is generally agreed that the ram, unlike the bull, does not play an important part in the transmission of vibriosis. In ovines, the digestive tract is most often the portal through which the infection enters.

In cows and sheep the disease, as a rule, readily wanes, conferring active immunity, which permits pregnancy to occur.

Bulls which are carriers and are apparently unaffected constitute the chief problem, because it is through these that the disease spreads to heifers and cows which have not yet acquired active immunity as a result of either previous mating with an infected bull, or of artificial insemination with contaminated sperm.

The diagnosis of vibriosis is based upon microscopic examination of smears or on cultivation of the vibrios from the cotyledons, amniotic fluid and stomach contents or internal organs of aborted foetuses. The agglutination test with vaginal mucus is more valuable than the test with blood serum, because the antibodies appear earlier and persist longest in the mucus.

As a measure of prevention and control of bovine vibriosis, newly acquired, sexually mature animals should be segregated from the herd until laboratory examinations have shown that they are free from infection. Bulls with a low fertility rate are suspect carriers of *Vibrio fetus* and should not be allowed to serve in the natural way. When artificial insemination is used, the diluted semen of suspected bulls can be rendered harmless by the addition of streptomycin. Before mating occurs, heifers should receive a preventive intra-uterine infusion of antibiotics.

In the light of the scarcity of published cases one might feel inclined to assume that *V. fetus,* which almost prevails universally in domesticated ruminants, very rarely affects human beings. However, because the disease is not characterized by a specific syndrome and because laboratory investigations of vibriosis are not done as a routine procedure, it appears that the limited number of established cases of human infection reflects a state of neglect, rather than the actual situation. To be valid, cultivation from the blood requires special technical care, and the serum agglutination test must be performed with properly selected vibrio strains.

The pathogenicity of *V. fetus* to *man* was first suggested by Verge who, in 1947, isolated this organism from a woman who had aborted, the foetus being 6 months old. Some 30 additional cases of human disease caused by *V. fetus* have since been recorded in the literature. These indicate a relatively high incidence in France (Ward, 1948; Vincent *et al.*, 1947, 1949, 1950; Weismann-Netter *et al.*, 1954; Thibault *et al.*, 1955; King, 1957, and others). All of these cases in France were adults between the ages of 31 and 74, comprising 17 males and only 4 females.

Vincent's cases seem to be of special significance, because there were among them 3 pregnant women, blood cultures from whom were positive. One of them aborted, the foetus being dead; another gave birth to a premature child that soon died, while the third, who received intensive therapeutic treatment, delivered at term a constitutionally weak infant. All 3 women had symptoms of pleuropneumonia.

In nearly all cases of human infection, the illness started with a sudden bout of remittent or intermittent fever. Chills, marked headache and malaise were often complained of. In most cases a generalised systemic infection occurred, which was sometimes accompanied by symptoms of bronchitis, pulmonary oedema and pleural effusion, or by slight disturbances of the digestive tract (nausea, diarrhoea or constipation). Some of the patients showed jaundice, while swelling of the liver and spleen and lymphadenopathy were also noticed. Almost half of the affected persons showed morbid manifestations of the central nervous system. There was general weakness and loss of weight. The duration of the disease varied from a few days to several months. In nearly all cases spontaneous recovery ensued.

Because of the absence of specific morbid characteristics, the diagnosis depends on the isolation of the *Vibrio* from the patient. Usually it was cultivated from the blood; it has been found once in the sero-sanguineous fluid obtained by puncture from the knee of an old man suffering from chronic traumatic arthritis at a time when he was affected by an acute attack of fever.

Several authors believe that *V. fetus* infection may be suspected in cases of septicaemia accompanied with thrombophlebitis (Kahler *et al.*, 1960; Jackson *et al.*, 1960; Beeson, 1961).

Very little is known of the epidemiology of vibriosis fetus in human beings. Among the cases recorded, only 4 individuals were directly exposed to infection by farm animals and 3 others reported a history of earlier contacts with animals. In a case of septicaemia described by Spink (1957) the patient was employed in a meat packing plant on the killing line. Direct transmissibility of *V. fetus* to man was demonstrated in the case of a laboratory worker who was handling cultures of the organism and developed a pustule on the cheek, from which the vibrio was recovered. In several instances pre-existing disease (rheumatic cardiopathy, chronic cirrhotic hepatitis, etc.) seemed to have served as predisposing factors in persons living in a contaminated environment. Twice the infection took place shortly after the extraction of teeth, which might suggest auto-infection with *V. fetus* that was part of the oral flora.

In a number of cases the patients responded favourably to therapy with chlortetracycline, chloramphenicol and dehydrostreptomycin. In view of our scanty experience, no final evaluation of antibiotic treatment is as yet warranted.

REFERENCES

AUGUSTE, C., R. BUTHIAUX and A. JACQUET, *Arch. Mal. Appar. dig.*, 43 (1954) 861.

BEESON, P. B., *The Yearbook of Medicine*, 1960, 62 Series, p. 63.

FRANK, A. H., *Animal Diseases, Yearbook, U.S.A.*, 1956, p. 224.

JACKSON, J. F., P. HINTON and F. ALLISON, *Amer. J. Med.*, 28 (1960) 986.

KAHLER, R. L. and HUNTINGTON SHELDON, *New Engl. J. Med.*, 262 (1960) 1218.

KING, E. O., *J. infect. Dis.*, 101 (1957) 119.

KING, S. and D. BRONSKY, *J. Amer. med. Ass.*, 175 (1961) 1045.

KNAPP, W., *Zbl. Bact. I. Abt. Orig.*, 161 (1954) 422.

KNAPP, W. and W. MASSHOFF, *Dtsch. med. Wschr.*, 79 (1954) 1266.

LAING, J. A., *F. A. O. Agricult. Studies, No. 32*, Rome (1956).

LEVI, M. L., *J. comp. Path.*, 60 (1950) 65.

LEVI, M. L., L. NEEMAN, L. KERSTEIN and R. TAMARIN, *Proc. XV Internat. Vet. Congr. I*, 2 (1953) 112.

MASSHOFF, W., *Dtsch. med. Wschr.*, 78 (1953) 532.

MASSHOFF, W. and W. DÖLLE, *Virchows Arch. path. Anat.*, 323 (1953) 664.

STEGENGA, TH. and L. J. TERPSTRA, *T. Diergeneesk.*, 71 (1950) 293.

TERPSTRA, L. J., *Bull. Off. int. Épiz., Rep. 19th Session* (1951) 1.

THIBAULT, P., J. GAILLARD, J. SECOND and R. CHATELAIN, *Bull. Acad. nat. Méd. (Paris)*, 139 (1955) 65.

TRUEBLOOD, M. S. and G. POST, *J. Amer. vet. med. Ass.*, 134 (1959) 562.

VERGE, J., *Rev. Path. comp.*, 47 (1947) 309.

VINZENT, R., *Presse méd.*, 57 (1949) 1230.

VINZENT, R. and ALLOY, *Rec. Méd. vét.*, 128 (1952) 541.

VINZENT, R., J. DELARUE and H. HERBERT, *Ann. Méd.*, 51 (1950) 23.

VINZENT, R., J. DUMAS and N. PICARD, *Bull. Acad. nat. Méd.*, 131 (1947) 90.

WARD, B. Q., *J. Bact.*, 55 (1948) 113.

WEISMAN-NETTER, R., P. THIBAULT, ROBERT LÉVY and L. SECOND, *Bull. Soc. méd. Hôp. Paris*, 70 (1954) 834.

WILLEMS, R., *Bull. Off. int. Épiz.*, 48 (1957) 690.

15

A. CH. RUYS

Rat bite fevers

Rat bites are sometimes followed by general infections, caused by the microorganisms which are usually found in infected wounds. In addition to these, two distinct clinical entities have been recognized, both of which are known as rat bite fever, although they are caused by different organisms.

In the Far East, many centuries ago, a specific disease was known which followed the bite of a rat; it was given the name sodoku (so = rat, doku = poison). In the 19th century, isolated cases of this typical rat bite fever were seen in both Europe and America. In 1900, Miyake gave an exact description of 11 patients suffering from sodoku, and this brought the disease to the attention of the medical profession outside Asia. At that time, the cause of the disease was still unknown. Later it was shown that the aetiological agent of sodoku is a spirillum.

After a period of much confusion it is now generally recognized that another microorganism *(Streptobacillus moniliformis, Haverhillia multiformis)*, which can also be transmitted by the bite of rats, causes a disease different from sodoku.

SODOKU

Sodoku is characterized, as a rule, by normal healing of the wound caused by the bite of the infected rat, without any treatment; but after an incubation period of approximately 3 weeks – a period which may vary from 1 to 5 weeks – the patient suffers from a bout of fever, often without prodromal symptoms. The attack lasts 2 or 3 days, the fever then subsiding, only to be followed a few days later by a recurrence of the attack. In benign cases, the intermittent fever with remissions may continue for no more than 4 to 5 weeks, whereas in the severer forms it may last from 2 to 3 months. If it is untreated, the disease rarely becomes chronic.

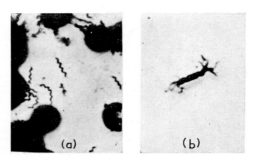

Fig. 28.   (a) *Spirillum muris* from peritoneal fluid. Giemsa stain. 1500x. (b) *Spirillum minus*. Löffler mordant staining method. 2000x.

Severe headaches and pain in the joints and muscles are frequent. Arthritis is rare. Usually, with the first attack – sometimes later – there is a generalized exanthematous eruption, which at first has a bluish macular aspect, but often becomes papular. The exanthema disappears with the fever and may re-appear with each new attack.

At the time of the first bout of fever, the healed bite-wound begins to show a characteristic circumscript bluish-red infiltration which is sometimes very painful. In some instances a central necrosis is present, although there is always little formation of pus. The regional lymph nodes tend to become swollen and tender and this is repeated more or less with each attack of fever. There are, however, also confirmed cases of sodoku which show neither exanthema nor reactions at the site of the wound.

During the attack, the blood picture is characterized by leucocytosis with a relative lymphopenia. The eosinophil cells then disappear, but they show a critical increase a few days before the fever rises again (Kuipers and Ruys).

The aetiological agent was first described in 1916 by Futaki and his co-workers, who demonstrated a spirochaete-like organism in the skin and lymph glands of a patient with sodoku. They succeeded in transmitting the disease, by means of the blood of the patient, to monkeys, mice, rats and guinea pigs. In their description, these authors mention the existence of flagellar structures at both ends of the organism (Fig. 28).

Although the flagella are rarely made visible by ordinary Giemsa staining, they can be easily seen by dark field illumination. Adachi, using a special staining method, proved that these structures consist of a bunch of flagella, a fact which is also sometimes visible in the darkfield (Zuelzer). They are demonstrated still better by Ruge's fixative and Löffler's mordant staining technique (Ruys). Because of these facts, and because the structure of the microorganism is rigid, it has been concluded that it belongs, as Zuelzer first suggested, to the bacteria and not to the spirochaetes. Carter had, already in 1887, exactly described the organism and had suggested the name *Spirillum minor*.

It is classified in the order of *Pseudomonadales*, in the family of the *Spirillaceae*, and has been named *Spirillum minus*. Two varieties are now-adays recognized, *i.e. var. morsus muris* found in rats, and the less virulent *var. muris*, found in mice. Some minor serological differences exist between these two varieties. Similar differences were found between strains obtained from wild rats and field voles in Japan. The strain from field voles proved less virulent in experimental infection of monkeys.

Attempts to cultivate *Spirillum minus* have so far been unsuccessful, although successive transfers through mice can be achieved with good results. This spirillum can sometimes be demonstrated microscopically in the dark field in fluid expressed from the infiltrated wound. Also, in smears fixed with methyl alcohol and stained with Giemsa solution, the spirilla can be easily recognized by their spirochaete-like appearance. In blood their number is often too limited to be demonstrated microscopically.

The best way to isolate this spirillum is to inoculate mice with blood from the patient taken on the day after the peak of the fever or with fluid from the wound or the infiltrated skin. In positive cases the spirilla are found in the blood and peritoneal fluid of the mice from the 5th or 7th day onwards. They can be easily recognized by dark field illumination, against which they appear as very motile, rigid microbes, 2–5 microns long, with two or more twists. They move by means of the action of the flagella. After a few days the number of the spirilla increases markedly, but later it gradually diminishes. The mice are little affected, but remain throughout life carriers of some spirilla in their blood and peritoneal fluid. At times and for short periods, very large numbers of the organism appear in the peritoneal cavity.

Chronically infected mice often have a staring coat and may show infiltrations of their oral and genital regions and the hair may be lost.

It should be mentioned, however, that white mice may have a silent infection with the less virulent variety, *Spirillum var. muris*. A thorough search in the darkfield may then reveal, in the blood or the peritoneal fluid of such animals, only a few spirilla. Carriers of this strain appear healthy and are immune to infection with the *morsus muris* variety (see below). It is, therefore, necessary to control all mice from the 5th day after the inoculation. Each primary infection with spirilla shows itself by a rapidly rising number of spirilla in the blood.

Guinea pigs react within 3 to 10 days of a subcutaneous inoculation, showing infiltration, enlargement of lymph nodes and fever, sometimes followed by conjunctivitis and, in a few cases, by keratitis. Many show loss of hair, especially that of the oral, scrotal and anal regions, and some show marked inflammation of subcutaneous tissue.

Spirillum minus may be found in the blood of apparently healthy, wild rats *(var. morsus muris)*. Mooser suggested that only those rats that were suffering from spirillar conjunctivitis could transmit the disease, the spirilla entering the wound through the lacrimal duct, the nose and the cleft lip of the rat. However, the author found in a number of observations that rats showing the organism in their blood (which proved to be able to transmit the disease by biting guinea pigs and other rats) did not suffer from conjunctivitis and that no spirilla were present in their conjunctival fluid or mouth.

Rats with negative blood failed to transmit the disease to other animals. It thus seems probable that in the act of biting the buccal mucosa is injured and that contamination may take place by the penetration of a small quantity of infected blood or fluid from subcutaneous tissue into the wound.

Wild rats, which were carriers of spirilla, did not, when they were kept in the laboratory for up to 5 months, show any clinical symptoms.

The percentage of wild rats found infected with *Spirillum minus* varies in different countries. In Japan, higher percentages of rats have been found positive (between 6 and 14) than is generally found elsewhere. In London, Coles was able to demonstrate the presence of *Spirillum minus* in only 1 out of 100 rats; on the other hand, Joekes (1925) claimed to have found the organism in the same town in 25% of the rats. The author isolated only 4 strains from 350 rats in Amsterdam (1926). Soesilo in Indonesia found 1 out of 30 rats infected, Heisch in Nairobi – 7 out of 44.

The bite of other animals does occasionally transmit the disease. For example, Reitzel described a patient suffering from sodoku which was attributable to the bite of a field mouse. Infections from the bites of cats, dogs, ferrets and weasels have been reported. These animals may have been primarily infected when they were hunting rats.

As to the prevention of the disease, extermination of rats, which are the main carriers, will minimize the chance of infection. Because of the small percentage of infected rats, rat bite fever has never been a serious hazard, except perhaps in trench warfare. Whether disinfection of the bite wound by iodine tincture is a satisfactory precautionary measure has yet to be ascertained.

Until it was replaced by penicillin and streptomycin, salvarsan was the treatment of choice for rat bite fever. In animal experiments, penicillin proved to be the more reliable of the two antibiotics.

HAVERHILL FEVER

Haverhill fever – the other rat bite fever – appears after a much shorter incubation period than sodoku.

The microorganism, which is the causative agent of this disease, can be isolated in pure culture from the blood. It has been described under several names: *Streptothrix muris ratti, Asterococcus muris, Actinobacillus muris, Streptobacillus moniliformis* and *Haverhillia multiformis*. The latter two names are now generally adopted.

The microorganism was probably cultured for the first time from a case of rat bite fever by Schottmüller (1914), who named it *Streptothrix muris ratti*.

The disease is characterized by sudden onset of high temperature, chills and general symptoms which appear within a few days, or sometimes within 48 hours, after the bite of an infected rat. The site of the wound heals without any complications and is not re-activated later in the course of the disease. A typical bluish-red exanthema, sometimes with a morbilliform appearance, soon becomes visible.

In some patients small pustular lesions develop. Shifting pains in the joints, intense muscular pains, and, in severe cases, arthritis also, may complicate the picture. Adjacent lymphatics and lymph nodes may be involved. After a short period, the fever generally subsides, although new bouts may occur. Sometimes the disease takes a more septic course, with toxic symptoms. Endocarditis is a serious complication. In untreated cases, the mortality rate is about 10%.

Infections with *S. moniliformis* may also occur without the bite of a rodent. As long ago as 1925, Levaditi *et al.* described this clinical picture in a member of their research team from whose blood a bacterium was cultured for which they suggested the name *Streptobacillus moniliformis*. No contacts with rodents were mentioned.

In 1926 in Haverhill (U.S.A.), an epidemic was described of a new disease called *erythema arthriticum epidemicum*. From the blood of 11 patients, a microorganism was isolated which was thoroughly studied by Parker and Hudson, who named it *Haverhillia multiformis*. Later it proved to be identical with *Streptobacillus moniliformis*. It is now generally recognized that Haverhill fever is the form of the disease in which the causative agent enters the body not through a lesion of the skin, but probably by ingestion of contaminated food. The source of the infection of the Haverhill epidemic was the consumption of raw milk.

Despite the fact that the clinical entities of the two forms of rat bite fever are easily differentiated, in some patients the picture is so confused that it is suggested that the bite of the rat could have transmitted both the causative agents, the streptobacillus and the spirillum. It is therefore necessary to employ, in every case of illness following the bite of a rat, techniques which will demonstrate both these microorganisms. So far, however, no proven case of such double infections has been recorded.

Streptobacillus moniliformis can be easily isolated from the patient's blood and skin lesions. Media enriched with blood, serum or ascitic fluid are required for its growth *in vitro*. On solid media, a high degree of moisture is essential.

Growth occurs both aerobically and anaerobically. The most characteristic feature of this non-motile, gram-negative microorganism is its extreme pleomorphism. Both slender small rods and, especially under unfavorable conditions, long, curved filaments with spindle-shaped or spherical swellings on them can be observed. True branching does not occur. The morphology is highly dependent on the medium and the age of the culture. In fluid media, growth occurs at the bottom, either in granular masses or with a more fluffy appearance, often with a clear supernatant fluid.

As to the epidemiology of the disease, little is known about its incidence among wild rats and other rodents. Strangeways (1933) isolated *S. moniliformis* from the nasopharynx of 4 out of 6 wild *rats*. Sometimes up to 50% of laboratory strains of white rats have been found to be infected, the animals carrying *S. moniliformis* in their nasopharynx without clinical symptoms. In Amsterdam, 2 out of 20 healthy white rats from the same batch (out of which one had caused human infection) were positive.

Sometimes the infected rats suffer from purulent lesions from which *S. moniliformis* is discharged.

Whereas *S. moniliformis* has been found repeatedly in apparently healthy rats, the infection in *mice* often seems to run a severer course.

Epizootics have been observed in wild mice, as well as in laboratory stocks of white mice.

Freundt (1956) described an epizootic in a strain of white laboratory mice with a high mortality and morbidity, which was characterized by general symptoms, polyarthritis, gangrene and spontaneous amputation of limbs. In feeding experiments the disease could be transmitted to other animals. It is suggested that in these cases the portal of entry was not through the intestines but through the mouth and throat. In experimental infections there was marked difference in the susceptibility of different experimental animals.

Often the disease is only recognized as a laboratory hazard after an accident has occurred. Treatment with large doses of penicillin and strepto-mycin has been recommended. In some cases a broad-spectrum antibiotic, such as chlortetracycline, should be administered to clear up the infection. Whether immediate disinfection of the wound will prevent development of the disease has yet to be proved. In the case of Lubsen *et al.* (1950) tincture of iodine did not work.

REFERENCES

ALLBRITTEN, F. F., R. F. SHEELY and W. A. JEFFERS, *J. Amer. med. Ass.*, 114 (1940) 2360.
ALTEMEIER, W. A., H. SNYDER and G. HOWE, *J. Amer. med. Ass.*, 127 (1945) 270.
BROWN, TH. M. and J. C. NUNEMAKER, *Bull. Johns Hopk. Hosp.*, 70 (1942) 201.
BIJLMER, J., *Antoni v. Leeuwenhoek*, 18 (1952) 246.
FUTAKI, K., J. TAKAKI, T. TANIGUCHI and S. OSUMI, *J. exp. Med.*, 23 (1916) 249.
FREUNDT, E. A., *Acta path. microbiol. scand.*, 38 (1956) 231.
HEILMAN, F. R. and W. E. HERRELL, *Proc. Mayo Clin.*, 19 (1944) 257.
HEISCH, R. B., *J. trop. Med. Hyg.*, 53 (1950) 33.
JELLISON, W. L., P. L. ENEBOE, R. R. PARKER and L. E. HUGHES, *Publ. Hlth. Rep. (Wash.)*, 64 (1949) 1661.
KUIPERS, F. C. and A. CH. RUYS, *Ned. T. Geneesk.*, 73 (1929) 1207.
LOMINSKI, I. R. W., A. S. HENDERSON and J. W. MCNEE, *Brit. med. J.*, (1948 II) 510.
LUBSEN, N., A. B. J. V. D. PLAATS and F. H. WOLTHUIS, *Ned. T. Geneesk.*, 94 (1950) 102.
MIYAKE, H., *Mitt. Grenzgeb. Med. Chir.*, 5 (1900) 231.
PLACE, E. H. and L. E. SUTTON, *Arch. intern. Med.*, 54 (1934) 659.
REITZEL, R. J., A. HAIM and K. PRINDLE, *J. Amer. med. Ass.*, 106 (1936) 1090.
ROBERTSON, A., *Ann. trop. Med. Parasit.*, 18 (1924) 157; 24 (1930) 367.
RUYS, A. CH., *Arch. Schiffs-u. Tropenhyg.*, 30 (1926) 112.
SOESILO, R., *Geneesk. T. Ned.-Ind.*, 66 (1926) 522.
SPRECHER, M. H. and J. R. COPELAND, *J. Amer. med. Ass.*, 134 (1947) 1014.
STRANGEWAYS, W. I., *J. Path. Bact.*, 37 (1933) 45.
ZUELZER, M., *Zbl. Bakt., I Abt. Orig.*, 85 (1921) 154.

16

J. VAN DER HOEDEN

Leptospirosis

Leptospirosis is probably the world's most wide spread contemporary zoonosis. It affects man and a very wide variety of animal species, the latter forming potential reservoirs of the causative agent and being sources for further propagation.

The history of this disease is quite recent. In 1916, almost simultaneously in Japan (Inado *et al.*) and in Germany (Uhlenhuth *et al.*) the spirochaetal aetiology of Weil's disease was recognized, after having been identified, 30 years previously, as a clinical entity *sui generis* (Weil, 1886: "Typhus biliosus nostras, a peculiar suddenly appearing infectious disease accompanied with fever, splenomegaly, icterus and nephritis").

From the wealth of newly acquired data collected during the last few decades by physicians, veterinarians, bacteriologists and epidemiologists it has been elicited that the agent causing Weil's disease and related parasitic organisms are of first rate significance as pathogens to animals and that they not seldom cause considerable harm to human health and welfare.

The causative organisms of leptospirosis belong to the genus *Leptospira* of the family *Treponemataceae* (Order *Spirochaetales*). The *Leptospira* which causes Weil's disease has been named *L. icterohaemorrhagiae* (syn. *L. icterogenes*). 2 years after the discovery of this *Leptospira* type another *(L. hebdomadis)* was identified as the cause of seven-day fever in Japan (Ido *et al.*, 1918); and in 1925 a third strain *(L. autumnalis)* was described as the agent of Japanese autumnal fever.

Continued research brought to light a great variety of leptospiral infections in almost every part of the world, including several already well known diseases of hitherto obscure aetiology. *L. pyrogenes* and *L.*

bataviae were first found in Indonesia in 1923 and 1926 respectively, *L. grippotyphosa* in the U.S.S.R. in 1928, *L. canicola* in the Netherlands in 1933, *L. australis A (Ballico)*, *L. australis B (Zanoni)* and *L. pomona* in 1937, and *L. hyos* in 1942 in Australia, *L. sejroe* in Denmark in 1939, *L. saxkoebing* and *L. ballum* in the same country in 1944. In the course of the following years more than 80 different types have been added to the list of pathogenic leptospirae.

Shortly after the discovery of the organism causing Weil's disease in man, Ido *et al.* (1919) found the same microorganism in 40% of grey rats in Japan. It is remarkable that it took several years before the wide distribution of pathogenic leptospirae among free-living and domestic animals was ascertained.

Whether the rather sudden establishment of the ubiquity of leptospiral infections resulted from actual extension of their dissemination in many parts of the world, or from the increased awareness of clinicians and bacteriologists, is still a matter of speculation. In several regions a wider dissemination of these organisms seems indeed to have occurred. The fact that a great part of the infections in animals can be discovered only by serological or cultural investigations may also have delayed their recognition. These subclinical or latent infections have a particular significance in the epidemiology of leptospirosis, because the affected animals are often carriers of the organisms for a long time and excrete the leptospirae in their urine. Data collected in Italian and Spanish rice fields, where, according to Babudieri (1958), before systematic preventive vaccination was initiated, the yearly toll of the disease among labourers ranged between 10 and 20 thousand, indicate how important leptospirosis is to human health. Its great extension among livestock in some parts of the world is illustrated by the estimate that, in the U.S.A. alone, the annual losses of animal industry due to this disease amount to more than 100 million dollars.

The discovery of saprophytic leptospirae *(L. pseudoicterogenes;* species: *biflexa,* Wolbach and Binger, 1914) antedates that of the pathogenic leptospirae (species: *interrogans*). Numerous and different strains are found almost everywhere in nature, particularly in water and humid soils.

All leptospirae are morphologically alike, *viz.*: a cylindrical proto-plasmic body twisted around a rigid axial filament. The organisms appear as very thin threads (3–30 micron length, 0.06–0.12 micron breadth) with close spiral coils and typical hooked or curved ends; they pass through certain kinds of bacterial filters (*e.g.* Seitz E. K.). It is very difficult to stain them, the most effective methods being either prolonged exposure to concentrated Giemsa solution or silvernitrate impregnation (Levaditi). The organisms are easily recognised by their peculiar manner of locomotion when they are observed by dark-field illumination.

Growth requires oxygen and a slightly alkaline medium. The optimal temperature for development is 28 to 30°. Multiplication is often considerably enhanced by the presence in the medium of bloodserum, and sometimes of haemoglobin, yeast extract or vitamin B_{12}.

Leptospirae readily die in an acid environment, or when there is a high grade of salinity, or bacterial pollution (water, sewage, soil, urine). They do not withstand desiccation.

The acidity of carnivore urine rapidly destroys leptospirae excreted from the kidneys and this occurs to some extent already while the organisms are in the bladder. This fact, and the presence of specific lysins in the urine of infected animals, may explain why leptospirosis is relatively rarely transmitted by dogs which are continuously shedding the parasitic organisms. The same may apply to interhuman infection. These factors, however, should not be regarded as constituting a safeguard against the contagiousness of such urines in general, especially when they are diluted with water, or are voided on alkaline soil.

In milk also, whether it is fresh, stored or pasteurised, pathogenic leptospirae soon degenerate and finally disappear by a lysin, which is a normal constituent of the milk of women, cows and goats. According to Kirschner and Maguire (1955) this lytic factor retains its activity up to a dilution of 1 : 32 or 64. Its harmful effect on pathogenic leptospirae, together with that of the specific immune lysins which are voided by infected animals, probably accounts for the fact that, in spite of frequent excretion of the organisms from cow's udders, milk-borne leptospirosis in man has not been recorded.

Investigations of the viability of leptospirae in the tissues of dead animals have yielded contradictory results, probably because of variations in the post-mortal pH and the antagonistic action of bacterial contamination.

Formerly, classification within the genus *Leptospira* was based on a great number of factors, but it has been found that the only feature that is sufficiently constant to be effectively used for its taxonomy is the antigenic structure. No valid classification of leptospirae can be based on their morphological, cultural or metabolic properties. Nor can the degree of virulence be satisfactorily used for this purpose. Serologically identical strains may differ considerably in their virulence.

At the present time the only method generally adopted for the differentiation of pathogenic leptospirae is the one introduced by Wolff and Broom (1954), which is based upon the principle of comparison of cross-agglutinin–absorption tests with sera of rabbits immunized against individual strains. This system, however, is merely of tentative value. Instead of speaking of "species" it has therefore been agreed to use the less committing terms "serological types", or "serotypes".

Serotypes having partially common antigenic structures are combined in "serogroups". By definition, two strains are considered as representing different serotypes if, after cross-agglutinin–absorption with adequate amounts of the heterologous strain, 10 or more % of the homologous antibody titre remains present in both antisera. From the serotypes (formerly called "complete" and indicated by AB) are distinguished "subserotypes" (formerly: "incomplete" biotypes, A), which differ from serotypes in that they leave, after cross-absorption with the heterologous strain, 10 or more % of the homologous titre in one antiserum, but less than 10% in the other. The arbitrarily chosen residual titre-limit of 10% does not exclude the eventual application of constant minor differences in epidemiological considerations.

The former belief that saprophytic "water leptospirae" might acquire pathogenic properties after passage through certain animal species, is now discredited. Some investigators, however, postulate that, under natural conditions, transition of one pathogenic leptospira serotype into another may be accomplished as a result of adaptation to the metabolisms of different host species. This would be shown by minor changes in the antigenic structure (Gsell, 1949; Kmety, 1954).

During the first week of the illness, the circulation of leptospirae in the blood can be demonstrated by direct dark-field microscopy, or by cultural methods or inoculation into susceptible test-animals. When few leptospirae are present, visible growth in culture media may take several weeks. The susceptibility of guinea pigs is restricted to only a few serotypes; hamsters and merions are more universally useful as test-animals.

Leptospirae may be found in the cerebrospinal fluid some days after their appearance in the blood. At about the end of the second week of the illness, the organism is usually present in the urine, the duration of its excretion in this depending on the kind of host species and the serotype involved. In cattle, urinary excretion of *L. pomona* has been observed for more than 4 months, in pigs for from 6 months to 1 year. Most infected sheep in New Zealand ceased shedding leptospirae after 2 or 3 months, although their persistence for as long as 9 months has occasionally been recorded (Webster and Reynolds, 1955). Leptospiruria in dogs may be continued for a very protracted period of time (*e.g.* $4\frac{1}{2}$ years, McIntyre and Seiler, 1953), whereas leptospirae are rarely found in horse's urine, where their short-lived appearance occurs at a rather late stage of the disease.

As a rule, rodents excreting leptospirae do not show signs of illness. Rats infected with *L. icterohaemorrhagiae,* mice with *L. saxkoebing* or *L. ballum* and voles with *L. grippotyphosa* were found to remain renal carriers for more than 1 year, sometimes even for the remainder of their lives. The majority of rodents shedding leptospirae are found in the older age group. According to Fühner (1950), human beings seldom excrete leptospirae for longer than 1 month, although Johnson (1950) recorded continued excretion of *L. pyrogenes (zanoni)* in the urine of a man 11 months after his recovery from the disease.

As opposed to the relatively small number of leptospirae to be found in the urine of herbivore carriers, their number in the urine of rodents, dogs and hogs is usually appreciably larger.

The diagnostic laboratory methods most commonly applied aim at detecting leptospiral antibodies in the blood-serum. For this purpose the method of choice is the agglutination test, this being eventually combined with the lysis reaction, the results of both usually being microscopically read. Antibodies react especially with the causative serotype, although not infrequently strong co-agglutination with other serotypes belonging to the same serogroup does occur. Newly born calves of infected cows may posses at birth a high antibody concentration, which dwindles to nil in the course of a few months. A small number of presumably intra-uterine transmissions of antibodies from infected mothers to their offspring has been recorded in literature. Moreover, Fennestad and Borg-Petersen (1957) showed that foetuses of cattle can become infected *in utero,* and that they themselves actively produce antibodies. Considerable passive transmission of antibodies to young calves may also occur in the colostrum and milk of infected cows.

Paradoxical seroreactions with heterologous serotypes are not infrequently encountered during the acute stage of the illness. Whereas the heterologous titer rapidly rises in the early stages and soon drops thereafter, the antibody concentration against the causative serotype gradually increases and ultimately surpasses the heterologous level. For this reason determination of the nature of the prevailing serotype by means of one test only done in the early stage of illness may be misleading.

No rational explanation has yet been given of the prolonged persistence of high-level seroreactions with *Leptospira* serotypes which, according to our system of classification, are not antigenically related to the causative strain. These heterogeneous titres are not infrequently higher than those obtained with the homogeneous strain. They may be a source of diagnostic error and may lead to incorrect epidemiological evaluation. Kméty (1954) recorded human infections with *L. icterohaemorrhagiae* in Czechoslovakia which displayed higher agglutinin values with *L. pomona* than with the causative serotype. The reverse has been reported by Faine and Kirschner (1953) in man in New Zealand and by Morse and Allen (1956) in cattle in the U.S.A. Strong cross-agglutinations with *L. autumnalis* and *L. hebdomadis* have been observed in cattle infected with *L. pomona* (Stoenner *et al.*, 1956).

The simultaneous presence of agglutinins for several serotypes has often been established in horses. Among 201 equines on a stud farm in Yugoslavia, Zaharija (1952) observed 125 (62%) with significant reactions for 2 to 5 different leptospirae. Exceptionally the multiplicity of agglutinins finds its explanation in double-infection. (Wiesmann and Suter, 1956: *L. pomona* and *L. hyos;* Smith and Doherty, 1956: *L. hyos and L. mini-szwajizak*, in man; the author, 1958: *L. canicola* and *L. szwajizak*, in hedgehogs).

Agglutinins and lysins often persist in blood and urine for a considerable period, the duration being determined both by the kind of host species and the leptospiral serotype. The author (1936) observed positive reactions with *L. icterohaemorrhagiae* in the sera and urine of persons in Holland, who had suffered from Weil's disease up to 20 years earlier. The possibility should not be excluded that repeated infections may have caused this continued high serotitre level. Naumann (1950) found significant agglutinin titres for *L. grippotyphosa* 3 years after recovery from mud fever. *L. pomona* agglutinins usually disappear more rapidly from cattle, although long lasting reactivity has also been recorded (Morse *et al.*, 1955). The sera of a large percentage of rats shedding *L. icterohaemorrhagiae* are entirely lacking in specific antibodies.

Among the leptospirae that are widely disseminated over the continents special mention should be made of *L. icterohaemorrhagiae, L. canicola* and *L. pomona.* Other serotypes are confined more closely to limited territories. Striking regional differences may be noticed in the incidence of serotypes, the largest diversity of strains having been encountered in Australia and south-east Asian countries (43 in Malaya). On the other hand, a much smaller range of serotypes is to be found in northern Europe (4 in England and in Holland).

Inability to resist desiccation renders leptospirae, when they are outside their hosts, extremely sensitive to the degree of humidity of the environment. In a general way, infection by the parasitic organism will occur only after having made direct contact with the urine or organs of carrier animals or with water, mud, humid soil or crops contaminated with such urine (Cane-cutter's-, Ricefield worker's-, Pea-picker's disease, Harvest fever). This accounts for the frequency of leptospirosis among butchers, slaughter-house and meat packing personnel, breeders of cattle and pigs

(Swine-herd's disease), veterinarians, sewerage workers, miners employed in a wet environment, anglers, fish trimmers and agricultural labourers working in heavily irrigated or inundated fields. In hot and dry climates with heavy dew formation, the urine of nocturnal animals, voided on soil and crops, is a hazard to workers in the field during the early hours of the day.

Multiple cases of leptospirosis usually occur among bathers and, still more, among persons who accidentally immerse themselves in canals, creeks or ponds. Outbreaks in bathing establishments are not uncommon. In most instances open waters are contaminated by rats or voles.

A large number of human infections also were connected with water polluted by the excretions of domestic animals. Mitov and Jankov (1956) recorded an outbreak of L. pomona infection among children bathing in a canal to which cattle and swine had access, 31 and 75 % of which respectively reacted significantly with this serotype. Misao et al. (1956) reported in Japan two water-borne outbreaks of canicola fever, involving 157 bathers in an area in which a large number of dogs carrying leptospira were found.

The foremost portal of entry for leptospirae is the skin, especially when it has been wounded, cut or abraded or has become soddened by long continued contact with water. The mucous membranes of the eyes, nose and throat are also susceptible.

Bites of dogs, rats, voles and ferrets have been recorded as preceding leptospirosis by 5 to 10 days.

In several instances it was believed that ingestion of contaminated water caused mass infection.

Jorge (1932) reported an epidemic of Weil's disease in Lisbon, which involved 126 persons who had drunk the water of a fountain, the cistern of which was heavily infested by rats excreting L. icterohaemorrhagiae. Rankow (1955) investigated an explosive outbreak in Yugoslavia which involved more than 390 men, of whom 8 died. L. icterohaemorrhagiae was supposed to have contaminated a public well which supplied drinking water to the area. Ianovich et al. (1957) observed, in a Russian town, 70 cases of canicola fever in persons drinking water from a defective pump which had most probably been contaminated by dog's urine, heavy rains having aided the transmission.

Rats, hamsters, mice and young dogs are easily infected, either by eating the organs of animals which were carriers of leptospirae, or experimentally by oral application of a fresh leptospira culture. Most probably the organisms enter the lymphatic tissues of the throats of these animals. In man, contaminated food may also be a source of infection. Direct interhuman transmission is very rare. Doeleman (1932) described such a case in a woman who acquired Weil's disease through coition; her husband, convalescing from Weil's disease, was excreting the organism in his urine.

Laboratory infections have been reported, as having resulted from pricking the skin with a contaminated needle or cutting it with a glass splinter, or they were acquired by sucking a culture through a pipette, or splashing it into the eyes, or by the bites or scratches of test animals.

In several regions of the world the absence of leptospirosis has been ascribed to acid soils and natural waters. Musaev (1960) found that in Azerbaijan (USSR) only one-sixth of the leptospirosis cases among livestock occurred on premises on which the soil was acid, as compared with the remainder which occurred on neutral or alkaline soils.

Outbreaks resembling epidemics have often occurred in swampy regions (*L. grippotyphosa* or *L. sejroe* in east European countries and Germany, causing mud fever, field fever, swamp fever, harvest fever, pea-picker's and hay-maker's disease). They were connected with field work, abundance of field rodents (especially voles), floods, heavy rains and other climatic conditions which contributed to the epizootic spread of infection among the local small-animal population and promoted transmission of the organisms to man. In tropical and subtropical regions the same applies to labourers in plantations which require abundant seasonal irrigation. This accounts especially for outbreaks of the disease in the workers on the ricefields in southern Europe and the sugar-cane cutters in Australia, many of whom work bare-footed on soil, which is heavily contaminated with the excretions of rodents.

In addition to the external factors which promote infection, internal conditions may contribute to the appearance of clinically evident lesions. Allergy to leptospirae seems to play an essential part in the establishment of certain local processes. The high frequency of significant seroreactions to pathogenic leptospirae in clinically healthy horses obviously indicates that many hidden or latent infections occur in these animals. One is inclined to correlate this fact with pathological processes of as yet undetermined origin.

As an example, equine periodic ophthalmia (recurrent iridocyclitis, moonblindness) may be mentioned. It is now almost generally believed that this is a leptospiral disease and that its aetiology is vested in an allergic reaction. The eye, sensitized in the acute stage of the illness, will be stimulated to a local tissue-reaction when the same allergen (serotype) is repeatedly introduced. According to Witmer (1954) persistence of the parasitic organism in the uveal tissue determines the focus of the ophthalmic lesions and relapses. In several instances leptospirae have been isolated from the aqueous humor of the affected eyes. This fluid also often shows a significant antibody concentration corresponding to the serotype in question.

The view just stated is supported by the discovery that relapses of moonblindness failed to take place when the horses were moved to an area free from pathogenic leptospirae, whereas return to the original environment brought back the ophthalmic attacks. Other pathological conditions, such as meningitis, haemorrhagic jaundice and haemoglobinuria in different host-species have also been ascribed to allergic sensitivity, and in these also localisation of the lesions is determined by the site of the latent focus of leptospiral infection.

Genetical factors do not apparently play any significant part in the pathogenesis of leptospirosis. The discrepancy in the statistics of the incidence of the disease may well be due to the different environmental conditions and modes of employment of the animals. The higher frequency of infection with certain leptospira serotypes in male persons as compared with females can generally be related to greater occupational exposure. This view is supported by the facts observed in *canicola* fever originating from contact with dogs, this contact being domestic rather than occupational, so that it affects approximately the same number of persons of both sexes. Likewise, the incidence of Weil's disease among male and female workers employed in the fish market in Aberdeen (Scotland) was about equal.

A bout of leptospirosis caused by a given serotype will confer immunity to later infections with the same strain. This contrasts with the increased susceptibility which apparently develops when subsequent infections are caused by certain other serotypes.

Infectivity and morbidity are greatly dependent on the serotype of the causative leptospirae; some serotypes are more pathogenic to man or certain animal species than others are. Whereas some leptospirae may produce a benign non-icteric disease, others provoke serious symptoms, which include marked jaundice and uraemia, and a relatively high death rate. However, under the influence of altered local conditions, the morbid reactions may undergo fundamental changes.

It is sometimes stated that *L. grippotyphosa* is in Europe, "the most anicteric" benign leptospirosis, but it causes serious illness in man with frequent incidence of icterus (70% in 1949–'50), and eventually death, in Israel. In that country, as well as in the U.S.S.R., the same organism also gives rise to severe outbreaks in cattle and goats, whereas in most other countries infection of these animals usually remains unobserved.

L. sejroe and *L. saxkoebing* infections, which are, as a rule, mild in Denmark, are in Italy more serious and sometimes fatal. In short, the antigenic structure of a leptospira strain is not always correlated with its pathogenicity.

It has been assumed that the variable pathogenicity is connected with the animal reservoirs to which the parasitic organism has adapted itself. The following examples may support this assumption.

Pet-dogs which are eliminating *L. canicola* are only very exceptionally a hazard to their owners, and rarely more than one case of *canicola*-fever is encountered in a family owing such animals. Neither clinical nor serological evidence of infection was found by the author among 38 persons working for long periods in the kennels of military and police dogs, more than 60% of which were affected by *L. canicola* and many of which were excreting the organism in the urine. Similarly, infection could not be established in 27 stable workers who were tending a large, heavily contaminated herd of cattle during an outbreak of leptospirosis – canicolaris, which had obviously originated from wide spread infection among jackals in the area. On the other hand, a large number of workers in various pigsties suffered from *canicola* fever (in one establishment 5 out of 7) although in most instances the swine, which significantly reacted and were excreting leptospira, did not exhibit clinical signs of the infection.

In addition to factors connected with the leptospirae and their carriers, the environment may have a definite influence on the course of the disease. In the last mentioned case, for instance, besides the massive excretion of leptospirae, which is characteristic of infected swine, the peculiar conditions prevailing in the pigsties doubtless played an important part in extending the incidence among the persons employed (unhygienic surroundings; frequent urinating of swine on concrete floors, which are abundantly splashed by water; intimate contact of the skin of hands, arms and bare feet of the workers with the heavily soiled animals and sties, etc.). Similar influences may also be at work in the epidemiology of leptospirosis caused by other serotypes.

As Burnstein and Baker (1954) have pointed out, quantitative factors are most probably of considerable importance in explaining the different results obtained by experiments on contact-infection. These authors noticed contamination of all healthy calves and pigs placed in a room together with infected swine for 12 to 45 days, whereas healthy pigs brought under similar conditions into direct contact with infected calves did not acquire infection.

Seasonally conditioned incidence is related to climatic factors and occupational exposure. Alterations of the ecological conditions brought about by man in a given territory may effect local situations which influence the epidemiology of leptospirosis. Reclamation of waste lands, afforestation, irrigation, draining, changes of crops or of agricultural methods are but some of the factors which may promote propagation of wild life, especially that of rodents, or drive away local fauna, or attract new species. By these influences the natural reservoirs of leptospirae, and consequently the epidemiology of leptospirosis can strikingly be altered in any given region. Outbreaks of leptospirosis have often been recorded during, or shortly after, excessive multiplication or mass-migration of rodents. Moreover, the moving of domestic animals from an infected herd to a non-infected place involves the risk of the introduction of carriers from which an outbreak may originate.

Picard (1954) recorded almost simultaneous occurrence of leptospirosis caused by the *ballum* serotype among the workers in the rice fields of the Rhône-delta in southern France and the Ebro-delta in Spain. He suggested that migrating birds acted as probable links between these remote outbreaks. Investigations of Babudieri (1958) have demonstrated the epidemiological importance of birds as carriers of leptospirae; he isolated *L. bataviae* from the organs of several species of wading birds in the Italian rice-fields. All the birds excreting leptospirae had migrated from Central Africa. By wading in contaminated water or ingesting mice infected with leptospirae, these birds may have become distributors of pathogenic leptospirae, so that they were, over long distances, links in the chain of infection between rodent-reservoirs and man. Experimental oral infection of the birds with *L. icterohaemorrhagiae*, *L. pomona* or *L. bataviae*, produced in them moderate agglutinin-titres and the pathogenic organisms were isolated from the bird's blood for 10 days after infection and from the faeces for 26 days. Experimentally infected ducks reacted in a similar way.

Because leptospirae circulate in the blood during the first stage of the illness, and because introduction of a few of the organisms into, or beneath the skin is sufficient to establish infection, it is conceivable that blood-sucking arthropods may also play a part in the epidemiology. Van Thiel (1948) successfully transmitted pathogenic leptospirae by means of mosquitoes, biting flies, body lice and bugs. However, no development of the organisms within the insects was noticed. Kunert and Schmidtke (1952) found viable leptospirae in the digestive tract of non-bloodsucking flies for a period of up to 26 hours after an infective meal. The organisms may adhere to the proboscis, or be excreted in the faeces or be regurgitated in the contents of the pro-ventriculus. Infected ticks have been occasionally found in nature. The author isolated *L. canicola* from *Rhipicephalus sanguineus* collected from a hedgehog in Israel. In southern Russia, *L.*

grippotyphosa was isolated from *Dermacentor marginatus,* parasitic on cattle in an endemic area. Although leptospirae may persist in ticks for a considerable time, the results of experimental transmission of the organisms by means of infected ticks have been contradictory. There are as yet no indications that ticks play an essential part in the epidemiology of leptospirosis. However, next to mammalian and avian hosts, they may constitute a reservoir in nature which is little influenced by atmospheric factors and consequently contributes to the survival of leptospirae under adverse environmental conditions ("maintenance vectors").

The most important sources of leptospiral infection are the long-term animal-carriers which shed the organisms from the kidneys along the urinary tract. Such state of carriership may exist without the hosts ever having shown clinical signs of infection. The distribution of leptospirae in the environment is directly connected with the number of animals excreting the parasitic organisms and with the local conditions favouring their maintenance outside the body.

A leptospira-serotype may be carried by animals belonging to various genera or species. Usually one of these represents the main reservoir in any particular region, others being secondary, or merely occasional carriers. The universal hosts of *L. icterohaemorrhagiae* are rats, especially *Rattus norvegicus;* various species of voles are the reservoirs of *L. grippotyphosa;* swine are the principal carriers of *L. pomona* and *L. hyos* and dogs of *L. canicola.* Under certain conditions the role of main host may be passed to another animal species; in addition to dogs, it has been shown for instance that jackals, pigs and hedgehogs may be reservoirs of *L. canicola.* Moreover, one animal species can be a carrier of different leptospira-serotypes.

The diversity of animal hosts of leptospira serotypes, as well as their world-wide distribution, are shown in Table XXIII.

The syndrome of leptospirosis is basically the same in both man and animals. Differences of the intensity of the pathological lesions and the frequency of their appearance are generally of a quantitative nature. Pathogenic leptospirae most often affect the liver and kidneys.

Whereas in rapidly progressing infections the liver is chiefly affected, in less acute infections the first lesions occur in the kidneys. The leptospirae often multiply in the lumina of the renal tubuli, where they actually live in colonies on the epithelial surfaces. Ocular manifestations occurring in an early stage of disease include conjunctivitis and injection of the

TABLE XXIII

WILD MAMMALIAN HOST ANIMALS OF *Leptospira* IN VARIOUS COUNTRIES *

Animals	Leptospira serotypes	Countries
Order: *Marsupialia*		
Fam.: *Didelphidae*		
Didelphis marsupialis (American Opossum)	*ballum, pomona, hyos, grippo, australis, autumnalis, mini georgia, -atlantae, ictero, "hebdomadis group".*	U.S.A.
D. azarae	*grippo, mini*	Brazil
	paidjan	Argentina
Paramelis nasuta (Long-nosed bandicoot)	*autumnalis, australis, kremastos*	N. Queensland
Trichosurus sp. (Australian opossum)	*medanensis*	N. Queensland
Thylacis obesulus (Rat kangaroo)	*kremastos, robinsoni*	N. Queensland
Order: *Insectivora*		
Fam.: *Erinacidae*		
Erinaceus europaeus,	*autumnalis*	Bulgaria, U.S.S.R.
E. roumanicus (Short eared hedgehog)	*australis (bratislava)*	U.S.S.R., Roumania, Bulgaria, Poland, Czechoslovakia, Scotland, Denmark, Italy
	australis (australis)	Israel
	pomona	Czechoslovakia, N. Zealand, Denmark
	bataviae	Bulgaria, Poland
	ictero, poi, sejroe	Czechoslovakia, Poland, Denmark
	grippo	Czechoslovakia, Poland
	canicola, mini (szwajizak)	Israel

* The data contained in Tables XXIII and XXIV are based upon mention of isolates in literature up to April 1963. Taxonomy of serotypes and – groups of the genus *Leptospira* mentioned in Table XXIII is found in the first 2 columns of Table XXIV. (The names *L. icterohaemorrhagiae* and *L. grippotyphosa* have been abbreviated *L. ictero* and *L. grippo*).

Animals	Leptospira serotypes	Countries
	ballum	Israel, Italy
	poi	U.S.S.R.
	sejroe	Czechoslovakia
	saxkoebing	Poland, Denmark, Italy
	pyrogenes	Australia
	autumnalis	U.S.S.R.
Hemiechinus auritus (Long-eared hedgehog)	canicola, grippo	Israel
Fam.: Soricidae		
Sorex araneus (Shrew)	poi	Czechoslovakia, U.S.S.R., Poland, Finland, Denmark
	grippo	Czechoslovakia, U.S.S.R., Poland
	sejroe	Poland
Fam.: Talpidae		
Talpa altaica (Mole)	poi, pomona	U.S.S.R.
Order: Chiroptera		
Cynopterus sp. (Fruit bats)	cynopteri, schüffneri	Indonesia, Andaman Islands
Myotis sp. (Brown mouse eared bats)	medanensis, wolffi	Malaya
Order: Edentata		
Dasypus novemcinctus (Armadillo)	pomona, canicola, autumnalis, sentoti, luisiana (hebdomadis group)	U.S.A.
Order: Lagomorpha		
Fam.: Leporidae		
Lepus europaeus (Brown hare)	grippo, australis, hyos	Czechoslovakia
Oryctolagus cuniculus (European rabbit)	sejroe	Hungary
Sylvilagus floridanus (Cottontail rabbit)	ballum	U.S.A.

Table XXIII (cont.)

Animals	Leptospira serotypes	Countries
Order: Rodentia		
Suborder: Sciuromorpha		
Marmota monax	ictero, ballum	U.S.A.
(Woodchuck, Groundhog)	pomona	U.S.A., Canada
Suborder: Myomorpha		
Fam.: Muridae		
Rattus norvegicus	ictero	all continents
(Brown-, sewer-, Norway rat)	bataviae	Europe, Indonesia, Malaya, Puerto-Rico
	pomona	Italy, Portugal, Hungary, Czechoslovakia, Yugoslavia, Roumania
	ballum	Italy, Spain, Portugal, Roumania, U.S.A., Canada, Israel, Puerto-Rico
	grippo, canicola	U.S.S.R.
	"hebdomadis"-group, autumnalis	Roumania
	hyos	Bulgaria
	pyrogenes	Australia
	sejroe	Poland
	saxkoebing	Hungary
	javanica	Indonesia, Malaya
	manilae	U.S.A., Puerto-Rico
	djatzi	Puerto-Rico
R. mülleri	ictero, pyrogenes, bataviae, australis, grippo, wolffi, hyos	Malaya
R. flavipectus	canicola, pyrogenes, autumnalis	China
R. rattus	ictero	all-continents
(Black-, house rat)	autumnalis	Malaya
	pyrogenes	Australia, Japan
	ballum, manilae	U.S.A.

Animals	Leptospira serotypes	Countries
R. alexandrinus (Roof rat)	grippo, mini (szwajizak)	Israel
	javanica, pyrogenes	Indonesia
	australis	Australia
	ictero, autumnalis	Asia, Africa, Europe
R. diardi (Indonesian house rat)	autumnalis	Indonesia
	javanica, bataviae, pyrogenes	Indonesia, Malaya
R. culmorum (Australian house rat)	australis	Australia
	javanica	Indonesia
R. brevicaudatus (Indonesian field rat)	javanica, bataviae, pyrogenes	Indonesia
	autumnalis	Malaya
R. exulans-concolor (Small rat)	schüffneri, benjamini, canicola, ictero, hebdomadis	Malaya
	javanica	Malaya, Indonesia
	australis	S.E. Asia, Australia, Europe
R. conatus	djasiman, hyos, autumnalis, malaya, pyrogenes, australis, grippo	Malaya
	ictero	Australia
R. bowersi	djasiman, hyos	N. Borneo
	autumnalis	Malaya
R. whiteheadi	mankarso	China
R. rajah	schüffneri, hebdomadis, javanica, hyos	Indonesia
Mus musculus (House mouse)	ballum	Malaya
	pomona	Denmark, Netherlands, Czechoslovakia, U.S.A., Germany, France, Israel, Czechoslovakia, U.S.S.R., Poland, Italy, Portugal
	sejroe	Denmark, Czechoslovakia, Poland, Finland, Italy
	australis	Australia, Poland
	saxkoebing	Denmark, Czechoslovakia, U.S.S.R.

References p. 273–274

Table XXIII (cont.)

Animals	Leptospira serotypes	Countries
	ictero	Poland, Czechoslovakia, U.S.A., Puerto-Rico
	grippo	Poland, Israel, Czechoslovakia, U.S.S.R.
	mini (szwajizak)	Israel
	hebdomadis	U.S.A.
	bataviae	Poland, Bulgaria,
	djatzi	Puerto-Rico
M. spicilegus (Gleaner mouse)	ballum	N. Spain, S. France
	sejroe	Denmark, Italy, Germany
	saxkoebing	Europe, E. Asia
M. brevirostris	pomona, sejroe	Italy
M. molessinus	ictero	Korea
Micromys minutus, (Harvest mouse, dwarf mouse)	bataviae	N. Italy, U.S.S.R., Finland, Czechoslovakia, Bulgaria
	ictero	Denmark, Czechoslovakia, Bulgaria, E. Asia
	grippo	E. Asia, Poland
	mini(mini), pomona	Bulgaria
	sejroe	Denmark
	bataviae	U.S.S.R.
Arvicanthis abyssinicus (Abyssinian mouse)	ndambari	Congo
A. niloticus (Striped mouse)	ictero	Turkey
Apodemus sylvaticus (Long-tailed wood mouse)	grippo	Germany, Czechoslovakia, N. Italy, U.S.S.R. Hungary
	sejroe	Germany, Czechoslovakia, N. Italy, Poland, Hungary
	saxkoebing	Germany, Czechoslovakia, Italy, Poland, Bulgaria

Animals	Leptospira serotypes	Countries
A. speciosus (Large Japanese field mouse)	*bataviae*	Italy, Czechoslovakia
	ballum	Portugal, Sardinia, U.K., Italy, Spain
	poi	Denmark, Poland, U.S.S.R.
	ictero, australis	Bulgaria
	autumnalis	E. Asia (Japan)
A. agrarius (Striped field mouse)	*grippo*	Czechoslovakia, U.S.S.R., Poland
	pomona	Czechoslovakia, U.S.S.R., Denmark, Bulgaria
	sejroe	Asia
	saxkoebing, ballum	Denmark
	bataviae	Bulgaria
	canicola	U.S.S.R.
	ictero	Korea
A. flavicollis (Yellow-necked field mouse)	*grippo*	Czechoslovakia, Hungary
	sejroe	Denmark, Italy
	saxkoebing	Denmark, Italy, Czechoslovakia, Yugoslavia
	poi	Denmark, Finland
	australis(jalna)	Czechoslovakia, Yugoslavia
	bataviae, sejroe	Czechoslovakia
A. microps Sigmidon hispidus (Cotton rat)	*ballum*	U.S.A.
Bandicota indica (Large bandicoot rat)	*australis(australis)*	Australia
Peromycus maniculatus (Deer mouse)	*ballum*	U.S.A.
Fam.: Cavidae Cavia aperae azarae C. pamparum (Cavy)	*ictero*	Brazil
	pomona	Argentina
Fam.: Microtidae Arvicola terrestris (Water vole)	*grippo*	European continent
	canicola	U.S.S.R.

Table XXIII (cont.)

Animals	Leptospira serotypes	Countries
Clethrionomys glareolus (Red backed bank vole)	grippo	Germany, Czechoslovakia, Denmark, U.S.S.R.
	australis(bratislava)	Czechoslovakia
	saxkoebing	Denmark
	poi	Denmark, U.S.S.R.
	ballum	U.K.
Ondatra (Fiber) zibethicus (Musk rat)	sejroe, saxkoebing	Poland, U.K.
	pomona	U.S.S.R.
Microtus arvalis (Common field vole)	grippo, ictero	U.S.A., Poland, Czechoslovakia
	grippo, ballum	Europe
	bataviae, pomona	U.S.S.R., Poland
	mini(mini)	Bulgaria
	saxkoebing	Germany, Italy, Denmark
	autumnalis, naam	Poland
	australis (jalna)	Czechoslovakia
	australis (bratislava)	Poland
	bataviae	Finland
M. agrestis (Field vole)	sejroe	Finland, Hungary, Poland
	sejroe	Denmark, Finland
	saxkoebing, pomona	Denmark
M. montebelloi	grippo	U.S.S.R.
	autumnalis	E. Asia
	ictero, sejroe, saxkoebing	Japan
M. guentheri (Levant vole)	hebdomadis	Japan, Congo
	grippo	Israel
M. pennsylvanicus	ballum	U.S.A.
M. hirtus	ballum	U.K.
M. oeconomus (ratticeps) (Root vole, Tundra vole)	grippo, hebdomadis group, poi	U.S.S.R.
	grippo, bataviae, poi	

Animals	Leptospira serotypes	Countries
Fam.: Cricetidae		
Cricetus cricetus	*grippo*	Germany, Hungary, Poland
(Common hamster)		
Fam.: Myocastoridae		
(Beaver rats)		
Myocastor coypus	*ictero*	Italy, U.S.A., Argentina
(Nutria)	*paidjan, zanoni*	U.S.A.
Order: Carnivora		
Fam.: Canidae		
Canisaureus	*canicola*	Israel
(Jackal)		
Urocyon cinereoargenteus	*australis, ictero, pomona, ballum*	U.S.A.
(Grey fox)		
Dusicyon gymnocercus	*canicola*	Argentina
(pampar fox)		
Vulpes vulpes	*ictero, sejroe, australis*	Czechoslovakia
(Common fox)	*grippo*	Czechoslovakia, U.S.A.
	pomona	U.S.S.R.
Vulpes fulva	*pomona*	U.S.A.
Fam.: Viverridae		
Herpestes javanicus	*javanica*	Indonesia
(Indian mongoose)	*ictero, djatzi*	Puerto-Rico
H. ichneumon	*ictero*	U.S.A.
	canicola	Hawaii
H. edwardsi	*ballum*	U.S.A.
	bataviae	Canada, Cuba, N. Queensland
Fam.: Procyonidae		
Procyon lotor	*australis, autumnalis, ballum*	U.S.A.
(Raccoon)	*mini (georgia), pomona, grippo,*	
	hebdomadis group, ictero, hyos, pomona, paidjan	Canada

Table XXIII (cont.)

Animals	Leptospira serotypes	Countries
Fam.: Mustelidae		
Mustela (Putorius) putorius (Polecat)	*grippo*	Czechoslovakia, Poland
M. erminea (Stoat)	*grippo, bataviae poi, sejroe*	Czechoslovakia, U.S.S.R. Denmark
M. nivalis (Weasel)	*grippo*	Czechoslovakia
Mephitis mephitis (Striped skunk)	*pomona, ballum, hyos, canicola, ictero, grippo, australis,* hebdomadis-group *(mini georgia)*	U.S.A.
Spilogale putorius	*ballum*	U.S.A.
Fam.: Felidae		
Lynx rufus (Bobcat, Wild cat)	*pomona, ballum, hyos grippo*	U.S.A. U.S.S.R.
Order: Artiodactyla		
Fam.: Suidae		
Sus scrofa (Wild boar)	*hyos*	Czechoslovakia
Fam.: Cervidae		
Cervus elaphus (Red deer)	*grippo, pomona, australis, bataviae*	Czechoslovakia
Cervus nippon (Sika deer)	*pomona*	U.S.S.R.
Capreolus capreolus (Roe deer)	*grippo*	Czechoslovakia
Dama virginiana (White-tailed deer)	*pomona*	U.S.A.
D. dama (Fallow deer)	*grippo*	Czechoslovakia

episcleral blood vessels. During convalescence, or long after clinical recovery, uveitis and iritis may develop.

The clinical symptoms exhibited in *cattle* are varied. Fever appears 1 to 2 weeks after infection and it usually lasts no longer than 4 or 5 days. The disease may either run a rapid course, develop more gradually, or remain clinically inapparent. At the onset there are general signs of illness, with utter depression, general weakness and loss of weight; sometimes watery diarrhoea exists for one or several days. In the acute form, haemolytic anaemia with a rapid fall of the haemoglobin index occur and these symptoms are associated with haemoglobinaemia and haemoglobinuria. The urine becomes dark red or almost black and contains albumen and bile-pigments.

Heavy jaundice indicates a serious development of the disease, while high urea-concentration is often a sign that death is to be anticipated in from a few days to a week. Histological examination of the liver shows focal necrosis, with minute round-cell infiltration around the smaller bile ducts and sometimes dissociation of the hepatic cords and areas of focal necrosis. The kidneys show interstitial nephritis and, in the acute phase, petechial haemorrhages. The pale kidney is often considerably enlarged and multiple white spots are scattered principally throughout the cortex. Microscopically there is diffuse and focal round-cell infiltration, particularly in the cortex, epithelial cells show necrosis and the distended tubules contain hyaline and cell casts. In the chronic stage, the white spots with distinct margins extend as wedges towards the center of the kidney. One of the early signs of illness is curtailment of milk production, which may lead to total agalactia.

During the febrile period the mammary secretion is thickened, yellowish or bloody. After clinical recovery the milk yield often remains below normal for several weeks and sometimes it is permanently impaired below the quantity originally secreted.

Abortion is among the more severe pathogenic side effects. It usually occurs at mid-term. The foetus, foetal membranes and umbilical cord are oedematous; prolonged retention of the foetal membranes is common.

The course of herd infections is subject to great variations. In one part of a country outbreaks with a mortality of 10 to 20% have been observed, whereas in another area the same organism may merely provoke inapparent infections, which are detectable by an increase in the number of cows which react serologically and a rise of their serotiters. Usually most subclinical infections are observed at the outset and towards the termination of the enzootics.

Since 1935, severe outbreaks of bovine leptospirosis have been repeatedly reported from the U.S.S.R. (Michin and Azinow). In 1946 *L. grippotyphosa,* the serotype which causes mud-fever in man, was identified as the agent of the disease in cattle (synonyms, used in the U.S.S.R.: *L. icterohaemoglobinuria, L. vitulina, L. icteroanaemia I)*. Similar enzootics occurred in Israel and other Middle Eastern countries *("L. bovis",* 1946). Serological evidence of bovine *grippotyphosa* infections has been reported from several European, Asiatic and African regions, Australia and Surinam.

In 1949, Sutherland *et al.* in Australia, demonstrated *L. pomona* as the cause of "red-water" (haemoglobinuria) among calves. Until then the cause of this disease was unknown, although Clayton *et al.* (1937) had already isolated in that country the same serotype from sick dairy farmers. *L. pomona* was also identified in swine herd's disease in Switzerland (Gsell, 1944). The wide distribution of *L. pomona* in the U.S.A. (original: "New Jersey strain") is shown by the enormous damage, already mentioned, that it causes to animal industry in that country.

L. pomona is also important in certain parts of the U.S.S.R. (synonyms: *L. icteroanaemia II, L.D.V.B., type Monjakov,* etc.). In several European countries, as well as in Canada, Argentina, New Zealand, China, and in the Congo it has been reported in cattle. *L. hyos* (synonym: *L. mitis Johnson),* first isolated from a man in Brisbane (1940), is like *L. pomona,* mainly found in swine, but it also affects cattle in Australia, Argentina, Germany, Belgium and other European regions. Several other serotypes have been found to be pathogenic to the bovines in various countries, *e.g. L. icterohaemorrhagiae* in Europe (since 1949), Argentina (synonym "*L. bonariensis*", 1947), New-Zealand, Central Africa (1955) and Japan (1956). High antibody titres for *L. sejroe* have been found in bovines in several parts of Europe and North America, and for the closely related *saxkoebing* serotype in Denmark, Switzerland and Italy. *L. hardjo,* which like the latter two serotypes, belongs to the *hebdomadis* serogroup, was isolated from cattle in Louisiana in 1960 (Roth *et al.*). These authors suggested that *L. hardjo* may be responsible for the frequency of antibodies against the *sejroe* serotype in North American cattle.

L. hebdomadis, L. australis A and *L. autumnalis* have been isolated from sick cows in Japan (1951). A serological indication of bovine infection with the first was recorded in Europe and Central Africa, with *L. bataviae* and *L. butembo* in Congo, with *L. ballum* and *L. poi* in Denmark (1956), with *L. mini szwajizak* in Israel (1959). *L. canicola* brought about serious outbreaks among cattle in Israel (1955) and has also been recorded in cases of bovine leptospirosis in the U.S.A., Denmark and East Germany.

Most leptospiral infections in *goats* may, although they often remain clinically undetected, acquire a serious character in some territories and may almost wipe out entire herds. In such outbreaks, which are characterized by intense orange-tinged jaundice and reddish to blackish urine, death may be expected after only a few days of illness. These symptoms are frequently associated with abortion.

Caprine leptospirosis caused by the *icterohaemorrhagiae* serotype was first recorded in Austria in 1937. Outbreaks of *grippotyphosa*-infection have been reported from the U.S.S.R. (1941) and from Israel (1953); heavy losses resulted. The *pomona* serotype has been found in North-American (1955) and Chinese goats. In the Congo (1956) serological evidence was found of caprine infection with *L. icterohaemorrhagiae*, *L. grippotyphosa*, *L. bataviae*, *L. hebdomadis* and *L. butembo* (1953).

In *sheep*, in which the disease follows a course similar to that seen in goats, the incidence of leptospirosis is lower.

L. pomona infection was recorded in ovines in New Zealand (1952), in the U.S.A. and Hungary (1958); *L. grippotyphosa* infection occurred in the U.S.S.R. (1949) and in Iran (1961),*L.ballum* infection in Argentina (1962). Significant titers for the *grippotyphosa* serotype were noted in Israel (1950) and East Germany (1957) and for *L. icterohaemorrhagiae* in West Germany (1951), Italy (1955), the Congo (1956), East Germany (1957) and Somalia (1960), for *L. sejroe* in Poland, for *L. bataviae* and *L. butembo* in the Congo.

Icterohaemorrhagiae agglutinins were found in dromedaries in Iran (1959); *L. grippotyphosa* in camels in South Kasachstan (U.S.S.R.). In Somalia (1960), antibody levels of diagnostic value were recorded in 11 of 61 dromedaries (6 against *L. grippotyphosa*, 2 against *L. icterohaemorrhagiae* and *L. canicola*, and 1 against *L. ballum*).

Leptospiral infection of *swine* has a world wide distribution. These animals are easily infected with various serotypes along different routes, but most swine either show slight pathologic symptoms or none at all. Frequently apparently healthy hogs excrete enormous numbers of leptospirae in the urine for extended periods of time, so that they are dangerous to susceptible domestic animals and to man. Conjunctivitis, fever, icterus, anaemia and haemoglobinuria are the most common symptoms in swine. Rather typical are meningitic and encephalitic signs (stiffness of the neck, incoordination, circling movements ("tourniquet") and hyperirritability). When these symptoms appear, the mortality may become very high. In the U.S.A. and the U.S.S.R. heavy losses are sustained from multiple abortions. Unthriftiness of young piglets is a frequent sequel to leptospiral infection. The lowered general resistance facilitates secondary infections, especially by salmonellae. At slaughter, a large number of whitish spots are found scattered in the cortex of the kidneys, and chronic infections cause scarring, shrivelling and focal fibrination.

In all 5 continents the serotypes most frequently encountered in swine are *pomona* and *hyos*. The former was originally described in Australia (1939), later in Argentina (syn.: "*L. suis*", 1944) and Indonesia (1948) and Peru (1960). *L. hyos* was isolated from pigs in Switzerland in 1948, in Australia in 1951 and Peru (1960). In Hungary 84% of the pigs reacted with *pomona* antigen (1956). *L. icterohaemorrhagiae* was recovered in England from icteric hogs (1951) and afterwards in several other countries. *L. canicola* infection of swine has been reported as an important source of human disease in Israel (1954), Roumania (1956), Czechoslovakia, Great Britain and U.S.S.R. (1957). It has also been observed in Portugal, Hungary and Switzerland. Furthermore, hogs may harbour several other leptospirae, *i.e. L. grippotyphosa, -poi, -autumnalis, -australis, -sejroe, -saxkoebing,* and *-ballum.*

As has already been mentioned (see p. 245), in several parts of the world a considerable number of clinically healthy *horses* show significant sero-reactions with the locally prevailing leptospirae. Bokori *et al.* (1958) reported an incidence of 5 to 70% in horses in various regions in Hungary. This high frequency led some investigators to look for a link with equine diseases of hitherto obscure origin, *e.g.* hypertrophic cirrhosis of the liver (Schweinsberger disease), Zdár disease (Pokorný) and chronic lymphang-itis (Schlossberger *et al.*). These aetiological relationships are, however, still hypothetical. Horses sometimes exhibit general symptoms common to acute or subacute leptospirosis. Bordjoski (1957) described an epizootic in Yugoslavia, which affected 52 horses with high fever, anorexia, polydipsy, conjunctivitis, meningismus, jaundice and oedematous swelling of the legs.

Jivoin (1958) reported sporadic cases and enzootic outbreaks among horses in Roumania characterized by hepato-renal, cardio-vascular and respiratory syndromes and digestive disorders. Most affected horses were icteric. Less frequent were urticaria, loss of hair, oedema on several parts of the body, abortion, irido-cyclitis and fatal meningo-encephalitis. The most characteristic equine lesion is moonblindness (periodic ophthalmia, see page 247), the leptospiral aetiology of which was discovered by Heusser *et al.* (1948) in Switzerland. This syndrome usually appears after a considerable latent period, as a non-purulent panophthalmia with a preponderance of uveitis and a tendency to relapse; sometimes total blindness results. In the outbreak in Yugoslavia cited above, 45% of the horses showed 2 to 8 months after the acute symptoms appeared, irido-cyclitis and pannous keratitis.

A significant titre of antibodies for *L. pomona* has often been observed in horses in the U.S.A. (1950), Germany (1951), Switzerland, France (1954) and Bulgaria (1959); for *L. grippotyphosa* in Israel (1952), Germany and Switzerland (1952), France (1954) and Poland (1956); and for *L. canicola* in Germany (1951), France (1954), Bulgaria, Israel and U.S.A. Occasionally there was serological evidence pointing to equine in-fection with *L. icterohaemorrhagiae, L. sejroe, L. australis A, L. hyos, L. saxkoebing, L. ballum, L. bataviae* and *L. salinem.*

Infections with *L. icterohaemorrhagiae* in *dogs* were recorded in Germany as early as 1916. 9 years later, Okell *et al.* established that "yellows" (enzootic jaundice), which is often observed in dogs in England and has a high mortality rate, is caused by the same organism. In 1933, Klarenbeek and Schüffner, in Holland, discovered that, another serotype, *L. canicola*, is the cause of the serious "Stuttgart's disease" of dogs. Leptospirosis affects dogs of various races and all age groups in almost every part of the world. Its higher incidence in male rather than in female dogs has been ascribed to their habits of licking the genitals and urine of the bitches.

The high incidence of *L. canicola* infection in the dogs of several countries, which may surpass 50%, usually remains fairly constant. The clinical manifestations of canine leptospirosis vary considerably. Many long standing infections remain unobserved by the owners, while the animals keep on excreting the organisms.

Gravest of all is the haemorrhagic form, which has a sudden onset with high fever lasting 3 or 4 days, general symptoms of malaise, intense depression and signs of dehydration, non-purulent conjunctivitis and episcleritis, congestion and haemorrhages of the skin and mucous membranes. Stomatitis, often complicated with ulceration, causes foul breath. The icteric form of canine leptospirosis takes an acute or subacute course. Frequent vomiting and constipation precede renal symptoms. In several instances jaundice appears in the first week of illness. With the exception of young puppies, icterus is much less frequently produced by *L. canicola* than by *L. icterohaemorrhagiae*. On the other hand, renal lesions are associated more often with *L. canicola* infections, which run either an acute, subacute or chronic course.

Stuttgart's disease is dominated by nephropathic signs (azotemial uraemia). Histological examination reveals vacuolar degeneration and necrosis of tubular epithelial cells, accompanied by a tendency to regeneration. The uraemic form is characterized by focal interstitial nephritis. The high incidence of chronic cirrhosis of the kidneys in old dogs has been considered to be a sequel of the leptospiral infections which frequently occur during early life.

Differentiation between infectious jaundice caused by *L. icterohaemorrhagiae* and Stuttgart's disease due to *L. canicola* cannot usually be based on clinical observations alone. Moreover, distinction between the two serotypes in the diagnostic serotests may be hampered by cross-agglutination of the animal's serum.

References p. 273–274

The following comparative ratios of the incidence of *L. canicola* and *L. icterohaem-orrhagiae* infections in canines have been reported. In England 8.5 to 1 (in Glasgow 40:0); in Germany 4.4 to 1; in Holland 23 to 1; in the U.S.A. 11 to 1; in Denmark 18 to 1; in Buenos Aires 83 to 1; in California 26 to 0; in Israel 240:0. The opposite was observed in Rome (1 to 26.5) and Honolulu (1 to 2). In evaluating these figures one should, however, take into consideration that they reflect only temporary situations, which are liable to great changes. In Indonesia, New Zealand and Australia the *canicola* serotype has only recently been detected and then only in very sparse distribution.

Serological evidence of infection with *L. hebdomadis* was found in dogs in Indonesia (1929), in the Congo (1953) and in Japan (1956); *L. bataviae* in Yugoslavia, Czecho-slovakia, Congo and in Peru (1958); *L. australis* in Indonesia, Japan (1951), East Germany (1955) and Congo; *L. autumnalis* in Japan and Malaya; *L. javanica* and *L. medanensis* in Indonesia (1935); *L. pomona* in New Zealand (1954), Indonesia, Central Europe, China and U.S.A. (1959); *L. grippotyphosa* in Israel and Congo (1953); *L. saxkoebing* in Yugoslavia, Germany (1954) and Denmark (1956); *L. sejroe* in the same countries and Hungary; *L. ballum* in East Germany and Yugoslavia; *L. kabura* and *L. butembo* in Congo (1942), *L. hyos* in Peru (1958), and *L. mini* in Israel.

In *cats,* in view of their intimate contact with mice and other potential rodent carriers of leptospirae, a high frequency of leptospirosis might be surmised. There exists, however, a considerable contrast between the incidence in domestic felines and canines. Experimental infection did not cause any signs of illness in the cats, although they may temporarily excrete the leptospirae. In accordance with their natural resistance, routine examinations in several countries seldom revealed leptospiral infection of the cat population.

Among cats in Denmark antibodies have occasionally been found against *L. ictero-haemorrhagiae, L. bataviae, L. saxkoebing* and *L. poi* (1956). A few instances of *L. canicola* agglutination were recorded in cats in Germany (1957). Infection with *L. grippotyphosa* was serologically demonstrated in a cat in Czechoslovakia. In England low agglutinin titres were noticed in a few instances, but attempts to isolate the organism failed. 3 cases of chronic interstitial nephritis were observed in cats which showed agglutinins for *L. canicola* in their serum (Hemsley, 1956). In Peru (1958) *L. canicola* and in the U.S.A. *L. pomona* (1962), were isolated from a cat. In contrast to other parts of the world, in certain Indonesian regions feline leptospirosis is not rare. Esseveld and Collier (1938) isolated several strains belonging to the *bataviae* serotype from cats in Djakarta (formerly: Batavia); the infection-rate increased with the age of the animals (25 to 30% of those weighing more than 1½ kg, reacted).

Outbreaks of leptospirosis in which *L. icterohaemorrhagiae* or *L. pomona* were involved have been reported several times from farms breeding *silverfoxes* (in England, 1934; in Germany, 1937; in Sweden, 1939; in

Poland, 1956). The disease, which chiefly affected young animals, ran a course similar to that of "yellows" of dogs and sometimes it decimated the stock.

Although *chickens* and other domestic birds can be infected experimentally, very slight or no pathological lesions are observed. For this reason no epidemiological importance has as yet been attached to poultry. The possible role of wild birds has been discussed on page 250.

With the exception of cats and poultry all domestic animals and especially dogs, swine and cattle, have been recorded as sources of leptospiral infections of *man*. In point of fact, most extended human infections are connected with natural reservoirs among wild rodents or other small field animals.

The incidence among human beings varies considerably in different parts of the world. From South Africa only a few sporadic cases have as yet been reported. On the other hand, in the jungle districts of Malaya, where one-third of the domestic animals and about one-sixth of wild rodents gave evidence of leptospiral infection, 35 % of the febrile diseases in foreign military personnel and 13 % of those in adult male non-European civilians, were caused by various serotypes of *Leptospira* (McCrumb *et al.*, 1957).

The incubation period in man varies between 1 and 2 weeks. The onset is sudden, with high fever, often accompanied by chills. Usually the fever runs a biphasic course; the first attack lasts 3 to 6 days and is followed, after an afebrile interval of 8 to 10 days, by a short relapse at a lower febrile level.

Other initial symptoms frequently encountered are hyperaemia of the conjunctival vessels and epicorneal injection without secretion, starting on the 3rd or 4th day, photophobia, heavy headache (an expression of meningismus) with increased tension of the clear liquor, myalgia causing acute attacks of pain especially in the calf muscles, relative bradycardia, sometimes bronchitic signs, renal irritation (albuminuria, and red- and white blood cells, hyaline and granular casts in the sediment), hypotony, and not seldom a scarlatine-like exanthema on the rump and thighs for a few days. Insomnia and depression or irritability may alternatively occur. Moderate hypochromic anaemia exists.

The course of human leptospirosis varies between a subclinical type and one that is very grave and fatal. The seriousness of the disease is proportionate to the intensity of the icterus and the disintegration of the

TABLE XXIV

OCCURRENCE OF DIFFERENT PATHOGENIC *Leptospira* SEROTYPES AND SUBSEROTYPES IN
HUMAN BEINGS IN VARIOUS COUNTRIES WITH MENTION OF YEAR OF FIRST APPEARANCE *

Serogroup	Serotype	Country
icterohaemorrhagiae	*icterohaemorrhagiae*	Japan (1914), in all continents
	incompleta	Denmark (1938), in all continents
	naam	Java (1936)
	mankarso	Sumatra, Malaya (1938)
	sarmini	Indonesia (1930)
	ndambari	Congo (1954)
	mwogolo	Congo (1946)
javanica	*javanica*	Malaya (1956)
	poi	Italy (1942), Denmark (1945), Malaya (1956)
	celledoni	Queensland (1953), Malaya (1957)
canicola	*canicola*	Netherlands (1934), in all continents
	schüffneri	Indonesia (1938), Andaman Islands (1939), Malaya (1958)
	benjamini	Sumatra (1937), Congo (1946)
	kamituga	Congo (1939)
	bafani	Congo (1946)
	kahendo	Congo (1946)
	malaya	
ballum	*ballum*	Denmark (1944), Netherlands (1948), Yugoslavia, Portugal (1951), Puerto-Rico (1960), Spain (1953), France (1954), Sardinia (1955), U.S.A. (1958), Italy, W. Germany (1959)
pyrogenes	*pyrogenes*	Indonesia (1923), Malaya (1928), Okinawa (1944), Japan (1951), Italy (1953), China (1960)
	zanoni	Queensland (1936), Italy (1942), Brazil (1954), Malaya (1956)
	robinsoni	Queensland (1951)
autumnalis	*rachmati* (*"autumnalis"*)	Indonesia (1923), Japan (1925), Malaya, Andaman Islands (1928), Indo China (1937), Thailand (1951), France, Germany, U.S.A. (1952), N. Borneo, Hungary (1955), China (1960)
	bangkinang	Indonesia (1937)
	sentoti	Sumatra (1937), Malaya (1958)
	djasiman	Indonesia (1937)
australis	*australis*	Queensland (1937), Switzerland (1946), Indonesia (1948), Germany (1950), Japan, S. Vietnam (1951), France, Indo-China (1952), Hungary, Madagaskar (1955), Malaya, Czechoslovakia (1956)
	muenchen	Germany (1953)
	bratislava	Czechoslovakia (1960)
pomona	*pomona*	Australia (1937), Switzerland (1938), Italy

* The classification is partly provisional.

Table XXIV (cont.)

		(1940), Argentina (1944), France (1945), Indonesia (1948), Hungary, Austria (1950), Yugoslavia, U.S.A., N. Zealand (1951), Spain (1952), Czechoslovakia (1954), Malaya, Chile (1956), Rumania (1957)
grippotyphosa	*grippotyphosa*	U.S.S.R. (1928), Andaman Islands (1931), Indo-China (1933), Germany (1938), Netherlands, Italy (1942), Denmark, Switzerland (1944), France (1945), Israel, Congo (1946), Cuba (1949), Austria, Hungary (1950), U.S.A., Spain (1952), Finland (1953), Czechoslovakia, Greece, Yugoslavia (1954), South America (1955), Malaya (1956), Rumania, Egypt (1957), Morocco, Iran (1959), Puerto Rico (1960)
hebdomadis	*hebdomadis*	Japan (1918), Indo-China (1938), Indonesia (1941), U.S.S.R. (1951), Okinawa (1952), Malaya (1954), N. Borneo (1955), Germany (1956)
	hebdomadis (nona)	Congo (1960)
	medanensis	Australia, Malaya (1954)
	wolffi	Indonesia (1937), Malaya (1954)
	hardjo	Sumatra (1938)
	mini-mini	Italy, Rumania (1941), Congo (1955)
	mini-szwajizak	Australia (1952), Israel (1959)
	mini-Georgia	U.S.A. (1960)
	kremastos	Queensland (1952), Jamaica (1957), Trinidad (1962)
	kabura	Congo (1946)
	kambale	Congo (1960)
	jues	Congo (1956)
	sejroe	Denmark (1939), France (1945), Switzerland (1946), Germany (1948), Austria (1950), Yugoslavia (1952), Finland (1953), Czechoslovakia (1955)
	saxkoebing	Italy (1941), Denmark (1944), Germany (1951), Hungary (1955), Spain (1960)
	borincana	Puerto-Rico (1959)
bataviae	*bataviae*	Indonesia (1926), Italy (1938), Congo (1946), Switzerland (1948), Denmark (1949), Viet-Nam (1950), Japan, Thailand, U.S.A., Puerto-Rico, Australia, Bulgaria (1951), Hungary, Indo-China (1952), Malaya (1954), Spain (1960)
hyos	*hyos*	U.S.S.R. (1938), Australia (1942), Argentina (1944), France (1950), Switzerland, Yugoslavia (1952), Italy (1953), New Zealand (1954)
	kisuba	Congo (1956)
cynopteri	*butembo*	Congo (1946)

kidneys. Soon after the initial symptoms, or at a later-stage, "aseptic" lymphocytic meningitis may develop, the liquor remaining clear. Jaundice, chiefly hepatic in origin, often follows the febrile period, at the end of the first week of illness. The bilirubin level of the blood is raised; urobilinuria also exists when icterus is not perceptible. A haemorrhagic diathesis is demonstrated by a tendency to sub-epithelial, sub-mucosal and sub-serosal bleedings, as well as by haemorrhages in organs and muscles. When interstitial nephritis develops, the urine contains albumin, hyaline and granular casts, erythrocytes and leucocytes; the output declines; in extreme cases anuria and uraemia may precede death. As a rule, the kidneys are normal after recovery.

Ocular complications, especially iritis, iridocyclitis and uveitis, usually appear at an advanced stage of the illness, or during convalescence or even up to a year after clinical recovery. In most cases complete restoration of health ensues, but a chronic condition, with turbidity of the corpus vitreum and reduced vision may develop. The recurrent form of panophthalmia, peculiar to equine leptospirosis, very seldom occurs in man.

According to Atkins (1955), migraine should be regarded as a rather frequent sequel to infection by L. icterohaemorrhagiae. This author found such a condition in 48% of persons who had formerly suffered from Weil's disease, as compared with only 12% in a control group.

In several countries an average mortality of 5 to 10% due to leptospirosis has been reported in man (in cases with intense jaundice up to 30% may succumb). In other regions the disease is practically always benign.

Table XXIV includes the most important leptospiral serogroups and -types which affected human beings in various parts of the world.

The spread of leptospirosis among domestic animals is greatly promoted by overcrowding on narrow, humid, in-sanitary premises or pastures, and by the addition of animals from infected herds to uninfected stock. Only animals which, after blood testing, have shown to be safe, should be permitted to join a serologically negative herd. In infected regions replaced ruminants should be segregated from "clean" local stocks for at least a month and retested before they are admitted. This measure should be carried out intelligently, because excretion of the leptospirae is usually much more limited than is the persistence of antibodies. Healthy animals, however, should not be allowed to share fields, watering places and feedlots with infected herds, and care must be taken that the water supply is not drained from soil on which infected animals are grazing. Domestic animals excreting *Leptospira* should be either eliminated from a herd, or slaughtered. If circumstances permit, all reacting animals in a herd should be separated from the non-reactors. Aborted foetuses and foetal membranes must be destroyed. Splashing of milk on the floor must be avoided and adequate drainage of muddy soil should be provided for. Rodents should be eradicated from sheds and pastures whenever there is a risk of leptospirosis. In certain regions the exclusion or extermination of other wild animals, such as shrews, hedge-hogs, jackals, foxes, skunks and wading birds, should also be considered. Man and domestic animals alike will benefit from such control measures. Workers on irrigated or flooded fields should be cautioned against direct contact with contaminated water or mud and should be advised to use high rubber shoes and gloves. In such environments the eradication of rodents, particularly before harvest time, is strongly recommended.

The same protective measures apply to labourers in other exposed professions, such as miners and sewerworkers. Special care should be exercised by butchers when they are slaughtering infected cows, goats, sheep or pigs.

Bathing may be hazardous in rat-infested areas and in natural waters to which dogs, cattle, swine and other domestic animals have access. Rat proofing of bathing establishments is by itself insufficient; water supplies must also be checked.

Small amounts of calcium chloride added to drinking water will rapidly kill leptospirae, while sodium hypochlorite has been recommended for the disinfection of premises and objects.

The literature on methods of eliminating the infection from urinary carriers by antibiotics is confusing. Because this treatment will be effective only during the early days of the illness, chronic infections would not apparently benefit from it. Nevertheless, prolonged administration of chlortetracycline or terramycin in the food of swine seemed to suppress *pomona*-infection. When it was given to infected pregnant sows, fewer abortions, a lower mortality rate among newborn pigs, increased weights at birth and weaning, and better health and thriving of the piglets were noticed (Baker *et al.*, 1957). Furthermore, very satisfactory results have been recorded in the treatment of acute Stuttgart's disease of dogs. For animal therapy, streptomycin, aureomycin, tetramycin and erythromycin have been especially recommended, preferably when some of them are combined. For dogs antibiotics have replaced the highly potent immune sera formerly used. The contradictory evaluation of antibiotics in human leptospirosis is mainly due to the fact that treatment was usually started at a much too advanced stage of the illness. It has been proved that beneficial results can be expected only if the antibiotics are given when the first symptoms appear and before the organisms have settled in the organs.

Preventive vaccinations have been carried out in Japanese coal miners since 1919. Tens of thousands of persons have been vaccinated and it is claimed that the results have been very satisfactory. In Great Britain, dogs were adequately protected against "yellows" by the injection of a killed suspension of *L. icterohaemorrhagiae* (Dalling and Okell, 1926). Large-scale vaccination programmes have been instituted as a result of recent advances in our knowledge of the importance in both Europe and North America, of leptospiral infections.

A successful trial was made in Spanish rice field workers in 1953 (Altava *et al.*, 1955) with formalin-killed *Leptospira* cultures. It was continued on a large scale by Babudieri in Italy and followed in the U.S.S.R. (Lioubachenko, 1958) and Poland (Parnas, 1959).

The immunity conferred by the introduction of leptospirae is strongest for the types employed. The most efficacious results are therefore obtained with vaccines prepared from single or combined *Leptospira* strains of the serotypes commonly prevailing in the region in which immunization will be carried out. In the U.S.S.R. the vaccine for human use contains *L. icterohaemorrhagiae*, *L. pomona* and *L. grippotyphosa*. Until 1959 more than 200,000 occupationally exposed persons had been vaccinated with good results. In Poland 2,500 subjects were treated with a similar product of *L. grippotyphosa* and *L. sejroe*.

More than 10,000 rice field workers were vaccinated in Italy with selected strains of *L. icterohaemorrhagiae* and *L. bataviae*, killed with formalin, yielding a very satisfactory outcome. The vaccine used in Spain contains *L. icterohaemorrhagiae* and *L. ballum*.

In Tunisia beneficial results are claimed from vaccination of cattle and sheep against *L. grippotyphosa* infection (Gayot, 1955). Mass vaccinations of animals have as yet been done only in the U.S.A. and the U.S.S.R. In the latter country more than 16 million domestic animals, including cattle, small ruminants, horses and silverfoxes, were vaccinated and optimal results were claimed. In the U.S.A., where only *L. pomona* is used for vaccine production, more than 1,500,000 cattle and swine had already been immunized in 1957. Various methods were used for the preparation of these "bacterins" *e.g.*: alternative freezing and drying (York and Baker, 1953), acid-heat extraction of living cultures (Hoag and Bell, 1955), and attenuation of the strain by passage through more than 500 embryonated eggs (Kenzy *et al.*, 1957).

In general, the campaign against leptospirosis in man and domestic animals must be approached from different angles. The main factors to be considered are associated with environmental, hygienic and geo-climatic conditions, the presence of water and the existence of persistent reservoirs of the causative organisms in wild and domestic animals.

REFERENCES

ALEXANDER, A., P. W. WETMORE, L. B. EVANS, H. JEFFRIES and C. A. GLEISER, *Amer. J. trop. Med. Hyg.*, 4 (1955) 492.
ALSTON, J. M. and J. C. BROOM, *Leptospirosis in man and animals*, Edinburgh–London, 1959, 367 pp.
ALTAVA, V., M. BARRERA, J. VILLALONGA, P. GIL, C. MARIN and B. BABUDIERI, *Rev. Sanid. Hig. públ. (Madr.)*, 29 (1955) 167.
ATKINS, J. B., *Brit. Med. J.*, (1955 I) 1011.
AUSTONI, M., *Le leptospirosi*, Torino, 1953, 715 pp.
BABUDIERI, B., in *Leptospirae and Leptospirosis*, Polish Acad. Sci., Warsaw, 1960, p. 88; p. 191.
BAKER, C. E., M. J. GALLIA, K. E. PRICE and E. A. WHITE, *Vet. Med.*, 52 (1957) 103.
BOKORI J., G. HIRT, L. KASZA and F. KEMENES, *Acta vet. Acad. Sci. hung.*, 8 (1958) 265.
FERNESTADT, K. L., Vet. Doct. Thesis, Kopenhagen, 1963.
FAINE, S. and L. KIRSCHNER, *N. Z. med. J.*, 52 (1953) 12.
FENNESTAD, K. L., Vet. Doct. Thesis, Copenhagen, 1963.
FENNESTAD, K. L. and C. BORG-PETERSEN, *Nature*, 180 (1957) 1210.
GAYOT, G., *Bull. Off. int. Épiz.*, 44 (1955) 143.
GSELL, O., *Rev. méd. Suisse rom.*, 69 (1949) 613.
HOAG, W. G. and W. B. BELL, *Amer. J. vet. Res.*, 16 (1955) 381.
HOEDEN, J. V. D., *J. infect. Dis.*, 103 (1958) 225; *Advanc. vet. Sci.*, 4 (1958) 277.
JOHNSON, D. W., *Med. J. Aust.*, 2 (1950) 724.
Joint Wld Hlth Org./F.A.O. Expert Comm. on Zoonoses, Second Rep., techn. Rep. Ser., No. 169 (1959) 83 pp.
KIRSCHNER, L. and T. MAGUIRE, *N.Z. med. J.*, 54 (1955) 560.
KMETY, E., *Zbl. Bakt., I. Abt. Or.*, 161 (1954) 382.
McCRUMB, F. R., J. L. STOCKARD and others, *Amer. J. trop. Med. Hyg.*, 6 (1957) 238.
McINTYRE, W. J. M. and H. SEILER, *J. Hyg.*, 51 (1953) 330.
MISAO, T., S. HIROYOSHI and others, *Amer. J. Hyg.*, 63 (1956) 294.
MORSE, E. V., V. ALLEN, A. F. KROHN and R. HALL, *J. Amer. vet. med. Ass.*, 127 (1955) 417.
MUSAEV, M. A., *Veterinarija*, 37 (1960) 22.
PARNAS, J., *Arch. exp. Vet.-Med.*, 13 (1959) 171.
SMITH, D. J. W. and R. L. DOHERTI, *Med. J. Aust.*, (1956) 643.

STOENNER, H. G., F. W. CREWS, A. E. CROUSE and others, *J. Amer. vet. med. Ass.*, 129 (1956) 251.
Symposium on the Leptospiroses, Med. Sci. Public., Washington, D.C., 1 (1952) 224 pp.
THIEL, P. H. v., *The Leptospiroses*, Leyden, 1948, 231 pp.
WEBSTER, W. H. and B. A. REYNOLDS, *N. Z. vet. J.*, 3 (1955) 47.
WITMER, R., *Amer. J. Ophthal.*, 37 (1954) 243.
WOLFF, J. W. and J. C. BROOM, *Docum. Med. geogr. trop. (Amst.)*, 6 (1954) 78.
YORK, CH. J. and J. A. BAKER, *Amer. J. vet. Res.*, 14 (1953) 5.
ZWIERZ, J., *Leptospirozy*, Warsaw, 1957, 320 pp.

CHAPTER II

RICKETTSIAL DISEASES

1

J. W. WOLFF

Introduction

Rickettsioses are febrile exanthematic diseases caused by rickettsiae, bacteria-like organisms which occur under natural conditions in arthropods. From these vectors the organisms can be transmitted to various animals and occasionally to man. Rickettsioses therefore, with three exceptions, belong to the zoonoses. The exceptions are epidemic typhus, its recrudescent form Brill-Zinsser disease and trench fever, which are diseases in which man is the only vertebrate acting as reservoir of the causal rickettsiae in nature.

Our knowledge of these organisms and of the transmission of the rickettsioses dates from 1909, when Ricketts described bacilliform organisms in the blood of patients with Rocky Mountain Spotted Fever. Several years later Rocha Lima (1916) found similar organisms in blood smears taken from typhus patients and also in smears from lice that had fed on patients with epidemic typhus. The names "*Rickettsia*" for the genus and "*Rickettsia prowazekii*" for the causal organism of epidemic typhus were coined in honour of Ricketts and von Prowazek, workers who both died of typhus when they were investigating this disease.

Later, in various parts of the world, it was found that other febrile exanthematous diseases are caused by different species of rickettsiae and are transmitted to man and animals by arthropods. In Table XXV these rickettsioses are grouped according to their vectors. The cause of Q-fever, although it is in many respects similar to the rickettsias, has been, because of its special biological characteristics, classified in a different genus, namely, *Coxiella*. This disease will be discussed in a separate chapter.

With regard to their morphology, growth requirements and biochemical reactions, rickettsiae occupy an intermediate position as a separate group of organisms between

TABLE XXV

RICKETTSIAL DISEASES IN MAN

Disease	Causal organism	Vector	Natural reservoir	Geographical distribution	Weil-Felix Reaction		
					OX-19	OX-2	OX-K
I. Louse-Borne							
Epidemic Typhus ⎱ Brill-Zinsser Disease ⎰	R. prowazekii	Pediculus humanus	Man	World-wide	++	+	—
Trench Fever	R. quintana	Pediculus humanus	Man	central and eastern Europe	—	—	—
II. Flea-Borne							
Endemic (Murine) Typhus	R. mooseri	Xenopsyllus cheopis and other rat-fleas	Rat	World-wide	++	+	—
III. Tick-Borne							
Spotted Fever Group (Rocky Mountain Spotted Fevers in U.S.A. and similar infections in Canada, Mexico, Brazil, Colombia and Panama)	R. rickettsii	Dermacentor andersoni and various other species of ticks	Ticks, rodents	western Hemisphere	+	±	—
Boutonneuse Fever, Kenya Typhus, S. African Tick-bite Fever, Indian Tick Typhus, Siberian Tick Typhus, N. Queensland Tick Typhus	R. rickettsii and R. conorii (R. sibericus, R. australis)	Rhipicephalus sanguineus and various other species of ticks	Rabbits, dogs and rodents	World-wide	+	±	—

Disease	Causal organism	Vector	Natural reservoir	Geographical distribution	Weil–Felix Reaction		
					OX-19	OX-2	OX-K
IV. Mite-Borne							
Tsutsugamushi, Scrubtyphus	R. tsutsugamushi (R. orientalis var. R. tamiyai)	Larvae of species of trombiculid mites	Mites, field rats, small mammals?	Japan, s. and s.e. Asia, western Pacific and N. Australia (Queensland)	−	−	+
Rickettsialpox	R. akari	Allodermanyssus sanguineus	Mus musculus (also rats in U.S.S.R.)	U.S.A., U.S.S.R. (Africa?)	−	−	−
Q Fever	Coxiella burneti	Air-borne infection in man	Sheep, goats, cattle, ticks, wild rodents	World-wide	−	−	−

References p. 282–283

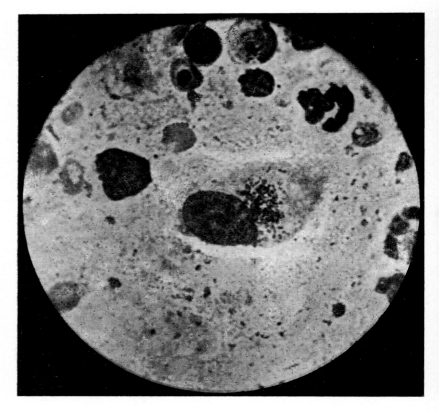

Fig. 31. *Rickettsia orientalis* in peritoneal fluid of an infected mouse
(Photo: Prof. J. W. Wolff; Institute for Tropical Hygiene and Geographical Pathology,
Royal Tropical Institute, Amsterdam)

the bacteriae and the larger viruses particularly those of the psittacosis-lympho-granuloma group (Fuller, 1959).

The morphology of rickettsiae has much in common with that of bacteria (Fig. 31); they are pleomorphic, coccobacillary structures with a cytoplasm and enclosed by a membrane. They do not stain well with ordinary bacterial stains, but require special techniques (Giemsa, Castañeda, Macchiavello). Under phase contrast microscopy or in stained preparations the organisms are bipolar and have a diameter of about 0.3–0.5 μ; but their size varies considerably within the same species and depends on the age of the organism, the animal host, and on environmental factors. Examination by electron-microscopy has shown that the granular material in the intermediate zone of the cell beneath the membrane is less dense than the similar layer in bacteria, and that the cytoplasm is denser.

Rickettsiae do not produce enzymes and do not grow on ordinary bacterial media.

Reproduction takes place by binary fission within the endothelial cells of the susceptible host, or in the body of the arthropod vector. Pathogenic rickettsiae are predominantly intracellular parasites, although Weyer (1954) has found extracellular multiplication of rickettsiae in the haemolymph of body lice.

In recent years techniques have been developed for the cultivation of rickettsiae in embryonated eggs (Cox, 1938), and in cells of tissue cultures. The growth rate of rickettsiae in tissue culture (mainly *R. tsutsugamushi*) seems to be much slower than that of bacteria.

Gildemeister and Haagen (1940) were the first to show that rickettsiae produce toxins which, in contrast to the exo- and endotoxins of bacteria, are exclusively found in *living* rickettsiae, their toxic action being lost by treatment with formalin or by heating to 60°. Mice are highly susceptible to these toxins and are killed a few hours after intravenous inoculation of suspensions of living rickettsiae. Toxins have been demonstrated in *R. prowazekii, R. mooserii, R. tsutsugamushi, R. rickettsii* and *R. conorii*, and neutralizing antibodies have been detected in sera from persons convalescent from, or vaccinated against, epidemic and murine typhus. The toxicity of certain species of rickettsiae can be reduced by ultraviolet radiation, or by the action of antibiotics (aureomycin).

The pathological changes in the organs of mice and rats after the inoculation of pathogenic rickettsiae are broadly similar to the pathology of the rickettsioses in man and larger animals. They are mainly localized in the cells of the vascular endothelial system. Increased capillary permeability occurs, with dilatation of the capillaries, and extravasation and concentration of the blood. Clarke and Fox (1948) showed that, in erythrocytes of rabbits and sheep placed in contact with suspensions of *R. prowazeki* and *R. mooseri*, haemolysis occurred, while Fuller (1959) demonstrated the appearance of intravascular haemolysis in rabbits inoculated with large doses of these two species of rickettsiae, a phenomenon not observed after inoculation with *R. tsutsugamushi*.

With the exception of *Coxiella burneti*, most rickettsiae are not very resistant to unfavourable conditions; they are killed by common antiseptics and heat (56° for 30 min). They are, however, far more resistant to dessication; *R. prowazekii* may remain viable in louse faeces for many months (Weyer, 1959a). Blanc and Balthazard (1940, 1944), in experiments with *R. mooseri* in the dried faeces of fleas preserved in vials over calcium chloride, found that the organisms remained viable for more than 7 years. Nevertheless, Weyer has pointed out that, under natural conditions in tropical and subtropical areas, the life span of rickettsiae is probably much shorter. *R. prowazekii, R. mooseri* and *R. quintana* in faecal matter of lice and fleas are more resistant than are *R. rickettsii* and *R. conorii* in tick faeces (Weyer, 1959b, 1961).

During the course of an infection with pathogenic rickettsiae specific antibodies appear in the blood serum of man and animals and these can be demonstrated by agglutination reactions and complement fixation techniques in which rickettsial antigens are used. However, before these diagnostic tools became available as a result of the preparation of pure suspensions of the various species of rickettsiae from yolk sac cultures (Cox, 1938), another serological test – the *Weil–Felix reaction* – had already been extensively employed. This test is an agglutination reaction for which suspensions of living or killed antigens of special strains of proteus bacilli (*Proteus* OX-19, OX-2 and OX-K) are used. These strains were isolated during the first World War in Rumania by Weil and Felix (1916) from the urine of patients with typhus fever and their antigens yielded diagnostically significant reactions with the serum of these patients. Later, Castañeda (1934) found that both *R. prowazekii* and *Proteus*-OX-19 possess a common carbohydrate antigen. Positive Weil–Felix reactions with the OX-19 and OX-2 strains of *Proteus* could also be demonstrated in the patient's sera during infections with endemic (murine) typhus and various spotted fevers, whereas in scrubtyphus (tsutsugamushi) the reaction is positive with antigens of the OX-K strain.

During the last decades, the action of antibiotics on rickettsiae has been studied extensively and it has been found that broad-spectrum antibiotics (chloramphenicol and tetracyclines) have excellent therapeutic value in the treatment of most of the rickettsioses, including epidemic typhus. In experiments with cultures of rickettsiae *in vitro,* Weyer (1951) found that chloramphenicol is less active than aureomycin and terramycin, while both antibiotics were inactive against *R. rickettsii.* The action of these antibiotics usually does not cause sterilization, but it inhibits the growth of the rickettsiae. Ultimate recovery from a rickettsial disease depends on the development of immunity.

GENERAL REFERENCES

BLANC, G., *Arch. Inst. Pasteur Tunis,* 36 (1959) 429.
BLANC, G.and M. BALTHAZARD, *Bull. Soc. Path. exot.,* 33 (1940) 25; *Arch. Inst. Pasteur Maroc,* 2 (1944) 658.
CLARKE, D. H. and J. P. FOX, *J. exp. Med.,* 88 (1948) 25.
COX, H. R., *Publ. Hlth Rep. (Wash.),* 53 (1938) 2241.
FULLER, H. S., *Arch. Inst. Pasteur Tunis,* 36 (1959) 311.
GILDEMEISTER, E. and E. HAAGEN, *Dtsch. med. wschr.,* 66 (1940) 878.
RICKETTS, H. T., *J. Amer. med. Ass.,* 52 (1909) 379.

Rocha Lima, D., *Arch. Schiffs-u. Tropenhyg.*, 20 (1916) 17.
Weyer, F., *Z. Tropenmed. Parasit.*, 3 (1951) 215; *Acta trop. (Basel)*, 11 (1954) 193; *Arch. Inst. Pasteur Tunis*, 36 (1959 a) 411; *Ergebn. Hyg. Bakt.*, 32 (1959 b) 73; *Z. Tropenmed. Parasit.*, 12 (1961) 78.

2

J. W. WOLFF

Louse-borne rickettsioses

a. Epidemic typhus

(Louse-borne typhus, typhus exanthématique, Fleckfieber, Tabardillo)

Since ancient times epidemics of typhus fever have been among the worst afflictions of mankind, especially during periods of war, famine, poverty, overcrowding and displacements of population groups forced to live under poor hygienic and sanitary conditions.

The first clinically recognizable descriptions of typhus as a distinct disease date from the middle of the 16th century, but it may be safely assumed that among the many pestilences which occurred in earlier centuries typhus played a major role. Thus Mac-Arthur (1959) gave new arguments for his conviction that the "Plague of Athene" described by Thucydides, which raged in 430 B.C. during the Peloponesian war, was an epidemic of typhus. The disease had up to the end of the 19th century, claimed many millions of victims in several parts of the world and its history is vividly described by Zinsser in his well-known classic "Rats, Lice and History" (1935). Typhus flared up again in Europe during the first world war; in Russia alone the number of cases between 1918 and 1922 has been estimated at 30 million, with 3 million deaths. During the last world war several epidemics occurred among the civil population in Europe and north Africa, especially in overcrowded areas and concentration camps, while relatively few cases were reported among military personnel, owing to better hygienic conditions and preventive immunization. After the war, cases of typhus continued to occur in many countries to which displaced people returned and had to live under poor sanitary conditions in devastated and bombed areas. In Japan and Korea, for instance, more than 26,000 cases were reported after the cessation of hostilities, with a mortality of 7–10%; but in Poland also, in the U.S.S.R. and in the Americas and Africa, a large number of cases of typhus fever have been recorded in recent years.

The studies of Charles Nicolle and his co-workers (1909) on the experimental transmission of typhus have shown that, under natural conditions, the human body louse, *Pediculus humanus corporis,* and also the head louse, *P. humanus capitis,* are the arthropod vectors of the disease, although experimentally *Phthirius pubis* can also transmit the disease (Weyer, 1952). The cause of the disease is *R. prowazekii* and man is its reservoir.

In recent years a few observations have been published which suggest that organisms resembling *R. prowazekii* can be found in animals too. Positive serological agglutination reactions with the antigens of *R. prowazekii* were observed in a number of domestic animals in Ruanda-Urundi (Giroud and Jadin, 1954) and Reiss and Gutfreund (1955, 1956), in Ethiopia, isolated strains of rickettsiae, which were, in laboratory experiments, similar to *R. prowazekii,* from goats and sheep and also from two species of ticks caught on domestic animals. Positive serological reactions for *R. prowazekii* were found in a significant number of zebu, sheep and goats. It was therefore suggested that in Ethiopia two cycles of typhus fever exist which can overlap, *i.e.:* man → louse → man and domestic animals → ticks → domestic animals. This animal cycle would bring epidemic typhus within the group of true zoonoses.

The life-cycle of the louse occurs entirely in the clothes and garments of its human host and all the developmental stages of the arthropod are susceptible to infection with *R. prowazekii.* Transovarial transmission of the pathogenic agent does not, however, occur.

The onset of the disease is acute after an incubation period of 10 to 14 days, with headache, general weakness, pains in various parts of the body, and high fever of 1 or 2-weeks duration. About the 4th day of illness a characteristic cutaneous rash appears which, during the following days, spreads from the body to the extremities. In severe cases death ensues during the second week of the illness.

The pathological lesions are characterized by a proliferation of the endothelium of the arterioles and capillaries, accompanied by thrombosis, haemorrhages and perivascular cell infiltrations. During the second week the Weil–Felix reaction for the antigens of Proteus OX-19 and OX-2 becomes positive.

After recovery from an attack of typhus a long-lasting immunity remains, although in a number of cases a recrudescence which is usually rather mild has been reported. This mild variety of typhus, called "Brill–Zinsser disease", occurs predominantly in immigrants from Poland and other countries of eastern Europe, who had suffered many years earlier from an attack of typhus in their native country (Brill, 1910; Zinsser, 1934). In the U.S.A. Murray and Snijder (1951) isolated strains of *R. prowazekii* from such patients, and in 1955, Price recovered *R. prowazekii* from a lymph node of a patient in U.S.A. who had undergone an operation and had immigrated from eastern Europe to the U.S.A. more than 20 years earlier. The factors which cause this recrudescence of typhus are still unsufficiently known.

In the control of typhus it is of primary importance to break the chain of transmission by killing of all the body lice. For this purpose the dusting of clothes with residual insecticides, such as DDT, has proved to be highly effective.

Shortly before the second world war a vaccine made from killed *R. prowazekii* (Cox's yolk sac vaccine) was developed. It was used on a large scale in army personnel during the war. In recent years immunization experiments have been carried out with a vaccine prepared from an avirulent strain of *R. prowazekii* (the "E-strain, Clavero and Perez Gallardo, 1943, 1944) and this has yielded promising results in endemic regions of Peru (Fox *et al.*, 1959).

b. Trench fever

(Wolhynia fever, Fünftagefieber)

First recognized as a separate disease during the first world war, when about 1 million cases occurred among soldiers in louse-infested areas of Europe, trench fever disappeared practically entirely in the years between the two wars. During the last world war a few epidemics occurred in Yugoslavia and in the Ukraine.

The disease is caused by *Rickettsia quintana*. The clinical symptoms of it are similar to those of a mild form of epidemic typhus. No mortality has been observed, but convalescence may be prolonged.

Immunity to reinfection is conferred after a first attack, but is probably not of life-long duration. No reliable serological diagnostic reactions are known; the Weil–Felix reaction is negative with all three strains of *Proteus*-X. It has not yet been possible to prepare antigens of *R. quintana* on a sufficiently large scale. At present, the best diagnostic procedure is that of xenodiagnosis.

The disease is transmitted from man to man by the body louse, *P. humanus,* just as epidemic typhus is (Weyer, 1954). When volunteers were experimentally infected, *R. quintana* appeared in the blood, sputum and urine. Xenodiagnosis has shown that the rickettsias can persist in the blood for very long periods after the fever has abated. The body-louse can transmit the disease from 5 to 10 days after it has taken a meal of infected blood and it remains infective for life (in contrast to *R. prowazekii,* which kills the louse), but does not transmit the infection transovarially to a second generation of lice. In the gut of the louse *R. quintana* is outside the cells. The usual laboratory animals are not susceptible to inoculation with *R. quintana,* but Rhesus monkeys have been experimentally infected (Mooser and Weyer, 1953).

REFERENCES

CLAVERO, G. and F. PEREZ GALLARDO, *Res. Sanidad Hig. publ.,* 17 (1943) 1; 18 (1944) 1.

FOX, J. P., A. MONTOYA, M. E. JORDAN, J. R. CORNEJO UBILLUS, J. I. GORCIA, M. A. ESTRADA and A. M. GELFAND, *Arch. Inst. Pasteur Tunis,* 36 (1959) 449.

GIROUD, P. and J. JADIN, *Bull. Soc. Path. exot.,* 47 (1954) 765.

MACARTHUR, W. P., *Trans. roy. Soc. trop. Med. Hyg.,* 53 (1959) 424.

MOOSER, H. and F. WEYER, *Z. Tropenmed. Parasit.,* 4 (1953) 513; *Proc. Soc. exp. Biol. (N.Y.),* 83 (1953) 699.

MURRAY, E. S. and J. C. SNIJDER, *Amer. J. Hyg.,* 53 (1951) 22.

PRICE, W. H., *J. Bact.,* 69 (1955) 106.

REISS-GUTFREUND, R. J., *Bull. Soc. Path. exot.,* 48 (1955) 602; 49 (1956) 946.

TAYLOR, R. M., J. R. KINGSTON and F. RIZK, *Amer. J. trop. Med. Hyg.,* 6 (1951) 863.

WEYER, F., *Z. Tropenmed. Parasit.,* 3 (1952) 302; *Médicine,* 38 (1954) 1267.

J. W. WOLFF

Flea-borne rickettsioses

Endemic typhus

(Murine typhus, Urban typhus, Shop typhus, Flea typhus, Rat typhus)

During the first decades of this century typhus-like fevers were described
under various names in the southern regions of the U.S.A., Mexico and
in other subtropical and tropical countries. The disease differed from
classical epidemic typhus in that it followed a milder course, caused
negligible mortality and in the fact that it was not dependent on contacts
between man and lice. Cases occurred mainly in the summer or autumn;
they were sometimes more frequent in urban than in rural areas (Malaya,
Sumatra) and in persons whose occupations could easily bring them to
rat-infested localities. Studies made in the U.S.A. and Mexico, where the
disease occurred in an endemic form, have shown that endemic typhus is
caused by a rickettsia, *R. mooseri* *, which is morphologically and antigenically closely related to *R. prowazekii*. In nature the brown rat, *Rattus
norvegicus,* is usually the reservoir of *R. mooseri* (Maxcy, 1929) which is
transmitted from rat to rat by the rat-flea, *Xenopsylla cheopis* (Dyer *et al.,*
1931; Mooser *et al., 1931*). Endemic (murine) typhus is therefore a
zoonosis in which the natural cycle is rat → rat–flea → rat, and human infections occur incidentally by means of the rat-flea.

---

* Recently Mooser (1959) has stated arguments for his contention that the name
R. typhi often used in American literature to designate the causal organism of endemic
typhus (see Bergey's *Manual of Determinative Bacteriology,* 7th ed.) is incorrect,
because the name *R. typhi* must be regarded as a synonym of *R. prowazekii*.

It is worthwhile recalling that the same process occurs in plague infection, which is transmitted to man by a similar mechanism. However, Dinger (in a personal communication) pointed out that in both diseases the epidemiological consequences are at variance. Plague infection in rats is usually fatal. The infected rat-fleas, loaden with plague bacilli, leave their murine host to prey on a human victim and thus inoculate the bacteria by the biting act. Murine typhus, on the other hand, is a sporadic endemic disease, not fatal to rats; the disease is enzootic and the fleas do not leave the rats' nests in large numbers. Moreover, the manner in which man is infected by the flea is far less effective, because the entire development of the typhus rickettsiae is intracellular and there is no multiplication in the gastro-intestinal tract of the flea. Because the flea's gastro-intestinal tract is covered with a strong hyaline membrane, which prevents the bursting of the cells filled with rickettsiae, no free rickettsiae are found in the stomach, so that the regurgitation mechanism plays no role. The only source of infection is the faeces, which contains only the few rickettsiae which may be released from ruptured epithelial cells of the Malpighian tubes. These faeces are introduced by rubbing into the bite wound or into the skin by scratching.

After an incubation period of 6 to 14 days the onset of the disease is acute, with symptoms similar to those of a mild attack of epidemic typhus, *i.e.* headache and a macular rash. Usually the fever does not last more than 10 to 12 days, and it ends by lysis. Recovery is rapid and uneventful. The mortality rate is very low. As in epidemic typhus, the Weil–Felix reaction for OX-19 and OX-2 becomes positive during the course of the disease as do also the complement-fixing reactions with antigens of *R. prowazekii* and *R. mooseri,* so that in regions where both rickettsioses are present, a differential diagnosis on clinical symptoms and serological tests alone is hardly possible. However, strains of *R. mooseri* can be isolated by the inoculation of white rats or guinea pigs with the patient's blood during the febrile period. In male guinea pigs the inoculation of *R. mooseri* causes enlargement of the scrotum with adhesions of the tunica vaginalis without development of necrosis, large numbers of rickettsiae being present in the cells of the tunica vaginalis (Mooser, 1928). This *Neill–Mooser tunica-reaction* is specific. In recent years other biological differences between *R. mooseri* and *R. prowazekii* have been found.

The therapy of the disease is the same as that of other mild rickettsioses, broad-spectrum antibiotics being of value. After an attack of the disease long lasting specific immunity develops.

In the rat, *R. mooseri* is present in the blood during the first week of infection, but the organisms can remain viable for long periods in the brain and other organs. It has been found that a large number of other rodents (*e.g.* the cotton rat, *Sigmodon hispidus,* and tropical species of rats) can be easily infected experimentally and occasionally they have been found infected in nature. This is also true of many other ectoparasites of rats (*e.g.* the rat-mite, *Ornithonyssus bacoti;* the rat-louse, *Polyplex spinulosus* and the rat-flea of temperate zones, *Nosopsyllus fasciatus*). In Indonesia natural infections were found in a trombiculid rat-parasite, *Ascoschöngastia indica* (Gispen, 1950), which does not, however, bite man.

In laboratory experiments body lice have been readily infected. In single instances the isolation of *R. mooseri* has been reported from lice, feeding on human hosts (Weyer, 1959). Therefore, in countries where louse infestation occurs and *R. mooseri* is present (Mexico, China, India), human infections might occasionally be caused by louse transmission. Epidemiologically this would be of minor importance as compared with the role of the flea vector (Fox, 1960), from which the infection is passed to man in the same way as in epidemic typhus *i.e.* by scratching and in-oculating the dry infected faeces into the skin. Despite the postulate that infection of man could be caused by food products contaminated with infected rat-urine, this mode of transmission has not yet been sufficiently substantiated.

During recent times it has been established that endemic typhus has a world-wide distribution in tropical and subtropical regions and in these regions the infection prevails in rats. In the southern U.S.A. thousands of cases were reported between 1940 and 1946. In the following years a sharp decline occurred and in 1957 the number of cases had dwindled to 114. This decrease coincided with, and was mainly due to, the extensive ratproofing of ware-houses and food premises and to the application of residual insecticides (10% DDT or other preparations) to rat-runs, followed by the poisoning of rats with rodenticides (Platt, 1958).

REFERENCES

DYER, R. E., A. RUMREICH and L. F. BADGER, *Publ. Hlth Rep. (Wash.),* 46 (1931) 334.
GISPEN, R., *Docum. neerl. indones. Morb. trop.,* 2 (1950) 223.
MOOSER, H., *J. infect. Dis.,* 43 (1928) 241; *Arch. Inst. Pasteur Tunis,* 36 (1959) 301.
PLATT, H. D., *Ann. N.Y. Acad. Sci.,* 70 (1958) 516.

4

Tick-borne rickettsioses

a. Spotted fever group

Tick-borne rickettsioses are widely distributed in various parts of the Western hemisphere, the Mediterranean region, eastern Europe and in several areas of the U.S.S.R., Africa, Australia (Queensland) and India. One of the most severe rickettsioses, *Rocky Mountain Spotted Fever*, belongs to this group. Clinical descriptions have been reported since the last decades of the 19th century. It occurred in a severe form in valleys on the Western side of the Rocky Mountains in U.S.A. (Bitterroot valley in Montana) and was later found to be present more sporadically and in a less severe form in localities of the eastern part. In later years similar infections were established in other parts of the U.S.A. and in Canada (Rocky Mountains), Mexico, Brazil, Columbia and Panama.

In 1906 and the following years studies by Ricketts, Wolbach and other workers have shown that the disease is caused by a rickettsia, *R. rickettsii*, which is transmitted from rodents to man by the wood tick, *Dermacentor andersoni* in western Montana, and by other species of ticks elsewhere. Ricketts also showed that the tick can acquire the infection in all stages of its development and that it remains infected for life and transmits the rickettsiae transovarially to the next generation.

In nature, various rodents and other small animals constitute reservoirs of the rickettsiae, the cycle being maintained by the immature ticks, which belong to different species according to the region in which the disease prevails. Man is infected incidentally by the bites of infected ticks.

The clinical symptoms vary from mild to extremely serious infections, with a case mortality rate up to 70%. They are in many ways similar to those of epidemic typhus, but the incubation period is shorter, the fever lasts longer and the rash has a different localization. After an incubation period of 4–8 days, during which vague prodromal symptoms may be present, the onset is abrupt, with high fever, severe headache, muscle

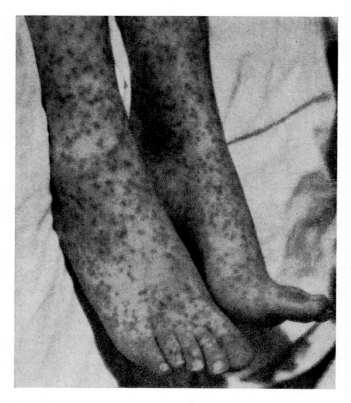

Fig. 32.   Skin rash (purpura) in Rocky Mountain Spotted Fever with confluent petechiae on purplish-red background.
(Photo: Ash and Spitz; from R. Simons, Handbook of Tropical Dermatology and Medical Mycology, Elsevier, Amsterdam, 1952)

pains and prostration, while cerebral symptoms may suggest encephalitis. Fever continues for 2 or 3 weeks. The clinical picture can be complicated by myocardial symptoms. Recovery begins with lysis of the fever, on which quick convalescence follows. The rash usually appears on the second to the fourth day of the illness; it begins at the ankles and wrists, but soon spreads over the entire body and becomes confluent with petechiae on a red-purplish background (Fig. 32). In the development of the rash, in severe cases, necrosis and gangrene of parts of the skin may develop. An attack of the disease confers permanent immunity.

The Weil–Felix reaction is positive for the *Proteus* OX-19 and OX-2 strains. Although in some cases higher titres with the OX-2 than with the OX-19 antigen have been reported, the reaction is not definitely specific as regards differentiation between epidemic and endemic typhus in areas where both infections prevail. For the differential diagnosis more rewarding results have been reported in recent years with toxin neutralization tests, complement–fixation with purified antigens of *R. rickettsii* and some other refined tests. It has been found that specific complement–fixation titres persist for 6 to 8 years after an attack.

The pathological lesions found in man and animals after experimental inoculation show a general infection of the endothelial cells of the small blood vessels with *R. rickettsii*. These are present in the blood during the first week and sometimes also during the first part of the second week. They can be demonstrated in skin sections. Typical of spotted fever rickettsiae is their invasion and multiplication in the nuclei of the endothelial cells of the small capillaries and invasion of the muscle cells of the media of arterioles, where they cause necrosis, haemorrhages and thrombosis (Pinkerton-Hass, 1932).

In experimental infections of guinea pigs with virulent strains a typical scrotal reaction occurs which is more severe than that caused by *R. mooseri* and differs from this in that necrosis and gangrene of the skin of the scrotum occur, while parts of earlobes and foot-pads may also become necrotic.

As in all rickettsioses, treatment with broad-spectrum antibiotics has yielded good results.

In nature this zoonosis is transmitted by various species of ticks, the immature stages of which feed on rodents and other small animals. The rickettsiae are inoculated with the saliva of the tick during the biting act. As the rickettsiae are present in all the tissues of the tick, infection of man may occasionally occur also by the crushing of ticks on the skin, or by contamination of the bite wound by the faeces of infected ticks. The viability of *R. rickettsii* in drie dtick faeces appears, however, to be much lower than that of other species of rickettsiae in the faeces of lice and fleas.

The main vector in the western part of U.S.A. is *Dermacentor andersoni*.

References p. 295

In other parts of the U.S.A., *D. variabilis* can transmit the disease, while several other tick species, among which are *Haemaphysalis leporis-palustris* and *Amblyomma americanum,* have been found occasionally infected in nature. Reservoirs of *R. rickettsii* have been encountered in a large number of wild rodents and small animals (wood rat, meadow mouse, deer mouse, cottontail rabbit and other rabbit species, squirrel, porcupine, weasel, etc.). In Brazil opossums and dogs have been found infected, while in Columbia the native monkey was found to be susceptible to inoculation with *R. rickettsii.* In most natural hosts the infection is not apparent and it is seldom fatal to these hosts.

b. Boutonneuse fever

(Fièvre boutonneuse, tick-borne typhus, exanthematous fever, Kenya typhus, South-African tick-bite fever, Fièvre escharonodulaire, etc.).

This rickettsiosis was first described as a clinical entity in Tunis by Conor and Bruch (1910). After an incubation period of 5–7 days, the onset is sudden with fever, headache and pains in the joints and muscles. In the majority of cases a small ulcer *(tache noire)* is present at the site of the bite of a tick; it has a black necrotic centre and a dark red peripheral area and is accompanied by enlargement and tenderness of the regional lymph nodes. A few days later a maculo-papular rash develops on the extremities, which spreads over the entire body. The disease is mild and as a rule the patient recovers after a short period of convalescence. During the disease, antibodies are developed against the *Proteus* OX-19 and OX-2 strains.

It was soon established that the disease is caused by a rickettsia, *R. conorii,* which is morphologically indistinguishable from, and antigenically closely related to, *R. rickettsii,* while animal experiments proved that there exists complete cross-immunity between Rocky Mountain Spotted Fever and Boutonneuse fever. There are, however, biological differences, because strains of *R. conorii* inoculated into male guinea pigs produce only minor scrotal reactions. In the Mediterranean countries the disease is transmitted by the dog tick, *Rhipicephalus sanguineus,* and dogs, especially puppies, appear to be the main reservoir of the disease.

In recent years, similar rickettsioses have been found in many other countries and these are transmitted by various species of ticks. In these regions, however, it is doubtful whether the dog is a reservoir. It has there-

fore been suggested that vertebrate hosts are not essential to the maintenance of the cycle of infection in nature. *R. conorii* can remain viable for
long periods in ticks (up to 18 months) without obviously harming these
vectors. The rickettsiae are transmitted transovarially to subsequent tick
generations.

Tick-bite fever in South Africa was at first considered to be a rickettsiosis
distinct from Rocky Mountain Fever (Pijper and Dau, 1930) but experimental studies in later years have shown that complete cross-immunity
is present between these two diseases. It has been shown that boutonneuse
fever in countries of the Mediterranean basin and in other parts of Africa
(Kenya tick typhus, Abessynian tick typhus, etc.) are essentially similar
infections although they are caused by antigenically slightly different
varieties of *R. conorii*. Various ticks can, however, transmit the disease
and, in addition to *R. sanguineus, Haemaphysalis* and *Amblyomma*
species may act as vectors in other countries.

A number of similar diseases have been described in other parts of the
world. In Queensland (Australia) cases of fevers resembling boutonneuse
fever have been observed since 1946 (Brody). These are probably transmitted by *Ixodes holocyclus*. Strains of rickettsiae *(R. australis)* isolated
from these cases were closely related, but not identical with *R. rickettsii*.
Positive serological reactions for the isolated strains were found in the
sera of a few marsupials (bandicoot, opossum) caught in the area in which
the patients lived.

In India similar infections were reported in 1917 by Megaw, who
suggested transmission by ticks. A strain of rickettsiae, isolated from *R.
sanguineus* and other tick species, was investigated in 1952 by Philip, who
found by animal experiments, a closer relationship to *R. conorii* than to
R. rickettsii.

In the U.S.S.R. extensive studies have been made in recent years of
Siberian tick typhus, caused by *R. sibericus*, which, according to Philip
et al. (1958), seems to be identical to *R. rickettsii*. The disease is transmitted
by ticks, the species of which varies, according to the region involved,
while small wild animals appear to be the reservoirs.

REFERENCES

BRODY, J., *Med. J. Aust.*, 1 (1946) 511.
PIJPER, A. and H. DAU, *J. trop. med. Hyg.*, 33 (1930) 93.
WOLBACH, S. B., *J. Amer. med. Ass.*, 84 (1925) 723.

5

Mite-borne rickettsioses

Scrubtyphus

(Tsutsugamushi, Kedani fever, Japanese river fever, Japanese flood fever, mite fever, rural typhus, etc.).

Even in the 17th century Japanese authors described fevers related to the bite of a sand mite. The first report in European literature on *tsutsugamushi* was published in 1879 (Baelz *et al.*). During the following years its aetiology and ecology were studied by Japanese workers, who discovered that the vector is the larva of a trombiculid mite, *Trombicula akamushi* and that the cause is *R. tsutsugamushi* (syn. *R. orientalis*) and the rodent reservoir, *Microtus montebelloi*. Later on other mites were found to be involved as vectors in other regions of Japan.

During the first decades of this century diseases resembling scrubtyphus were encountered in several countries of South and South-East Asia and on islands in the Western Pacific.

In Sumatra, Schüffner separated the disease from typhoid fever as a definite clinical entity, during an epidemic of typhoid and typhoid-like fevers among the labourers of a tobacco plantation, where new crops were planted regularly in areas covered by scrub. In some cases the Widal reaction failed to show positive results, while blood cultures also remained negative. Moreover, in about 80% of the cases a primary eschar was present on some part of the body, with swollen regional lymph nodes and a skin rash. Schüffner pointed out the similarity of this form of 'pseudo-typhoid' to tsutsugamushi and surmised that a mite was the vector (Schüffner and Wachsmuth, 1909). In 1921 a survey was published with epidemiological notes on 300 cases of this disease observed between 1908 and 1920 (Schüffner, 1921). During the following years extensive studies were conducted on scrubtyphus in Sumatra and Java.

Walch and Keukenschrijver (1935) found that the disease was transmitted by the larva of a mite, *T. deliensis*. In following years it was shown that usually, during the course of the illness, antibodies against the *Proteus* X-K strain developed, that mice were very susceptible to experimental inocculation of infective material and that the causal *Rickettsia* could be cultivated on embryonated hen or duck eggs (Kouwenaar and Wolff, 1939). Between 1930 and 1940, cases of scrubtyphus were also reported from other parts of Indonesia and from the Philippines, India and Burma.

During the second world war severe outbreaks of scrubtyphus occurred among allied troops on the islands of the Western Pacific and in parts of China, Burma, Assam, India and Malay, with a total of more than 18,000 cases and a death rate which varied in single outbreaks from 0.6–35%. These casualties stimulated, during and after the war, extensive studies of various strains of *R. tsutsugamushi*, of the species of vector-mites, and of the rodent hosts and the treatment and control of the disease. After it was found that broad-spectrum antibiotics were highly effective, and repellents had been developed against the arthropod vector, the number of cases of scrubtyphus decreased rapidly.

The disease is characterised by a sudden onset, after an incubation period of 10–14 days, with fever, headache, enlargement of lymph nodes and a primary ulcer, often at the sites of close contact between the skin

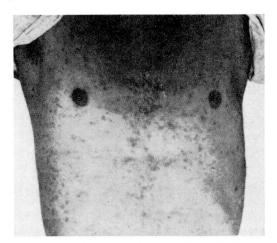

Fig. 33. Macular rash and ulcer in scrubtyphus (from R. Simons, Handbook of Tropical Dermatology and Medical Mycology, Elsevier, Amsterdam, 1952).

References p. 299

and clothes. This primary eschar is not always present. Clinical symptoms can resemble those of typhoid fever. In the majority of cases a rash develops between the fifth and eight day of the illness, with macular spots on the body surfaces (Fig. 33), spreading to the arms and legs. In severe cases the rash may become maculo-papular, in other cases it may remain very superficial and may disappear in a few days. If the infection is fatal, death usually occurs during the second week, with symptoms of pneumonia, encephalitis or circulatory failure. The death rates differ in various outbreaks, but they have been reported, in some instances, to be as high as 40–50%. However, after the introduction of antibiotic therapy, mortality has become negligible.

The pathological lesions are the same as found in other rickettsioses.

In scrubtyphus the Weil–Felix reaction has proved to be a very useful diagnostic test, because in most cases OX-K-agglutinins appear in the sera of patients during the second week of the illness and attain maximum titres in the third week, after which the titre rapidly declines. Complement–fixation tests have yielded less reliable diagnostic results, because the strains involved may be antigenically different from that of the antigen used. This is also the reason why attempts to vaccinate exposed individuals with killed suspensions of *R. tsutsugamushi* were not always successful. The best method of diagnosis is the isolation of *R. tsutsugamushi* by inoculation of the patient's blood, taken during the febrile period, into white mice.

Studies on experimental infection in human volunteers showed that after an attack, immunity against infection with the same strain of *R. tsutsugamushi* lasts for several years. However, it must be remembered that antigenic differences exist between various strains of *R. tsutsugamushi* isolated in different epidemics.

The disease is transmitted by the larvae of mites which require body fluid for their development. The larvae of the mites feed chiefly on rats or other rodents. Man is only incidentally infected.

Studies by Sasa and co-workers (1957) indicate that most probably the mite is stimulated to bite by the carbon dioxide expired by the host. In this active stage the larvae showed a negative geotaxis and proceeded to the top of the object (grass blades etc.) on which they were present. Like other acarines, the infected mite is a lifelong carrier of *R. tsutsugamushi* and passes on the infection to the next generation transovarially. In different countries various species of mites and rodents have been found infected in nature. Surveya in Malaya, New-Guinea and Burma showed tha tfoci of infection may be limited by a number of ecological and climatic factors to a very small area. (Audy *et al.*, 1951, 1958, 1961).

Prophylactic measures were very successful in military campaigns at the end of the second world war. They consisted of treatment of garments with repellents (dimethyl- and dibutyl-phthalate, benzylbenzoate, etc.), field sanitation (burning and clearing of bush and treatment of the ground with dieldrin or lindane), and rat-destruction with rodenticides (warfarin, Antu, etc.).

REFERENCES

AUDY, J. R. and J. L. HARRISON, *Trans. roy. Soc. trop. Med. Hyg.*, 44 (1951) 371.
KOUWENAAR, W. and J. W. WOLFF, *Proc. Sixth Pacific Science Congr.*, V, 1939, p. 633.
SASA, M., H. TANAKA, Y. UENO and A. MIURA, *Jap. J. exp. Med.*, 29 (1957) 31.
SCHÜFFNER, W., *Proc. Fourth Congr. F.E.A.T.M.*, II, 1921, p. 334.
WALCH, E. W. and N. C. KEUKENSCHRIJVER, *Arch. Schiffs-u.Tropenhyg.*, Beiheft, 29 (1925) 420.

6

J. W. WOLFF

Rickettsialpox

(Rickettsiose vésiculaire, Gamasorickettsiosis vesicularis)

Although this disease is mite-borne, its clinical symptoms, and the characteristics of the causative organism, *R. akari* (Huebner *et al.*, 1946), are more closely related to the rickettsioses of the spotted fever group than to scrubtyphus. The disease was first described as a new rickettsiosis in 1946 by Huebner *et al.* in New York city and independently by other workers in the U.S.A.

Clinically the symptoms resemble those of a mild form of endemic typhus, with acute onset of fever, chills, severe headache, pain in the back and the presence at the site of contact with the mite vector, of a red papule which develops into a black eschar (Fig. 34), and may resemble a vaccinia pox. Nearly always a maculo-papular rash develops a few days after the appearance of fever. There is no special pattern of distribution and after some days, vesicles are formed which quickly dry and disappear without scarification. In most cases slight leucopenia exists during the first week of the disease. In the cases observed in U.S.A. no deaths were recorded. The Weil–Felix reaction remains negative for both OX-19 and OX-K antigens. Convalescence is without sequelae.

Rickettsialpox has been reported in urban residents of dwellings infested with house mice *(Mus musculus)*. Mice (and rats in the U.S.S.R.) are the reservoirs of *R. akari* in nature. The vector is a mouse parasite, the mite *Allodermanyssus sanguineus*, from which strains of *R. akari* have been isolated on several occasions. In contrast to the trombiculid vector of scrubtyphus, this mite does not need body fluid in the larval stage, although its nymphs and adults are blood-sucking parasites.

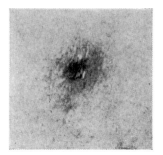

Fig. 34. Primary lesion (eschar) in rickettsialpox.
(Photo: Rose – N. York; from R. Simons, Handbook of Tropical Dermatology and
Medical Mycology, Elsevier 1952)

Infections resembling rickettsialpox have also been found in town populations in the U.S.S.R. (gamasorickettsiosis vesicularis), where they are transmitted by several species of *Allodermanyssus*, which are parasites on rats and mice. Serological evidence of related diseases has been reported from equatorial- and South-Africa.

The biological characteristics of *R. akari* and *R. dermacentronoxus murinus* (the name given to the causative agent in the U.S.S.R.) show close relationship to *R. conori* of the spotted fever group. These rickettsiae also multiply in the nuclei of endothelial cells and cross complement–fixation tests showed that both strains of rickettsiae were closely related to *R. mooseri*.

Treatment with broad-spectrum antibiotics is of therapeutical value. Protective measures should aim at the eradication of rats and mice from urban centres.

REFERENCES

HUEBNER, R. J., P. STAMPS and C. ARMSTRONG, *Publ. Hlth Rep. (Wash.)*, 61 (1946) 1605.
HUEBNER, R. J., W. L. JELLISON and C. POMERANTZ, *Publ. Hlth Rep. (Wash.)*, 61 (1946) 1677.

7

Z. EVENCHIK

Q-Fever

Q-fever is an acute communicable disease of animals and man caused by a rickettsia. In animals the infection usually is clinically not apparent, but in man it frequently causes a systemic disease.

Q-fever was first recognized as an entity *sui generis* in 1935 when it appeared epidemically among slaughterhouse workers in Queensland (Australia). The causative agent was isolated by Derrick in 1937. He called the disease Q-fever (Q stands for query) and the organism *Rickettsia burneti*. About the same time, Davis and Cox isolated from wood–ticks *(Dermacentor andersoni)* in Montana, U.S.A., a filtrable *Rickettsia* which they called *R. diaporica*. Comparative investigation by Dyer, Burnet and Freeman (1939) showed that *R. diaporica* is identical with *R. burneti*, and thus proved that the agent of Q-fever is present in North America. During the following years the observation of human infections was restricted to Australia. But in 1944, outbreaks of atypical pneumonia among allied troops in Italy were identified as Q-fever and were recognized as being identical with "Balkan Grippe", which had occurred during the preceding winter season in Greece, and was characterized by broncho-pneumonia (Caminopetros). Gradually the disease was identified in various parts of the world.

Simultaneously a number of outbreaks were recorded in Amarillo (Texas) among slaughterhouse personnel (Cox *et al.,* 1947), in Chicago meat packing houses (Shepard, 1947), and in California, where it was found to occur endemically (Lennette and Berge, 1947). Up to 1955, Q-fever had been recorded in 51 countries in all continents (Kaplan and Bertana, 1955). Remarkable was the total absence of the disease from certain territories, *e.g.* New-Zealand, Sweden, Norway, Finland, Denmark and Ireland. The relatively scanty importation of livestock into these countries may account for this fact.

R. burneti is a pleomorphic, intracellular organism. Its has a rod-like to cocco-bacillary form and measures 0.25–0.5 micron. It easily stains by the Giemsa or Macchia-vello methods, taking a purple colour by the first method and a red colour by the second. In smears from animal tissue or the yolk sac of infected eggs, the organism occurs in large cytoplasmatic masses. Electron microscopic pictures of *R. burneti* show no morphological differences between it and other rickettsiae. It passes through Berkefeld N filters and other membranes with a pore diameter of 400 millimicrons. Unlike other rickettsiae, *R. burneti* does not react with the X-antigens of *Proteus* and does not produce a cutaneous rash in human beings. Because of these differences Phillip (1948) proposed the creation of the new genus, *Coxiella*, for the causative agent of Q-fever. The name *Coxiella burneti* is now generally accepted and is listed in Bergey's *Manual of Determinative Bacteriology*.

Characteristic for *C. burneti* is its great resistance to various physical and chemical influences. It remains viable in milk and water at room temperature for several days and can be preserved in the frozen state at $-20°$ or $-70°$ as well as after lyophilization.

Lennette *et al.* (1949), found that pasteurization at 61.5° for 30 minutes destroyed the organism in only 95% of the examined milk samples. According to Babudieri (1953) low pasteurization is not sufficient to free the milk from viable *C. burneti*. Huebner *et al.* found that heating of milk at 71.5° for 15 minutes destroys the *Coxiella burneti* present in it. *C. burneti* is killed by 0.2% formalin within 24 hours and by 0.4% phenol after several days. In faeces the organism may retain its infectivity for 586 days (Phillip, 1948), and in dried blood for 186 days. In dry air and in desiccated urine, faeces, placenta or other materials from infected animals, *C. burneti* survives for a considerable time.

C. burneti can be cultivated in embryonated eggs, or in tissue cultures, and can be maintained in ticks and laboratory animals. If *C. burneti* is inoculated into the yolk sac of 6 to 8 days old embryonated eggs, death of the embryo usually occurs after incubation at 37° for 7–9 days. Infected yolk sacs provide very useful material for seed inocula, and for the production of diagnostic antigens and vaccines. In ticks multiplication takes place in the epithelial cells of the intestines, a fact which explains the high concentration of the organism in the faeces of ticks. Several laboratory animals are suitable for experimental work with *C. burneti*. These include guinea pigs, mice, hamsters, rabbits and monkeys. The infection does not cause apparent symptoms in any laboratory animals, excepting the guinea pig, in which a strong reaction with high fever may develop.

Under natural conditions infection of domestic animals is usually not clinically detected. After invasion of the blood stream of cows, sheep and goats, the organism settles in the mammary glands, supra-mammary lymph nodes and placenta. The infection may last for many months or years and usually rickettsiae are for a long time excreted in the milk. Although a very large number of rickettsiae are found in the milk, the milk-yield is usually not decreased. By inoculation of massive doses of *C. burneti* into the lactiferous ducts of a cow, Bell *et al.* (1949) succeeded in producing acute mastitis with a systemic reaction of brief duration. During the acute stage of the disease *Coxiella* was present in the blood and after recovery of the host it persisted in the milk. Experiments with calves fed on infected milk showed excretion of *Coxiella* in their stools. Babudieri (1953) demonstrated the possibility of experimental infection with *C. burneti* via the conjunctiva, provided that a large number of organisms is used. When pregnant cows were inoculated intradermally, the organism was subsequently recovered from the milk, urine, and placenta. The organism was isolated from the blood, milk and placenta of a cow infected intranasally, and complement–fixing antibodies appeared in the serum of this cow. In spite of the high concentration of *Coxiella* in the placenta of infected animals of various species, abortion is almost restricted to *goats*. Caminopetros in Greece and Kishperger and Wiesmann in Switzerland, isolated *C. burneti* from the milk and placenta of goats during the epizootic occurrence of abortions among these animals. In Israel, the organism was obtained from the placentae of aborting sheep. Lennette *et al.* showed that naturally infected sheep harbour *C. burneti* in the placenta, amniotic fluid, faeces and milk. Experimental studies proved that sheep can be infected by the intravenous route as well as by the respiratory tract (Abinanti, 1953). From these experiments it was deduced that sheep infected by the respiratory tract, excrete *C. burneti* only after parturition. The same is probably true for goats. In both these animals the organisms appeared in the placenta and milk. In infected sheep and goats Caminopetros in Greece reported bronchopneumonia.

Although natural infection with *C. burneti* usually does not provoke any symptoms of disease in domestic animals, it is capable of causing a rather serious illness in *man*.

The incubation period, varying from about 2–4 weeks, is followed by sudden onset of high fever (39–40°), with chills, malaise, severe headache and muscular pains, especially in the limbs. After a few days a mild, dry cough ensues, accompanied by pain in the chest. The febrile period lasts for several days up to 2 weeks. In practically every patient pneumonitis develops, which is similar to that seen in primary atypical pneumonia. As a rule, physical signs are lacking, but the roentgenogram is almost pathognomonic. The segmental or lobal infiltrations, common in Q-fever, persist after the patient's clinical symptoms have disappeared. The disease should not be regarded as being a purely respiratory illness. Hepatic involvement, including slight jaundice, has been noticed in numerous severe cases. A status typhosus has also been reported. Thrombophlebitis, pleurisy, and pleural effusions are rare complications. The skin lesions seen in some other human rickettsioses do not occur. Convalescence is rapid and recovery is complete; the mortality is very low, except in elderly persons, among whom deaths have been reported.

General laboratory investigations are of little avail in the diagnosis of Q-fever. The Weil–Felix reaction is negative. The ultimate diagnosis of infection by *C. burneti* can be established only by isolation of the causative organism or by serological methods.

When a respiratory disease occurs in a person occupationally associated with livestock, their products or excretions, Q-fever should be suspected. The history of the illness and its clinical picture cannot by themselves warrant the diagnosis. Because the symptomatology in man and animals is not specific and since the infection is often clinically not apparent, laboratory tests are needed to ensure diagnosis.

C. burneti is eliminated in the urine and excretions of sick and convalescent persons. It can be recovered from the blood, urine and sputum. Babudieri (1954) isolated the organism from the milk of a woman who had suffered from Q-fever 7 months earlier. Syruček *et al.* (1958) cultivated *C. burneti* from the placentae of three women, who had suffered from the disease 2 to 3 years previously.

C. burneti is commonly found in the milk, placenta and spleen of infected animals. For its isolation guinea pigs, hamsters, mice or embryonated eggs are usually used. The organism may be identified by staining smears from the yolk sacs of inoculated eggs or from the spleens of the infected test animals. Guinea pigs which develop fever are sacrificed and spleen material is transferred to another animal. Every animal must be tested serologically for the presence of specific complement-fixing or agglutinating antibodies, about a month after the inoculation.

The most widely employed serological methods are the complement–fixation (c.f.) and the agglutination test. The antigens of choice are prepared from yolk sac cultures of selected *Coxiella* strains (Nine Mile, or Henzerling). The complement-fixation test is only exceptionally positive during the first week of the illness, the number of positive reactions rising from 65 to 100% between the second and fourth week after infection. The complement–fixing antibodies may reach a high titre and may persist at this level for many months, or years.

In infected animals these serological reactions usually remain positive for a shorter period than they do in man. Nowadays many investigators prefer the agglutination test, because it is easier to perform and simpler to read. During the last few years microscopic slide agglutination by the method of Babudieri, and capillary tube agglutination by the method of Luoto, have been introduced. Both techniques are simple, economic, rapid to perform and more sensitive than the complement–fixation test (Lennette). Agglutinating antibodies appear during the first week after the onset of the disease and give a positive test at this time in 50% of cases, a percentage which rises to 100 within 2 to 4 weeks.

The serological reactions with antigens of Q-fever are highly specific and no cross-reactions occur with the sera of persons suffering from other rickettsial diseases: Q-fever positive sera do not react with Weil–Felix antigens.

In cows the detection of specific agglutinins in milk whey is a valuable and sensitive method of survey. In sheep, positive whey reactions are obtained only in cases in which *C. burneti* is excreted in the milk. In Italy an allergic palpebral test is used for the diagnosis in cows and sheep. The reaction appears 3 to 4 days after the application of the allergen and persists for several days. Allergic tests have been found positive even in infected animals with negative serological reaction.

Q-fever usually occurs as an occupational disease affecting persons who handle livestock and raw animal products or come into contact with the animal excretions. It is, therefore, common among farm labourers and slaughterhouse workers, or individuals who live within a short distance of infected dairy-farms, goat-pens or markets. In some outbreaks, in which many of the patients had not been in direct contact with domestic animals, there was evidence that these patients had drunk raw milk or had lived beside roads frequented by livestock. Several cases have been reported in factories in which the source of infection was dust adhering to the infected wool or hair derived from animals.

Q-fever occurs in epidemic outbreaks mostly in villages, occasionally also in towns. It remains limited within an area, frequently taking the form of an endemic infection, with isolated cases which have no direct mutual connection. The persistence of the infection in such a region is largely due to the facts that infected animals excrete the organisms for a long time and that *C. burneti* is highly resistant to environmental influences. It can survive for a long time in the organs of animals, especially in the udder, spleen, liver and kidneys. Probably most human cases of Q-fever are contracted by inhalation of contaminated air. The consumption of raw milk containing *C. burneti* can also play an important role in causing the disease. *C. burneti* remains viable for several days in contaminated milk, butter, cheese or cream, and the ingestion of these foodstuffs may also be a source of infection. From the epidemiological point of view, the respiratory tract is much more important as a portal of entry than the alimentary tract. One of the richest sources of infection with *C. burneti* is the placenta which, like the amniotic fluid, contains enormous numbers of rickettsiae. After delivery, the abandoned placenta may be dragged away or devoured by dogs or other animals and this may contribute considerably to the spread of the disease. The dust of desiccated placental tissue, post parturition discharge, urine, faeces and sputum of infected animals may be carried by the wind over rather great distances. The incidence of human cases in endemic regions like California and Greece reaches its maximum during the calving and lambing seasons, most probably as a result of inhalation of the dust from dried, infected placentas abandoned in the fields. Butchers and other persons handling slaughter products are highly exposed to infection.

Inhalation of dust from contaminated straw has also been mentioned as a possible source of infection. Epidemic outbreaks in Italy among soldiers sleeping on straw, and cases of Q-fever among workers after unpacking machinery padded with straw of suspect origin in Switzerland and the U.S.A., seem to indicate that this material may play a part in the spread of the disease.

The epidemiological role of ticks as vectors of *C. burneti* has not yet fully been clarified. Under certain conditions they may play a part in the transmission of the infection to domestic animals. Such ticks evacuate large numbers of rickettsiae in their faeces, which may, after drying, contaminate the environment. However, their importance to human epidemiology, in Europe at least, seems to be very slight. Many outbreaks of Q-fever among human beings have been reported where ticks could reasonably be excluded as vectors of *C. burneti*. Lennette (1952) did not consider that these arthropods were responsible for the spread of the infection in California. It should, however, be kept in mind that many species of ticks have been found naturally infected with *C. burneti*. Investigations have shown that the organism may pass from the larva to the nymph and then to the adult stages of all the species of ticks tested, although only in *Ornithodoros moubata* was the infection carried over to the next generation (Davies, 1943; Weyer, 1953).

The great variety of animals from which *C. burneti* has been isolated makes it difficult to determine the principal host of the organism in nature. Furthermore, there exist several alternative ways of spreading of the organism from one host to another. A simple cycle including animals and ticks has been demonstrated in Australia, where Derrick and Smith (1939) found that a large number of bandicoots *(Isoodon torosus)* were infected with *C. burneti*. At the same time the investigators isolated the organism from many ticks *(Haemaphysalis humerosa)* collected from these animals. They suggested a close association between bandicoots and ticks in the maintenance of *C. burneti*. Blanc *et al.* (1947) in Morocco isolated *C. burneti* from *Rhipicephalus sanguineus*, *Rhipicephalus bursa* and *Hyalomma marginatum*. In Montana, U.S.A., *Dermacentor andersoni* was found to be a reservoir of Q-fever rickettsiae, but the isolation of the organism from these ticks was not accompanied by the recovery of *C. burneti* from the small animals on which these ticks are normally parasitic. In California the ear-tick, *Otobius mégnini*, was the only ectoparasite found to be infected with *C. burneti*. However, as an Argasid tick it remains on one host only and no evidence, therefore, exists of its role in the transmission of the infection. Blanc *et al.* (1947) found that a gerbil, *Meriones shawi*, and a mountain rabbit were naturally infected with *C. burneti*. Babudieri and Moscovici reported the isolation of *C. burneti* from a pigeon and obtained serological evidence of the infection in another pigeon and a goose. Giroud and Jadin recorded, in an endemic area in Belgian Congo, natural infections in pigs and in human body lice. The rickettsiae killed the lice in a few days and consequently, according to these authors, the lice probably do not contribute much to the spread of the infection from man to man. Serological investigations in Pakistan and Egypt indicated the possibility that camels are infected with *C. burneti*. In Israel the author established the presence of significant serotitres for *C. burneti* in 11 out of 145 hedgehogs *(Erinaceus europaeus* and *Hemiechinus auritus)* caught in the fields. From numerous records it is clear that *C. burneti* is maintained in nature in various small animals and several arthropods. However, the demonstration of a relationship between these natural reservoirs of Q-fever and its spread among domestic animals and man requires further research.

Several cases of laboratory infection have been reported; these were caused by inhalation of infected and aerosoled yolk sac material handled by unexperienced workers, or by merely working in a room in which infected test animals were housed. Direct inter-human infection is a very great exception. Patient-to-patient infection of Q-fever in a hospital was reported by Siegert in 1950.

It is difficult to evaluate the therapeutic value of antibiotic treatment for human Q-fever, because of the great variation in the severity and duration of the untreated disease. According to Clark and Lennette, treatment with large doses of aureomycin significantly reduced the duration of the fever. Other antibiotics, such as oxytetracyclin or chloromycetin, sometimes combined with the first mentioned antibiotic, are also used. Penicillin, streptomycin and sulfonamides have not been found effective.

Preventive measures against Q-fever are directed towards protection of man against contamination by animal carriers or infected animal material, and towards the direct destruction of sources of infection. Effective Q-fever prophylaxis depends mainly on adequate knowledge of its epidemiology under the environmental conditions of a given region. Precautions must be taken to prevent direct contact between man and possible sources of infection. The immunization of slaughterhouse workers, dairy workers or other persons exposed to infected animal material may be desirable. It must, however, be borne in mind that in certain persons the Q-fever vaccine may provoke serious side-effects (*e.g.* haemorrhagic nephritis) and it must, therefore, be used with caution.

In areas in which the disease is endemic, special prophylactic measures should be applied. A large proportion of the milk from local dairies may contain living *Coxiella,* and boiling or adequate pasteurization of this milk is a necessity. Pasteurization for a short time at a high temperature is recommended. Under certain circumstances prohibition of removal of animals through, or from, infected areas should be made compulsory. If it is known that Q-fever is present in a region, a survey must be extended to all kinds of animals and to those persons, who have contact with infected materials. Milk and blood samples must be collected and investigated for the presence of *C. burneti* or its specific antibodies.

Q-fever is an example of a zoonosis of significant importance for human beings and of minor or even negligible interest to animal industry. Like several other zoonoses, Q-fever is a challenge to both the veterinary and medical professions. Epizootiological studies carried out with comprehension of the different local conditions and intensive surveys of the

References p. 310

disease by laboratory methods may provide a solution of the problems involved.

REFERENCES

Babudieri, B., *Advances in the Control of Zoonoses, W.H.O./F.A.O. Monogr. Ser.*, 25 (1953) 157.

Bell, E. J., R. R. Parker and H. G. Stoenner, *Amer. J. publ. Hlth*, 39 (1949) 478.

Blanc, G., L. A. Martin and A. Maurice, *C. R. Acad. Sci. (Paris)*, 224 (1947) 1673.

Caminopetros, J., *Proc. 4th intern. Congr. trop. Med. and Malaria*, 1948, p. 441.

Cox, H. R., *Amer. J. trop. Med.*, 20 (1940) 463.

Hoeden, J. v. d. and Z. Evenchik, *Arch. Inst. Pasteur Tunis*, 36 (1959) 571.

Huebner, R. J., *Publ. Hlth Rep. (Wash.)*, 63 (1948) 214.

Huebner, R. J., W. C. Jellison, M. D. Beck and F. P. Wilcox, *Publ. Hlth Rep. (Wash.)*, 64 (1949) 499.

Kaplan, M. M. and P. Bertana, *Bull. Wld Hlth Org.*, 13 (1955) 829.

Lennette, E. H., W. H. Clark and B. H. Dean, *Amer. J. trop. Med.*, 29 (1949) 527.

Parker, R. R., E. J. Bell and H. G. Stoenner, *J. Amer. vet. med. Ass.*, 863 (1949) 55; 864 (1949) 124.

Philip, C. B., *J. Parasit.*, 34 (1948) 457.

Smith, D. J. W. and E. H. Derrick, *Aust. J. exp., Biol. med. Sci.*, 18 (1940) 1.

Stoker, M. G. P. and B. P. Marmion, *J. Hyg. (Lond.)*, 50 (1952) 1; *Bull. Wld. Hlth Org.*, 13 (1955) 781.

Syruček, L., O. Soběslavský and I. Yutvirsh, *Ž. Mikrobiol. (Mosk.)*, 2 (1958) 29.

CHAPTER III

VIRAL DISEASES

A. Neurotropic viral diseases

B. Arthropod-borne animal viral diseases

C. Myxoviral diseases

D. Miscellaneous viral diseases

A. Neurotropic viral diseases

1

Rabies

The cause of rabies is a filterable virus which has, as a rule, a predilection for nervous tissues. The virus is approximately 125 millimicrons in diameter and can be destroyed by the adding to suspensions of infected tissue, varying concentrations of formalin, phenol, bichloride of mercury, mineral acids and bases, and other disinfectants. Rabies virus remains viable for long periods of time when bits of infected tissue are stored in 50 % glycerol–saline or pure glycerol at 4°; at this temperature, lyophilized suspensions will also keep. Another method of storage preferred is the freezing of suspensions and storage of them at –30° to –60°. The keeping qualities of the virus in the frozen state are greatly enhanced if 20 % tissue suspensions are prepared, and substances rich in protein of amino acids are added, such as serum, sterile milk, or egg yolk. The resistance of the virus to physical and environmental influences is variable and depends in a large measure on the breaking up of the infected host tissue. Usually, however, the organism's resistance can be described as being quite labile. The virus is destroyed easily by sunlight and heat and its infectivity becomes negligible when it is exposed to ordinary environmental conditions of light, heat and air. This property has a practical application in that fomites have not been known to play a part in the transmission of the virus. For this reason, it is not felt necessary to carry out extensive disinfection of rooms, furnishings, or any objects which might have become contaminated with the saliva of a rabid animal.

In 1804, by transmission experiments in dogs, Zinke first found the cause of rabies in saliva. Magendie and Breschet were the first to demonstrate in 1813 that the cause of rabies was the same in man and dogs, when they were able to infect dogs with saliva from a human patient. In the 1880's, Pasteur's classical work threw a new light on methods of working with the virus in the laboratory. It was this work which established the modification of viruses by serial passage through a definite tissue system of an animal species. Pasteur gave the term "street virus" to the rabies virus found in nature. He was able to modify this virus by intracerebral serial passages through rabbits. The incubation period became shorter with succeeding passages, until it reached a point at which this period became fixed and he therefore named this newly modified agent the "fixed virus". In contrast to the long and variable interval of the street virus, the fixed virus, as a rule, cannot form Negri bodies and is more strictly neurotropic in character. Since it has become more highly adapted to neural tissue, fixed virus has lost its tropism for salivary gland tissue, even when it is introduced by the peripheral route.

As is done with other neurotropic viruses, the standard measurement of the ability of rabies virus to multiply and destroy nerve tissue in the living animal is carried out by intracerebral inoculation of varying dilutions of suspensions of infected tissue into young adult laboratory white mice.

Either natural, or artificial, infection of an animal with the rabies virus stimulates the production of specific antibodies, which may be detected by complement-fixation (CF) or serum neutralization (SN) tests. The complement-fixation test is usually not used, because of the difficulty of obtaining good, stable, standard antigens from infected tissues, and because the CF antibodies do not persist very long. Serum neutralizing antibodies, however, persist for much longer periods, the SN test is the serological test of choice for confirmatory identification of the virus and for determining antibody levels in man and animals for epidemiologic purposes, as well as for measuring the antigenic response of vaccines.

The mouse is the animal of choice in rabies experiments, but other animals, such as guinea pigs, hamsters, rabbits and dogs, are frequently used. Hamsters are gaining in popularity because of their high degree of susceptibility by peripheral routes of infection (Koprowski, 1949). Adaptation of the virus to chicken embryos was accomplished by Kligler and Bernkopf (1938) by the chorioallantoic route, and later by Dawson (1941) by intracerebral inoculation of the embryo. Koprowski and Cox (1948) were able to effect serial passage of the virus in chicken embryos by yolk sac inoculation. This yolk sac technique was used by Powell and Culbertson (1950) for adapting the virus to duck embryos. Recently, Kissling (1958) has been able to adapt rabies virus to hamster kidney tissue culture; although there was evidence of virus multiplication, cytopathogenic effects were not detected.

Unlike most other pathogenic animal viruses, distinct or separate immunologic types or strains of rabies virus have never been identified by the methods at present known for establishing such differences. Thus, virus strains isolated from cases of rabies transmitted by vampire bats in Latin America are immunologically indistinguishable by cross-protection, CF or SN tests from strains isolated from rabies transmitted by dogs or foxes.

The incubation period of rabies is extremely variable and is generally long. In all species of lower animals clinical rabies presents much the same picture. The average incubation period in *dogs* is 3 to 8 weeks, but, as in man and in other susceptible animals, this period can be very different. In dogs it has ranged from 10 days to 6 months. It is rarely less than 2 weeks or more than 4 months. The clinical course of the disease in dogs can be divided into three phases, the prodromal, the excitative, and the paralytic. The term "furious rabies" refers to animals in which the excitative phase is predominant and the term "dumb rabies" to those cases in which the excitative phase is extremely short or absent and the disease progresses quickly to the paralytic phase. In the prodromal stage, which lasts 2 to 3 days, the animal may exhibit a subtle change of temperament. Highly strung dogs may become more affectionate than usual, whereas ordinarily affectionate animals may shy away from their owners and become snappy and irritable. During this phase, there is a slight rise in temperature, dilatation of the pupils, and a sluggish corneal reflex. The excitative phase, which lasts from 3 to 7 days, is the one during which signs of the disease are most easily recognized. The dog becomes increasingly irritable, restless, and nervous. In the early part of this stage it may shun people and hide in dark places, under furniture, or in closets. It shows exaggerated responses to sudden stimuli of sight and sound. Excitability, photophobia, and hyperesthesia may become apparent. It may snap at insects and imaginary objects. Often there is a tendency to eat unusual things like sticks, straw, stones, and soil. Restlessness increases, and the animal develops an urge to move and roam. At this time, it may begin to wander aimlessly through town and countryside, all the time becoming more irritable and vicious; it is at this stage that the animal is most dangerous because of its tendency to bite anything that it encounters, be it man, animal or inanimate object. If the dog is confined at this stage of the disease, it will bite at chains or the bars of a cage or kennel (Fig. 35), breaking its teeth or inflicting severe trauma on its oral tissues. In most cases, there is a characteristic change in the bark, which is caused by paralysis of the laryngeal musculature. There is difficulty in swallowing, due to spasms, and eventual paralysis of the muscles of deglutition, which causes the animal to drool saliva (Fig. 36). Sometimes heavy, rapid respiration through the mouth will cause frothing of the drooling saliva. Convulsive seizures and muscular incoordination are apparent towards the end

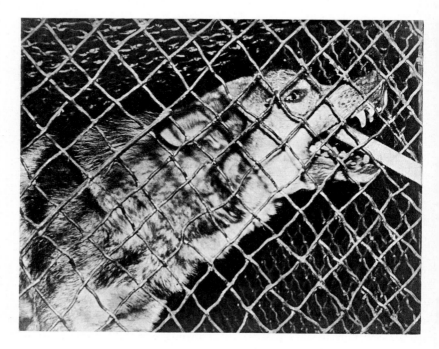

Fig. 35.   Dog in furious stage of rabies.
(Photo: Marvin Carter, Memphis, Tenn.)

of this stage. If the animal does not die during one of the convulsive seizures, it enters into the paralytic stage, during which the disease progresses from muscular incoordination to paralysis of the entire body and thence to coma and death. The clinical course of the disease characterized by the excitative phase may last as long as 10 days, including the prodromal phase, but rarely as long as 12 days.

The paralytic stage begins almost immediately if the excitative phase is either quite short or entirely absent. The clinical course of the paralytic stage is less spectacular and is therefore often difficult to diagnose. This is the form referred to as *dumb rabies*. The most characteristic sign of this form of the disease is the so-called "dropped jaw", caused by paralysis of the muscles of mastication, which makes it impossible for the animal to eat or drink. Paralyzed, too, are the pharyngeal muscles, causing drooling of saliva. Often the animal emits a choking sound, which leads

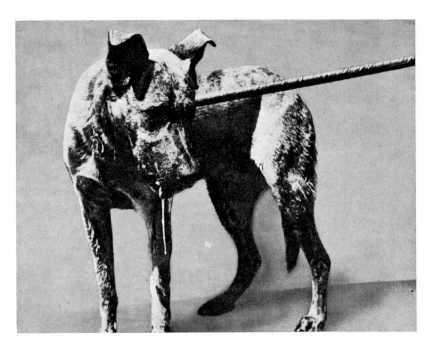

Fig. 36.   Dog in paralytic stage of rabies.

the owner to believe there is a bone stuck in the throat. After initially affecting the head and neck region, the paralysis soon becomes generalized over the body, and death ensues from the second to the fourth day after the onset.

The disease in dogs and *cats* is similar and is generally characterized by viciousness and excitation. Swift movements and erratic behavior are more marked in rabid cats than in dogs, and their bites are considered more dangerous, because they are generally of the deep puncture type.

Rabies in *cattle* generally assumes a furious form. As this stage of the disease becomes apparent, there is restlessness, nervousness, and there may be some indication of pruritus. The animal becomes aggressive and will move about violently, pawing, and butting into other animals and objects. In some cases, the affected animal cannot retain saliva. The most striking signs are fits of bellowing, general straining, and tenesmus. Although cattle may thrash about violently, they rarely bite. As the disease enters the paralytic stage, the first signs are weakness in the hind legs, followed by paralysis of the muscles of locomotion. Death comes after a period of complete paralysis and prostration.

As in cattle, rabies in *horses* and *mules* is characterized by excitation. They become very restless, excitable, and vicious. They often kick, paw, and bite other animals or moving objects, and sometimes themselves. Frequently the ears stand erect and the lips are drawn back with loss of saliva. Dysphagia is marked. Paralysis soon extends from the head and neck region to the muscles of locomotion; and death ensues after the animal has become recumbent and prostrate.

Rabies in *sheep* and *swine* is not seen as often as it is in other livestock, although the clinical course is similar, with restlessness, nervousness, hyper-excitability, and spasms of muscle groups followed by paralysis and death.

In *man*, the incubation period averages from 30 to 60 days, with a range of 2 weeks to 5 months. In rare instances, human cases have been reported in which the incubation period was as short as 10 days and as long as 8 months. The early stages of the disease are marked by prodromal symptoms of headache, malaise, slight elevation of temperature, nervousness, and anxiety. In the majority of cases, there is a sensation of tingling, pain, or burning around the site of the bite. This occurs quite early in the course of the disease. As the disease progresses, there is an increase in anxiety and nervousness, with development of increased sensory reactions, excitability, hyperesthesia, and generalized pressor syndrome. There is an increased tendency to move, and the patient often lashes about in bed. The symptom most often associated with human rabies is the so-called hydrophobia or "fear of water" phenomenon. This is due to the painful spasms of the pharyngeal muscles which occur when fluids are swallowed. Subsequent

conditioned reflexes related to swallowing will similarly cause these pharyngeal spasms, so that the patient tends to shun fluids brought to him. By
the same token, he avoids swallowing his saliva, which often drools from
his mouth. Although these swallowing symptoms are not constant, they
occur frequently enough to make them the most characteristic of the
disease in man. The increased anxiety is often associated with a feeling
of impending death. As the excitation phase develops, there may be
convulsive seizures. In rare cases, maniacal symptoms and violence with
biting, kicking and sudden lashing of the body may be elicited. Generally
there are relatively relaxed periods between those of excitation, during
which the patient is quite lucid. Most patients die during the height of an
episode of excitation, but in some the disease may progress to generalized
paralysis, and the patient may expire in prostration.

Rabies elicits no gross characteristic pathologic alterations which can
be seen during post-mortem examination. The histopathologic lesions of
the central nervous system are inflammatory in nature and are very much
like those seen in other infections. As a rule, there is more damage to the
pons, medulla, brain stem, and thalamus than to other parts of the brain.
This is probably associated with the fact that the virus is contained in
greatest concentration in these parts. The changes which can be seen
include nuclear and cytoplasmic degeneration of the neurons, neuronophagia, and diffuse gliosis. Often one can see evidence of petechial hemor-
rhage around the blood vessels, as well as perivascular, lymphocytic
cuffing found in so many infections of the central nervous system. The
well-differentiated accumulation of glial cells (so-called Babes nodules)
which one sometimes sees throughout the brain, and the marked neuronal
degeneration and lymphocytic infiltration in the dorsal root and cranial
nerve ganglia, cannot be considered pathognomonic, because these
changes may also be found in other encephalitic diseases.

In 1903 Adelchi Negri reported the pathognomonic lesion of rabies,
namely, the characteristic inclusion body which bears his name. The
Negri body is found in the cytoplasm of the neurons. It is generally
rounded and acidophilic and has a mottled matrix; staining with most
differential red-blue stains reveals that it contains characteristic, basophilic, internal granules. Examination of brain tissue for the presence of
Negri bodies has evolved as an important standard procedure in the
laboratory diagnosis of rabies.

Over the years the pathogenesis of rabies has been widely studied. The evidence of most experimental investigation shows that the virus travels in a centripetal direction from the point of entry in the area of the wound along nerve trunk pathways to the central nervous system. Infection of the salivary glands depends upon whether the virus moves in a centrifugal direction to the salivary glands via the nerve trunks. It is thought that the spread of the virus by neural pathways is related to the degeneration of the myelin sheaths and the general demyelination which is seen in the white matter in various stages of the disease.

Recently, Schneider *et al.* (1958) reported the isolation of microscopic corpuscular elements from a sedimentable fraction of salivary glands from rabid carnivores.

Rabies is diagnosed by recognition of its characteristic clinical, pathological, and virological features. The animal suspected of being rabid should be captured and confined and the disease should be allowed to progress until the animal dies. Premature killing of such animals will reduce the accuracy of the laboratory diagnosis, because the development of Negri bodies in the brain is directly related to the duration of the clinical illness. If circumstances necessitate destruction of the animal, care should be taken not to mutilate the head, because damage to the brain will render it less useful for diagnosis. After decapitation in the field, the head should be cooled promptly and kept cold; wherever possible, it should be delivered by messenger, or by express freight, via rail, air or road. It should be put into a tin or other suitable water tight metal container, which should be tightly closed. This receptacle, in turn, should be put into a large, watertight, metal container, cracked ice being put between the inner and outer containers. The use of dry ice in packing the head should be avoided if microscopic diagnosis is desired, because freezing the specimen often distorts and tears the brain tissue; furthermore, the time required for thawing causes delay in diagnosis.

Either histological sections of brain tissue blocks or fresh tissue applied to a slide by the impression or smear technique may be microscopically searched for Negri bodies. For histologic sections, the staining techniques which have given the best results are those of Schleifstein (1937), Stovall and Black (1940), or Lillie's (1948) modification of Stovall's method. Most diagnostic laboratories are not equipped to prepare histologic sections. A film of fresh brain tissue, properly applied and stained, is just as accurate for purposes of diagnosis and is manifestly simpler, quicker, and less costly.

For the impression or smear technique the stain of choice is Sellers' (1954).

The Negri body is well differentiated by Sellers' stain as a body coloured magenta or heliotrope (purplish pink) with well stained dark blue to black, basophilic, internal bodies. All parts of the nerve cell stain blue, and the interstitial tissue stains rose-pink. Erythrocytes stain a copper color (orange, tinged with red) and they can be easily differentiated from the reddish magenta of the Negri bodies.

The Negri body varies in shape, although it is generally rounded. Its size also varies greatly; it is usually within the limits of 0.24 to 27.0 microns.

The Negri body lies within the cytoplasm of the neuron. Classically, it is found between the nucleus and one corner of the neuron, or in the prolongation of the cell body. It should, however, be stressed that the intracytoplasmic position of the Negri body can be expected with reasonable consistency only in histological sections of the brain. In the simpler tissue techniques, the histological pattern is disturbed, so that it is difficult to discern the outline of the nerve cell, and one may very often see well formed Negri bodies which appear to be entirely outside the neuron. Thus, Negri bodies which satisfy the requisites of morphological identification, whether they seem to appear inside or outside the neuron, are sufficient to establish a positive diagnosis.

The most striking characteristic of the Negri body is its internal structure. The matrix of the Negri body is acidophilic, and contained within it are small inner bodies (Innenkörperchen), *i.e.* basophilic granules which stain dark blue to black. The size of these inner granules generally varies from 0.2 to 0.5 micron. Rarely, an orderly arrangement of the inner granules, as in a rosette design, may be seen. For purposes of diagnosis, it is sufficient to recognize these granules as part of the inner structure of the Negri body, regardless of their number or pattern of distribution. Although Negri bodies may be found in any portion of the grey matter rich in neurons, they are most often found in the hippocampus (Ammon's horn) and are often abundant in the cerebellum and cerebral cortex. These are the three areas studied in routine examinations.

Because other types of inclusion bodies may sometimes resemble Negri bodies, they may be mistaken for them. This is particularly true of the dog, fox, skunk, cat, and laboratory white mouse. These inclusions which are not Negri bodies all have the same staining characteristics with Sellers' stain and cannot be differentiated from one another by the techniques described above. The important point is that Negri bodies have a very definite internal structure characterized by basophilic inner granules; they have a heterogeneous or mottled matrix, are not highly refractile, and have a definite purplish tinge. In these respects they differ from the inclusions which are not Negri bodies.

Hottle *et al.* (1951), in their electron microscopy studies, found no particles in the Negri body which could be recognized as elementary bodies of the virus. Lepine and Croissant (1951) interpreted the Negri body as a cellular reaction around the virus particles. Cytochemical studies (Wolman and Behar, 1952) indicated that the inclusions might be virus particle aggregates.

On the basis of their studies of rabies virus antigens by the fluorescent antibody technique, Goldwasser and Kissling (1958) reported that the Negri bodies are of viral origin.

Negri bodies are not always demonstrable in the brains of rabid animals, and, in these cases, attempts must be made to isolate the virus by using laboratory mice. Surveys of rabies cases have shown that 10 to 15 % of the cases proved positive by mouse inoculation had been missed by direct microscopic examination of the brain for Negri bodies (Johnson, 1942; Leach, 1938; Damon and Sellers, 1941).

The white mouse is the animal preferred, because it is inexpensive, so that several animals can be used for each specimen, and because of the relatively short incubation period of street virus infection in the mouse and the constant and typical signs and consistent production of Negri bodies in this animal (Webster and Dawson, 1935). The test is carried out by the intracerebral inoculation of 0.03 ml of a 10 to 20% suspension of the suspected tissue into each of 5 mice per specimen. Tissue sections from the hippocampus, cerebral cortex, cerebellum, and the pons–medulla area are pooled for preparation of the suspended inoculum; thorough sampling of these areas on both sides of the brain is important, because of the possible variability of the distribution of the virus.

Contaminated or decomposed specimens treated with antibiotics can be injected into animals without affecting the virus. Emulsions to which are added 500 to 1000 units of penicillin and 2 mg of streptomycin per ml of tissue suspension, or their equivalents of other antibiotics, are ready for inoculation after 30 minutes at room temperature.

Diagnosis of rabies in an animal does not always mean that the saliva is infective; for this reason the mouse inoculation test of the submaxillary salivary glands of biting animals, for the presence of virus, provides definitive evidence of whether or not a bite has entailed a risk. Isolation of the virus from the salivary glands also provides important epidemiologic information.

In cases in which other viral encephalitides are suspected, the serum neutralization test is valuable as a specific confirmatory procedure. In these cases, suspensions of the tissue in question are mixed with immune stock serum and tested in mice with the usual negative and immune controls.

After the work of Goldwasser and Kissling in 1958, the fluorescent antibody test was used on a series of naturally infected salivary glands by Goldwasser et al. (1959) and on brain specimens sent into health department laboratories for rabies diagnosis by McQueen et al. (1960). Carski (1960) and Wilsnack (1960), developed and refined the test. The test is being adopted as a supplementary diagnostic tool by an increasing number of laboratories, particularly in the United States and Israel. The test allows direct, visual observation of the specific antigen–antibody reaction.

It is based on the microscopic examination of tissue specimens for specific fluorescent staining, when the tissue has been placed in contact with *conjugate,* the name given to antirabies serum which has been "tagged" by the addition of a fluorescent dye.

Examination of the slide containing a simple impression of the suspected tissue after fixing, staining and washing, is similar to any other microscopic examination, except that a source of ultraviolet light and a specialized system of filters and condensers are used.

Investigations of the fluorescent antibody test have shown that this diagnostic method, when it is properly done, can establish a highly specific diagnosis on test specimens within a few hours and that there is a high degree of correlation between this test and the mouse inoculation test.

In the United States, there were 4,083 laboratory confirmed cases of rabies during calendar year 1959, e.g. 1,119 reported in dogs, 292 in cats, 1915 in wildlife, 751 in farm livestock and 7 in man. There was a decrease of 731 cases from the total number of cases reported for the previous year and 524 of this smaller number of cases were in dogs.

The geographical distribution of rabies in the United States has remained substantially the same for several years past (Fig. 37).

The biggest increase in incidence was in New York State, which reported 478 cases in animals in 1959, as compared to 261 cases during 1958. This increase was the result of an epizootic of fox rabies in 7 counties of western New York State which was previously free from rabies and represents the worst outbreak in the State since 1946.

RABIES—REPORTED LABORATORY CONFIRMED CASES
U. S., BY STATE; 1959

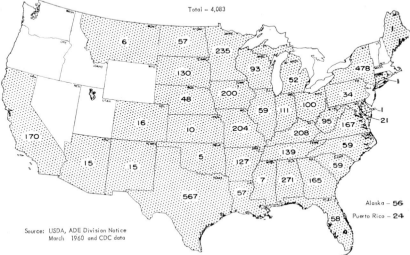

Fig. 37. Distribution of rabies cases in the U.S. in 1959.

References p. 345

In 1946, a national rabies control programme was begun by the Communicable Disease Center, U.S. Public Health Service, consisting of research, technical consultation, and training activities. During the 15-year period since that time, 33 State Health Departments have established veterinary public health programmes and have organized rabies control. Progress achieved in control during these past 15 years is reflected in the annual number of cases, in the whole of the U.S.A. (see Table XXVI).

TABLE XXVI

CASES OF RABIES IN THE UNITED STATES *

Year	Dogs	Wildlife	Cats	Livestock	Man	Total
1946	8384	956	455	1055	22	10,872
1959	1119	1915	292	751	7	4,083

* Agricultural Research Service, U.S. Department of Agriculture; Communicable Disease Center, U.S. Public Health Service.

Similarly, human deaths have dropped from 22 in 1946 to 7 in 1959, a decrease of 68%. Although the dog still accounts for most of the cases and remains the most important vector of the disease, the striking decline in canine cases from 8384 in 1946 to 1119 in 1959 (86%), in spite of a greatly increased dog population, is eloquent testimony to the success of organized rabies control programmes throughout the United States during this 15-year period. In sharp contrast to the decrease in canine rabies, the reported number of wildlife cases has doubled.

Canada remained relatively free from rabies for about 10 years, until a small focus of infection was discovered in the Northwest Territory in 1947. By 1952–53, the disease had swept south from the arctic region and had set off a serious epizootic of wildlife and dog rabies in the western province of Alberta and in parts of British Columbia and Saskatchewan. By 1957 this western Canadian region was rid of the disease and the following year new areas, which were heavily affected, principally by fox rabies, were reported from the province of Ontario.

A recent report of the Pan-American Health Organization gives the incidence for 1958 in 22 areas in the Western Hemisphere. From these areas 7,724 cases of rabies in animals were diagnosed and reported. More than 100 cases were recorded in each of the following countries: Argentina, Brazil, Canada, Chile and Peru; the United States, Guatemala,

Nicaragua and Venezuela reported more than 50 cases each. Although no information was provided for Mexico, a report sent to the World Health Organization indicated that, in 1958, 747 captured animals in the Federal District were positive for rabies. Similarly 81 positive animal cases were reported by the National Institute of Hygiene of Ecuador. Dogs have been most often incriminated as the source of rabies in man and other animals. The other animal most often reported with this disease in the Americas is the *cow*. Uruguay reports that it has been free from rabies for more than 20 years. Brazil, Mexico, the United States, French Guiana, and Trinidad have reported incidents involving the transmission of rabies by *bats*. In 1958, 186 human cases of rabies were reported and in five countries (Brazil, Columbia, Mexico, Peru and Venezuela) there were reports of 10 or more human deaths from this cause.

In 1959, the Veterinary Public Health Unit of the World Health Organization sent out a survey questionnaire on the status of rabies to nearly 300 laboratories, institutes, health organizations and veterinary departments in 108 different countries and territories. Replies were received from 223 rabies control organizations from 89 countries. The incidence figures requested were for the calendar year 1958.

The survey has shown that rabies is present in 62 countries, but there were no replies from 20 countries. There were 26 countries which reported that they were at that time free of rabies. These were:

Australia	Cyprus	Luxembourg	Portugal
Austria	Denmark	Federation of	Singapore
Basutoland	Guadeloupe	Malaya	French
Belgium	Hong Kong	Martinique	Somaliland
North Borneo	Iceland	Netherlands*	Sweden
Republic of	Ireland	New Zealand	Switzerland
China (Taiwan)	Japan	Norway	United Kingdom
			Uruguay

* A few cases of rabies have occurred among man, dog and cat in Amsterdam and vicinity in 1962 (Ed.).

Dunker (1958) reviewed the incidence of rabies in several West European countries during recent years. Table XXVII presents a comparative summary of rabies cases in various wild and domestic animals in these areas.

TABLE XXVII

INCIDENCE OF RABIES IN WEST EUROPEAN AREAS

	Countries				
	West German Republic			Austria	Italy
	Years				
Animals	1955	1956	1957	1950–1956	1950–1956
Foxes	1172 (52.9%)	1044 (69%)	1578 (67.4%)	244 (5.2%)	
Deer	366 }(22.5%)	267 }(20%)	312 }(16.8%)	—	
Other wild animals	134	76	84	125 (2.6%)	
Cats	200 (8.9%)	130 (8.6%)	147 (6.2%)	363 (7.6%)	155 (4.3%)
Dogs	144 (6.4%)	69 (4%)	131 (5.6%)	3946 (82.8%)	2971 (84.2%)
Cattle	172 }(9.2%)	110 }(8.4%)	90 }(4.2%)	— }(1.2%)	215 (6%)
Other livestock	32	16	9	56	197 (5.5%)
Total	2227	1712	396	4634	3538

Table XXVIII gives the number of rabies cases in man as compared with that of animals in Italy and Spain.

TABLE XXVIII

	Periods	Animals	Man
In Italy	1947–1951	8232	275
	1952–1956	1575	22

		Dogs	Cats	Man
In Spain	1951–1953	1217	48	38
	1954–1956	1172	146	24

A total of 947 deaths from human rabies (82 in treated and 845 in untreated persons) were reported from 65 countries. The greatest toll of human lives was reported from India, the Philippines, Mexico, Thailand and Egypt. The total number of persons who received vaccine treatment in these 65 countries was 487,728, and paralytic side-reactions attributable to the vaccine occurred in 49 persons.

The reports from 69 countries indicated that the dog can be considered to be the main vector of the disease in most countries. Wild animals, however, have begun to play an increasingly important role in the transmission of the disease. For instance, the fox is more important than the dog as a vector of the disease in Canada, Poland and Germany. In the United States, skunks have been shown to be important vectors and bats are important in the Americas.

Rabies is principally a disease of such carnivorous or biting animals as *dogs, foxes, jackals, skunks, wolves, cats,* and *coyotes,* although all warm-blooded animals are susceptible to rabies. The disease is found in the Arctic regions, as well as in the temperate and tropical countries of both hemispheres. Climate and season have no direct influence on its occurrence, and it may be present in enzootic or epizootic proportions during any time of the year. Its incidence in animals is highest during those seasons when movement and contact among them is greatest and, in the United States, this is generally during the autumn shuffle of fox populations, when family groups break up, or during late winter or spring, when wild carnivores move about in search of food, and mate.

A prerequisite to infection is the entry of the rabies virus into a wound.

Practically all cases of rabies occur as the result of the entry of saliva laden with the virus into a wound caused by the bite of a rabid animal. It is possible also for infection to occur when infected saliva comes into intimate contact with pre-existing, fresh, open wounds. This danger is present when owners try to remove what seems to be a "bone in the throat" of a choking rabid dog, or try to relieve what appears to be "choke" signs in a rabid cow. Instances of infection due to other means, such as indirect exposure via fomites, are so rare that they are negligible. There are no reports in the medical literature of infection through the alimentary tract, and this is not possible unless there are open abrasions of the gastro-intestinal mucosa.

Attempts to infect laboratory animals by feeding them with suspensions of rabies virus have failed. Similarly, negative results have been obtained after feeding experimentally infected white mice to susceptible dogs and foxes, although later it was possible to infect these animals successfully by parenteral routes. Although it has been reported that the milk of rabid cows occasionally contains rabies virus, ingestion of infected milk is not considered to be a normal mode of infection. Arthropods play no role in the transmission of rabies, and, indeed, there is no evidence of viraemia in animals infected naturally or artificially (Bell *et al.*, 1957; Kissling, 1957).

Animals naturally infected may emit the virus in the saliva in quantities sufficient to account for the natural spread of rabies. Virus is found in the salivary glands in animals dead of rabies in 54 to 90% of the cases; its prevalence is slightly higher in foxes and skunks than in dogs. The titer of virus in positive salivary glands varies from a trace to as high as $10^{6.8}$. In dogs, the excretion of virus in the saliva occurs after the onset of the clinical disease, but because the prodromal signs are so obscure, a few days may elapse between isolation of saliva from daily test samples and the appearance of the classical, frank signs of rabies. For this reason it is recommended that biting animals in which rabies is suspected should be confined under clinical observation for 10 days. This period allows a generous margin of safety; if the confined animal remains clinically well during this period, it is certain that it was not infectious at the time of the bite.

Rabies is fatal. No *man* has recovered from the disease after clinical symptoms have begun. In general, the same can be said for lower animals, although a few cases have been reported in which dogs have recovered from the disease after signs of rabies developed (Starr *et all*, 1952). However, these are so rare that they are medical curiosities. Therefore, the disease is considered to be invariably fatal in all species after symptoms have become evident.

Attack rates in man vary, from 3 to 50%, according to the part of the world in which the exposure occurs and the type of biting animal. A worldwide average of 15% is most widely accepted as the rate of rabies deaths among untreated persons bitten by rabid animals. Although accurate figures are not available, there seem to be species differences in relative susceptibility to infection. Among domestic animals, cattle are among the most susceptible species in the wide host range. Factors which influence the probability of infection are the presence and quantity of virus in the saliva of the biting animal, the severity of the bite, and the possible interposition of clothing. Thus, bites in the region of the head, neck, and face are the most dangerous, next those on the extremities (hands, feet, arms, legs), and least those on the trunk. The duration of the incubation period in the rabies victim is likewise related to the part of the body bitten and the portal of entry of the virus. Cases characterized by unusually short incubation periods most often occur after severe bites, particularly in the region of the head. These factors are now believed to be governed by differences in the relative richness of the peripheral nerve supply to various parts of the body, rather than by the distance of the bite from the central nervous system.

Rabies is more infective to younger than to older animals; and this is probably also true of man. In the 10-year period 1944–1954, more than half the total human rabies deaths in the United States were in children under 15 years of age. Children, of course, are more likely to be bitten and this accounts largely for the greater incidence among them. It is difficult to assess the relative importance of a possible increased, inherent susceptibility of the lower age groups.

Rabies in wildlife and the disease as it is found in domestic dogs, particularly in urban areas (Johnson, 1948), are the two epidemiologic types that can be recognized throughout the world. There are no antigenic differences between these types; they are classified in this manner on the basis of natural spread of the disease. In certain rural areas where rabies is enzootic, this epidemiological differentiation may not always be so distinct. Factors which influence the presence of both types simultaneously in a given area are the frequency or degree of contacts between wild species and domestic dogs, the relative size of the population and the immunological status of both groups.

With the success of the control of rabies of dogs, attention has been centered on what seems to be an increase in the spread of the disease among various species of wild animals. In addition to the very obvious fact that rabies in wild animals may cause huge losses of livestock, there are also public health aspects of the problem of sylvatic rabies. Of primary significance are the reports of direct exposures of man to rabid wild animals. During the past several years, 20% of the human deaths from rabies in the United States have been caused by the bites of rabid wild animals, principally foxes and skunks. Studies of rabies in these wild species indicate that, sooner or later, the disease spills over into canine populations, from which the hazard is greater because of man's closer association with dogs. There is general agreement that, if rabies is to be eventually eradicated, or brought to a controllable minimum, the reservoir of the virus in the country's wild fauna must necessarily be included in scientifically devised control operations.

At present in the United States, the principal wildlife vectors of the disease are the grey fox (genus *Urocyon*), the red fox (genus *Vulpes*), the small spotted skunk (genus *Spilogale*) and the large striped skunk (genus *Mephitis*). The distribution of this wildlife rabies in the U.S.A. is shown in Fig. 38.

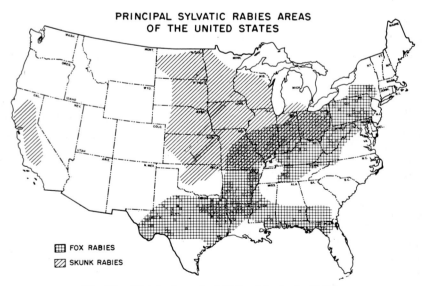

PRINCIPAL SYLVATIC RABIES AREAS
OF THE UNITED STATES

FOX RABIES
SKUNK RABIES

Fig. 38. Distribution of wild life rabies in the U.S.A.

The current high incidence of fox rabies in the United States seems to have begun in 1940, and the great increases in skunk rabies in the upper Mississippi and Missouri Valleys seem to be only about 5 or 6 years old. To be sure, fox rabies was reported in Massachusetts about 1800, in Alabama in 1890; and skunk rabies in Kansas in 1871 (lit.: Sandoz, 1954).

Even though *coyote* rabies ravaged the mountains and prairies of the Far West several decades ago, the current picture of rabies in the U.S.A. has not incriminated the coyote to any appreciable extent. The only important focus of rabies in the *raccoon* in recent years has been reported from Florida.

Endemic rabies in *arctic foxes* has plagued the islands and mainland of Alaska, the Yukon, and the northwest territories of Canada. Fox and wolf rabies has swept southward through western and central Canada during the past few years, creating one of the largest rabies problems in the history of the country.

In the spring of 1950 the *mongooses* of Puerto Rico were incriminated as the principal vectors in an epizootic of rabies, with dogs and farm animals responsible for secondary transmission. This was the first major rabies outbreak in the western hemisphere attributed to the Indian mongoose.

At present western Europe, especially western Germany, is experiencing serious outbreaks of fox rabies (see Table XXVII). The important vector in Eastern Europe is still the *wolf*. Wolf rabies extends down the Caucasus to the Caspian Sea; in Iran, attacks by rabid wolves are still responsible for the loss of many human lives.

The mongoose has not been reported as a serious vector of rabies in India, although it abounds in its native land and, as has been mentioned above, it has been the principal transmitter of rabies in Puerto Rico. In India, the *jackal* is the most important wild vector. The jackal is also the principal sylvatic transmitter of the disease in the eastern Mediterranean region and in eastern and central Africa. In the South African veld a wide variety of *meerkats* and *mongooses* keeps the disease going.

The Communicable Disease Center (CDC) at present has many research projects under way which study the natural behavior of rabies in wild animals in the U.S.A. Preliminary results of these investigations have shown that there may be some evidence that subclinical immunizing infections occur in wild animals in nature.

References p. 345

Serum antiviral substance (neutralization of at least 32 LD_{50} of rabies virus by un-diluted serum) has been found in 12 out of 262 (4.6%) fox bloods tested, in 11 out of 196 (5.6%) raccoon sera, in 2 out of 185 (1.8%) oppossum sera, in 5 out of 27 (18.5%) bobcat sera, and in 7 out of 48 (14.5%) skunk sera. These animals came from areas with a recent history of fox rabies outbreaks; this is in contrast to completely negative antibody results obtained by SN tests from nearly 300 animals taken from known rabies-free areas. There may be evidence of a relationship between the demonstration of antibodies and the time of the outbreak. Out of 670 individuals of all species tested, 1.6% showed antibodies before an epizootic peak, whereas 5.2% were serologically positive after an epizootic peak, and 5.1% were serologically positive in enzootic areas. Thus serum surveys of wild animals in nature could possibly be used, in conjunction with population density surveys, for predicting epizootics of rabies with greater accuracy than with either of these methods alone.

75% of the submaxillary glands of naturally infected foxes contain rabies virus. In no instance have salivary glands been found infected without concurrent infection of the central nervous system, a fact which indicates that the fox can transmit the disease as a symptomless carrier. The transmitting potential of foxes, however, is high, as is shown by the facts that it was found that experimentally infected foxes experience long periods of illness, and that daily testing of saliva showed that it contained rabies virus for long periods of time (in one individual for 17 days). Positive saliva swabs were obtained from 7 out of 24 experimentally infected foxes and from one of these it was obtained from 1 to 3 days before classical, clinical signs were observed.

A rabies virus survey of over a 1,000 small wild rodents trapped in high enzootic and epizootic fox rabies in New York and Georgia revealed no evidence of infection, a fact which confirmed previous reports that these species do not serve as reservoirs of the disease in the wild.

Helmboldt and Jungherr (1955) reported canine distemper in wild carnivores which exhibited clinical signs that simulated those of rabies.

The transmission of rabies by *bats* was first established in 1916 (Haupt and Rehaag, 1921), during an outbreak of a severe paralytic disease of cattle in Brazil. In Trinidad 89 persons died between 1929 and 1935 of a disease characterized by an ascending paralysis. The early cases were diagnosed as bulbar poliomyelitis. At the same time, an epizootic of a fatal paralytic disease in cattle was occurring and this was thought at first to be botulism. The work of Pawan and Hurst (1931, 1932, 1936) is a well-documented, epidemiologic classic in the establishment of this outbreak of fatal paralytic disease in man and cattle as rabies caused by the bites of infected bats. The principal vector involved in these outbreaks was the vampire bat *(Desmodus rotundus murinus)*, and this species remains as the most important vector of rabies in many parts of Latin America today.

Vampire bats are found from northern Argentina and southern Brazil northward to about a 100 miles south of the Rio Grande River in Mexico; those in Trinidad came over from the northern coast of South America. They are not known to occur in the United States or in the eastern Hemisphere. Vampire bats are haemophagous. They inflict, with their highly adapted, sharp incisor teeth, small, crater-like wounds in the skin of their victims and lap the escaping blood with a long, well-developed tongue. It has been shown that vampire bats can, on occasion, transmit rabies as true, symptomless carriers.

Vampire bat rabies continues to be a great problem in most of the South American countries and Mexico. Malaga–Alba (1958) stated that it is the most frequent cause of death from rabies in South American native cattle and estimated that the damage due to it during 1956 was about 1 million head of livestock, which represented an economic loss of about 80 million dollars. The hazard of human attacks by vampire bats is present when persons sleep out of doors or in unscreened buildings in enzootic areas; the vampire bat will feed on man when livestock sources of blood meals are not readily available. A total of 117 human deaths have been reported from Trinidad, Mexico, and British Guiana. Programmes for the destruction of vampire bats by dynamiting and gassing caves, and bat-proofing abandoned dwellings and tree hollows, have proved temporarily successful in some countries; these measures seem to have been most successful in Trinidad, but it is almost impossible to carry them out in some of the rugged mountain areas of the Sierra Madre mountain ranges in Mexico. The most effective method for controlling the disease in livestock in recent years has been vaccination of cattle with high egg passage (HEP) Flury chicken embryo vaccine. In Mexico alone, over 5 million head of cattle have been vaccinated with the HEP Flury vaccine in mass immunization programmes. These programmes have reduced paralytic cattle rabies to occasional sporadic cases in the enzootic areas (Malaga-Alba, 1958; Camargo, 1955).

In the vampire bat rabies areas of Latin America investigators have found evidence of rabies in a variety of nonhaemophagous bats; several species of frugivorous and insectivorous bats have been found infected during outbreaks of bat rabies. Bat rabies in the United States was unknown until June 1953, when the virus was isolated from a yellow bat (*Dasypterus floridanus*), which had bitten a child in Florida. Since this first reported case, about 500 cases have been diagnosed in bats from 30 States in widely diverse geographic areas of the United States (Fig. 39), and from one province in Canada (British Columbia) and, recently, from Yugoslavia and Turkey. 4 species of tree-living or solitary bats and 20

species of colonial or cave-dwelling bats have been so far implicated.
All are insectivorous. The greatest number of isolations have been made
from the Mexican free-tailed bat *(Tadarida brasiliensis mexicana)* in the
southwestern United States. The largest number of examinations have
been made in Texas (approximately 2500 with 73 of them positive), New
Mexico (3000 with 89 positive isolations), Oklahoma (1071 with 2 positive)
and Florida (approximately 5600 with 46 positive). The remaining rabid
bats were either reported from smaller survey areas, or were isolated
cases diagnosed in public health laboratories and reported through the
usual channels, a source which reflects an increasing awareness of the
presence of bat rabies among disease-control authorities and the general
public.

So far 5 human rabies deaths have been attributed to transmission from
rabid insectivorous bats in the United States and there has been one
record from India.

One case occurred in Big Spring, Texas in 1951 and was investigated retrospectively
and reported by Sulkin and Greve in 1954. The biting had occurred when a woman
picked up a moribund bat along the roadside. In 2 human deaths attributed to bat

**STATES WHICH HAVE REPORTED BAT RABIES
WITH DATE OF FIRST ISOLATION**

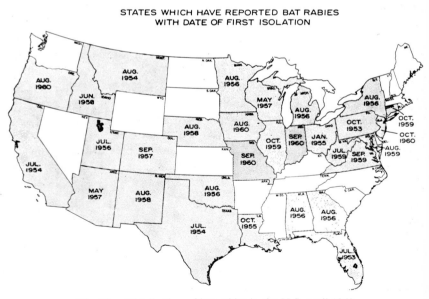

Fig. 39.   Distribution of bat rabies in the U.S. until 1960.

transmitted rabies, evidence points to contraction of the disease in a Texas bat cave and in both of these cases no known history of a bite could be elicited. The earlier case (1956) was that of a Texas State Health Department scientist, who had been working in the cave on a bat rabies research project. The other case occurred in 1959 when a mining engineer spent some time in the cave on a prospecting assignment for a bat guano mining company. A case reported in 1959 from Wisconsin occurred after a man was bitten on the lobe of his ear. The remaining case was the only one thus far which could be unquestionably attributed to the bite of a known rabid bat in California in 1958 (Lennette *et al.*, 1959, Humphrey *et al.*, 1960). In this case, a woman was bitten when she picked up a moribund silverhaired bat *(Lasionycteris noctivagans)* in her back yard. Rabies virus was isolated from the bat. Two months later, the woman became ill and died after symptoms strongly suggestive of rabies. Rabies virus was isolated from her brain at autopsy by the California State Health Department.

It has been possible to infect experimentally several species of animals, including bats, with virus isolated from naturally infected bats by peripheral routes, but in most instances this has been accomplished with difficulty. It is of interest that experimentally infected bats often exhibit furious signs of the diseases (Fig. 40). So far it has not been possible to transmit the disease by inducing rabid bats, the saliva of which was known to be infectious, to bite adult animals in the laboratory. However, Bell in 1959 and Constantine in 1960 succeeded in transmitting rabies to suckling mice and hamsters respectively, by the bites of infected bats.

The problem of asymptomatic rabies is one of many in the epizootiologic puzzle of the disease in insectivorous bats. It is well established that their chiropteran cousins, the vampire bats in Latin America, can transmit the disease for long periods of time without showing signs of illness. It has been suggested that this symbiotic host–virus relationship may be also present in the insectivorous bats. During current studies by the Communicable Disease Center in caves of the southwestern United States, rabies virus has been isolated from 0.5 % of 2,478 apparently normal bats tested in pools of 3 and 4, and from 14.6 % of 199 individually tested bats, which were collected in flight. Rabies virus was detected in the salivary gland, but not in the central nervous system, of 5 out of the 13 rabid bats in the first sample, and in 14 of the 29 rabid bats in the second sample; these bats remained clinically normal until they were killed for testing. The data thus far obtained, although suggestive, do not conclusively prove that there are, in the U.S.A., asymptomatic insectivorous carrier bats.

Infection rates in the respective samples of moribund and abnormally behaving bats were 8.7 and 76.0 %, in sharp contrast to the infection rates of 0.5 and 14.6 % in clinically normal bats. Some of the infected bats exhibit convulsions and spasmodic contraction of the abdominal muscles. Vicious biting of one bat by another was observed in one instance; however, most of the sick bats showed signs of paralysis. Monthly samples of bat sera were tested for SN antibodies, and an average of 21.3 % of a total of 1588 bats were found to have significant levels of antibody, with a range from 14 to 40 %.

Native wild carnivores (grey foxes, silver foxes and coyotes) developed rabies after they had been kept for approximately 1 month in bat-proofed and arthropod-proofed cages within a large bat cave in southwestern United States. Circumstances of this field study indicate bat-to-carnivore

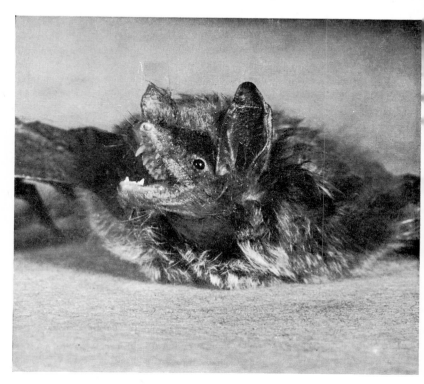

Fig. 40.   Pipistrel bat in furious stage of rabies.

transmission by a non-bite route and support consideration of an airborne medium as the mechanism of rabies transmission under the conditions existing in this cave at the time of the study.

Once the clinical disease develops, there is no known treatment for rabies. Wounds of exposed persons are locally treated and immuno-specific, biological therapy (Pasteur treatment) is carried out. In persons bitten by rabid or suspected animals, the wound should be thoroughly irrigated as soon as possible with soap or detergent solution (Shaughnessy and Zichis, 1943, 1954). In deep, narrow punctures which cannot be cleansed it may be necessary to use strong mineral acids such as nitric acid. On the basis of practical observations, immediate suturing of these wounds is contraindicated. Experimental evidence obtained from laboratory animals has shown that infiltration of hyperimmune rabies antiserum into the tissues around and beneath the bite wound is, when it is feasible, effective in the prevention of rabies (Erzogovac, 1956; Perez-Gallardo *et al.*, 1957).

A variety of human post-exposure rabies vaccines are available today; the most widely used of them are the Semple vaccine (1919), a phenolized fixed virus, and an ultra-violet irradiated fixed virus vaccine; each of these is given in 14 divided, subcutaneous doses, one dose being given daily. An adequate level of immunity develops about 14 days after treatment is initiated. Both the Semple and ultra-violet irradiated vaccines are suspensions of central nervous system tissue containing inactivated or "dead" virus. A similar, inactivated, CNS virus vaccine is that of Hempt (1925), which is treated with ether and phenol, and is used in some European countries.

The human antirabies vaccines, made of suspensions of living, fixed virus, that are used in the United States today are the Sellers (1923) and Harris and Shackell (1911) vaccines. They are used on a modified, daily dosage regime which varies from 7 to 21 days, according to the site and severity of the bite. In some parts in the world the original "dried cord" method of Pasteur is still used for preparation and administration of rabies vaccine.

Over the years, one of the very real problems in the specific biological therapy of exposed persons has been the inefficacy of vaccine for the treatment of severe bite cases, especially in those cases in which the region of the head has been involved, or, when the incubation period has been too short to allow for the development of active immunity. This problem has now largely been overcome by the production of hyperimmune rabies antiserum, which can be administered to confer sufficient passive immunity during the critical early period before the vaccine can stimulate active protection. Convincing experimental evidence, obtained by challenging laboratory animals and by antibody studies in man, has established the value of this hyperimmune antiserum, provided that it is followed by the usual course of vaccine treatment. These findings were corroborated by a limited field trial sponsored by the World Health Organization in Iran, where only 1 out of 13 persons died of rabies after they had been severely bitten in the region of the head by a rabid wolf and had been treated with serum and a course of vaccine, whereas 3 out of 5 individuals similarly bitten by the same wolf and treated with a course of vaccine alone succumbed to rabies (Baltazard and Bahmanyar, 1955).

In recent years attention has been drawn to the occasional occurrence in exposed persons of postvaccinial encephalitis, and neurological and paralytic complications following the administration of the prescribed series of rabies vaccine treatments. These reactions are believed to be tissue-specific, isoallergic phenomena which are apparently not related to the rabies antigen present, but rather to some encephalitogenic component of the nervous tissue in the vaccine. They occur most frequently after the seventh inoculation and most often in persons who have had previous Pasteur treatment. Reports on the frequency of these complications vary as follows: 1 in 527 (Cook et al., 1955), 1 in 600 (Pait and Pearson, 1949), 1 in 2025 (Appelbaum et al., 1953), 1 in 7200 (Sellers, 1948), 1 in 8500 (McKendrick, 1940). Experiments are at present proceeding in search of new approaches which will lead to an effective vaccination regime without the danger of damage to the central nervous system. In the meantime, the promiscuous administration of antirabic inoculations should be discouraged and each case should be carefully judged in the light of the particular circumstances under which the individual was bitten.

The Fourth Report of the Expert Committee of the World Health Organization on Rabies (1960) includes a detailed chart which should serve as a valuable guide in establishing indications for vaccine treatment of exposed persons.

In order to avoid the nerve tissue vaccines currently employed, work has been carried out to produce new vaccines prepared by the inoculation of embryonated duck eggs. One is a single-passage, fixed-virus vaccine grown in developing duck embryos which has been inactivated by the addition of beta-propiolactone. It has been shown that this new duck embryo vaccine elicits a good serum neutralizing antibody response and it is now being marketed under licence in the United States for human use (Peck et al., 1955, 1956; Greenberg and Childress, 1960). The other new vaccine now undergoing field trials is a living, modified, virus vaccine (Flury-strain) grown in chicken embryos; it differs from the Flury-strain, canine vaccine in the serial, egg-level passage used. The dog vaccine is produced from the 14th to 15th egg passage, and is designated as the low egg passage (LEP) vaccine, whereas the human vaccine is made from the 180th to 190th passage, and is known as the high egg passage (HEP) vaccine. Serum neutralization studies have shown that a single, 0.2-ml intradermal dose of avian embryo vaccine produced good antibody response in volunteers with a history of previous Pasteur treatment (Fox et al., 1955, 1956, 1957; Koprowski, 1956; Tierkel, 1958; Fox, 1958). There is thus an indication that booster inoculations of this material may be adequate for post-exposure vaccination in persons previously treated, *i.e.,* in those in whom the hazard of postvaccinal complications would be greatest if a series of nervous tissue vaccines were used.

This work suggests that prophylactic pre-exposure booster inoculations at certain specified intervals can be recommended for high-risk groups such as veterinarians, laboratory workers, dog wardens, predator control specialists, etc.

A practical vaccine for dogs was not developed and used successfully in the field until the early 1920's, even though much of Pasteur's original work with vaccines was done on the canine disease.

This was the vaccine of the Japanese workers Umeno and Doi (1921), a phenolized, rabbit brain product. It was not until Habel (1940) developed a standard mouse potency test for Semple-type vaccines that intrinsic improvement in vaccines occurred. The Semple-type vaccine used for dogs is a 20% heat-inactivated and phenol-treated, fixed-virus, brain emulsion of equine, caprine, or ovine origin for inoculation in single doses of 5 ml. It is known variously as phenolized, nervous tissue or Semple vaccine. The first significant experimental contribution to our knowledge of the duration of immunity in dogs following rabies vaccination was made by Johnson (1945) of the Rockefeller Foundation. The result of this work indicated excellent protection in dogs for 1 year after a single dose of this phenolized vaccine. It was on the basis of this work and subsequent field trials that the single-dose method of canine rabies vaccination was put into universal practice as an integral part of rabies control programmes.

In recent years one of the most important advances in the field of rabies immunization has been the development of a modified, living-virus vaccine (Flury-strain) produced in chicken embryos (Koprowski and Cox, 1948). The strain of virus in this vaccine was named after a young human rabies patient in Georgia from whom it was isolated at autopsy.

The isolated virus was passaged serially by Johnson through 136 1-day-old chicks by the intra-cerebral route, and was subsequently adapted to chicken embryos by Koprowski and Cox by the yolk sac route of inoculation. It was observed that continuous serial passage of this strain through embryonated chicken eggs attenuated the virus and rendered it nonpathogenic to laboratory animals and dogs after 40 to 50 egg passages, when it was inoculated peripherally. It was further seen that the virus became so modified in character that it thrived in the entire developing chicken embryo, and could be isolated from all of the tissues of this embryo. The facts that it could be inoculated safely by peripheral routes and that its pantropic character in the embryonated egg made the entire embryo a rich source of the virus, led to tests of the immunizing power of the egg-adapted Flury-strain. A preliminary study by Tierkel *et al.* (1949), and extensive trials by Koprowski and Black (1950, 1952) showed that the strain has a high level of immunizing capacity in dogs. Comparative studies of the duration of the immunity, done by experiments on dogs at the Communicable Disease Center, U.S.

Public Health Service, have shown that the Flury-strain, chicken-embryo vaccine is significantly superior to the older types of inactivated-virus, nervous-tissue vaccines for periods of at least 3¼ years between vaccination and experimental exposure (Tierkel *et al.*, 1953). Field experience with this vaccine has corroborated the results of the controlled tests (Kaeberle, 1958). The reports of the Expert Committee on Rabies of the World Health Organization, in 1954 and 1957, recognized that a single intramuscular injection (in the posterior thigh muscles) of the chicken-embryo LEP vaccine (Flury-strain) produces excellent immunity in dogs for at least 3 years and this Committee recommended the use of this vaccine in mass-immunization programmes. The live canine LEP-(Flury strain)-vaccine is prepared as a 33% whole-embryo emulsion for intramuscular inoculation of single doses of 3 ml. A similar egg-adapted, modified living virus-vaccine was developed by Kemron in Israel from the "Kelev" strain, originally obtained from a naturally infected dog. Although this vaccine confers good protection in dogs and cattle, the duration of immunity beyond 1 year has not been ascertained.

Further studies have shown that pups can be vaccinated successfully as early as 3 months of age with LEP-Flury vaccine, although the animals in these experiments were challenged after relatively short postvaccination periods (Kissling and Edison, 1955; Kaeberle, 1958; Dean, 1956). Thus, in areas which have successfully eliminated rabies, but are faced with the constant danger of its reintroduction, a prophylactic regimen for dogs can be visualized as being somewhat similar to smallpox vaccination in human populations; dogs are vaccinated with chicken-embryo vaccine at 3 months and 1 year of age, followed by booster vaccinations 3 to 4 years later. It should be emphasized, however, that this procedure by no means precludes the necessity of carrying out intensified, mass canine vaccination campaigns in areas of enzootic or epizootic rabies.

Cats may be effectively vaccinated with either phenolized, nervous-tissue vaccine or chicken-embryo (Flury) vaccine. A recent study carried out by the New York State Health Department showed that phenolized vaccine and both LEP and HEP Flury vaccine conferred significant protection in adult cats; protection with the phenolized vaccine was greater than that induced by either LEP or HEP Flury chicken-embryo vaccines (Dean, 1956; Kaeberle, 1958). Vaccination of kittens under 6 months of age is not recommended. Although rabies in cats occurs in enzootic areas, the cat is not considered to be an important vector of the disease. There is no evidence that rabies persists among cats in areas in which the disease has been successfully eliminated from dogs and wildlife vectors. For this reason, cats are rarely included in mass vaccination programmes. When, however, rabies occurs in cats, these animals are clearly a public health menace, and cat owners are encouraged to have their animals vaccinated for their own protection.

In cattle, phenolized vaccines have been used sporadically throughout the years. There is little or no information on the efficacy of this vaccine, except that obtained from informal field observations made by practising veterinarians on individual cases and herds. Outside the vampire bat rabies areas of Latin America, experience of pre-exposure vaccination practices in cattle is meager. In one study Gomez *et al.* (1955) found that a single dose of 30 ml of 33% of chloroform-inactivated, nervous-tissue vaccine protected cattle challenged 1 year after vaccination, whereas 15 ml of the same vaccine did not.

The success of Flury, living-virus, chicken-embryo vaccine in dogs led to trials of it in cattle. The early use of the LEP Flury vaccine in cattle seemed to show that it could be used effectively to protect against subsequent exposure to rabies. However, field use of the LEP vaccine showed that it may cause inoculation infection with paralysis and sometimes death in cows. Because of these observations, the use of LEP Flury vaccine was discontinued in this highly susceptible species. This experience prompted the development of the HEP–Flury vaccine which proved innocuous for all species of animals tested. In its 1957 report, the Expert Committee of the World Health Organisation on Rabies recommended the use of HEP vaccine for cattle and suggested that a second dose of this vaccine, administered 30 days after the first, may have a booster effect and provide more complete protection. Pre-exposure vaccination of cattle is most widely practised by official agencies in the heavily infected, vampire bat rabies areas of Latin America, where it is at present the most effective method of controlling bovine paralytic rabies. Although individual herd owners have been having their valuable cattle vaccinated in highly enzootic sylvatic rabies areas of the United States, mass vaccination of cattle, as an official State-wide program, has not been found economically feasible (Dean, 1956).

In addition to cattle, other species of animals have been shown to be susceptible, occasionally, to vaccine virus infection by the LEP–Flury vaccine. Because it has been used widely with safety in dogs and cats, veterinarians have administered this vaccine to skunks and foxes which had been tamed as household pets and have found that these wild species will occasionally succumb to LEP–Flury vaccine. Studies carried out in these vaccine-infected animals failed consistently to demonstrate infection of the salivary glands or "reversion" of the modified virus to a natural or virulent state. In view of this experience, it is recommended that wild pet animals, such as skunks, be vaccinated with HEP-Flury vaccine or phenolized nervous-tissue vaccine. Data on controlled experiments concerning the antigenic efficacy of rabies vaccines in species other than dogs, cats, and cattle are at present grossly inadequate.

Although vaccination of dogs after they have been bitten by a rabid animal, was practised for many years, it has little practical value, because, in many cases, too much time elapses between the bite and the opportunity for vaccination. Good results have been obtained when hyperimmune antiserum has been given and has been followed by 3 dose courses of Flury vaccine. The need for the immunization of dogs after they have been bitten is diminishing with the extension of mass vaccination programmes and with the increase in the number of pre-exposure canine vaccinations reported throughout the country. The principal value of postexposure vaccination nowadays is its use as a single inoculation booster in previously vaccinated dogs which have been bitten by rabid animals.

The ultimate solution of the rabies problem depends on the control and eventual elimination of the disease from animal populations. This may be accomplished by setting up transmission barriers, *e.g.,* by animal vaccination, the elimination of stray dogs, and the reduction of excessive numbers of wildlife vectors. Extensive laboratory research and field projects have proved that these techniques can successfully eradicate the disease from a given area, provided that they are integrated into a carefully planned and well-executed programme.

Field demonstrations have proved that local programmes work best when they are carried out on a wide basis. Local control should include the following basic activities: (1) Mass vaccination of dogs. This should be carried out intensively on a schedule that aims at the vaccination of all owned dogs within the shortest possible time. In the face of a serious outbreak, at least 70% of the entire dog population of the area should be vaccinated within 2 to 3 weeks. This is best carried out by enlisting all the available veterinarians of the region in an organized canine-vaccination campaign. Dramatic demonstrations of the efficacy of mass immunization programmes have been reported from several countries of the world, such as Malaya (Wells, 1954), Israel (Kaplan *et al.,* 1954), the United States, and others. In the U.S.A., a number of mass immunization campaigns have been effective in eliminating rabies from large cities. Excellent examples of these were the campaigns in Memphis in 1948 where 23,000 dogs (Tierkel *et al.,* 1950) (Fig. 41), and in Houston in 1954, where 45,000 dogs (Tierkel, 1956) were vaccinated within a single week.

(2) Elimination of all stray dogs. Mass vaccination will not reach the stray or owner-less dog, which remains a potential threat in the transmission of rabies. Licensing or registration of all dogs is often a valuable adjunct.

(3) Reduction of excess numbers of wildlife vectors. Outbreaks of rabies in wild animals usually occur when the population of the species affected becomes particularly dense in a given area. Organized trapping and poisoning programmes are the most effective methods of reducing this overpopulation to a safe level.

Other important measures are restraint of dogs while the control campaign is under way, and insistence on a continual and energetic publicity campaign. Essential to the success of the programme is good organization under veterinary, medical and public health control, with the fullest use of all the technical resources in the community. If a human death from rabies occurs, a complete epidemiological investigation should be carried out.

(4) Management of animals known to have been exposed to infection. Whenever new cases of rabies appear in the community, it is important that information be obtained regarding the exposure of other animals. All dogs and cats bitten by an animal known to be rabid should be: *a,* destroyed immediately; *b,* if the owner is unwilling to destroy the exposed animals, they should be placed in strict isolation in a kennel for 6 months; *c,* if the animal has been vaccinated previously within 1 year with nervous tissue vaccine, or within 3 years with chicken-embryo vaccine, it must be revaccinated and restrained (on a leash or in confinement) for 30 days.

The coordination of control measures is the keynote of a successful, State- or

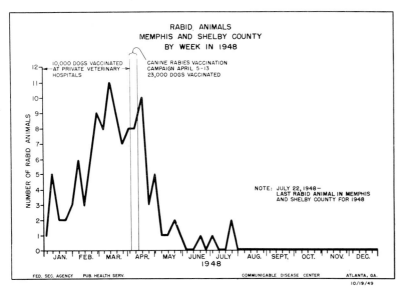

Fig. 41.   Results of preventive vaccination against rabies of dogs in the Memphis region of Tennessee.

References p. 345

Province-wide rabies control programme. Experience has shown that this is best effected by delegating the administration of such a programme to a qualified veterinarian trained in public health work at the State or provincial level. The development of a programme under the State Public Health veterinarian can insure an effective uniformity of control among the local health authorities. In his capacity as controller of the programme, the Public Health veterinarian acts as a liaison officer between the Public Health, Wildlife, and Livestock Disease control agencies. He arranges for regular exchange of information on control with neighbouring States. The Health Department veterinarian is responsible for collecting and evaluating epidemiological data on human exposure and on infection in animals and man.

Meyer (1954) has stated that no general measure has proved so effective as quarantine for preventing the establishment of the disease in rabies-free countries. Australia, New Zealand, the Hawaiian Islands, Great Britain, and the Panama Canal Zone have been successful in ensuring their rabies-free status by imposing strict quarantine regulations on all imported dogs and cats. In the United Kingdom, where there is a 6-months quarantine regulation, rabies has occurred, since the regulations were put into effect in 1919, in 22 imported dogs during quarantine. From time to time, pressure is brought on the authorities in these countries to relax the regulations for the convenience of owners of pets. In each instance, so far, the rabies control officials, after thorough investigation and evaluation of these procedures, have elected to continue the rigid enforcement of quarantine. It is felt that the lowering of the safeguards would invite the added danger of introducing the disease into the wild fauna of the area. One of the most dramatic illustrations of this danger is the sad experience of Puerto Rico, where the disease became firmly established in the mongoose population of the island in 1950 (Tierkel *et al.*, 1952). Mongoose rabies continues to be a major and costly Public Health problem in Puerto Rico, which previously had been one of the world's rabies-free areas.

The report of the WHO Expert Committee on Rabies (1960) recommends that countries free of rabies prohibit the importation of dogs and cats or subject them to a prolonged period of quarantine, preferably 6 months, at the port of entry.

REFERENCES

APPELBAUM, E., M. GREENBERG and J. NELSON, *J. Amer. med. Ass.*, 151 (1953) 188.

BALTAZARD, M. and M. BAHMANYAR, *Bull. Wld Hlth Org.*, 13 (1955) 747.

BELL, J., *Science*, 129 (1959) 1490.

BURNS, K. F., C. F. FARINACCI, T. G. MURNANE and D. F. SHELTON, *Amer. J. publ. Hlth*, 46 (1956) 1089.

CARSKI, T. R., *Communic. Dis. Center Publ.*, 1 (1960) 64.

CONSTANTINE, D. G., *unpublished Communic. Dis. Center Rep.*, 1957 and 1960.

CONSTANTINE, D. G., *Rabies transmission by non-bite route*, in the press, 1962.

DEAN, D. J., *Working Document WHO/Rabies*, Nos. 56, 57, 58 (1956).

DUNKER, S. M., *Thesis*, Frankfurt/Main, 1958, 61 p.p.

ENRIGHT, J. B., W. W. SADLER, J. E. MOULTON and D. G. CONSTANTINE, *Proc. Soc. exp. Biol. (N.Y.)*, 89 (1955) 94.

ERZOGOVAC, D. T., *Wien. tierärztl. Mschr.*, 43 (1956) 288.

FOX, J. P., *Ann. N.Y. Acad. Sci.*, 70 (1958) 480.

FOX, J. P., H. KOPROWSKI, D. P. CONWELL, J. BLACK and H. M. GELFAND, *Bull. Wld Hlth Org.*, 17 (1957) 869.

GOLDWASSER, R. A. and R. E. KISSLING, *Proc. Soc. exp. Biol. (N.Y.)*, 98 (1958) 219.

GOLDWASSER, R. A., R. E. KISSLING, T. R. CARSKI and T. S. HOSTY, *Bull. Wld Hlth Org.*, 20 (1959) 579.

HUMPHREY, G. L., G. E. KEMP and E. G. WOOD, *Publ. Hlth Rep. (Wash.)*, 75 (1960) 317.

JOHNSTON, R. V., J. W. NEWBERNE, C. J. YORK, G. R. BURCH and A. H. BRUECKNER, *J. Amer. vet. med. Ass.*, 130 (1957) 61.

KAPLAN, M. M., Y. GOOR and E. S. TIERKEL, *Bull. Wld Hlth Org.*, 10 (1954) 743.

KLECKNER, M., *unpublished Communic. Dis. Center Rep.*, 1958.

KLIGLER, I. J. and H. BERNKOPF, *Proc. Soc. exp. Biol. (N.Y.)*, 39 (1938) 212.

KOPROWSKI, H., *Canad. J. publ. Hlth*, 40 (1949) 60.

MCQUEEN, J. L., A. L. LEWIS and N. J. SCHNEIDER, *Amer. J. publ. Hlth*, 50 (1960) 1743.

NEHAUL, B. B. G., *Amer. J. trop. Med. Hyg.*, 4 (1955) 550.

PECK, F. B. Jr., H. M. POWELL and C. G. CULBERTSON, *J. Amer. med. Ass.*, 162 (1956) 1373.

SELLERS, T. F., in T. R. HARRISON (Ed.) *Principles of Internal Medicine*, 2nd. ed., New York, 1954, p. 1106; *W.H.O. Monogr. Series*, No. 23, (1954) 32.

SHARPLESS, G. R., J. BLACK, H. R. COX and J. M. RUEGSEGGER, *Bull. Wld Hlth Org.*, 17 (1957) 905.

STARR, L. E., T. B. CLOWER, C L. BROMLEY. and C. F. ROUTH, *Vet. Med.*, 49 (1954) 366.

TIERKEL, E. S., *Working Document WHO/Rabies*, No. 26 (1956).

TIERKEL, E. S. and H. D. NEFF, *Publ. Hlth Service Publ.* U.S. Govt. No. 568 (1957).

TIERKEL, E. S., H. KOPROWSKI, J. BLACK and R. H. GORRIE, *Amer. J. vet. Res.*, 10 (1949) 361.

TIERKEL, E. S., L. M. GRAVES, H. G. TUGGLE and S. L. WADLEY, *Amer. J. publ. Hlth*, 40 (1950) 1084.

TIERKEL, E. S., G. ARBONA, A. RIVERA and A. DE JUAN, *Publ. Hlth Rep. (Wash.)*, 67 (1952) 274.

TIERKEL, E. S., R. E. KISSLING, M. E. EDISON and K. HABEL, *Proc. 90-th Ann. Meeting Amer. vet. med. Ass.*, Toronto, 1953, p. 443.

WELLS, C. W., *Bull. Wld Hlth Org.*, 10 (1954) 731.

World Health Organization, Expert Comm. on Rabies, *W.H.O. Technical Rep.*, Second Rep. No. 82 (1954); Third Rep. No. 121 (1957); Fourth Rep. No. 201 (1960); *World Survey on Rabies, Mimeographed Rep.* (1960).

2

H. S. FRENKEL

Aujeszky's disease

(PSEUDORABIES, INFECTIOUS BULBAR PARALYSIS, MAD ITCH)

Aujeszky's disease is a disorder in cattle, swine, dogs, cats and a number of other animal species, caused by a specific virus. It has been reported in almost all European countries and a large section of the middle-western States of North America.

Aujeszky, a Hungarian physician and veterinarian, differentiated the disease as a separate morbid entity in 1902. Probably it is of world-wide distribution and was known in early times. Nikolitsch argued that an epidemic ailment among the Germanic soldiers, prevailing in the year 553, and extensively described by the Byzantine historian Agathias, must have been pseudorabies. According to Hanson, a similar disease occurred in the United States as early as the beginning of the nineteenth century.

The most prominent symptom is pruritus (Fig. 42) which can be so severe that it results in serious lesions of the skin and underlying tissues.

The incubation period varies from 3 to 6 days. The symptoms also vary according to the animal species. Weariness, refusal of food, and a facial expression of fear at the onset of the disease are characteristic signs in *cats* and *dogs*. The affected animal often changes its attitude, licking the wounded spot on the skin. Extensive excoriations and even deep skin lesions may develop within a few hours.

Dogs may display symptoms similar to those of rabies, but, although they attack other dogs more eagerly, they are wary of attacking man. They show inability to swallow, and paralysis of the glossopharyngeous nerve results in a flow of saliva from the mouth. As a rule, but not in every instance, there is a slight rise of temperature. Death occurs almost without exception within 24 to 36 hours.

Cattle show spasmodic contraction of the masticatory muscles. They are inclined to rub or chafe the skin of the muzzle or other parts of the head. The skin on both sides of the thorax may be so intensely chafed, scratched or bitten that the hair is completely rubbed off and a red, transudating and bleeding surface is left. Perspiration, gnashing of teeth, tympanitis and paralysis of the pharynx are associated symptoms. In most cases death occurs within 48 hours. Fever is present only at the beginning of the illness.

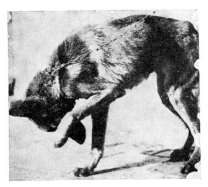

Fig. 42.   Pseudorabies in a dog; intense itching.

In *sheep* the clinical picture is slightly different. The symptoms observed are chafing of the lips and nibbling of wool, with ensuing progressive general weakness. Because of paralysis of the pharynx, saliva runs out of the mouth; the foamy character of the saliva may be due to its admixture with fluid derived from lung oedema. Death usually follows within 24 hours.

The disease in *horses* begins with feverishness, excitation and anorexia. The animals are readily excited and frightened. Pruritus, resulting in energetic rubbing of various parts of the skin, chiefly of the head, muscular tremor, clonic spasms, paralytic feebleness are observed. According to Lourens, horses die within 3 days, although recovery is more frequent as compared with carnivores and cattle. Sometimes the disease runs a benign course.

In *swine* the clinical picture may be much varied (Akkermans, 1963). Aujeszky's disease can spread very quickly among these animals; at times more than 50% of a herd may become involved within 6 to 8 days.

However, the disease is benign, with low fever, accompanied by unsteadiness and sometimes vomiting. The course may be so mild that it escapesnotice when the swine are not closely watched. On the other hand, theinfection may be severe and acute encephalomyelitis may then develop. This severe type occurs mostly in unweaned piglets. Occasionally diarrhoea with chocolate coloured faeces is observed. When this happens, the animal dies in 4 to 6 days.

Jackals, hedgehogs and *rodents* (rabbits, guinea pigs, mice and rats) are susceptible to experimental infection. This may be easily accomplished by feeding the animals with organs containing the virus.

Not much is known of the process of natural infection, though it is possible through skin-wounds and by the oral route. Rats may introduce the virus into swineherds, the pigs developing the disease when they eat diseased rats. Aujeszky's disease is transmitted to other susceptible species on the farm by hogs which may themselves be asymptomatic.

The mode of transmission of infection among animals has not yet been elucidated. Saliva can hardly be the vehicle, because it is almost virus-free, unless it is mixed with oedematous pulmonary fluid. Skin parasites have been incriminated (Kern), but it was not possible to confirm that they actually can transmit the infection.

Infection by the oral route is likely whenever the meat and viscera of diseased animals are eaten or when water contaminated by infected blood or urine is drunk.

The development of the disease is briefly as follows: The virus multiplies first in the subcutaneous or submucous tissue in and around the primary site of infection. From there it enters the bloodstream, in which, it is believed, the virus rapidly increases. The viraemia involves the bloodcirculatory system in the pathological process and inflammatory symptoms develop in the central nervous system.

Post mortem examination of the central nervous system reveals hyperaemia of the brain and meninges. In the medulla oblongata and in some spots in the pedunculi, there are, in addition to hyperaemia, transparent greyish-red foci.

The histopathological changes are: capillary and more extensive haemorrhages and extravasation of blood into the perivascular lymph sheaths of the veins. Besides these haemorrhages, which destroy the nervous tissue, vascular and perivascular cellular infiltrations are to be seen. Polymorphonuclear leucocytes do not appear. Most of the infiltrating cells resemble plasma cells. Cytoplasmic or intranuclear inclusion bodies are absent. No Negri-bodies are observed in the ganglion cells of the Ammon's horns.

Traub successfully grew the virus in tissue cultures from the testicular cells of rabbits and guinea pigs. He also cultivated it in chick embryos.

When brain, containing the virus, is examined by the electron microscope, it shows somewhat spherical particles with a diameter of between 90 and 100 millimicrons.

Monkeys are susceptible to intracerebral infection. When they were infected intradermally or rectally they showed slight nervous symptoms and some scratching, but rabbits inoculated with the brain tissue of these monkeys did not show any evidence of infection.

The susceptibility of man for the virus is very low. So far only 4 cases of human infection have been mentioned in literature. Von Rátz (1913) reported on 2 boys who had developed pruritus after wounding their hands during autopsies of animals infected with pseudorabies; but the evidence that these cases were real Aujeszky's disease was insufficient. In 1938 Tuncman (Istanbul) described 2 cases of human infection. The first case was that of a laboratory technician who cut a finger while manipulating the carcass of a rabbit which had died of pseudorabies. 2 to 3 hours later, he felt very severe pruritus in the wounded finger. Soon the arm and the body became affected by intense itching. After 6 hours, rapid recovery began. The second case was a female worker who soiled her hands with the organs of animals which had died of pseudorabies. 18 hours later she suffered from itching in the hand which spread to the arm, shoulder and back. When these symptoms were treated, the itching disappeared; however, she still complained of headache, weakness, an urticarial rash on the feet, an aphthous eruption on the gums and pain in the knees.

In neither of the above cases was blood serum taken for examination for the presence of neutralizing antibodies, nor was any demonstration of the causative agent attempted. Further, an incubation period as brief as those stated in these cases has not been observed either in natural or experimental infections of susceptible animals. For these reasons none of these cases can with certainty be considered to have been genuine cases of Aujeszky's disease in man.

References p. 350

REFERENCES

AKKERMANS, J. P. W. M., *Vet. doct. Thesis,* Utrecht, 1963, 128 pp.
AUJESZKY, A., *Zbl. Bakt. I. Abt. Orig.,* 32 (1902) 353.
BURGGRAAF, A. and L. F. D. E. LOURENS, *T. Diergeneesk.,* 59 (1932) 981.
FRENKEL, H. S., *T. Diergeneesk.,* 59 (1932) 1429.
GALLOWAY, I. A., *Vet. Record,* 50 (1938) 745.
HANSON, R. P., *J. Am. vet. med. Ass.,* 124 (1954) 259.
NIKOLITSCH, M., *Arch. Hyg. (Berl.),* 140 (1956) 241.
REAGAN, R. L., M. P. HARMON, W. DAY and A. L. BRUECKNER, *Amer. J. vet. Res.,* 13 (1952) 581.
REMLINGER, P. and J. BAILLY, *La maladie d'Aujeszky,* Paris, 1938.
SHAHAN, W, W. KNUDSON, W. SEIBOLD and W. DALE, *N. Amer. Vet.,* 28 (1947) 440.
TUNCMAN, Z. M., *Ann. Inst. Pasteur,* 60 (1938) 95.

3

Lymphocytic choriomeningitis

Lymphocytic choriomeningitis is a viral infection occurring in mice, guinea pigs, dogs and monkeys. Humans in contact with these animals may also become infected. The name is derived from the characteristic pathological finding of a lymphocytic infiltration of the chorioid plexus in the brain.

Armstrong and Lillie, in 1934, isolated the virus for the first time from the brain of a monkey which had been inoculated with human tissue. They recognised the presence of a hitherto unknown agent and described its properties and pathological effects. In 1935 Rivers and Scott recovered the same agent from the cerebrospinal fluid of several human cases of aseptic meningitis. Also in 1935, Traub reported the occurrence of the virus in white laboratory mice.

According to filtration experiments with collodion membranes, the virus has a diameter of 35 to 60 millimicrons. Seitz EK filters do not retain it. A smaller particle is also produced during the multiplication of the virus and this is identical with the "soluble" antigen used in the complement-fixation test. The virus can be preserved in 50% glycerin, by lyophilisation, or by freezing at $-70°$. White laboratory and wild grey mice, various species of rats, guinea pigs, dogs and monkeys are susceptible to experimental infection. The virus has been grown in embryonated hens' eggs and in tissue cultures.

Natural infection with the virus has been observed in various species of mice, guinea pigs, dogs and monkeys. In many instances the infection occurs asymptomatically or in the form of a short febrile episode. Virulent strains may cause severe and fatal disease. Latency, and the occurrence of carriers which retain the virus for extended periods, or even for life, are special characteristics of the infection.

References p. 355

Of great interest are the observations of Traub on the epidemiology of the infection in a colony of white mice. 50% of the mice were found infected, but symptoms of the disease, such as emaciation, somnolence or retarded growth, were present in only 20%. Mortality in the infected colony was 2 %. It was possible to isolate the virus from the spleen, liver and kidneys of the infected animals by inoculating organ suspensions intracerebrally into virus-free mice or guinea pigs. The virus could also be found in the blood, urine, semen and nasal secretion. In mice carrying the virus it was possible to activate the infection by intracerebral inoculation of sterile broth. In intracerebrally inoculated mice, after an incubation period of 3 to 13 days, a fatal meningo-encephalitis developed. Such animals sat in a huddled position and frequently developed chronic convulsions. They died in a typical posture with rigid extension of the hind legs.

The age at which animals came in contact with the virus had a decisive effect on the subsequent course of the infection. If mice were infected *in utero* or shortly after birth, the virus caused a mortality which, with virulent strains, reached 60%, but usually it was much less. In surviving animals the virus persisted throughout life, but caused no symptoms. In animals which were infected when they were several weeks old, the carrier state did not last so long.

Intracerebral inoculation was usually fatal, while peripheral inoculation produced no signs of disease and a solid immunity developed thereafter.

The virus has frequently been isolated from naturally infected *grey mice (Mus musculus);* these animals probably represent the most important reservoir for human infection.

In *guinea pigs* both natural and experimental infection can cause considerable mortality, which is preceded by diarrhoea, emaciation and extreme weakness. The virus is present in all the organs and in the blood, but it disappears after recovery of the animal.

In *dogs* asymptomatic infection seems to be the rule. An especially virulent strain, when it was inoculated into a young dog, caused fever, paresis and incoordination of the hind legs.

In *monkeys* natural infection is usually not accompanied by clinical signs, but there are some reports of monkeys which did exhibit symptoms. An outbreak in monkeys with severe involvement of the respiratory tract has been described. Intracerebral inoculation of monkeys results in a serious meningo-encephalitis with somnolence, tremor and paralysis. The mortality varies with the strains of virus employed. The cerebrospinal fluid contains up to 1,500 white cells, most of them lymphocytes. The virus was present in the blood and in all the organs.

In *man,* in addition to symptomless infection, three different types of the disease have been described. These are:

(1) An influenza-like syndrome, which is probably the most frequent result

of the infection. The symptoms are not specific and the aetiology can be revealed by laboratory examination only.

Characteristic is the case of a laboratory technician who was infected while working with the virus. He developed fever, which reached a maximum of 39.8° and lasted for 5 days. Prostration, anorexia and pains in his arms and back, especially severe in the lumbar region, were the main symptoms. Recovery was protracted, but complete. There was a marked leucopenia with 45% of neutrophils, 50% of lymphocytes and 5% of mononuclear cells. The virus was isolated from blood taken on the fifth day of the illness. Neutralizing antibodies were demonstrated several months later (Armstrong, 1941).

(2) A meningeal type of the disease has been observed by many investigators. In some cases it was the result of laboratory infections or it occurred in patients inoculated with the virus for therapeutic purposes (Lépine et al., 1937). In the experimental disease, fever first appeared after 36–48 hours, accompanied by symptoms resembling those of influenza. The temperature then went down and several days later meningeal signs, such as a stiff neck, headache and vomiting appeared. The disease frequently caused a marked loss of weight. Recovery, though it was always complete, took many weeks. The spinal fluid was clear, but contained up to 3,000 white cells, mainly lymphocytes. The virus was isolated from the blood and spinal fluid (Farmer and Janeway, 1942).

(3) A meningo-encephalitic syndrome represents the severest type of the disease. Somnolence, tremors and paralysis are present. Recovery is slow. Fatal cases in laboratory workers have been observed. The virus was isolated at autopsy from the central nervous system and the lungs.

In a few aetiologically proven human cases which came to autopsy, meningoplexal infiltration by lymphoid and small numbers of other cells with invasion of some cerebral vessel sheaths, occasional focal gliosis and cerebral oedema were the main findings. Frequently these changes were minimal. In addition to cerebral oedema, haemorrhages were found below the dura mater and in the lungs, kidneys and intestines. Much more characteristic are the findings in animals. Lymphocytic infiltration of the chorioid plexus, the pia mater and the vessels of the brain were regularly observed. The lungs showed congestion, oedema and a serous exudate. In mice and guinea pigs an enlarged spleen and severe degenerative changes in liver and kidneys have been noted (Lillie, 1950).

The virus can be isolated, by intracerebral inoculation into white mice or guinea pigs, from the cerebrospinal fluid, blood and internal organs. In view of Schwartzman's observation that the virus is firmly bound to the erythrocytes, whole blood rather than serum should be used for isolation attempts. Demonstration of a rise in the antibody titer is diagnostically significant. Neutralizing antibodies may not be present before 6–8 weeks after onset of the disease. They persist without a considerable drop in titer for many years. Complement-fixing antibodies appear earlier and show a more rapid decline.

It is difficult to assess the frequency of the infection in the human population. Only a few serologic surveys have been carried out. Without laboratory examination the diagnosis cannot be made.

Among 2,000 sera examined at random in the United States, 10% were found to possess neutralizing antibodies. In most of the reacting individuals no history of a nervous disease could be elicited. Their immune response may have been due to an aetiologically unrecognised influenza-like type of the disease, or to subclinical infection (Armstrong).

The presence of the virus has also been reported from various European countries and from Japan.

Person-to-person spread of the virus has never been recorded. Probably, all human infections are acquired by direct or indirect contact with infected animals, among which virus-carrying house-mice seem to be the most frequent source. Carriers have been trapped in 5 out of 6 houses in Washington D.C., where cases of lymphocytic choriomeningitis had occurred. Because mice excrete the virus in their urine and other secretions, gastrointestinal infection of man by contaminated food, and air-borne infection by dust in contaminated habitats, may occur. The virus may also enter through abrasions on the skin or through the conjunctiva. Laboratory infections of persons handling supposedly normal mice, dogs and monkeys have been reported. The possible presence of the virus in monkey tissues is of special importance when the latter are processed in vaccine production. Special investigations for detection of the virus have to be included in the safety controls of poliomyelitis vaccine.

Infected ticks carry the virus throughout their life cycles. Transmission to guinea pigs by infected nymphs of wood-ticks and by mosquitoes *(Aedes aegypti)* have been recorded. These observations suggest that man can probably be infected also by blood sucking arthropods (Shaughnessy and Milzer, 1939).

Preventive measures against the spread of lymphocytic choriomeningitis should pay attention chiefly to the eradication of mice and to making it impossible for them to infest human habitations. Laboratory personnel who handle monkeys, mice and dogs should use special care to protect themselves from infection.

No specific therapy for this disease is known. Spinal puncture often brings relief from the severe headache and from other symptoms due to increased spinal pressure.

REFERENCES

ARMSTRONG, C., *The Harvey Lectures*, 36 (1941) 5.
FARMER, TH. W. and C. A. JANEWAY, *Medicine (Baltimore)*, 21 (1942) 1.
LÉPINE, P., P. MOLLARET and B. KREIS, *C. R. Acad. Sci. (Paris)*, 204 (1937) 1846.
LILLIE, R. D., in: *The Pathogenesis and Pathology of Viral Diseases*, New York, 1950.
MAURER, F. D., *J. nat. Cancer Inst.*, 20 (1958) 867.
RIVERS, T. M. and T. F. M. SCOTT, *Science*, 81 (1935) 439.
VAN ROOYEN, C. E. and A. RHODES, *Virus Diseases of Man*, New York, 1948, 1051 pp.
SCHWARTZMAN, G. H., *J. Immunol.*, 48 (1944) 111.
SHAUGHNESSY, H. J. and A. MILZER, *Am. J. publ. Hlth*, 29 (1939) 1103.
TRAUB, E., *Science*, 81 (1935) 298.

B. *Arthropod-borne animal viral diseases*

1

Introduction

The viruses causing arthropod-borne animal diseases are characterized by their ability to multiply in arthropods and to infect a wide range of mammalian and avian hosts. The arthropod acts as a vector and becomes infected by ingesting vertebrate's blood in which the virus is circulating; thus, viraemia in the vertebrate is essential for the infection of the arthropod vector. Transmission of the infection to other vertebrates, including man, is by the bite of the infected arthropod. Infection of the arthropod vector may also occur by transovarian transmission as happens among the ticks which transmit viral diseases. Although these viruses are transmissible to man through arthropod vectors, transmission occurs from animal to man, rather than from man to man. In most instances, man plays no essential role in the biological cycle. Equines also are probably only accidental hosts for some of the viruses (western and eastern equine, and Japanese encephalitis). Birds, both domestic and wild, though they usually do not exhibit signs of disease, appear to be the essential link in the transmission of many of the viruses here considered.

The viruses included in this chapter are only a few of the viruses belonging to the arthropod-borne group which numbers at present more than 150 different and distinct types. They were chosen primarily on the basis of their clinical importance in man and in certain domestic animals.

The members of the group have a wide geographical distribution and have been reported from various parts of the world. Some are widespread in occurrence, others are confined to limited and recognized foci. The three *equine* types have thus far been established mainly from the western hemisphere. Two of these, the western and eastern equine encephalitides, occur in both northern and southern America; Venezuelan equine encephalitis is known only from South America. St. Louis encephalitis occurs principally in the U.S.A., Japanese encephalitis in the Far East, Murray Valley encephalitis in Australia and West Nile virus infection in the Middle East and Africa. More detailed information about the geographical distribution of the various viruses is given with the descriptions of the characteristics of the various types.

Some of the arthropod-borne viruses are closely related immunologically, while others show no cross-reactions. Immunological overlapping has been reported in the past among various members of the group and recently Casals and Brown (1954) have demonstrated the existence of distinct and sharply defined immunological groups. This was done by means of the haemagglutination (HA) and haemagglutination-inhibition (HI) reactions and the majority of the arthropod-borne animal viruses have been classified by these immunological tests into three major groups designated A, B and C. The classification here adopted of the various members of the arthropod-borne animal virus group is based on these methods. In addition to the HA reaction other immunological tests have been widely employed in the classification of these viruses, namely, the complement-fixation (CF) and neutralization (NT) tests. These serve at present mainly for the further subdivision of the main immunological groups. By means of CF and NT tests, members of groups A and B have been subdivided into subgroups, such as, for example, the St. Louis, Japanese and Murray Valley encephalitis, West Nile fever (SLE, JE, MVE, WNF) subgroup and the tick-borne subgroup; the latter, in addition to the fact that all the viruses in it are transmitted by ticks, is composed of antigenically closely related viruses. This immunological overlap has many important implications. First, it should be closely observed in the laboratory diagnosis of diseases caused by members of the group, both in typing of the isolates and in the antibody response. Secondly, it may be a determining factor in the geographical distribution of the various types. And finally, common antigens may be of use in the prophylactic immunization of man and domestic animals against the various diseases caused by these viruses.

All members of the group are neurotropic and will produce severe encephalitis in Swiss mice, particularly in newly-born ones, inoculated by the intracerebral route. The Venezuelan equine, Russian spring-summer and louping ill viruses are also virulent for the mouse by peripheral routes. The *equine* viruses are neurotropic in guinea pigs, rabbits, mice and hamsters, and will produce disease in numerous species of mammals when they are inoculated intracerebrally. They will cause infection in the embryonated hen's egg and several will kill the embryo in it.

All are small viruses, ranging in size from 15 to 45 millimicrons. They are unstable at room temperature and are best preserved in the frozen state at −70° or by lyophilization. Normal animal sera have a definite protective action against them. Most of them are easily inactivated by sodium desoxycholate, formaldehyde and ultraviolet light.

The clinical features of the diseases caused by these viruses may range from mild abortive infections to severe and fatal encephalitis. Subclinical infections are, with certain members of the group, also very common. Details of the diseases caused in humans and certain domestic animals are given with the descriptions of the other characteristics of the various members of the group. Diagnosis is made by isolation of the virus, chiefly from the CNS and, in some instances, from the blood, and by serological methods (HI, CF and NT).

The ecological and epidemiological aspects vary widely for the different members of the group and are discussed separately for each virus. The general epidemiological concept, which applies to the majority of these agents, but especially to the mosquito-borne virus diseases included in this chapter, is that infection is maintained in nature by a vertebrate–arthropod–vertebrate cycle. The infection in these vertebrate hosts is characterized by a viraemia without evident signs of the disease. The "spill-over" of these viruses into human and equine populations is probably incidental, but undoubtedly it presents an important public health and economic problem, particularly because the death rates associated with certain members of the group are high.

N. GOLDBLUM

Group A arthropod-borne viral diseases

a. Western equine encephalitis
(Synonyms: *Epizootic equine encephalomyelitis; WEE*).

Western equine encephalitis occurs in the western hemisphere and in nature affects primarily equines and man. Epizootics in horses and mules have been reported on numerous occasions in the U.S.A. during the last century. During the 1930's and 1940's, WEE has been a major veterinary problem in many western states in the U.S.A., causing thousands of deaths in equines. Severe cases of encephalitis as well as abortive and inapparent infections have also been reported in humans during epizootics and in interepizootic periods. Probably the most extensive human outbreak occurred in 1941 in the U.S.A. and Canada; it affected thousands of individuals and caused a large number of deaths. In addition to these countries, WEE has been reported from Argentina and other South American countries. In the U.S.A. the disease is at present confined to endemic foci in the western States along the Pacific Coast.

The causative agent of WEE was first isolated by Meyer, Haring and Howitt in 1930 from the central nervous system of horses. By studies on filtration through gradocol membranes, and by electron microscopy and ultracentrifugation, it was estimated that the size of the WEE virus is 25–40 millimicrons. It is unstable at room temperature and can be best preserved in the frozen state at $-70°$, or by lyophilization. The virus is readily inactivated by formaldehyde in the cold. It can be established by any route of inoculation in most of the common laboratory animals and it grows in embryonated hen's eggs.

The virus multiplies, causing cytopathic effects and forming plaques on chick embryo cell culture monolayers (Dulbecco, 1952).

WEE virus has a wide host range. In addition to its isolation from horses and mules, the virus has been recovered in nature from squirrels, deer, pigs and birds. Experimental infection has been induced in goats, calves, pigs and dogs. Mice, hamsters, rats, guinea pigs and rabbits are all highly susceptible to experimental infection by the intracerebral route; when mice are inoculated with mouse-adapted strains, they develop severe encephalitis and die within 2 days after inoculation with high virus concentrations.

Horses and *mules* are the domestic animals most frequently affected. Horses of all ages are susceptible, but in endemic areas young horses succumb most frequently to the disease. Older horses are frequently found to be immune, presumably as a result of previous abortive or subclinical infections. The incubation period of the disease in the horse varies from several days to 2 weeks. The onset of clinical symptoms is abrupt. There is usually an early stage of fever ("minor illness"), during which the virus multiplies in non-nervous tissue and may be recovered from the blood during a number of days. Following this phase, the horse becomes hypersensitive, and tremors, neck rigidity and spasms ensue. This stage is followed by encephalitis, progressive paralysis (Fig. 43) and death within 2–5 days. Death rates are about 27 %. The pathological features

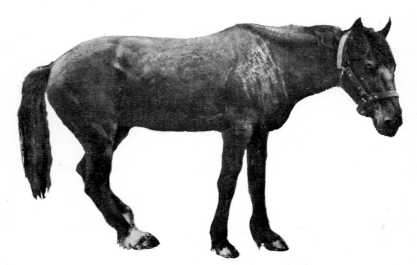

Fig. 43.   Arthropod borne virus encephalitis in a horse (paresis of hind legs).
(Photo: Dr. E. S. Tierkel, Atlanta, Ga.)

are characterized by lesions in many parts of the central nervous system. The meninges are oedematous and show mononuclear infiltration. There is nerve cell degeneration. Perivascular cuffing is frequent and there are characteristic and focal lesions in the brain and cord.

Meyer described the first human cases in 1938 and Howitt (1938) isolated the virus from the central nervous system of a man who died of the infection. The incubation period in man is about 1 week, but ranges from 4 to 21 days. The onset is sudden, with headache, chills, fever, nausea and vomiting. Pain and stiffness of the neck may occur. In many cases more pronounced neurological disturbances appear, such as insomnia, confusion, drowsiness, nystagmus, tremor and paralyses. Davis (1940) described cerebral atrophy, blindness, defects of speech and partial hemiplegia. The acute phase lasts on the average 1 week, recovery in most cases being complete. However, in some patients, and especially in infants, sequelae are left. The death rate is about 10%.

Mild human cases, which resemble non-paralytic poliomyelitis, have been reported. In addition, inapparent infections are frequently observed in certain areas.

Laboratory diagnosis is made by isolation of the virus, or by serological tests. Although WEE virus is present in the blood during the stage of viraemia, attempts to recover the virus from the blood have not, in most cases, been successful. The virus is most frequently recovered from the central nervous system in fatal cases. The best method to isolate the virus is by intracerebral inoculation of suspensions of tissue from the central nervous system into young or adult mice. The virus is harvested from the brains of mice dying of encephalitis and is identified by neutralization or complement-fixation tests. In equines and humans recovering from the disease, complement-fixing, neutralizing and haemagglutination-inhibiting antibodies appear within 7–10 days, and a rise in antibody titer may be demonstrated during convalescence.

WEE is most prevalent during the summer months (between May and September) and is predominantly a rural disease. It has rarely been reported from urban areas. It occurs most frequently in irrigated areas, such as the Yakima Valley in the State of Washington. There is strong evidence that the virus is transmitted to equines and man by the bites of mosquitoes. Although WEE virus has been isolated in nature from various species of culicine mosquitoes, *Culex tarsalis* is presumably the main vector in the western United States. Laboratory-bred mosquitoes of this species can be readily infected experimentally (Hammon and Reeves, 1947). *Culex tarsalis* feeds on mammals, as well as on birds, but shows a predilection for the latter. Experimental infection of birds by the bite of infected mosquitoes results in a viraemia with a high titer, which lasts for several days without obviously affecting the health of the birds. Although WEE virus has been isolated from bird-mites, their importance in the transmission cycle of the virus in nature is doubted. It is at present generally believed that the natural transmission of the virus is through a bird–mosquito cycle, although no definite species of bird can be specifically incriminated as its major host. Both equine and human infections are tangential or dead-end infections and probably play no role in the maintenance of the virus in nature.

WEE may be controlled either by directly attacking the mosquito vector or by active immunization of equines and man. The former is undoubtedly the method of choice, thanks to the recent development of residual insecticides. It has been used extensively in certain endemic areas of WEE (Reeves, 1951). However, owing to the complex problems of the vectors and their divergent bionomics, the use of insecticides has not always been very successful.

Excellent results have been obtained in the prevention of the disease in equines by using the formalized chick embryo vaccine developed by Beard *et al.* in 1938. In horses, this vaccine, administered intradermally in 2 doses of 1 ml at weekly intervals or in 10 ml doses given subcutaneously produces immunity for about 1 year. It has been widely used since its introduction and seems to have caused a marked reduction in the incidence of the disease. Active immunization of humans has not been practised on a large scale; it has been rather limited, and has been especially given to occupationally exposed groups, such as laboratory workers engaged in the production of vaccine or research on the virus.

There is no specific treatment for the disease in either equines or man. Good medical care is of great importance.

b. Eastern equine encephalitis
(Synonyms: *Epizootic equine encephalitis; EEE*).

Eastern equine encephalitis occurs in the western hemisphere and causes disease in equines, birds and man. It is enzootic on the eastern seaboard of the U.S.A. and extends from New England in the north down to Mexico. Outside the U.S.A., EEE infection has been reported from Canada,

Panama, Mexico, Cuba, Brazil and the Dominican Republic. Epizootics in equines have often been accompanied by outbreaks of encephalitis in man. Thus, during an epizootic that occurred in southern Louisiana in the summer of 1947, more than 14,000 horses and 15 people were affected at the same time. Similarly, during an outbreak that occurred in the Dominican Republic in 1948–1949, the incidence in humans coincided with that in horses, mules and donkeys (Eklund, 1951).

EEE was first recognized as an aetiological entity in 1933 by Ten Broeck and Merril and by Giltner and Shahan, who succeeded in isolating a virus from the brains of horses which had died of encephalitis. The virus was first recovered from the central nervous system of fatal human cases by Fothergill *et al.,* and by Feemster in 1938. It was also isolated from naturally infected pheasants (Tyzzer *et al.,* 1938) and pigeons (Fothergill and Dingle, 1938). EEE virus is probably spherical and measures 40–47 millimicrons. Its physicochemical properties are in general similar to those of WEE virus.

The host range of EEE virus is similar to that of WEE virus, but the eastern virus seems to have a greater power of invasiveness than the western virus has. Horses, goats, calves, pigs, dogs and sheep are all susceptible to experimental infection. Horses may be infected intracerebrally and intradermally (Meyer, 1933). Quantitative studies on the experimental infection of horses indicate that inapparent infections may be produced with low doses of EEE virus and lethal infections with high doses (Kissling *et al.,* 1954). The host range in laboratory animals includes mice, hamsters, guinea pigs and rabbits. The results of peripheral infection in mice depend, as Sabin and Olitsky (1938) showed, on the age of the mice. These workers noted that, as the age of the mice increased, there was a gradual decrease in susceptibility to infection by the intraperitoneal route. Thus, 15-day old mice were found to be highly susceptible to intraperitoneal infection, while at 3 months of age none of the infected mice died.

In addition to mammals, various species of *birds* were found to be susceptible to experimental infection; certain species succumb to a fulminating disease, while others develop no signs of infection, but show viraemia with low or high titers (Schaeffer and Arnold, 1954). EEE has been found in nature in pigeons and phaesants. Fothergill and Dingle (1938) isolated EEE virus from a pigeon which died during an outbreak in Massachusetts in 1938. Tyzzer *et al.* (1938) isolated EEE virus from 4 sick phaesants in Connecticut. Beaudette and Black (1948) have reported 13 outbreaks among pheasants raised in New Jersey during the period 1938–1946.

The disease in *equines* has been most thoroughly studied in horses. Ten

Broeck *et al.* (1935) were able to demonstrate the presence of EEE virus in the blood of naturally infected horses before the onset of clinical signs. The incubation period is short, ranging from 36 hours to 4 days. Two major clinical patterns are recognized. One is characterized by the appearance of fever, often bi-phasic, and symptoms of involvement of the central nervous system, such as depression, progressive incoordination, rocking motions, convulsions and prostration, which may terminate fatally or lead to recovery with or without sequelae. The other is a short-term fever, usually with a single rise in temperature without noticeable involvement of the central nervous system. In addition, subclinical infections, accompanied by a low titer viraemia, have been noted. Death rates during the various epizootics (Massachusetts, 1938; Louisiana, 1947 and the Dominican Republic, 1948–1949) have been very high, approaching 90%. The pathological findings in horses are in general similar to those found in WEE infections and are characterized by a primary nerve cell degeneration and infiltration; however, lesions of the central nervous system are more intense and extensive, showing focal and diffuse gliosis, perivascular round-cell infiltration, oedema, chromatolysis of neurons, and cytolysis and phagocytosis of glial cells.

The clinical features of the disease in *man* were first described from the outbreak in Massachusetts (1938). The incidence of the disease in children is high and very frequently runs a severe and fatal course. During the outbreaks in Massachusetts and Louisiana, 70% of the cases were in children under 10 years of age and the death rate was 65–70%. The onset is sudden with fever, restlessness, drowsiness, vomiting and malaise; stiffness of the neck and back, and convulsions occur. Death ensues in 3–8 days after the onset. In some cases which recover, spastic paralyses remain as sequelae. The pathological changes were described by Wesselhoeft *et al.* (1938) as consisting mainly of lesions of an acute disseminated encephalomyelitis in the basal ganglia, pons and medulla; congestion of meningeal vessels is frequent. Infiltration of the subarachnoid space and perivascular cuffing are a prominent feature. Nerve cell degeneration and a slight neuronophagia are also characteristic.

Diagnosis of the infection can be made only by laboratory methods. The virus may be isolated from the brains of fatal human, equine or avian cases. Neutralizing and complement-fixing antibodies appear during convalescence, and a distinct rise in antibody titer is evident about 10 to 14 days after the onset. It has been found that complement-fixing antibodies persist for up to 2 years after the illness. Sera collected after the outbreak of EEE in the Dominican Republic showed a high incidence of antibodies in both human (up to 17.3%) and equine (over 50%) sera.

Outbreaks of EEE occur mainly in the late summer months in rural areas and small towns. Our knowledge of the natural history of EEE is still incomplete. It is generally believed at present that the virus is maintained in nature by means of a bird–mosquito–bird cycle and that its transmission to equines and man is only occasional and incidental. However, there are certain gaps in our understanding of the exact cycle. The virus has been isolated on a number of occasions from wild birds (Kissling *et al.*, 1954). The same authors have also found that birds may be infected experimentally and may develop a subclinical viraemia. EEE virus has also been isolated from several species of naturally infected mosquitoes and quite frequently from *Culiseta melanura*. It is possible that the latter mosquito is responsible for the bird-to-bird cycle, but, because this mosquito is strictly zoophilic, it will not transmit the infection to man. It is highly probable that the species of mosquito which transmits the virus to man is different from that which maintains the virus in the bird-to-bird cycle in nature. Species of *Aedes* were strongly incriminated in the outbreak which occurred in the Dominican Republic (Eklund *et al.*, 1951). EEE virus has been isolated from bird mites (Chamberlain and Sikes, 1955), but their role in the cycle in nature is considered to be of minor importance.

The bird most commonly infected in the eastern United States, is the ring-necked pheasant and large epizootics among *pheasants* have occurred on numerous game farms in New Jersey and Connecticut. It appears that transmission of the virus from pheasants may be direct, without the intervention of an arthropod vector (Jungherr *et al.*, 1958).

Control measures are similar to those used for WEE. A formalinized vaccine prepared by Beard *et al.* (1940 has been successfully used for the prevention of the disease in equines. This vaccine has also been used for the immunization of human subjects who are occupationally exposed to infection.

No specific treatment has shown to be of any value, but good medical care is of great importance. Death rates depend to a large degree on adequate medical and nursing care.

c. *Venezuelan equine encephalitis*
(Synonyms: *Peste loca; VEE*).

Venezuelan equine encephalitis is caused by a virus which is similar in its properties to WEE and EEE viruses. It is primarily a disease of equines, but has been reported from man, in whom it causes a relatively mild, non-fatal illness. VEE infection is limited to South and Central America (Venezuela, Colombia, Trinidad, Ecuador, Panama and Brazil). The virus was recovered from the brains of horses which died of encephalitis and Beck and Wyckoff and Kubes and Rios (1938) found that it is an anti-genically distinct entity.

The virus has a wide host range, being highly pathogenic to horses, sheep, goats, rabbits, guinea pigs and mice. Mice of all ages are highly susceptible by extraneuronal routes of infection and not less so by intra-cerebral inoculation. Neutralization tests can be carried out in adult mice by the peritoneal route.

The virus multiplies well in the embryonated hen's egg and can be recovered from the yolk sac, chorioallantoic membrane and the embryo. It has been grown in certain cell cultures, on which it has a cytopathogenic effect.

Although epizootics have been observed and recorded (Venezuela, 1938; Trinidad, 1943), the information available about the clinical picture of the natural disease in *horses* is inadequate. The disease in experimentally infected horses is characterized by fever, weakness, progressive depression, diarrhoea and often death. Typical signs of involvement of the central nervous system are: continuous chewing motions, circling, pressing of the head against the wall, restlessness and muscle spasms. However, the disease in horses is not consistently an encephalitis. Some horses develop a febrile illness from which recovery is complete, others an inapparent infection with high virus titers in the blood.

The pathological findings in horses are principally vascular. No special gross lesions are seen, the liver is pale and the mucous membranes are congested. Microscopic lesions show mainly changes in the bone marrow, haemorrhages in the spleen and lymph nodes, necrotic foci and inflammation in the pancreas, and degeneration of the liver. In the brains of horses which die of encephalitis only minimal changes are observed; neuron damage is slight, but marked vascular lesions occur, such as: haemorrhages with leucocytic infiltrations, swollen endothelial cells, perivascular oedema and congestion of the meninges.

The course of the disease in *man* has been mainly studied in numerous cases of accidental laboratory infections. Casals *et al.* (1943) recovered the virus from the blood and upper respiratory tract of a laboratory worker suffering from a mild febrile illness. Lennette and Koprowski

(1943) described a number of laboratory infections. Persons infected during laboratory investigations usually exhibit signs and symptoms of a mild disease with fever, headaches and gastrointestinal disturbances; symptoms of involvement of the central nervous system are rare. The duration of the disease is short – a few days to 1 week – and recovery is complete. Two human cases of naturally acquired acute and fatal encephalitis have been described from the outbreak in Trinidad (Randall and Mills, 1944).

Laboratory diagnosis is made by isolation of the virus and by serological tests. In VEE infection in man, the virus may be frequently isolated from the blood and nasopharyngeal washings. In fatal equine cases the virus can be recovered from the brain by mouse inoculation. During convalescence, neutralizing, complement-fixing and haemagglutination-inhibiting antibodies develop and can be measured quantitatively.

The ecology and epidemiology of VEE is not well known. The mosquito *Mansonia tillitans* seems to have been the most important vector in the outbreak in Trinidad. It has also been shown that this mosquito can transmit the virus in the laboratory. Chamberlain *et al.* (1956) were able to infect birds by subcutaneous inoculation and to transmit the virus from bird to bird by the bite of experimentally infected mosquitoes. Infection of this kind is characterized by viraemia of low titer and the absence of symptoms. Experimental infection of horses results in viraemia of high virus titer which may be adequate to infect mosquitoes, a fact which makes mosquito transmission from horse to horse possible. This might suggest an epizootiology of VEE different from that of the two North American equine encephalitides. Other outstanding observations are that horses are highly susceptible to experimental intranasal infection, that they shed virus from the nose, mouth, eyes, urine and milk, and that they can infect by contact (Kissling *et al.* 1956). These findings suggest that mammals may be important in the epidemiology of VEE and that transmission may occur without the aid of an insect vector.

A formalin-inactivated vaccine prepared in chick embryos has been used in Venezuela for the immunization of horses (Kubes and Rios, 1938). In 1947, Randall *et al.* prepared a partially purified and effective vaccine for prophylactic use in man. Although it was shown by sensitive animal tests that the vaccine is safe, a number of individuals who received the vaccine developed infections and VEE virus was isolated from the blood and throat washings of several of them. It seems, therefore, that man is more susceptible to the virus than laboratory animals are.

3

N. GOLDBLUM

Group B arthropod-borne viral diseases

Mosquito-borne viral diseases

First subgroup: *SLE, JBE, MVE–WNF complex.*

The inclusion of these diseases in a single subgroup of group B arthropod-borne viral diseases is based chiefly on the close antigenic relationship between the viruses which cause them. These viruses also share a number of other properties and, with certain minor exceptions, closely resemble each other in their host range and pathogenesis in experimental infection. Otherwise, they differ widely in their geographical distribution, clinical manifestations and their ecology and epidemiology. St. Louis encephalitis (SLE) has not been known to occur outside the western hemisphere; Japanese B encephalitis (JE) has been widely distributed in the Far East; Murray Valley encephalitis (MVE) has been almost invariably restricted to Australia and New Guinea, and West Nile fever (WNF) has been found to occur mainly in Africa and the Middle East. Thus, excepting India, where both JE and WNF have been shown to coëxist, our knowledge of the world distribution of these four viruses indicates that infections by each of them occur in widely, but strictly limited, areas of the world.

Although it has been shown that all four members of the subgroup cause encephalitis in man, their degree of neurotropism is variable and their clinical spectra are extremely wide. It is highly probable that these viruses stem from a common "ancestor" and that local ecological conditions have resulted in the differences nowadays known in the pathological pictures they produce and their epidemiology.

All four viruses resemble each other closely in their properties. They are small viruses, which range in diameter from 15–50 millimicrons. They are labile at room temperature and are best preserved in the frozen state at $-70°$ or by lyophilization. Animal sera have a distinctly protective effect on the virus titer. All are inactivated by heating to 56° for 30 minutes, and by 0.1 to 0.2 % formaldehyde. Like other arthropod-borne viruses, they are highly susceptible to the action of sodium desoxycholate and to ether. They all possess a haemagglutinin which is stable at pH 9.0, the activity of which can best be demonstrated by the use of the erythrocytes of the 1-day old chick (Chanock and Sabin, 1953; Casals and Brown, 1954).

The experimental animal of choice is the white mouse. Infant mice are more susceptible than adult mice. The most sensitive route of inoculation is the intracerebral one. After 3–4 days of incubation, mice inoculated with a high virus concentration develop tremors, convulsion, ataxia and paralysis and die within 1–3 days. The virus multiplies rapidly in the brain and reaches concentrations of 10^8 to 10^9 mouse LD50. Hamsters are highly susceptible to MVE and WN viruses by the intracerebral and peripheral routes of infection, less so to SLE and JE (Hammon and Sather, 1956). All four agents multiply in the developing chick embryo after inoculation by various routes.

Various domestic and wild birds, when they are inoculated by peripheral routes, develop inapparent infections which are frequently associated with viraemia and antibody response.

Because diagnosis on clinical grounds only is not reliable, it has been necessary to supplement it with laboratory tests. In SLE, JE and MVE, virus isolations have been made mainly from the tissues of the central nervous system in fatal cases. In WNF, virus has been isolated from the blood in a great number of cases (Marberg et al., 1956; Goldblum et al., 1957). Laboratory diagnosis rests essentially on the demonstration of a rise in the titer of the specific antibodies. In the majority of infections, complement-fixing (CF) and neutralizing (NT) antibodies develop during convalescence. It has been shown that the CF antibody titers disappear after varying periods of time, while NT antibodies persist for long periods, presumably for life.

a. St. Louis encephalitis (Synonym: SLE)

The first recorded outbreaks of St. Louis encephalitis in the U.S.A. occurred during the summers of 1932 and 1933, and were fully documented in a U.S. Public Health Service Report (1935). A recurrence of the disease followed in 1937 and the disease thereafter spread in the central and western U.S.A. Muckenfuss et al, and later Webster and Fite (1933) succeeded in isolating the virus which causes the disease. At present, SLE virus is widely disseminated throughout vast areas of the U.S.A. and has a predominantly rural distribution in the western U.S.A., while it is mainly urban in the mid-western States. Epidemics have occurred during the summer months almost every year in the Yakima Valley, Washington.

The clinical picture of the disease varied in the different outbreaks. The incubation period ranges from 4–21 days. The onset is usually sudden, with severe headache and fever. In many cases the course of the illness is relatively benign. In others it is characterized by symptoms of varying intensity, involving the central nervous system, such as: nuchal rigidity, nausea, vomiting, restlessness, irritability, tremors and mental confusion. Convulsions often occur and are more common in children than in adults. The death rate has been approximately 20%. Inapparent infections, followed by the development of immunity, have been very common. WEE and non-paralytic poliomyelitis must be considered in the differential diagnosis of SLE. Infections due to SLE and WEE have occurred simultaneously in the same localities.

The pathological changes are almost entirely restricted to the central nervous system. There is acute inflammation and congestion of the meningeal and cerebral blood vessels and perivascular haemorrhages occur. Perivascular cuffing is regularly found. Cellular infiltration, necrosis of neurons and neuronophagia are prominent features.

The principal vector in the western U.S.A. is the mosquito *Culex tarsalis,* which frequently feeds on avian species and on man (Hammon *et al.,* 1951). Other mosquito species have also been incriminated as vectors in different outbreaks, chiefly *Culex pipiens* and *Culex quinquefasciatus.* Virus was isolated from mosquitoes of the two latter species during the 1954 Texas epidemic (Beadle *et al.,* 1957). The role of mites in the natural cycle is still problematical. Evidence has been brought forward that both domestic fowls and wild birds are important sources of the virus in nature. SLE virus has been isolated from several species of naturally infected wild birds. Chamberlain *et al.* (1957) and Kissling (1958) were able to infect experimentally several species of birds in which viraemia and inapparent infections were produced.

No specific treatment is as yet available. Prophylactic immunization by means of vaccines has been tried, but is impracticable for general use. The best prevention is through vector control.

b. Japanese encephalitis (Synonyms: Japanese B encephalitis; JE; JBE)

JE has been found to occur in widely dispersed areas in the Far East and in the Pacific. Infection has been recognized in Japan, Korea, Okinawa, the Philippines, China and far eastern USSR. Recently, Work and Shah (1956) have shown that JE also occurs in the south of India. Serious outbreaks of encephalitis caused by JE virus occurred in many areas of the Far East, both among indigenous inhabitants and among U.S. soldiers during World War II. The outbreaks of JE have been particularly confined to the summer months, August and September. In tropical areas, however, the disease is prevalent throughout the year.

The clinical picture and pathology resemble in many ways SLE. However, JE runs in general a more severe course, is characterized by slower convalescence and a higher incidence of sequelae and a higher death rate. The most common sequelae have been mental impairment and paralyses. Death rates have varied in the different outbreaks and in various agegroups, and have been estimated to range between 20 and 80%. Antibody studies have indicated the existence of a large number of inapparent infections as compared with overt disease. Approximately 1000 subclinical infections occur for each case of clinically recognized illness.

A wide variety of domestic animals, domestic fowls and wild birds develop inapparent infections which are frequently associated with viraemia. A high incidence of antibody was found in the blood of *horses, pigs* and *cattle*. Naturally infected horses may develop encephalitis and epizootics occur among them. In Japan, a high incidence of stillbirths in *swine* has been associated with outbreaks of JE in *man* and in horses, and virus has been isolated from piglets during such an outbreak (Burns, 1950). 94% of young pigs near Tokyo developed antibody to JE during the summer (Scherer *et al.,* 1959).

JE infection is mosquito-borne. JE virus has been recovered from several culicine mosquitoes, chiefly from *Culex tritaeniorhynchus,* which is probably the only vector in Japan (Buscher *et al.,* 1959). It has, however, been found that the vectors vary in different areas in the Far East. The important role of *wild birds* as the reservoirs of the infection in nature has been demonstrated in Japan by Buscher (1956). Although it is, like the North American equine encephalitides and SLE, believed that JE is naturally transmitted through a wild bird–mosquito cycle, the role of mammals and especially pigs in the natural cycle may be of greater importance than is suspected at present.

No specific treatment is known. Formalin-inactivated mouse-brain and chick embryo vaccines have been developed and used for the prevention of the disease (Sabin *et al.*, 1943; Smadel *et al.*, 1947), but it has been difficult to assess their efficacy. Hammon (1961) has recently reported the development of an attenuated vaccine.

c. Murray Valley encephalitis
(Synonyms: Australian "X" disease; MVE)

It is at present generally believed that Murray Valley encephalitis and Australian "X" disease are designations of the same disease. Australian "X" disease was first reported from an outbreak of encephalitis in Australia during the summer of 1917 and 1918 (Cleland and Bradley, 1917). It reappeared in epidemic form in 1922 and 1925. Unfortunately, the strains of the virus which had been isolated from fatal cases during these outbreaks were lost and could not be compared with the isolates of Murray Valley encephalitis virus recovered from a later outbreak in 1951. No further outbreaks have been reported since 1951. Evidence for the occurrence of infection with MVE virus has been obtained only from Australia and New Guinea. The virus has been recovered from the brains of fatal cases by French (1952) and by Miles *et al.*, (1951).

The clinical picture and pathology of MVE resemble closely those of JE. A large percentage of the cases during the 1951 outbreak occurred in children below the age of ten and the death rate was high. Antibody studies indicate that, as in JE, a high proportion of inapparent infections occur for each case of overt illness. Neutralizing antibodies have been found in wild and domestic birds and in various mammals (Anderson *et al.*, 1952; Miles and Howes, 1953). However, MVE virus has not yet been isolated in nature from any vertebrate except man. Nor has MVE virus been isolated from any naturally infected mosquitos, although it has been shown that various mosquito species can transmit the virus in the laboratory (McLean, 1953 and 1957). *Culex annulirostris* is incriminated on epidemiological grounds as the main vector and it is believed that the cycle in nature is a wild bird–mosquito cycle similar to that of SLE and JE.

d. West Nile fever (Synonym: WNF)

Following the initial isolation of West Nile virus (WNV) in 1937 by Smithburn *et al.* from the blood of a native woman in Uganda, this virus was again isolated by Melnick, Paul *et al.,* (1951) from the blood of 3 children living near Cairo, Egypt. In 1951 and 1952, it was shown that overt infection of West Nile aetiology occurred in Israel (Bernkopf *et al.,* 1953) and extensive investigations have been carried out in Egypt and Israel in order to elucidate the pathogenicity, the immunology and the epidemiology of West Nile virus infection.

The experience gained from the investigations of the pathological importance of WNV suggests a wide clinical spectrum of infection, ranging from a mild abortive illness to severe encephalitis. The incubation period is 3 to 6 days. The onset of the disease is sudden and the "typical" cases are characterized by fever, generalized lymphadenopathy and a rash. Additional common findings are severe headache, general malaise, ocular pains, a flushed face and gastrointestinal disturbances (Marberg *et al.,* 1956). In a small percentage of cases, meningeal involvement occurs and recently it was shown that WNV is the cause of severe encephalitis in aged persons. There are usually no sequelae and no fatalities.

WN virus has been isolated from about 20 % of the blood of febrile children and from patients suffering from WN fever during the acute phase on the first to the fourth days after the onset (Goldblum *et al.,* 1954, 1957). The duration of the viraemia is approximately 6 days.

Complement-fixing (CF) and neutralizing (NT) antibodies develop during convalescence from WN fever. CF antibodies appear shortly after the onset of the disease, rise to maximal levels in 2–3 weeks, remain at a high level for several months and then fall slowly to a very low titer by the end of 30 months. Homologous neutralizing antibodies develop somewhat later, reach maximum levels in 2–3 months and persist at the same level for 2–2.5 years, and probably for life. During convalescence heterologous antibodies to Japanese encephalitis and St. Louis encephalitis are found, but these do not persist for long periods of time and by the end of 2.5 years they have disappeared.

It was found that the seasonal incidence of infection is confined to the summer months – May through October – with a peak in July and August. Proof of this seasonal incidence was based on frequent virus isolations from human blood during these months, on the occurrence of outbreaks of the disease in the summer, and on the high conversion rates from CF negative to positive during the summer season.

The epidemiology of WN infection has been studied mainly in Egypt and almost all the data available on the natural transmission of the infection and on the source of virus in nature stem from these studies (Work *et al.*, 1953 and 1955; Taylor *et al.*, 1956). WN virus has been isolated twice from pigeons and once from a crow; one of the pigeons was ill and virus was isolated from its brain, spleen and blood. A survey of neutralizing antibodies of the common mammalian and avian species in the WN endemic areas showed a high percentage of positive results among the domestic quadrupeds and among most of the avian species, especially the hooded crow and the house sparrow. The potential importance of birds was further demonstrated by their great susceptibility to experimental infection with WN virus. High titers of virus, ranging between 3.5 to 8 logs, were found in the blood of the hooded crow and the house sparrow. The duration of the viraemia in these two species was shown to be as long as 6 days. Although the death rate is high among experimentally infected crows, a large number of immune crows were found among specimens collected in the late summer and winter, a fact which shows that many of them survive infection. Isolation of WN virus from the blood of a hooded crow in the field, the high incidence of immunity found in crows caught in endemic WN areas, and the susceptibility of this species to experimental infection all suggest that the hooded crow is the most probable reservoir of infection in nature.

The link between human and avian infection was sought in blood sucking arthropods. During a 3-year period of study, 1952 to 1954, Taylor *et al.*, (1956) examined more than 78,000 specimens, grouped in 1953 pools, for the presence of virus. Mosquitoes made up about two-thirds of the specimens and pools. WN virus was isolated in 17 instances and only from mosquitoes. Although sometimes mixed pools were used, it was calculated that 12 of the isolations were made from *Culex univittatus* and 5 from *Culex antennatus;* relatively to the number of specimens, WN virus was recovered 5 to 10 times more frequently from *C. univittatus* than from *C. antennatus*. Isolations of WN virus from mosquitoes were made during the summer months, July to September.

All these findings and additional observations on the bionomics of mosquitoes, and on the incidence of immunity to WN virus among crows in areas with varying WN endemicity, constitute strong evidence that mosquitoes are the principal, if not the only vectors, and that *birds* are the main reservoirs of this virus in nature (Taylor *et al.*, 1956). *Man,* in turn, becomes infected by the bites of mosquitoes which have fed on infected birds. Infections of domestic *quadrupeds* are probably tangential or dead-end infections. The problem of the overwintering of the virus remains unsolved, although circumstantial evidence points to a process of retarded transmission by mosquitoes that remain active during the winter months. The possibility cannot be excluded that the virus is transported over long distances by migratory birds.

e. *Yellow fever*

Yellow fever has been known to occur in two main epidemiological forms. The first is the classic or urban yellow fever which is transmitted by *Aëdes aegypti,* its cycle in nature being man–mosquito–man. The second is jungle or sylvan yellow fever, with a cycle involving wild animals and mosquitoes, human infections being incidental only. This chapter will deal with the latter form of yellow fever; it was recognized some three decades ago, and occurs in endemic and epidemic form.

Since Reed and his coworkers (1900) found that urban yellow fever is mosquito-borne, wide antimosquito campaigns in South America and the United States have resulted in the almost complete disappearance of this type of the disease. The reappearance of yellow fever in the late twenties and early thirties in widely scattered areas of South America indicated that infection transmitted by *Aëdes aegypti* is not the only epidemiological form. Definite proof of this assumption was obtained during a rural outbreak of yellow fever which occurred in Vale do Canaan, Brazil, in 1932. No *Aëdes aegypti* was found during this epidemic. The outbreak was followed by others in various South American countries from which *Aëdes aegypti* was absent. Thus, a second epidemiological entity was recognized, which is now known as sylvan or jungle yellow fever. It has been shown that it is almost entirely limited to persons who have close contacts with the jungle and live in close proximity to forests or are engaged in woodcutting or the clearing of trees. Incidental human cases have been found during epizootics among jungle animals, and neutralization tests have proved that wild monkeys frequently possess antibodies to yellow fever virus. At present there is a consensus of opinion that jungle yellow fever is basically a disease of forest-dwelling primates and there is circumstantial evidence which implicates marsupials as reservoirs in certain areas. Among blood sucking arthropods, evidence for the transmission of jungle yellow fever has been found only in certain species of mosquitoes. In vertebrates the infection is never chronic, nor is a carrier state known to occur among them. Transmission and the persistence of the infection in nature depends on an unbroken chain of self limited infections, which are partly lethal, in vertebrates which infect successive generations of mosquitoes.

At present jungle yellow fever is recognized in numerous countries of South America and Africa. Recently, extensive outbreaks have also been recorded from various countries in Central America. According to Soper (1943) jungle yellow fever is probably the original epidemiological type, while the variety transmitted by *Aëdes aegypti* is a development of "recent" times.

The viral aetiology of yellow fever was definitely proved by Reed and Carrol in 1902. However, it was not until the late twenties, when yellow fever virus was transmitted to laboratory animals, that extensive studies of the characteristics of the virus could be undertaken.

Yellow fever virus is one of the small viruses, ranging in diameter from 17 to 25 millimicrons. It is extremely labile and is readily inactivated by heat and antiseptics. Normal animal sera have a definite protective effect on the virus titer. The virus can best be preserved in the frozen state at $-70°$ C, or by desiccation.

Strains of yellow fever virus isolated from nature show both viscerotropic and neurotropic properties and differ widely in their pathogenicity to animals. Some are highly pathogenic to *Rhesus* monkeys, causing a fatal infection due to acute necrosis of the liver; other strains cause subclinical infections, the only manifestation being viraemia. All strains of yellow fever virus produce encephalitis, which can be best demonstrated by the use of the white mouse.

All species of monkeys so far tested were found susceptible to experimental infection with yellow fever virus. Guinea pigs are susceptible to intracerebral inoculation; rats and rabbits are refractory to experimental infection. Intracerebral passage of a strain of yellow fever virus in mice results in loss of the viscerotropic properties of the virus and an increase in its neurotropism. Such strains no longer cause visceral disease in monkeys, but will produce encephalitis. This method has been widely used to modify the virulence of yellow fever virus (Theiler, 1930). Such a strain, known as the French neurotropic strain, is used at present for the immunization of man against yellow fever. More profound attenuation of yellow fever virus was achieved by prolonged cultivation of it in tissue culture. Lloyd *et al.* (1936) succeeded in growing yellow fever virus in mouse embryonic cell cultures and later in minced chick embryo cells. A marked loss of virulence was thus obtained and this strain, known as 17D, grown in the developing chick embryo, is at present used extensively for human vaccination.

Infection with yellow fever virus is followed by the development of complement-fixing, neutralizing and haemagglutination-inhibiting antibodies. These antibodies can be measured quantitatively. The neutralization test in mice has been widely used for the determination of immunity to yellow fever throughout the world (Sawyer and Lloyd, 1931).

The incubation period of yellow fever in *man* ranges from 3–6 days. The severity of the disease may vary from a mild to a severe, fulminating infection. Inapparent infections accompanied by development of immunity are probably also common, as is shown by the frequent occurrence of antibody in certain areas of South America and Africa. The onset of the disease is usually sudden, with a continuous high temperature. Severe cases of yellow fever are usually characterized by two stages: a stage of congestion and one of stasis. During the first stage, nausea, vomiting, constipation, aches, and pain in the epigastrium and limbs are common features. The face is flushed, the eyes injected and haemorrhages may occur. The two stages of the disease are often interrupted by a fall of temperature. In the second phase there is a marked tendency to haemorrhage; jaundice may commence and vomiting of black coloured blood and suppression of urine are common. Prostration, anuria, jaundice and epigastric pains may increase in severity and death may follow. Most deaths from yellow fever occur during the fourth to tenth day of illness. Mortality may range from 5–40 %. The outstanding pathological findings are degeneration of the liver, the kidney and the heart. Multiple haemorrhages in various organs, and especially in the mucosa of the stomach and intestines, are commonly found. Necrosis, fatty degeneration of the liver and congestion and degeneration of kidney tissue are characteristic findings.

The most prominent and diagnostically valuable microscopic lesions are in the liver. These are characterized by extensive necrosis, fatty degenerative changes and minute haemorrhages throughout the liver parenchyma. There is no evidence of inflammatory reactions, either in the liver, or in the kidneys.

Laboratory diagnosis of yellow fever is made by isolation of the virus or/and by serologic tests. Virus can be isolated in the acute phase from the blood during the first 4 days of illness. The easiest and most promising method for isolation of the virus is by intracerebral inoculation of serum into mice, which develop typical signs of encephalitis. Identification of such an isolate as yellow fever virus is made by the neutralization test in mice, using yellow fever-immune animal serum. If virus isolation fails, diagnosis is based on the demonstration of a rise in specific antibody concentration during convalescence. The complement-fixation or mouse neutralization tests are both adequate for this purpose. However, in the interpretation of the results of serologic tests one should bear in mind the existence of cross reactions with other group-B arthropod-borne viruses. Post-mortem diagnosis is made by the examination of sections of the liver and is based on the presence of typical microscopic lesions.

Jungle yellow fever is endemic and "migrating" epidemic in wide areas of the interior mainlands of South America and of Africa. In its endemic form, cases are mainly confined to adult males who enter the forest or are engaged in clearing the jungle. They are infected by the bites of mosquitoes carrying yellow fever virus. In South America, various species of the genus *Haemagogus,* and especially *Haemagogus spegazzini* and its varieties, are incriminated as vectors. The infection in the jungle is maintained by a monkey – mosquito – monkey cycle and man is accidentally infected by the bite of a mosquito. Yellow fever neutralizing antibodies were found in a considerable proportion of monkeys in the jungle. In addition to monkeys, various species of marsupials were also found to have neutralizing antibodies against yellow fever virus, and it is suspected that they may serve as reservoirs of the virus, especially in regions where monkeys are rare or absent (Bugher *et al.,* 1944). The epidemic type of jungle yellow fever spreads through the South American continent, causing outbreaks of varying severity. One such prolonged epidemic in Brazil was described by Soper (1938). During recent years, jungle yellow fever has also spread across Central America (Costa Rica, Nicaragua, Honduras and Guatemala), causing local outbreaks (Soper, 1955). The epidemic waves coincided with a high death rate among monkeys.

In Africa, the arthropod vectors responsible for the maintenance and transmission of jungle yellow fever are different from those found in South America. The principal cycle involving monkeys and mosquitoes is similar. *Aëdes africanus* is incriminated as the main vector. However, though *Aëdes africanus* is probably the mosquito responsible for the maintenance of the cycle in nature, it does not transmit the infection to man. Another mosquito, *Aëdes simpsoni,* presumably transmits the virus from monkeys to man. In both South America and in Africa, jungle yellow fever may initiate secondary cycles of infection in which *Aëdes aegypti* plays a major part.

In contrast to urban yellow fever transmitted by *A. aegypti,* anti-mosquito measures will not control jungle yellow fever. For this reason active immunization with attenuated yellow fever vaccine is the only method of prophylaxis. At present the two kinds of attenuated vaccine just mentioned, the French neurotropic and 17D, are used. The former is applied extensively by the French in Africa; although it has been shown that it is an excellent immunizing agent, this vaccine may occasionally produce fatal encephalitis (Macnamara, 1953). The 17D vaccine strain has been used in South America in mass vaccination campaigns and has proved to be an extremely valuable form of protection against yellow fever.

f. Wesselbron virus infection

Wesselbron virus infection has been recognized as a disease of sheep and man in South Africa. The virus causes abortion and death in pregnant sheep and death in newborn lambs. Our knowledge of the disease in man is limited to one naturally acquired, and several laboratory infections. The virus was first isolated in 1955 by Weiss *et al.* (1956) from the tissues of a naturally infected lamb. Shortly thereafter, two additional strains were isolated by Smithburn *et al.* (1957) during an expedition in Tonga-land; one strain was recovered from the blood of a native member of the expedition personnel and the other from a pool of *Aëdes (Banksinella) circumluteolus* mosquitoes.

Wesselsbron virus is 30 millimicrons in size and was found to belong serologically to group-B arthropod-borne viruses (Casals, 1957). It is pathogenic to infant and adult mice by the intracerebral route. Guinea pigs and rabbits are resistant to infection. Experimentally infected vervet monkeys exhibit no clinical signs, but may show viraemia of low titer and a marked antibody response.

The clinical picture of the single naturally acquired infection in man was mild, and characterized by fever, headache, pains in the back, bones and joints, and disturbance of vision; the laboratory-acquired infections were more severe and convalescence was prolonged. Subclinical human in-fections are probably common, as is shown by the prevalence of antibodies to the virus in various areas of South Africa. A high incidence of antibody was also found among sheep and cattle.

Second subgroup:

Tick-borne viral diseases (Russian spring–summer complex)

Despite the fact that the viruses included in this subgroup and the diseases caused by them differ in many respects, they are treated as a single group for a number of reasons. First, they are all transmitted by ticks of the family *Ixodidae,* although this is not the only method by which they are transmitted. Secondly, they are all closely related antigenically and some of them are, according to certain authors, almost indistinguishable by various immunological tests. According to Olitsky and Casals (1959), this "is, at present, a confusing and poorly understood subject". This is truly so, in spite of the fact that a vast amount of literature has accumulated on the subject, especially during the last decade. However, since some of these disease entities have been recognized only quite recently, it is hoped that the problem will be clarified when more knowledge has accumulated. A great deal of confusion has been caused by differences in nomenclature, especially with regard to the so-called central european or biphasic meningo-encephalitis. This disease has been recognized in numerous European countries and in the western U.S.S.R. after World War II. Russian authors (Smorodintsev, 1958) regard the latter as related to, but not identical with, the previously recognized Russian spring–summer encephalitis, and differentiate between the "paralytic form" (Russian spring–summer encephalitis) and the "biphasic meningo-encephalitic form".

The disease entities included in this subgroup vary widely in their geographical distribution, in their pathogenicity to man and other vertebrates and in their tissue tropisms, vectors, modes of transmission and cycles in nature. Russian spring–summer encephalitis has been the cause of a very severe form of encephalitis and paralysis in man in forest areas of the Asiatic U.S.S.R. Central european meningo-encephalitis has been found in various European countries, including the western U.S.S.R.; during recent years it has been responsible for widespread outbreaks of meningo-encephalitis in Czechoslovakia, Austria and Yugoslavia (Hloucal, 1949; Krejci, 1949; Richling, 1955; Kmet *et al.,* 1955). Louping ill has been known for over a century, primarily as an epizootic disease of sheep in Scotland and northern England, and not as a particular cause of disease in man. Omsk haemorrhagic fever reported from Siberia, and Kyasanur forest disease recently recognized in India, differ from the infections just mentioned in their clinical features in man, which are characterized by haemorrhages without apparent involvement of the central nervous system. It is probable that all these diseases are caused by strains of a virus which are antigenically identical, but show variations produced by ecological conditions which have resulted in differences in their pathogenicity to man and animals.

The properties of these strains, their host range and laboratory diagnosis will be treated together, while the clinical picture in man and domestic animals, pathology and epidemiology will be dealt with separately.

The causative agents are small viruses ranging in diameter from 15–25 millimicrons. They are sensitive to ultraviolet light and are readily inactivated by heat. They can be preserved in the frozen state, or by lyophilization. Pond et al. (1953) have studied the immunological relationship between 4 strains of Russian spring–summer encephalitis, the virus of louping ill and the Czech strain of meningo-encephalitis. The results of the neutralization tests in mice suggest that these 6 strains belong to the same serologic group. The serologic deviations were very slight; they indicated that louping ill virus differed no more from the other strains tested than did one strain of Russian spring–summer encephalitis from the other. Immunization of mice with a killed Russian spring–summer encephalitis vaccine produced resistance to challenge with the heterologous strains. Pond and Russ (1955) also tested the immunological relationship of 2 isolates from Austria and Yugoslavia to other members of the tick-borne subgroup. The results of intraperitoneal neutralization tests in mice indicated that these 2 isolates are neutralized to the same extent by sera from rabbits immunized against each of 4 typical strains of Russian spring–summer encephalitis, louping ill virus and Czech encephalitis virus. It was therefore concluded that these 2 agents are strains of the Russian spring–summer encephalitis group of viruses. It has also been shown that Omsk haemorrhagic fever and Kyasanur forest disease are caused by strains of viruses closely related, if not identical, with the virus of Russian spring–summer encephalitis (MacLeod et al., 1956; Konowalchuk et al., 1957; Work, 1958).

All these strains are pathogenic to the white mouse by the intracerebral route. All except louping ill virus are also pathogenic to white mice by the intraperitoneal route. Monkeys vary in their susceptibility according to the strain and the route of inoculation. Rabbits and guinea pigs are resistant, although Soviet investigators found that guinea pigs show a certain degree of susceptibility (Smorodintsev, 1958). Sheep are susceptible by intracerebral inoculation to louping ill and Russian spring–summer encephalitis viruses. Certain strains have been grown in the embryonated hen's egg and in certain cell cultures.

Laboratory diagnosis is based on isolation of the virus, or/and serologic tests. Virus can be isolated from the blood in the early stages of the disease and from the central nervous system in fatal cases. A rise in complement-fixing and neutralizing antibodies can be demonstrated during convalescence.

a. *Russian spring–summer encephalitis (RSSE)*

The virus of Russian spring–summer encephalitis (RSSE) is the cause of severe encephalitis in *man* in the forest areas of Asiatic USSR. Geographically it occurs in a continuous band which extends across the northern Siberian and Russian territory. The main victims of the disease are persons working in virgin forests (foresters, lumbermen, hunters and road builders). RSSE was first recognized, and its aetiology established, by Silber *et al.* (1938). During subsequent years, Russian authors have made thorough investigations of the clinical picture, epidemiology and ecology of the disease.

The incubation period varies from 8–18 days. The onset is abrupt and is followed by fever, severe headache, nausea, vomiting and pain in the cervical region. The development of meningeal symptoms, such as neck rigidity, Kernig's and Brudzinski's signs, is rapid. The patients are tired and somnolent and may have epileptic convulsions. Paralyses of the muscles of the limbs, neck and back are common. Some patients develop flaccid paralyses and atrophy of the muscles in the shoulder region. In some the bulbar centers are affected and such patients become comatose and have difficulty in swallowing and breathing. Fatal course results from involvement of the respiratory center. Death occurs 4 to 7 days after the onset and the death rate fluctuates between 5 and 30%. Aftereffects are found in approximately 20% of the patients, the most common ones being paralysis and atrophy of the muscles of the neck and shoulder girdle.

The duration of the acute symptoms varies from 5 to 7 days, but the period of recovery is prolonged and may last up to 2 months. The clinical variations are numerous; they range from mild, abortive cases, through benign meningeal, to fatal bulbar forms. Spinal cell counts range from 25 to 100 cells, mainly lymphocytes and there is an increase in protein in the cerebrospinal fluid. RSSE virus is present in the blood and in the spinal fluid during the acute stage of the disease.

The pathological picture is that of an "acute non-suppurative meningo-polio-encephalomyelitis" (Smorodintsev, 1940). The meninges are inflamed, and there are severe inflammatory and degenerative changes in the brain and in the spinal cord. The severest lesions occur in the grey matter of the spinal cord and medulla. There is an acute perivascular infiltration of blood vessels in the brain, with a diffuse round cell accumulation in the grey matter. The degenerative changes in the neurons of the medulla and spinal cord range from early chromatolysis and loss of Nissl substance to complete necrosis and neuronophagia. Small focal haemorrhages in the grey matter are frequently observed.

The epidemiology of RSSE is characterized by a well demarked seasonal incidence. The first cases appear in April and their number reaches an epidemic peak in late May or early June and subsides at the end of June. Most cases occur among adult males. The disease is intimately associated with occupations which expose man to infected ixodid ticks. The main vector is *Ixodes persulcatus* and the mode of transmission is by the bite of the tick. Approximately 75 % of the patients give a history of tick bite 8–18 days before the onset of the illness. Ticks infected with RSSE virus have been collected from endemic areas of the disease. RSSE virus has been recovered from ticks by mouse inculation, or by allowing ticks to feed on mice. The tick may become infected at any stage of its metamorphosis (larva, nymph or adult male or female). Once the female tick has been infected, she will transmit the virus transovarially to her offspring. This has been followed through several generations of ticks (Chumakov *et al.,* 1945). The natural hosts of *Ixodes persulcatus* are forest animals, particularly rodents, which probably constitute the reservoir of the virus in nature. RSSE virus has been isolated from a number of *wild rodents* and neutralizing antibody has been found in certain rodent species. It is possible that, in addition to rodents, *birds* may be important in the natural cycle of infection, especially by their dissemination of infected ticks. RSSE is thus primarily not a disease of man. Infection of man is incidental, because he does not play a part in the natural cycle of the virus.

The use of protective clothing and tick repellents is recommended for the control of the disease. According to Russian investigators, local tick control is effective for a period of at least 1 week. A formalin-inactivated mouse brain vaccine has been used in the U.S.S.R. with favourable results.

b. *Central european or biphasic meningo-encephalitis*

This disease has been recognized in many Central European countries

(Czechoslovakia, Germany, Yugoslavia, Austria, Hungary, Poland, Bulgaria), and in Sweden, Finland and European U.S.S.R. Widespread epidemics in man have been reported from Czechoslovakia, Yugoslavia and Austria. According to Russian investigators, infection in *man* occurs not only through the bite of the tick, but also by drinking infected goat's milk (Smorodintsev, 1958).

The description of the clinical features of the disease is based chiefly on the reports by Bedjanic *et al.* (1955) on an outbreak in Yugoslavia, and on the work of Grinschgl (1955) in Austria and Smorodintsev in the U.S.S.R. (1958). In general there is a considerable diversity of clinical phenomena, both in different countries and in different patients during the same outbreak. In Yugoslavia and in European U.S.S.R., the outcome of the disease has always been favourable, without either deaths or permanent impairment of the central nervous system; not one of 2,500 patients observed by Smorodintsev and his associates in the U.S.S.R., died of the disease. The disease in Austria resembles to a certain degree RSSE, especially the paralytic cases in which involvement of the shoulder-girdle occurs. The death rate of the disease in Austria is lower than that of RSSE, amounting to 4.6% only. Typical cases of Central European meningo-encephalitis are characterized by meningeal and encephalitic symptoms, and by a biphasic temperature curve. The prodromal stage with its mild clinical course is followed by an afebrile interval which often simulates complete recovery; but after this most patients enter a more severe meningo-encephalitic stage.

The incubation period of the disease is variable and ranges between 4 and 21 days. The first stage is characterized by a short influenza-like illness with benign meningeal symptoms. The onset is sudden, with fever, headache, vomiting, anorexia, abdominal pains and a flushed face; a stiff neck and Kernig's sign are usually present. The blood picture usually shows leucopenia. After 3 to 5 days the temperature falls to normal and the disease enters a quiescent period which lasts from 4 to 20 days. The onset of the second, meningo-encephalitic stage is relatively sudden and some of its characteristics are high temperature, severe headache and frequent, sometimes incessant, vomiting. The milder cases show somnolence and mental confusion, while in the more severe cases coma and delirium occur. In some patients there are obvious encephalitic and encephalomyelitic signs, such as tremors, nystagmus, diplopia, retention of urine, transient paralysis of the face, and paralysis of the shoulder-girdle region and upper extremities, which are flaccid and resemble the condition seen in paralytic poliomyelitis. Grinschgl (1955), found that 71.5% of the 304 patients he studied were "meningeal", 23.5% paralytic and 5% encephalitic. The blood picture during the meningo-encephalitic stage shows a definite neutrophilic leucocytosis. In the spinal fluid there is an increase in the number of cells, up to 400 per μl, and also in the protein contents. This stage usually lasts 1 week. Clinically, RSSE differs from central european meningo-encephalitis by the absence of a prodromal stage, by a more severe clinical course, a higher death rate and more frequent paralyses especially in the shoulder region.

The pathological picture is that of an acute encephalitis with pronounced changes in the grey matter. There is infiltration and ganglion cell damage in the region of the spinal cord, medulla oblongata and pons. The anterior horns of the cervical medulla are particularly affected. Characteristic findings are: extensive vascular reactions, foci of inflammation, perivascular cuffing, degeneration of the ganglion cells consisting of chromatolysis and complete destruction with neuronophagia. Inflammatory changes in the cerebellum are a typical finding.

The epidemiology of central european meningo-encephalitis is characterized by a number of specific features. It has a distinct seasonal incidence; cases start to occur in April, increase in number in May and June, reach a peak in July and decline in October. It also shows a typical age distribution, most of the cases occurring in young or middle-aged persons and very seldom in young children or old people. Maximum morbidity has been confined to the ages between 11 and 30 years. Another epidemiologic feature is that the majority of the patients inhabit rural areas. In Yugoslavia, over 90% of the cases occur among peasants and villagers, and of these more than half occur among woodsmen or their families; no spread from man to man has been noted and in the great majority there has been only one case per family. Tick bites appear in the history of the majority of the patients. This is especially so in patients coming from towns and entering the endemic areas for a short stay. The most important tick vector is *Ixodes ricinus* and the infection in nature is presumably maintained by a cycle in wild rodents. In Yugoslavia the main route of transmission is through the bite of infected ticks (Kmet *et al.*, 1955). However, in other European countries, and especially in the U.S.S.R, the drinking of milk from *goats* bitten by ticks in pastures seems to be an important route of transmission, in addition to direct tick bite (Smorodintsev *et al.*, 1953) This has been proved by isolation of the virus from the milk of naturally or experimentally infected goats (van Tongeren, 1955–56). In various regions of the U.S.S.R., one way of infection may prevail over the other. In certain areas, up to 70 % of cases were found to have been infected through goat's milk. There are distinct differences in the epidemiology of the disease in the U.S.S.R., according to the mode of transmission. The "tick-borne" disease is sporadic, has an incubation period of 8–20 days and affects chiefly adults; the "milk-borne" disease has the character of a "family-group" outbreak, with an incubation period of 4–7 days, and affects children as well as adults. It is thought that a severe outbreak which occurred in Rojniava, Czechoslovakia, in 1951 with 660 cases was "milk-borne".

Prophylaxis is based on the control of ticks and the boiling of goat's milk. Workers exposed to tick bites, and especially woodcutters in endemic areas of the disease, should use protective clothing impregnated with tick repellents. Destruction of ticks by various methods is recommended in the U.S.S.R. for the control of the disease.

c. *Louping ill*

Louping ill is primarily a disease of sheep epizootically occurring in Scotland, and northern England and Ireland. It is of considerable economic importance, because of the losses it causes among sheep in the affected areas of the British Isles. Human infections have been mainly limited to laboratory personnel although the number of naturally acquired infections has been very small. Recently, it has been shown that human cases which clinically resembled poliomyelitis were due to the louping ill virus (Likar and Dane, 1958).

The disease in *sheep* almost always runs a diphasic course. The incubation period is 3–4 days. During the prodromal period there is a rise in temperature and the virus can be recovered from the blood by mouse inoculation. With the advent of the second attack of fever, signs of invasion of the central nervous system appear. The typical symptoms are champing of the jaws, tremors, paresis of the limbs and cerebral ataxia. The mortality in severe cases is very high. However, many mild, abortive and inapparent infections occur. This has been demonstrated by the fact that many animals on infected farms have been found to be immune, presumably owing to previous unrecognized or mild infections. The pathological picture in sheep is that of an acute encephalomyelitis. The meninges show congestion and infiltration. In the cerebral cortex there is perivascular cuffing and degeneration of nerve cells. The most pronounced changes can be found in the cerebellum, in which there is an enormous destruction of nerve cells.

Louping ill infection of *man* was first demonstrated by Rivers and Schwentker (1934), in whose laboratory several cases occurred among persons engaged in studying the virus. Numerous laboratory infections have also been reported among persons who had skinned sheep, or had harvested sheep tissues (Edward, 1948). Probably, some of these patients were infected through the respiratory tract. The incubation period in man is from 2–8 days. The typical course of the disease is biphasic. The prodromal phase is characterized by fever, malaise, headache and backache, with pain behind the eyes, which has been a striking phenomenon and is made worse by moving the eyes. This phase lasts approximately 1 week and is followed by the disease proper, in which central nervous system manifestations occur. These include stiffness of the neck, vomiting, drowsiness, mental confusion, photophobia and diplopia. The spinal fluid may contain up to 60 cells per microliter. Infection in man may be limited to the first phase only, or it may have a diphasic course. Usually it is mild, without sequelae or death, but recovery may be slow. A number of laboratory infections have presumably been inapparent and have been recognized only by positive complement-fixation reactions (Edward, 1948).

Epizootics occur mainly in the spring and early summer. The role of the tick, *Ixodes ricinus,* in the spread of louping ill virus among *sheep,* has been conclusively proved. Larval ticks become infected by engorging on the blood of infected sheep and transfer the infection to other sheep. The virus was recovered from naturally infected ticks that had fed on sheep during the prodromal phase of illness. The infection can be transmitted to sheep by the bite of nymphal ticks. Sheep appear to constitute the main reservoir in nature and the cycle is thus limited to sheep and ticks.

Human prophylaxis rests mainly on the use of protective clothing during the handling of infected sheep or their carcasses. A formolized vaccine has been successfully used to control the disease in sheep. It is prepared from the tissues of infected animals. Subcutaneous inoculation of this vaccine in sheep results in the production of neutralizing antibody.

d. Kyasanur forest disease

Our knowledge of Kyasanur forest disease is as yet incomplete. The main available data are confined to information obtained during a recent fatal epizootic in *monkeys* in the state of Mysore, India, with which a prostrating febrile illness in *man* has been associated. The clinical, virological and epidemiological features of the disease have been extensively studied by Work and his collaborators (1957–1959). Strains of a virus closely related, if not identical, to Russian spring–summer encephalitis virus were isolated from infected monkeys and humans. It is believed that Kyasanur forest disease is of fairly recent origin in India.

Clinically Kyasanur forest disease displays many of the features of Omsk haemorrhagic fever. The incubation period is approximately 5 days. The onset is sudden, with fever, headache, low back and limb pain, severe prostration and inflammation of the conjunctivae. These are followed by vomiting and diarrhoea. The cervical lymph glands are often enlarged. In severe cases, epistaxis, bleeding from the gums and stomach, as well as haematemesis and melaena occur. A papulo-vesicular eruption on the soft palate is frequent and is, when it is present, highly patho-gnomic. In all the cases studied neither neurological involvement, paralyses, nor muscle weakness have been seen. However, mental confusion and drowsiness have been observed. Fever may be high and prolonged, and the illness may be severe with dehydration and general prostration. The febrile period ranges from 5–14 days. The disease may display a biphasic course; 1–2 weeks after termination of the first febrile period, fever may recur and last up to 1 week. A persistent leucopenia is usually found. The virus has been isolated repeatedly from the blood during the acute phase of illness. Recovery is slow but there are no sequelae. Death may occur from internal haemorrhages or shock. The death rate is approximately 10%.

Human pathology, based on a few cases only, showed haemorrhages and consolidation of the lungs and massive haemorrhages in the gastro-intestinal tract. The main histological changes were found in the liver and kidney. No histological evidence of damage to the central nervous system has been obtained.

The outstanding feature in the epidemiology of the disease is the involvement of wild monkeys. Fatal epizootics in wild monkeys have attracted attention to the disease. Human infection, often fatal, occurred among the inhabitants of villages adjacent to forest areas in which dead monkeys had been found. The majority of human infections were in young adult males. The peak of the epidemic was during the months of April and May. The infection is transmitted by ticks of the genus *Haemaphysalis;* the most important vector is probably *Haemaphysalis spinigera* (Trapido *et al.,* 1959). Pools of the larvae and nymphs of species of *Haemaphysalis* collected in infected areas have repeatedly yielded the virus. Neutralizing antibody was found in the blood of *small wild mammals,* especially rodents, in these areas and it is assumed that they play an important role in the natural cycle of infection.

4

N. GOLDBLUM

Ungrouped arthropod-borne viral diseases

Rift Valley fever (Enzootic hepatitis)

Rift Valley fever is a severe acute illness of sheep and cattle associated with a high death rate. The disease in man runs a relatively mild course. Human infection is accidental and only persons in close contact with diseased animals or infected tissues contract the disease. Rift Valley fever was first described by Daubney et al. (1931) from an epizootic in Kenya, which involved large numbers of lambs and ewes; the mortality among newborn lambs attained 95%. Another extensive epizootic occurred in South Africa in 1951 with an estimated 100,000 deaths in sheep and cattle and 100 human cases (Joubert et al., 1951). The disease has been recognized in Kenya, Uganda, Sudan and South Africa. It has not been reported outside the African continent.

The virus was isolated by Daubney et al. from the tissues of infected sheep. It is one of the smallest viruses, ranging in diameter from 23 to 35 millimicrons. It is readily destroyed by heat, and can be best preserved at $-70°$, or by lyophilization. The virus is highly infective for sheep, cattle and goats (Findlay, 1932). Mice and hamsters are extremely susceptible to experimental infection by any route of inoculation. In infected mice the virus can be recovered from the liver and blood. Mice dying from the infection have extremely high blood titers, up to 10^{10} LD_{50}/ml (Mims, 1956).

The disease in mice is characterized by acute destruction of the liver, with massive lobular necrosis of the hepatic cells, congestion, haemorrhages and infiltration of the sinusoids.

By serial, intracerebral passage of the virus in mice a neurotropic variant has been obtained (MacKenzie and Findlay, 1936). This strain produces fatal encephalitis in mice without liver necrosis. Rift Valley fever virus grows well in embryonated hen's eggs. It has also been cultivated for a number of passages in minced chicken embryo tissue culture.

The disease in *sheep* runs an extremely rapid course. The incubation period is from 2–6 days. The onset is abrupt and the characteristic signs of the disease are weakness, loss of appetite, vomiting, diarrhoea and nasal discharge. Most of the infected ewes abort. Death usually occurs within 24 hours of the onset of symptoms.

In *cattle* the disease is less severe and less fatal, but pregnant cows abort.

The virus has a selective affinity for the parenchymal cells of the liver and the most striking pathological finding is focal liver necrosis. Small white foci of necrosis, surrounded by minute haemorrhages, are found evenly distributed throughout the liver. The parenchymal cells show characteristic eosinophilic hyaline degeneration and intranuclear inclusions.

Man is highly susceptible to infection. Natives employed in herding sheep during the epizootic in Kenya suffered from a short febrile illness (Findlay, 1932). Many farmers and veterinary medical officers contracted the disease during the 1951 outbreak in South Africa. The virus is extremely infectious to laboratory personnel. Nearly 20 laboratory infections are on record; human infection occurred with a virus strain that had been through over 300 passages in mice (Sabin and Blumberg, 1947).

The incubation period of Rift Valley fever in man is from 4–6 days. The disease in man is characterized by a sudden onset, general malaise, a flushed face, headache, backache and muscle pains, nausea and vomiting. Epigastric pains and photophobia are frequent. The fever is of the "saddle-back" type and lasts for a few days. Leucopenia is a characteristic feature of the disease. Retinal complications and loss of vision are not uncommon (Freed, 1951; Shrire, 1951). During the outbreak of the disease in South Africa, patients complained of blurred vision or even blindness, which developed after the end of the acute illness. It persisted for several months, but gradually improved and returned to normal.

Laboratory diagnosis is made by virus isolation or by serologic tests. The virus can be isolated from the blood by subcutaneous or intraperitoneal inoculation of mice. Identification of the isolated virus as Rift Valley virus is made by histologic examination

References p. 392–393

of the liver, or by the neutralization test in mice, using Rift Valley fever immune serum. Serological diagnosis is based on the demonstration of a rise in specific neutralizing or complement-fixing antibodies, which appear early after the onset of illness. Infected mouse liver may be used as antigen in the complement-fixation test.

Very little is known of the epidemiology of the disease. It is believed that mosquitoes transfer the infection to domestic animals. Circumstantial evidence of insect transmission was obtained during the epizootic in Kenya.

There is no evidence however of person to person spread, nor that man is infected by an insect vector. Smithburn *et al.* (1948) isolated Rift Valley fever virus from 6 lots of mosquitoes caught in the forest in Western Uganda. The mosquitoes included 6 species of the genus *Erethmapodites* and 3 of the genus *Aëdes*. It is believed that these infected mosquitoes play a role in the maintenance of the cycle of the virus in wild animals and that domestic animals become infected by blood-sucking arthropods. During the 1951 epizootic in South Africa, *Culex theileri* and *Aëdes caballus* were the 2 most prevalent species, but it was not possible to establish which species was responsible for the outbreak (Gear *et al.*, 1955).

For prophylaxis, the wearing of rubber gloves and protective masks during the handling of tissues of infected sheep or cattle is recommended. Stringent precautions for laboratory workers dealing with the virus are imperative. The mouse neurotropic strain developed by Smithburn (1949) and submitted to further passage in egg culture has been used extensively with very good results for the vaccination of sheep and cattle in South Africa.

GENERAL REFERENCES
ON ARTHROPOD-BORNE ANIMAL VIRAL DISEASES

BEADLE, L. D., *Publ. Hlth Rep.*, 74 (1959) 84.
BLASKOVIC, D. J., *Hyg. Epidem. Microbiol. Immunol., Prague*, 3 (1959) 132.
CASALS, J., *Trans. N.Y. Acad. Sci.*, 19 (1957) 219; *Bull. Wld Hlth Org.*, 24 (1961) 723.
CASALS, J. and L. V. BROWN, *J. exp. Med.*, 99 (1954) 429.
CLARKE D. H. and J. CASALS, *Amer. J. trop. Med. Hyg.*, 7 (1958) 561.
CHAMBERLAIN, R. W., *Ann. N.Y. Acad. Sci.*, 70 (1958) 312.
FIELDS, W. S. and R. J. BLATTNER, *Viral Encephalitis Symposium*, 5th Ann. Sci. Meeting Houston Neurol. Soc. Texas, Springfield, 1958.
HAMMON, W. M., *Amer. J. trop. Med.*, 28 (1948) 515; *Yale J. Biol. Med.*, 34 (1961–62) 304; *Publ. Hlth Rep.*, 76 (1961) 806.
HESS, A. D. and PRESTON HOLDEN, *Ann. N.Y. Acad. Sci.*, 70 (1958) 294.
HURLBUT, H. S. and J. L. THOMAS, *Virology*, New York, 12 (1960) 391.
KISSLING, R. E., *Ann. Rev. Microbiol.*, 14 (1960) 261.
MILES, J. A. R. *Bull. Wld Hlth Org.*, 22 (1960) 339.

PHILIP, C. B. and W. BURGDORFER, *Ann. Rev. Entomol.*, 6 (1961) 391.
PORTERFIELD, J. S., *Bull. Wld Hlth Org.*, 24 (1961) 735.
PORTERFIELD, J. S., M. C. WILLIAMS and J. P. WOODALL, *Nature*, 188 (1960) 252.
REEVES, W. C., *Amer. J. Publ. Hlth*, 41 (1951) 678.
RIVERS, T. M. and F. L. HORSFALL, *Viral and Rickettsial Infection of Man*, 3rd ed., 1959.
ROOYEN, C. E. VAN and A. J. RHODES, *Virus Diseases of Man*, 1948.
SABIN, A. B., *Arch. ges. Virusforsch.*, 9 (1959) 1.
SCHAEFFER, M., R. E. KISSLING and R. W. CHAMBERLAIN, *Amer. J. Publ. Hlth*, 48 (1958) 336.
SMORODINTSEV, A. A., Tick-borne spring – summer encephalitis, in E. BERGER and J. L. MELNICK (Eds.), *Progress in Medical Virology*, I., 1958.
STRODE, G. K., *Yellow Fever*, 1951.
World Health Organization, Techn. Rep. Ser. No. 219, *Arthropod-borne Viruses*, Geneva, 1961, p. 68.
WORK, T. H., Russian spring – summer virus in India, in E. BERGER and J. L. MELNICK (Eds.), *Progress in Medical Virology*, I, 1958.

C. Myxoviral diseases

1

H. BERNKOPF

Influenza

A number of interesting relationships between myxoviruses responsible for respiratory diseases in man and diseases in animals have been revealed by both epidemiological and laboratory examinations.

It has been reported that Sendai virus, for some time called influenza D-virus, which causes pneumonitis in newborn children and an influenza-like disease in adults, occurs in swine and wild mice in Japan, and that it has been isolated from these animals (Francis *et al.*, 1959).

Parainfluenza virus 3, another human pathogen of the myxo-group, was isolated from cases of shipping fever and respiratory disease in cattle (Abinanti *et al.*, 1960).

The type-A group of influenza viruses, all the members of which possess the same "soluble" complement-fixing antigen, includes a number of viruses pathogenic for animals, such as fowl plague, and influenza of swine, horses and ducks (Andrewes and Workington, 1959). No transfer of these viruses from animal to man has as yet been observed. The relationship of swine influenza to human influenza has been the subject of laboratory investigation and speculation for many years. Epidemics of swine influenza were first noted and described in 1918 in U.S.A. in the wake of the human pandemic of influenza in 1918–'19. It has been suggested that the human virus had at that time entered a new host and had caused the illness in swine, in which it has remained ever since, although it has now disappeared from the human population. This hypothesis has found some support in the finding of antibodies to swine influenza in the sera of people who had gone through the pandemic of 1918–'19, but not in those of younger people who were born after the epidemic had come to an end.

During the outbreak of Asian influenza in 1957, serological examinations were carried out in many countries to detect a possible animal reservoir of the new antigenic variant. Results were generally negative (Kaplan and Payne, 1959). Only in Japan, antibodies to Asian influenza were reported to exist in swine.

These observations tend to confirm a relationship between human and animal pathogens in the myxogroup of viruses. Continued study of possible cross-connections may bring to light further relationships of epidemiological interest.

REFERENCES

ABINANTI, F. R., R. J. BYRNE, R. L. WATSON, L. J. POELMA, F. R. LUCAS and R. J. HUEBNER, *Amer. J. Hyg.,* 71 (1960) 52.
ANDREWES, C. H. and G. WORTHINGTON, *Bull. Wld Hlth Org.,* 20 (1959) 453.
FRANCIS, TH., in TH. M. RIVERS and F. L. HORSFALL (Eds.), *Viral and Rickettsial Diseases of Man,* 3rd. ed., 1959.
JENSEN, K. E., E. MINUSE and W. W. ACKERMANN, *J. Immunol.* 75 (1955) 73.
KAPLAN, M. and A. PAYNE, *Bull. Wld Hlth Org.,* 20 (1959) 465.
KUROYA, M., N. ISHIDA and T. SHIRATORI, *Yokohama med. Bull.,* 4 (1953) 217.

2

H. BERNKOPF

Newcastle Disease

Newcastle disease is an acute systemic infection of fowls with primary involvement of the respiratory and nervous system. The name stems from the town Newcastle-on-Tyne in England, where the virus was first isolated by Doyle in 1927, one year after Kraneveld in the Dutch East Indies had given the first clinical description of the disease in poultry.

Since its original detection in the Far East, the disease has been encountered in all parts of the world in which laboratory studies on the identification of the virus have been carried out.

From filtration experiments the diameter of the virus (NDV) has been estimated to vary between 80 and 120 millimicrons. Electron microscopy has revealed that the virus in isotonic solution is spherical, but in hypertonic solutions filamentous and sperm-shaped particles appear.

A characteristic of the virus is its high resistance to detrimental factors in the environment. In chicken down and dust the virus may, at ordinary temperatures, remain active for many weeks. Refrigerated infected carcasses and other material containing the virus are infective for months. Ordinary disinfectants, such as phenol or formalin, have to be used at high concentrations to sterilize infected material, or premises in which infected animals have been kept.

The virus is classified with the group of myxoviruses, which includes also the viruses of influenza and mumps. It shares with these viruses a number of biological properties, such as growth in the allantoic sac of fertilized eggs and haemagglutination of chicken erythrocytes.

While no significant antigenic variation of the virus has been described, strains with various gradations of virulence exist, varying from those which cause only subclinical or very mild symptoms to strains which kill 90% of adult birds.

Chickens and *turkeys* are susceptible to the virus in nature. Sea birds have been suspected of introducing the infection into islands, and the virus has indeed been isolated from cormorants and gannets. Experimental infection has been successful with all the avian species tested, as well as with mice, rabbits, guinea pigs, hamsters and monkeys. Although natural infection of the calf and cat has been described, this seems to be a rare event.

The designation *avian pneumo-encephalitis* well describes the main pathological findings in infected birds. The disease occurs in an acute and a subacute form. In its acute form, after an incubation period of 4–11 days, the onset is sudden, with drowsiness, rapid respiration and fever. Diarrhoea, watery discharge from the beak and eyes, and respiratory distress, are the main signs of the disease. Opisthotonus, convulsions and paresis may also develop. Usually, death occurs within 1 week. While the acute form can be readily recognized by clinical examination, greater difficulty is experienced in diagnosing subacute infections. Here clinical symptoms may be few or absent, and mortality is low.

Young birds are more susceptible than older birds are and the death rate is higher among them. A constant feature in older birds is a sudden drop in egg production, often preceded by the laying of misshaped, soft-shelled or shell-less eggs. Pre-infection laying habits may never be attained again. Respiratory changes, such as sneezing, coughing, or a rattling noise in the throat, may be observed. Sometimes there is a slight watery discharge from the eyes and nostrils and a greenish diarrhoea. Affected birds are less inclined to feed and generally appear dull and listless. The morbid picture is not specific and can be differentiated only by laboratory investigations from other respiratory infections of the chicken.

Virus is present in the blood, muscles and all other organs. It is excreted in the faeces and is found in the secretions of the respiratory tract. The virus has been demonstrated in the air exhaled by infected birds. Fertilized and infertile eggs laid by chickens during the acute stage of the disease may contain virus.

On post-mortem examination of mild cases, little or nothing abnormal is observed. Common lesions are focal necrosis and haemorrhages in the viscera, particularly in the respiratory and alimentary tract. There may be excess of mucus in the trachea and interstitial pneumonia. The central nervous system may show haemorrhages, areas of degeneration, and necrosis of neurons, especially in the vestibular, reticular and cerebellar nuclei and in the Purkinje cells.

In contrast to the systemic character of the disease in birds, the virus in *man* generally causes only conjunctivitis. After an incubation period of 1–4 days, irritation and lacrimation of the infected eye are the first signs. The lesion frequently remains one-sided. Hyperaemia of the conjunctival blood vessels and swelling of the subconjunctival tissue appear in both the conjuctiva bulbi and tarsi. The lid may become oedematous and inflammatory symptoms become more severe. In about half the cases the preauricular lymph-node on the infected side is palpable. In some cases, fever, headache and other constitutional symptoms appear. The conjunctivitis usually lasts for 3–5 days, or, in severe cases, for 2–3 weeks. The cornea is not affected. Recovery is spontaneous and complete (Burnet, 1942; Anderson, 1946; Yatom, 1946).

Generalized infections, with low fever and mild influenza-like symptoms, with or without conjunctivitis, have also been reported. A case of mild encephalitis and another with virus pneumonia, both with isolation of the ND-virus, have been described. Recovery of the virus from 3 cases of haemolytic anaemia has also been reported. In the latter cases laboratory contamination with this very resistant virus had to be considered (Hanson and Brandly, 1958).

This virus may, in view of its relationship to such well-known human pathogens as the influenza and mumps viruses, be able to develop new pathogenic properties for man. It is of interest in this connection that the virus has been cultivated in cultures of human embryonic lung. It must be stressed, however, that so far, man-to-man transfer has never been observed. All human infections with NDV have been acquired by direct exposure to infected birds or to materials containing the virus. Infection has occurred by splashing virus directly into the eye, or by transmission by contaminated hands. The chief sufferers have been farmers, veterinarians, people engaged in the poultry industry, housewives handling infected animals and laboratory workers. Infection is thus a definite occupational hazard.

The laboratory diagnosis is based on isolation of the virus or demonstration of the antibodies.

The virus may be isolated from the blood, carcass and eggs of infected animals and from the conjunctival or naso-pharyngeal washings, tears and saliva of humans. There are also reports on isolation of the virus from human blood, urine and lung tissue. If it is suspected that any material contains the virus, it is inoculated in the allantoic sac of developing chick embryos. The embryo dies from the infection, frequently after the primary inoculation and always after one or two passages from egg to egg. The allantoic fluid contains the virus in high concentration. Infection is demonstrated by the fact that infected allantoic fluid will agglutinate red blood cells and by the inhibition of haemagglutination by specific immune serum.

For serological diagnosis the presence of a high titer of antibodies is necessary, or, preferably, a rise of antibody titer in the blood. The techniques of haemagglutination-inhibition, complement-fixation and virus-neutralization can be used for this purpose.

In man infection does not always lead to the production of antibodies. Considerable confusion has been caused by the existence of non-specific neutralizing and haemagglutination-inhibiting substances in human serum. In addition to a factor which is abolished by heating the serum for 30 minutes to 56°, cross reactions with mumps virus may lead to erroneous interpretation of serological tests. It is possible that the capacity of certain mumps antisera to neutralize NDV is a variable host response. The possibility has also been discussed that certain mumps virus strains share a common antigen with some strains of NDV (Evans, 1955). An unexplained phenomenon is the property of certain sera from cases of infectious mononucleosis and viral hepatitis to agglutinate red cells which have been treated previously with NDV (Florman, 1949). Serological tests should be carried out only with sera which have been inactivated and shown not to contain mumps antibodies. For diagnostic purposes it is preferable to isolate the virus under conditions which exclude laboratory contamination.

In outbreaks of the acute form of the disease, compulsory slaughter and destruction of all birds of the infected flock, together with thorough disinfection of the premises and the imposition of restriction of movements of the birds, and other suitable quarantine measures, have usually been successful in preventing further spread of the infection. It is more difficult to control the subacute form of the disease. Widespread immunization of birds is the only alternative to a "stamping out" policy. Both inactivated and live vaccines are used. Strongly attenuated strains serve for the latter purpose. The least virulent form of the virus can be given to day-old chicks by the respiratory route, either by dusting or by aerosols. Strains of slightly more virulent character are inoculated subcutaneously or intramuscularly into 4–5 weeks old chickens. A combination of preliminary injection of an inactive virus-preparation followed by infection with a live attenuated strain is also employed. Although in this way immunity of a very high degree can be produced, revaccination of breeding fowls is indicated.

Cleanliness, the wearing of protective goggles and protective clothing, especially during dusting and the application of aerosols are obvious methods of preventing human infection.

No specific antiviral drugs are known at present. Treatment is symptomatic only.

REFERENCES

ANDERSON, S. G., *Med. J. Aust.*, 1 (1946) 371.
BURNET, F. M., *Med. J. Aust.*, 2 (1943) 313.
CALLENDER, E. R., *Vet. Rec.*, 70 (1958) 907.
EVANS, A. S., *Amer. J. publ. Hlth*, 45 (1955) 742.
FLORMAN, A. L. *J. Bact.*, 57 (1949) 31.
HANSON, R. P. and C. A. BRANDLY, *Ann. N.Y. Acad. Sci.*, 7 (1958) 585.
HOWITT, B. F., L. K. BISHOP and R. E. KISSLING, *Amer. J. publ. Hlth*, 38 (1948) 1263.
JUNGHERR, E., R. E. LUGINBUHL and L. KILHAM, *Science*, 110 (1949) 333.
LÉPINE, P., P. ATANASIU and M. G. GAREAU, *Ann. Inst. Pasteur*, 79 (1950) 193.
YATOM, J., *J. Amer. med. Ass.*, 132 (1946) 169.

D. Miscellaneous viral diseases

1

F. DEKKING

Psittacosis and Ornithosis

Psittacosis is a disease of birds transmissible to man. As such it was recognized in 1874 by Juergensen and 6 years later by Ritter in Switzerland, who very appropriately, named the disease pneumo-typhus. Since then numerous small epidemics have been repeatedly described in Europe, all of them connected with psittacine birds.

From the source of infection in a large Paris epidemic in 1892, Nocard isolated a gram-negative, mobile rod, named by him *Bacillus psittacosis*. This was later recognized to be *Salmonella typhimurium*, which is frequently found as a concomitant organism in the disease in birds (see p. 135).

The pandemic of 1930 stimulated renewed attempts to isolate the aetiological agent, and these resulted in the independent discovery of the virus by various workers in Europe and the U.S.A.

This pandemic started in 1929 in Argentina, where so many cases of a severe influenza-like disease were obviously connected with sick parrots that even the general public could not remain insensitive to the risk of keeping these pets. When a very popular actress died of psittacosis, the sales of these birds virtually came to a standstill and the bird traders hastily exported their stock to Europe and the U.S.A. Although the epidemic had been mentioned in the weekly reports of the International Health Office, no country took any measures to counteract this infectious invasion, the result being that it was estimated that 200 to 500 patients had been infected, the death rate among them being about 20%. Later in 1930 an import ban on psittacine birds was imposed in all the countries involved. Since that time the infection has been recognized as being endemic in virtually all species of the domestic and wild birds investigated, all of which represent a potential source of infection for man.

The agent of psittacosis belongs to the psittacosis–lymphogranuloma group of viruses, a large and constantly expanding group of related viruses which infect an extensive range of animal species (with the exception of arthropods) and cause a variety of clinical diseases in these possible hosts.

TABLE XXIX

THE MOST IMPORTANT "VIRUSES" OF THE PSITTACOSIS–LYMPHOGRANULOMA GROUP

| Virus | Natural host | Other hosts | Experimental infection | | | | | Sensitivity to sulfon-amides |
| | | | Mice | | | Chick embryo | | |
			i.n.	i.c.	i.p.	Yolk sack	Chorio-allantois	
Psittacosis	psittacine and other birds	man	+	+	+	+	+	—
Ornithosis	pigeons and other birds	man	+	+	—	+	+	—
Lymphogranuloma group of viruses	man	none	+	+	—	+	—	+
Trachoma	man	none	—	—	—	+	—	++
Inclusion blennorrhea	man	none	—	—	—	+	—	++
Mouse pneumonitis	mouse	none	+	—	—	+	—	+
Cat pneumonitis	cat	man?	+	—	—	+	—	—
Enzootic abortion of ewes	sheep	man?	±	—	—	+	—	—
Sporadic bovine encephalomyelitis	cattle	man?				+	—	?

i.n. = intra nasal
i.c. = intra cerebral
i.p. = intra peritoneal.

There is a growing tendency to relate the organisms of this group to the rickettsiae rather than to the viruses. In addition to their relatively large size and their sensitivity to certain antibiotics and sulfonamides, they differ from the viruses by the presence of ribonucleic acid (RNA) as well as of deoxyribonucleic acid (DNA), constituting their genetic material, whereas "true" viruses contain either the one or the other but not both of them.

In accordance with Moshkovsky (1945), Bergey's Manual of Determinative Bacteriology (1957) classifies the psittacosis–lymphogranuloma group of organisms in the order of *Rickettsiales*, the family of *Chlamydiaceae* and the genus *Miyagawanella* ("*M. psittaci*", "*M. ornithosis*").

All the members of the group have a number of properties in common. Morphologically they are indistinguishable: the elementary body is round, with a diameter of 450 mμ; it shows up well with the Giemsa stain and with several other methods used in the examination of *Rickettsiae* (Castañeda and Machiavello stains); it is easily observed through an oil immersion objective. They share a group-specific heat-resistant antigen, mostly carbohydrate in nature, which is one of the best complement-fixing antigens known in virology. They multiply very well in the yolk sack of the chick embryo, most of them producing strain-specific toxins. Corresponding to their large size, they possess rather complicated enzyme systems, and are therefore sensitive to many chemotherapeutic agents. All are sensitive to aureomycin and other tetracyclines, some to penicillin, and even to sulfonamides. They are however, resistant to even high concentrations of streptomycin. Most of the members of this group have a remarkable tendency to cause, under both natural and experimental conditions, latent infections in different hosts.

Some members of the psittacosis–lymphogranuloma group are exclusive pathogens of man (the "viruses" of lymphogranuloma venereum, trachoma, and inclusion conjunctivitis); the avian "viruses" (psittacosis and ornithosis) frequently infect man; human infections with the other mammalian "viruses" may be possible, although they have been proved only in 2 instances; these were cases of infections with the viruses of enzootic abortion of ewes, and of bovine encephalomyelitis respectively, and both were laboratory infections.

Immunologically the members of this group can be distinguished only by rather delicate and complicated techniques. Specific neutralization tests are possible with sera prepared in roosters (other animal species being unsatisfactory in this respect), and neutralization of strain-specific toxin can be demonstrated in mice. Infection with most members of this group gives rise the to formation of complement-fixing antibodies, which can only be clearly demonstrated with the potent group-specific antigen: no strain-specific diagnosis can be made by this means. The purely local infections with the viruses of trachoma and inclusion conjunctivitis only cause very low titers. It is very unlikely that the agent of cat scratch disease is, as has sometimes been suggested, a member of the group, because complement-fixing antibodies to the group-antigen are found infrequently and, even when they are found, the titer in patient ssuffering from this generalized infection is low.

After infection with one of the "viruses" of this group true immunity probably does not appear. Resistance to re-infection seems to be based on persistence of the virus somewhere in the body. Re-infection is possible after the body has freed itself of the virus, or it may be endogenous if the equilibrium between the host and the parasite has been disturbed.

Although it may be assumed that spontaneous infections of birds with psittacosis virus frequently occur, as a rule the virus has a low virulence for these hosts. Probably under natural conditions the young birds are infected in the nests; they may or may not become ill, but they either carry the virus indefinitely, or liberate their tissues from the agent, and thereby become again susceptible to infection. Transmission of the virus through infected eggs has never been proved. If a carrier is exposed to adverse conditions, such as capture, overcrowding, transport or lack of food, active disease may develop. There are then, however, no specific clinical signs or symptoms by which psittacosis in birds could be recognized. A diseased bird may have ruffled feathers and be weak and emaciated. A common symptom is diarrhoea with soiled vent feathers. In pigeons respiration may be audible. At autopsy, no specific signs of infection can be found. Very often the spleen is enlarged and friable, but the virus has been frequently isolated from spleens of normal size. The liver may show focal necrosis, or a chamois decoloration. Sometimes the air sacks contain yellow patches of exudate, in smears of which the virus can be demonstrated. Pneumonia is rarely, if ever, observed.

In a fair proportion of impression smears from the spleen, the liver and air sack exudate stained by the above mentioned methods, virus can be demonstrated. From organs found positive in this way, virus can always be isolated with ease. A negative smear, however, does not exclude the presence of the virus and, as the microscopical examination of the smears is rather time consuming, isolation of the virus is the method of choice.

In infected birds, virus will be present in the spleen, the liver and also in the kidneys, by which it is probably excreted.

Pieces of these organs are pooled and ground into a 20% suspension in ordinary broth, to which streptomycin (about 500 µg per ml) should be added. From the pooled organs isolation of the virus is possible by primary injection into the yolk sacks of 7-day-old chick embryos. Most workers however consider that mice are more sensitive than eggs for this purpose. Intracerebral and intranasal infection routes are the most adequate methods, but psittacosis virus can also be readily isolated by intraperitoneal inoculation alone. The agent of ornithosis found in most non-psittacine birds will never kill mice by this route, so that these animals should be inoculated intracerebrally or intranasally. Better results are obtained if, in addition to the very small amount of material that can be injected intracerebrally, about 0.5 ml is injected intraperitoneally. In the author's experience intranasal infection of mice is a quicker and better method, which gives slightly more positive results. Some protection of the laboratory worker should be provided, the risk connected with this method being obvious. This risk, however, should not be overestimated: during 12 years of continuous use of these viruses by this method, the author has never observed a case of laboratory infection. Mice infected intranasally should be killed after 1 week and the material passed twice in this way before a negative result can be reported with confidence. Mice inoculated by the combined intraperitoneal–intracerebral method should be killed after 2 weeks and similarly 2 blind passages should be made before a negative report can be given. Virus can be demonstrated by staining the organs of infected mice; it will be found most abundantly in the lungs and impression smears made from the abdominal contents after removal of the abdominal wall. For brain material the Machiavello stain is superior to the other two methods.

Frequently infected birds develop complement-fixing antibodies to psittacosis virus. The production of these antibodies is, however, erratic and unpredictable. They may be formed only after several months or even not at all, and may persist for several years, their persistence being dependent on the presence of latent virus which maintains the infection. Virus is sometimes found in abundance in birds with negative serological tests, and virus isolation may be negative in birds showing highly significant titers in the complement fixation reaction (sometimes up to 1:4,000). Thus in individual birds the complement-fixation test is of a very limited value as an aid to diagnosis: a negative result does not exclude either active infection or shedding of infective virus, while a positive result may be nothing more than the footprint of an infection which has taken place several years previously, or just a sign that the bird is a carrier. So, a positive serological test has about the same value as a positive tuberculin test in humans: it means only that infection has taken place, but no information is obtained about the time when it occurred. The complement-fixation test, although of limited interest in individual cases, can, however, provide valuable information in group investigation. By this means it is possible to prove or disprove the presence of infection in flocks of birds, aviaries, or pigeon lofts. If all the birds show negative serological reactions, infection is highly improbable; if, on the other hand, even a few birds in a large flock show titers of 1:20 or higher, the whole group must be considered infected.

For the examination of sera of psittacine birds the direct complement-fixation test can be used. Sera of some other species of birds (ducks, turkeys and chickens) apparently contain only incomplete antibodies, which fix antigen but not complement in the direct test, and can only be demonstrated by using the indirect or complement-fixation inhibition test (Rice, 1948). Some workers reported that, with pigeon sera also, more positive results were obtained by using the indirect rather than the direct method. The author could not confirm these observations when he found that several hundreds of pigeon sera consistently gave identical results with both tests. These discrepancies might be explained by the properties of the different antigens. Recently a special antigen has been prepared which makes possible the use of a simple direct test, even with chicken serum. In mass surveys an intradermal test may be useful.

Psittacosis infection in *man* can be most successfully diagnosed by clinical and serological investigations. The incubation period in the human being is from 6 to 15 days. The disease is characterized by an infection of the upper respiratory tract and results chiefly in an atypical pneumonia, although cases of bronchitis without lung involvement have also been described. Even slighter symptoms may result from the infection. In severe cases, the picture is dominated by the toxic condition of the patient: this is the classic *pneumo-typhus* of Ritter. Most patients complain of very severe headache, some are comatose, others may be mentally confused and almost in a psychotic condition. Usually the ailment is diagnosed as typhoid fever, because physical signs of pneumonia are either lacking or very slight. X-ray examination, however, can show dense triangular shadows, which may be migrating in character. A dry cough may develop, but usually little or no sputum is produced. In contrast to typhoid fever, the blood sedimentation rate is usually very high. There may be considerable rise of temperature and profuse sweating. Even when the fever is high, the pulse rate is relatively slow.

As far as laboratory diagnosis is concerned, it is in principle possible to isolate the virus from the sputum or throat washings and from the blood in the early stage of the disease and from the lungs or spleen at autopsy. In practice, however, the chances of success are generally very small, because most specimens are obtained either too late in the disease, or after the patient had already started on a course of chemotherapeutic treatment. The method of choice for the diagnosis of psittacosis in man is therefore the complement-fixation test, with two samples of serum, one taken early in the course of the disease, the second 14 to 21 days later. A fourfold or greater rise in the titer provides acceptable evidence of infection. The finding of a high titer (128 or more), in a single serum sample taken in the convalescence period, has a limited diagnostic value, because it is known that such high titers may persist for 8 years or longer. Further, in man the development of complement-fixing antibodies is erratic: some patients may show very high titers even on the third or fourth day of the illness, while in others antibodies may be completely lacking until the third week after the onset of clinical signs, after which time they consecutively rise to a significant titer of 128 or more. For these and other reasons the results of complement-fixation tests should be critically appraised.

Low titers (up to 32) are very often found in healthy bird fanciers, or even in people with no known bird contacts, and with no history of psittacosis as a disease. On the other hand, infections with other agents of the psittacosis–lymphogranuloma group, especially with lymphogranuloma venereum virus, may also give rise to a high titer of complement-fixing antibodies, and even to rising titers brought about by another febrile disease, which probably appear on the basis of an anamnestic reaction.

In the diagnosis of psittacosis, therefore, the serological, clinical and epidemiological data should always be considered together. In contrast to lymphogranuloma venereum, intradermal testing is of no value in psittacosis.

The treatment of choice is aureomycin; if it is given in an adequate dosage, the temperature will become normal in 24 to 36 hours. This fall can almost be used as a diagnostic sign; if it does not occur, psittacosis is highly improbable.

Since the introduction of chemotherapy the death rate seems to have diminished considerably, but this may be more apparent than real, because nowadays the diagnosis of the less severe and atypical cases is made more frequently than it formerly was. Death is often caused by heart failure, especially due to a myocarditis which is probably toxic in origin. Infected birds excrete the virus with their droppings and nasal-pharyngeal secretions. The virus is rather resistant to desiccation, and remains, after it has dried, infective for rather a long time. The virus is most effectively disseminated through the air when birds clean their feathers of dried excreta, or when they are busy scratching the floor of their cages. On the other hand, incredibly intimate contacts do exist between sentimental bird fanciers and their pets, and infection is often acquired in this way. Psittacosis is an occupational disease of workers in the bird raising and trading industry and of those working in plants in which contaminated feathers and intestines are the main sources of infection.

Although until 1930, only psittacine birds were recognized as being sources of this infection, it soon became clear that many other species carry the virus. In the Faroe Islands epidemics of psittacosis broke out each year during the season when young fulmar petrels are caught as food. In these islands women who prepare the birds are far more often infected than are the men who catch them. It was also found that wild and domestic pigeons were extensively infected in the U.S.A., France, England, the Scandinavian countries, Czechoslovakia, Israel and the Netherlands. In this last country the carrier pigeon is the most frequent source of infection (Table XXX).

TABLE XXX

PROBABLE SOURCES OF INFECTION OF PSITTACOSIS PATIENTS IN THE NETHERLANDS

Years	Budgerigars	Pigeons	Canaries	Parrots	Other birds	Unknown	Bird trade	Total Nr. of patients
1953	2	23	11	1	6	22	—	65
1954	13	11	2	2	49	17	10	77
1955	48	23	1	5	42	26	5	118
1956	15	21	12	8	27	30	5	117
1957	8	25	12	2	15	17	1	73
1958	16	43	16	5	35	44	4	142
1959	17	43	20	4	21	38	3	127
1960	17	28	12	6	7	19	—	68 *

* Total numbers do not add up rightly because sometimes there are multiple sources of infection.

It can be postulated that massive breeding of birds inevitably carries the risk of psittacosis. Huge epizootics have been described on farms raising budgerigars, turkeys or ducks. It was found that domesticated ducks were infected on a large scale in the U.S.A. and Czechoslovakia and that they frequently infected the personnel who handled them.

Because the infection has been found in many different species of wild birds (pigeons, sparrows, egrets, petrels, etc.), these birds may account for the fairly large number of patients who have no known history of contacts with birds.

On the other hand systematic and searching questioning is often necessary to unravel the history of contacts with birds; 1 patient strongly denied such contact for days, until he suddenly remembered his daily habit of visiting a public square to feed the pigeons. To him (and to many others), such action does not constitute "contact with birds".

Once again it should be stressed that apparently healthy birds may be as infectious as very sick ones.

As a rule, man to man infection is rare in psittacosis, although patients are known to have carried the virus in their throats for 8 or more years. Such cases do, however, occur sporadically. On the other hand, it might be possible that some strains of psittacosis virus have attained a certain degree of adaptation to man. Several small outbreaks have been described, with well proved interhuman infection-chains involving 8 or more patients, with high mortality. The strains involved in these events seem to be slightly different from the ordinary bird strains, although nearly identical strains have been isolated from egrets in Louisiana, where a similar human outbreak had been recorded previously.

In the Netherlands the most remarkable aspect in the epidemiology of the last 10 years has been that almost all cases are solitary, while the classical family outbreaks are extremely rare, representing only a few percent of the total number of infections. Furthermore, most family outbreaks are still caused by psittacine birds. Budgerigars, however, from which psittacosis virus is readily isolated, rarely infect more than one member of the family. Infection in children is not so rare as has been generally supposed: about 5 % of the patients are younger than 16 years of age.

The only effective way of preventing psittacosis infection in man is to discourage the habit of keeping birds as pets at home. In the meantime the importation, raising and trading of birds should be made as difficult as possible by practical legal measures. In some states the importation of birds is permitted only for scientific purposes, or for keeping them in zoological gardens, while it is further restricted to one bird per family or per person entering the country.

Eradication of psittacosis from bird farms is extremely difficult. Medicated food, containing tetracyclines, sometimes meets with success, but healthy carriers may remain in such a flock and discouraging failures have been described. The most effective measures probably are a high standard of husbandry and segregation of the flock in small units which are strictly kept apart. Unemotional recognition of the risk of psittacosis by the bird breeder is a prime requisite for successful control.

REFERENCES

BEAUDETTE, F. R. (Ed.), *Psittacosis, Diagnosis, Epidemiology and Control*, New Brunswick, N.J., 1955, 240 pp.

BEAUDETTE, F. R. (Ed.), *Progress in Psittacosis Research and Control*, New Brunswick, N.J., 1958, 271 pp.

BEDSON, S. P., *Brit. med. Bull.,* 9 (1953) 226.

MEYER, K. F., in T. M. RIVERS (Ed.) *Virus and Rickettsial Infections of Man*, Philadelphia, 1948; *Bull. Wld Hlth Org.,* 20 (1959) 101.

RICE, C. E., *J. Immunol.,* 59 (1948) 365.

WENNER, H. A., *Advanc. Virus Res.,* 5 (1958) 40.

2

F. DEKKING

Cowpox and Vaccinia

Cowpox is a virus disease of cows transmissible to man and *vice versa*. Since Jenner (1798) proved that infection with cowpox protects man against smallpox, this disease has received considerable attention. Much speculation has been given to the origin of bovine pox disease, and, while Jenner thought that it might have some connection with horsepox, later investigators favoured the theory that cowpox was the result of infection with variola virus of human origin. Some outbreaks of cowpox which coincided in time with a smallpox epidemic seemed to substantiate this conception. At the beginning of this century, when in western Europe vaccination of man was almost universal, while smallpox very rarely occurred, the theory became popular that cowpox was in reality a retro-vaccination, *i.e.* infection of cows with vaccinia virus from a human source.

Ledingham (1935) was the first to point out that cowpox might be a disease *sui generis,* and this view was later confirmed by modern virus investigation.

It seems that some mammalian species, such as sheep, pigs, horses, rabbits, camels and mice, have their own characteristic pox viruses. Of these, sheep, mouse and rabbit pox are severe, generalised infections which are often lethal. The latter two can cause troublesome enzootics among laboratory animals. Human infections with sheeppox and horse pox (Fig. 44) have been described, but no modern virus investigation on these subjects has been reported. Infections of man with mouse pox and rabbit pox have apparently never occurred, in spite of close laboratory contacts with these animals.

The agent of cowpox belongs to the viruses of the pox group, the members of which cause vesiculous exanthemata in various animals. They all share a characteristic

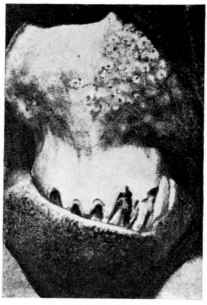

Fig. 44.   Horse pox (stomatitis pustulosa) on the upper lip of a horse.
(Photo: Institute for Veterinary Virus Diseases, State University, Utrecht)

morphology: the infective particle is large (200–350 millimicron) and has a brick-like, quadrangular form with rounded edges. There are important immunological differences among the different sub-groups, but most mammalian pox viruses are immunologically classified in the group to which the cowpox virus belongs. This includes: *Poxvirus variolae,* the virus of the human pox disease; *Poxvirus officinale* or *vaccinia,* the virus used for smallpox vaccination; *Poxvirus bovis,* the "wild" cowpox virus; *Poxvirus muris,* the virus of *Ectromelia* or mouse pox; and the recently discovered monkey poxvirus, which has not yet received an official name.

The members of this restricted group all share a very strong antigenic component; they all grow on the chorioallantoic membrane of the chick embryo, with the formation of characteristic pock-like lesions, as well as in the cells of tissue cultures of widely different origin. All give rise to the formation of acidophilic cytoplasmatic inclusion bodies (Guarnieri bodies) in many or even all of the infected cells. They are all resistant to ether. All members of the group can infect other species besides their natural hosts, but the *vaccinia* virus alone has a very wide and almost indiscriminate host range. Continuous passage of the other members of this virus group in a strange host only rarely succeeds.

The viruses of vaccinia and cowpox can infect both man and cattle, and the lesions caused by these infections are almost indistinguishable, a fact which has given rise to the speculations mentioned above.

Infection with these viruses mostly occurs through existing lesions (even slight ones) of the skin. After an incubation time of 2–7 days, a papule is formed which quickly develops into a vesicle, the contents of which become purulent within a few days. If the resulting pustule is broken, an ulcer-like lesion may develop, which ultimately heals under a scab. Apart from this local lesion, the infected individual *(man* or *cattle)* is generally ill, sometimes with very high fever. In man lymphangitis and swollen regional lymph nodes are frequently found, but as a rule, no viraemia occurs and generalization of the infection is exceedingly rare.

In cows the lesion is almost exclusively found on the teats, whereas in man any conceivable localization is possible. *Vaccinia* and *cowpox virus* have been isolated from the human eyes, the nose, lips and vulva, although the most frequent localization is the hand. In most places the infection in man gives rise to a typical vesicle with central "delle" which is generally easily recognizable. The lesions on the finger rarely appear as vesicles, because their character is strongly modified by the peculiar anatomical structure of the tissues (Fig. 45). In the thick callous skin, especially of farm workers, vesicle formation is virtually impossible. In such cases the finger lesions are indistinguishable from whitlow or paronychia, and they are very often erroneously diagnosed as such. The occupation of the patient and epidemiological enquiry will often disclose the true nature of the disease, while isolation of the virus provides the final diagnosis. By this method it has been possible to prove that infection with cowpox

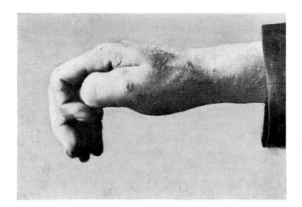

Fig. 45. Spontaneous vaccinia pustule on finger of a milker.
(Photo: Institute for Veterinary Virus Diseases, State University, Utrecht)

References p. 418

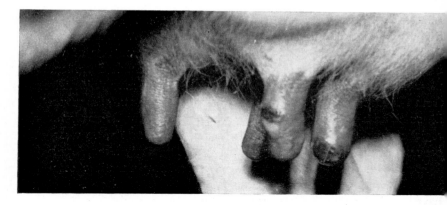

Fig. 46.   Vaccinia pustules on teats of a cow.
(Photo: W. A. Zijp, de Rijp)

virus carries the risk of postvaccinal encephalitis (Schreuder *et al.,* 1950.) The original aspects of the lesions on the teats of cows (Fig. 46) are often quickly lost, as a result of continued milking in spite of the infection; sometimes severe deformations develop.

The diagnosis can be substantiated by examining smears prepared by taking material obtained by scratching the bottom part of the vesicle and staining it by appropriate methods. These smears, if they are prepared in the early stages of vesicle formation, will show the presence of numerous elementary bodies (Paschen), and the absence of multinucleated giant cells, which are found only in the vesicles caused by *herpes* and *varicella* virus.

The virus can be cultured from vesicle fluid, but even the crusts of old lesions will often yield virus if they are taken and transported with proper care, and if no antiseptics have been applied to them. The egg membrane is the medium of choice, because the pocks formed are fairly typical for both *vaccinia* and cowpox. While *vaccinia* mainly attacks ectodermal cells and gives rise to proliferation with the formation of large pocks (2 to 4 mm in diameter) with a necrotic centre (Fig. 47(3)), cowpox virus attacks mesodermal cells as well, and the smaller lesions (1 to 2 mm), which are purely proliferative in nature, are bright red in colour, due to haemorrhages from the diseased blood vessels (Fig. 47(1)). These differences are striking and quite specific and they allow an accurate diagnosis in any outbreak of cowpox, in man as well as in cattle. The haemorrhagic lesions of cowpox virus are similar to those caused by rabbit pox, and also to those caused by most strains of neuro-vaccinia. However, immunologically there are slight, but definite, differences between these virus strains.

From cowpox virus, as well as from the other two haemorrhagic pox viruses, white variants have been obtained on the egg membrane (about 1 % of the pocks being white and non-haemorrhagic) (Downie *et al.,* 1952). These white variants (Fig. 47(2)) can be

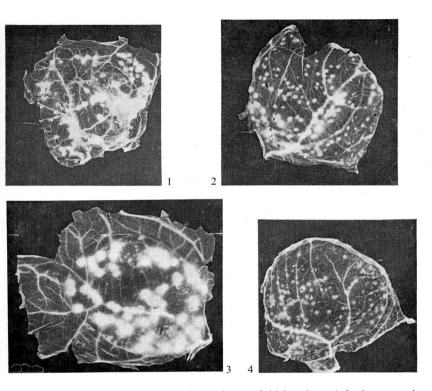

Fig. 47. Pox viruses on chorioallantois membrane of chick embryo. 1, Lesions caused by cowpox virus; 2, lesions caused by the white variant of cowpox virus; 3, lesions caused by *vaccinia* virus; 4. lesions caused by extromelia virus. (Photos: Dr. F. Dekking, Laboratory of Hygiene, University of Amsterdam)

obtained in pure form and can be subcultured readily. The character of the white lesions, however, and their antigenic make-up, are different from those of *vaccinia* virus.

Both *vaccinia* and cowpox virus can be readily isolated in many different tissue culture systems, and possibly this method is more sensitive for primary isolation of the virus than cultivation on egg membrane. Slight differences may be noted in the cytopathic effect, but, when lesions are stained, cowpox virus is easily recognized by the impressive number and size of the inclusion bodies found; infection with *vaccinia* virus gives rise to much smaller and less numerous inclusion bodies in the infected cells.

Although a very large number of different *vaccinia* strains is used for smallpox immunization all over the world, there does not exist one single strain of which the pedigree is known for certain. For some strains it is claimed that they are derived from variola virus. However, all supposed transformations of variola virus into *vaccinia*, by repeated passage on the bovine skin, have taken place in vaccine institutes, and it can be supposed that *vaccinia* virus is present almost anywhere in these institutes. In this way, even tapwater might be "transformed" into *vaccinia* virus by simple passage on to the skin of cattle. All attempts at such transformation under well-controlled conditions and strict aseptic precautions have failed. Continuous passages of variola virus in eggs or tissue culture of bovine epithelium do not alter the characteristics of this virus which seems, according to the author's as yet unpublished investigations, to breed true for at least 30 passages in these media. Continuous passages of variola virus in hosts other than man or the monkey have not been possible.

On immunological grounds it is improbable that *vaccinia* has been derived from genuine cowpox virus, and the origin of *vaccinia* virus has, in spite of much endeavour, remained an unsolved riddle of virology.

Natural cowpox virus seems to be endemic in most west European countries, and outbreaks have been studied and described in England, Austria, the Netherlands, Germany and France. In Holland, the infection is mostly introduced into the herd by a newly acquired cow and is spread by the act of milking. Transmission of the virus by insects is a highly probable theoretical possibility, but has never been proved, either by epidemiological analysis or by experimental research.

Cowpox is one of the rare animal diseases in which man is the principal vector. The infection is transmitted nearly exclusively by milking. We know of several cases in which the disease was introduced into a herd by an infected farmer. This is always so if *vaccinia* virus is the agent of infection and if either the farmer or one of the members of his family has been recently vaccinated. Although the disease caused by *vaccinia* virus in cows is as a rule more severe than that caused by cowpox virus, the infectivity of *vaccinia* virus seems to be lower. Out of 43 outbreaks investigated by the author, no virus was isolated in 7; in 8 outbreaks *vaccinia* virus was the cause, in 28, cowpox virus. In all cowpox outbreaks, not one cow of the herd escaped infection, while in all vaccinia outbreaks some of the cows always remained healthy.

There seems to be no definite seasonal incidence but epidemics appear to be slightly more frequent in the winter, when closer contacts occur between the stabled cows.

It might be possible to prevent outbreaks of natural cowpox by vaccinating all young cows with *vaccinia* virus (on the ear or in the perineum). However, apart from the risk of spreading the infection to other cattle or even to man, this measure does not seem to be economically feasible, and, considering the fairly low incidence of the disease, it might not even be advisable. A simple preventive measure consists in milking newly bought cows last of all for at least 2 weeks. If infection has started in a herd, the infected cows should be milked after the healthy ones, and the hands, teats and utensils should be washed with an antiseptic, the cheapest and probably most effective (certainly in cold weather) being a 1 to 2% aqueous solution of caustic soda. If an outbreak of cowpox has occurred in a herd, no unvaccinated persons should be allowed to milk the cows, because the infection in man frequently takes a severe course and even carries the risk of encephalitis. On the other hand, doctors should be aware of the hazard which a vaccinated person carries in transmitting the infection to cows as long as the vesicle has not healed; a vaccinated person must be considered infective till he has lost the scab of his pustule. No freshly vaccinated person should be allowed to milk cows, and no one milking cows should have close contact with vaccinated children or adults. Frequently women have carried vaccinia virus from their vaccinated children to the udder of the cow.

Repeated benign infections of the hand with vaccinia or cowpox virus in vaccinia-immune people is possible. Vesicle formation on the hand (from which virus can be isolated) may be seen while vaccination elsewhere on the body gives rise to nothing more than an "immediate reaction". This phenomenon is unexplained (Horgan).

No specific therapy of vaccinal lesions is available, although in cases of spreading infection due to agammaglobulinaemia, vaccinia hyperimmune gamma globulin may be useful. Lesions should always be kept dry and adhesive bandages should not be put on too close to the vesicle, because secondary lesions may develop in the macerated skin beneath the adhesive tape.

References p. 418

REFERENCES

BLANK, H. and G. RAKE, *Viral and Rickettsial Diseases of the skin, eye and mucous membranes of man*, Boston, Toronto, 1955, 285 pp.

DOWNIE, A. W. and DUMBELL, *Ann. Rev. Microbiol.*, 10 (1956) 237.

DOWNIE, A. W. and D. W. HADDOCK, *Lancet*, 262 (1952) 1049.

FENNER, F. and F. M. BURNET, *Virology*, 4 (1957) 305.

HORGAN, E. S. and M. A. HASEEB, *J. Hyg. (Lond.)*, 43 (1943) 273.

LEDINGHAM, J. C. G., *Proc. roy. Soc. Med.*, 29 (1935) 74.

SCHREUDER, J. TH. R., TH. G. VAN RIJSSEL and J. D. VERLINDE, *Ned. T. Geneesk.*, 94 (1950) 2603.

3

F. DEKKING

Contagious pustular dermatitis (Contagious ecthyma, sore mouth, orf)

Orf is a worldwide virus disease of sheep (sometimes of goats), which occasionally infects man. Because of its size and morphology, the virus obviously belongs to the pox-group. Numerous elementary bodies can be demonstrated in smears prepared from scrapings of the lesions it causes. These elementary bodies, like those of smallpox or *vaccinia*, stain well by Paschen's or Gutstein's methods. Some workers have demonstrated antigenic cross-reactions in the complement–fixation and neutralisation tests with *vaccinia* and *ectromelia* virus (Webster, 1958). Like the virus of *variola*, the virus of CPD is extremely resistant to adverse conditions, and in the laboratory it may survive for many years in dried scabs.

Under natural conditions sheep, goats and chamois are found infected. Experimental infection of rabbits has been possible up to 22 passages (Abdussalam, 1957), but mice and guinea pigs are resistant. On the chorioallantoic membrane of the chick embryo characteristic pin-point lesions are produced after inoculation of material from sheep or man, but after further passages infectivity for the egg membrane is lost rather quickly, and no more than 5 passages have been possible.

In *sheep*, after natural or experimental infection, a red papular lesion develops, on which a scab is very soon formed. Vesicle or pustule formation is rare; the character of the lesion is predominantly proliferative and sometimes it causes a protrusion of 1 to 2 cm above the normal level of the skin. After 1 to 4 weeks the scabs drop off, and as a rule no scar remains, because the lesion does not penetrate the basal layer of the epidermis. There is no viraemia and, if general symptoms are present, these are mostly caused by the feeding difficulties in lambs, in which the lesions are mostly located on the lips (Fig. 48). In ewes the teats are mostly affected, but lesions elsewhere on woolless skin are sometimes seen.

Sometimes the infection spreads to the mouth or extends further to the lung and even to the rumen. If secondary infection with *Necrobacterium*

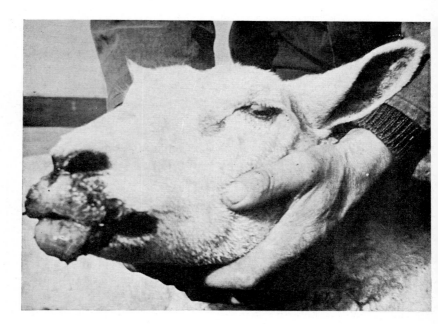

Fig. 48.   Ecthyma ovis. (Photo: Dr. P. H. Bool, Amsterdam)

develops, severe ulcerations and generally very poor condition of the animal may ensue.

In *man* the lesions are found mostly on the hands, but infection of any other region of the skin is possible. After an incubation period of 2 to 7 days, an indolent, itching, papular lesion develops, with a diameter of 5 to 30 mm. This lesion is sharply delineated, dark red in colour, with a greyish centre, and may look vesicular or pustular; it is solid to the touch. If the scab, which develops rather quickly, is taken off, clean, fleshy, but rather sodden tissue is found. Adenopathy is mild or absent and no general symptoms arise. The lesion heals in 2 to 4 weeks.

The epizootiology of contagious ovine ecthyma is not quite clear. Mostly the outbreaks occur in the spring, when the lambs are put to pasture. Infection occurs preponderantly in lambs 4 to 5 months old, rarely in those 1 to 2 weeks old. Scabs left on the soil in the fall or winter have been found infective next spring and this may explain the mechanism by which the virus survives the inter-epizootic period. An infection has been described on the knee of a boy who had fallen in an infected meadow a few days previously (Ward, 1956).

Man is mostly infected when he attempts to assist the feeding of diseased lambs; this explains the predominant localization on the fingers. Butchers are sometimes infected. The virus, however, has low infectivity for man (Pask, 1951). Inter-human infection has never been described, nor has infection of sheep by man been observed.

Immunity in sheep and man is strong and probably lasts a lifetime. In experimentally infected rabbits, however, it is very weak and does not remain present for longer than 6 months.

Prevention is possible by inoculating lambs with a virus-suspension prepared from powdered dried scabs. This inoculation is followed by the development of normal lesions, and thus should only be applied in areas in which the disease is endemic.

No specific therapy is known. As the lesions are indolent and leave no scar after healing, they are best left alone and the scab should not be taken off. A mildly antiseptic ointment may be used: for sheep 3 % phenol in vaseline has been recommended, while for man *Ung. hydrar. ammon. dil.* might speed recovery (Graham Bonnalie).

REFERENCES

ABDUSSALAM, M., *J. comp. Path.*, 67 (1957) 145; 217; 305.
BLANK, H. and G. RAKE, *Viral and Rickettsial Diseases of the skin, eye and mucous membranes of man*, Boston, Toronto, 1955, 285 pp.
GRAHAM BONNALIE, Correspondence, *Brit. med. J.*, (1951) 1265.
LIESS, B., *Zbl. Bakt.*, *I Abt. Orig.*, 185 (1962) 289.
Newsom's sheep diseases, Vol. II, Baltimore, 1958.
PASK, V. M., *Med. J. Aust.*, II (1951) 628.
WARD, C. W., *Med. Wld (Lond.)*, 84 (1956) 25.
WEBSTER, R. G., *Aust. J. exp. Biol. med. Sci.*, 36 (1958) 267.

4

F. DEKKING

Milkers' nodules

This disease is often described in the older literature as cowpox, while evident outbreaks of cowpox have been mistaken for milkers' nodules. There are however clear cut clinical and aetiological differences between these two ailments. Milkers' nodules in both cow and man, are slowly developing, indolent papules, 5 to 20 mm in diameter, and they are not surrounded by inflammatory reaction (Figs. 49 and 50). The incubation period is about a week, the development of the lesions taking from 4 to 6 weeks. The lesions heal without leaving a scar. They are greyish or bluish-red, and when they are cut, some clear fluid may ooze out, but true blisters are never formed. In cattle and man the general well-being remains unaffected.

Although some authors favour an allergic origin of this affection, it is possible experimentally to effect serial chains of infection in cattle as well as in man. Electron-microscopically the "virus" belongs to the pox-group, but, as with other members of this group (for instance *Molluscum contagiosum*), it is impossible to transmit the infection to the usual laboratory animals, or to provoke the formation of pox-like lesions on chick-embryo membranes. Evidently the virus is not related to the *variola-vaccinia* group, because it is possible to infect animals which have been vaccinated against cowpox and are highly immune against that virus. On the other hand immunity against homologous reinfection is only slight, and no immunity against infection with vaccinia or cowpox virus exists in convalescent animals. It has been proved experimentally that reinfection with milkers' nodules is possible 1 month after the original nodules have healed.

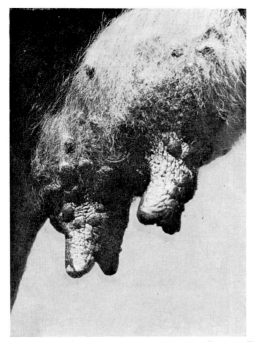

Fig. 49.   Milker's nodules on udder and teats of a cow (Israel).

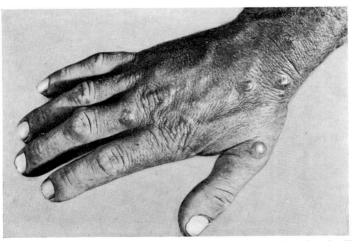

Fig. 50.   Milker's nodules on hand of man milking the cow mentioned under Fig. 49.

References p. 424

Recently from milkers' nodules of a young man a virus has been isolated which causes cytopathic changes in bovine and non-bovine cell culture. Serial passages of this virus could only be made in the cells of bovine origin (Friedman-Kien *et al.*, 1963).

Electron microscopy showed elementary bodies measuring 120–280 millimicrons, with spiral structure, resembling the virus particles of orf and bovine papular stomatitis. There was no immunological relationship with vaccinia virus.

The epidemiology of milkers' nodules is like that of cowpox: cows may infect man, man may act as vector. Unlike cowpox, however, chronic infection or rather reinfection can occur in a herd, because of the lack of immunity.

As this is a very benign disease, general health and milk production remaining unimpaired, there is no need for the application of special sanitary or therapeutic measures.

REFERENCES

BERGER, K., *Zbl. Bakt., I. Abt. Orig.*, 162 (1955) 363.
BLANK, H. and G. RAKE, *Viral and rickettsial diseases of the skin, eye and mucous membranes of man,* Boston, Toronto, 1955, 285 pp.
FRIEDMAN-KIEN, A. E., W. P. ROWE and W. G. BANFIELD, *Science,* 140 (1963) 1335.
KAISER, M., *Wien. klin. Wschr.,* 64 (1952) 669.

5

J. VAN DER HOEDEN

Vesicular stomatitis

Stomatitis vesicularis (sore mouth) is a virus-disease which principally affects equines and cattle; it occurs less frequently in swine, and only exceptionally in man.

In South Africa outbreaks which occurred among horses as early as 1884 have been retrospectively regarded as vesicular stomatitis (VS). Several cases were observed in the U.S.A. and Canada in 1916, and, during World War I, the infection was transferred to Italy, Great Britain and France by the importation of army horses from America.

The disease has not been observed in sheep, or it has been found extremely rarely in them, although sheep can be infected experimentally. Susceptibility to VS-virus has also been established in mice, rats, guinea pigs, hamsters, ferrets, chinchillas and chickens. The causative agent was detected by Cotton, in 1925. This virus (VSV) produces in cattle symptoms having much in common with those caused by the virus of foot and mouth disease (FMD), for which it is easily mistaken. The virus particles of VS, however, differ considerably in size from those of FMD, the first measuring 70–90, the second 10–12 millimicrons. Moreover, FMD virus does not affect horses. Cotton (1926) differentiated two distinct immunological virus types of VSV and called them *New Jersey* and *Indiana*, respectively.

The earliest recorded outbreaks of vesicular stomatitis occurred mainly in *horses* and *mules*. During the last three decades in the U.S.A. *cattle* have been chiefly affected. At present VS prevails sporadically or enzootically in several parts of North- and Latin America, while it has practically disappeared from Europe. The first outbreak among *swine* in 1943 which involved about 50% of 1,500 animals, was observed in Missouri (Schoening and Crawford). Since 1952 the distribution of VS among pigs has considerably increased. Enzootic outbreaks of VS occur particularly in hot climates; in moderate climates they usually remain restricted to the summer months and quickly subside when frost sets in.

The incubation period of the disease is short, averaging from 2 to 5 days. Symptoms start with fever and dullness, which are rapidly followed by the appearance of superficial blisters on the mucous membranes of the tongue and other parts of the mouth; exceptionally they spread to the adjacent skin of the lips and in swine they often affect the snout. As in FMD, smacking of the lips, refusing food and marked drooling of ropy saliva from the mouth are constant signs.

The thin-walled vesicles soon rupture, giving rise to superficial ulcers which tend to coalesce so that large areas of the epithelial surface of the tongue are pushed off. Ordinarily these erosions are covered with fresh epithelium within a week and the lesions have completely healed after about a fortnight. Exceptionally, secondary bacterial infections delay the healing process.

In cows the lesions may spread to the skin of the teats and cause mastitis with temporary loss of milk secretion. Moreover, cattle and swine suffer from lesions on the feet, which are particularly extensive in the inter-digital spaces, and are, especially in swine, complicated by secondary bacterial infection. Serious damage is caused by *Necrobacterium necrophorus*. Not infrequently pigs are lamed and sometimes sloughing of the hoof ensues.

The virus is found in the blood during the febrile stage of the illness and is densely concentrated in the blisters. This makes the saliva a most important source of infection for 5 or 6 days after the development of the vesicles.

Data based on the results of complement-fixation and virus neutralisation tests revealed that the infection is much more widespread than could be inferred from the incidence of active disease.

In the State of Wisconsin epizootics of VS have been observed at intervals of about 10 years, involving thousands of cattle and horses (Hansen and Karstad, 1958). In the south-eastern States each summer numerous scattered cases occur among swine. Serological surveys in Georgia revealed the presence of antibodies against the New Jersey type of VSV in about 45% of domestic swine, 50% of cattle, and 80% of horses and mules. Of the wild fauna tested, about 83% of feral swine, 48% of raccoons and 60% of deer showed positive reactions. 30% of the human population reacted.

The disappearance of the disease at the onset of frosty weather suggests that biting arthropods possibly play a part in the epizootiology of VS. Ferris *et al.* (1955) reported mechanical transfer of the virus for 1 to 3 days by the stable fly *(Stomoxys calcitrans)*, 6 different species of *Tabanids*, 3 species of *Chrysops* and 4 species of mosquitoes.

Despite the high infection rate of the human population in enzootic areas, clinical symptoms are rarely observed in *man*. The disease takes an influenza-like course and is self limited. The first cases, comprising three persons working on VS-research in England, were recorded by Burton in 1917. They were followed in 1945 by three cases in men who had handled lesions on the teats of cows in Colorado (Heiny) and by five other cases among laboratory workers in Wisconsin (Hanson *et al.*, 1950).

55 of a total of 100 laboratory personnel at the Beltsville institute of veterinary research showed serological evidence of infection either with the New Jersey or with the Indiana virus type. 31 of these persons (57%) recorded clinical symptoms which suggested infection with VS (Patterson *et al.*, 1958). It is, however, probable that among the "asymptomatic" reactors there may have been individuals whose attacks were erroneously taken to be influenza.

The incubation period of New Jersey-type infections in man was 2 to 6 days, and that of the Indiana-type infections 2 to 18 days. Usually the onset was sudden, marked by fever lasting about 24 hours, with abundant sweating and sometimes chills and headache. Pain in the muscles of the limbs, general weakness and dizziness followed. About one third of the patients suffered from sore throat with swollen lymph nodes, especially the cervical and submaxillary glands.

Slightly raised blisters with enflamed bases appeared on the buccal surfaces of the lips. Itching conjunctivitis, probably due to splattering of infected material during laboratory operations, was observed in 20% of the cases.

The course of the ailment, without exception, was benign, the symptoms subsiding after 2 or 3 days, although general weakness persisted longer. Complications have not been reported. In about 10% of the cases the disease had a diphasic character, the symptoms just mentioned returning after an interval of 4 days.

Infection seems to be restricted to persons who come into actual contact with the saliva of affected animals, or with cultures of the virus. Patterson *et al.* (1958) reported positive serum tests with VSV in 95% of exposed laboratory workers, in 100% of persons who regularly handled infected animals, and in 70 veterinary trainees who had worked in contaminated environments. On the other hand, the sera of people who had not come into contact with VSV did not react. These authors supposed that the virus most probably enters by the nasopharyngeal and ocular routes. The virus may also penetrate through abrasions of the skin.

The virus was isolated from the blood of an infected laboratory worker at the Plum Island Laboratory by Fellowes et al. (1955). Although encephalitic symptoms have not as yet been reported in man, their rare appearance in animals indicates a certain grade of neurotropism of the virus.

There is no evidence of transmission of VS from man to man. However, infection as a result of laboratory contacts with the virus and among the rural population in regions in which the disease prevails in livestock and wild animals, seems to be quite common.

In view of the benign course and rapid recovery from the disease, only symptomatic treatment is indicated.

Measures of prevention of the spread of vesicular stomatitis include the removal of newly infected animals from the herd and their isolation for 3 weeks, until recovery is completed. Disinfection of contaminated premises and objects by washing and spraying with a 2% solution of lye (sodium hydroxide) is indicated. Humans who handle recently infected animals or virus cultures should wear protective clothing and rubber gauntlets. The eyes must be protected by spectacles.

REFERENCES

FELLOWES, O., G. T. DIMOPOULLOS and J. J. CALLIS, Amer. J. vet. Res., 16 (1955) 623.
FERRIS, D. H., R. P. HANSON, R. J. DICKE and R. H. ROBERTS, J. infect. Dis., 96 (1955) 184.
HANSON, R. P. and C. A. BRANDLY, Amer. J. publ. Hlth, 47 (1957) 205.
HANSON, R. P. and L. KARSTAD, Vet. Med., 53 (1958) 17.
HANSON, R. P., A. F. RASMUSSEN, C. A. BRANDLY and J. W. BROWN, J. Lab. clin. Med., 36 (1950) 754.
HEINY, E., North Am. Vet., 26 (1945) 726.
KARSTAD, L. H., E. V. ADAMS, R. P. HANSON and D. H. FERRIS, J. Amer. vet. med. Ass., 129 (1956) 3771.
PATTERSON, W. C., L. O. MOTT and E. W. JENNEY, J. Amer. vet. med. Ass., 133 (1958) 57.
RASMUSSEN, A. F., C. A. BRANDLY and J. W. BROWN, J. Lab. clin. Med., 36 (1950) 754.

6

J. VAN DER HOEDEN

Pseudovesicular stomatitis of bovines

Since Mollaret *et al.* (1953) described human cases of disease caused by the agent of bovine pseudo VS, more attention has been paid to this specific infection in animals.

In *cattle* the eruption is localised on the mucous membranes of the lips, palate and muzzle (Fig. 51), exceptionally on the tongue. The feet and udder are not affected. The lesions start as small, whitish, round papules, which are firmly attached to the tissues and reach 1 to 2 cm in size and often coalesce. They are surrounded by a red zone. Later on they dry up and become cicatrized, attaining a yellowish-brownish colour, not infrequently with a shallow depression at the center. If secondary bacterial infection occurs, ulcers may develop, which are covered with brown crusts or pseudomembranes. The small papules on the tongue are papillomatous, granulomatous or nodular. Usually no general sign of disease is noticed, but a rise of the body temperature may occur for about 24 hours. Vesicles like those formed in FMD or VS and lesions like milker's nodules do not appear.

The disease, which is highly contagious among *cattle,* was thoroughly studied by Mollaret *et al.* during outbreaks in western France. Out of 180 bovines examined, 140 were affected. Sheep and horses seemed to be only slightly susceptible to the virus or were not affected at all. The characteristic lesions developed after experimental infection and the results of serological and virus neutralisation tests, differentiated this virus from the viruses of FMD, VS, vaccinia and ovine ecthyma.

Mollaret *et al.* reported 4 *human* infections which occurred within a year's time in the Central Laboratory of Veterinary Research of the Ministry of Agriculture in Alfort (France), where the virus of pseudovesicular stomatitis was studied. From the blood of these patients a virus was isolated which corresponded in every respect with the virus found in bovines. In guinea pigs it caused stomatitis with gingival ulcers or death within 19 days. Suckling mice and young rabbits (Fig. 52) reacted similarly to material taken from infected cows or from the human patients. When serum, taken from these patients was injected intradermally, or was rubbed into scarifications of the skin of sheep, pustules resulted. The blood of the human patients produced typical lesions in a calf.

As in cattle, the course of the disease in *man* is benign.

After an asymptomatic incubation period of approximately 7 days, fever, general symptoms resembling those of influenza and viraemia are present for about a week. A remission lasting 3 to 4 days may simulate recovery,

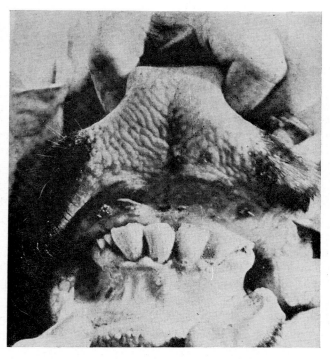

Fig. 51.   Lesions on lip and gum of cow in first stage of bovine pseudovesicular stomatitis infection.
(From: P. Mollaret, L. Salomon and Mme. L. Salomon, 1953; courtesy, La Presse Médicale, Paris).

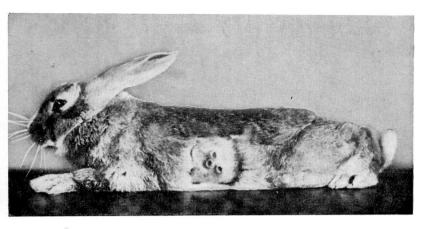

Fig. 52. Lesions on skin of a rabbit inoculated with virus of bovine pseudovesicular
stomatitis.
(From: P. Mollaret, L. Salomon and Mme. L. Salomon, 1953; courtesy, La Presse
Médicale, Paris).

but is followed by a renewed period of fever with signs of acute meningitis.
In this stage herpes eruption and transitory enlargement of lymph nodes
and spleen have been observed and the viraemia still continues. Even
about 1 month after the onset of the disease, the virus was found in the
patients' blood. Noteworthy is intracranial hypotension. The cell type in
the cerebrospinal fluid is purely lymphocytic. Slight buccal and pharyngeal
lesions have been observed from the fifth day of the illness onwards.
Although the few cases as yet observed of human infection with the virus
of pseudovesicular stomatitis concerned only laboratory workers, it is
probable that persons occupationally exposed to cattle suffering from
this disease, run a risk of becoming infected too.

In cases of so-called sterile lymphocytic meningitis, attention should be
paid to the possibility that the disease may be pseudovesicular stomatitis.

REFERENCES

MOLLARET, P., L. SALOMON and MME L. SALOMON, Bull. Soc. Méd. Hôpit. Paris, 69
(1953) 923; C. R. Acad. Sci. (Paris), 236 (1953) 2555; Presse méd., 61 (1953) 1615;
1645.
SALOMON, L. and MME L. SALOMON, C. R. Acad. Sci. (Paris), 237 (1953) 112.

H. S. FRENKEL

Foot and Mouth Disease
(Stomatitis aphthosa epizootica, Aphthae epizooticae)

The infectious nature of foot and mouth disease (FMD) was recognized about two centuries ago. In ruminants and swine it is accompanied by fever and is characterized by the presence of blisters on the hairless skin and hornifying mucous membranes. Sites of predilection in ruminants are the mucous membranes of the tongue, especially its upper part, the palate, the dental plate, the lips and the hairless skin around and between the claws. Furthermore, blisters are to be seen on the mucous membrane of the rumen, especially on the pillars, on the skin of the teats of cows in lactation, on the muzzle and, rather exceptionally, on the hairless skin margin around the bases of the horns.

The virus of foot and mouth disease was discovered by Löffler and Frosch (1898) and was the first viral cause of an animal disease to be established.

The disease runs a bi-phasic course: the first phase includes incubation and the appearance of one or more primary blisters, usually in the oral cavity (Fig. 53); the second phase, which is associated with high fever, is characterized by viraemia, dissemination of the virus to the points of predilection and the development of secondary blisters. The blisters are mostly haematogenous in origin. Those on the teats (Fig. 54) are most often due to infection caused by the contaminated hands of the milker.

In addition to the localizations mentioned above, the virus may also develop non blister-like lesions in the heart and the skeletal muscles. This is mainly observed in very young animals, although adults may show inflammation and degeneration of the muscles as well.

The disease, when it is not complicated by secondary infections, is benign.

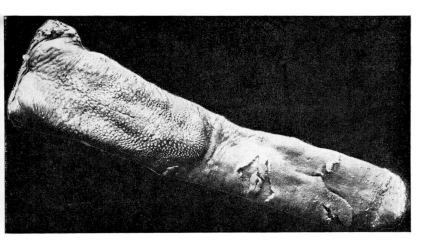

Fig. 53.   Foot and Mouth disease; ruptured blisters in the mucous membrane of cow's tongue. (Photo: Institute of Veterinary Pathology, State University, Utrecht)

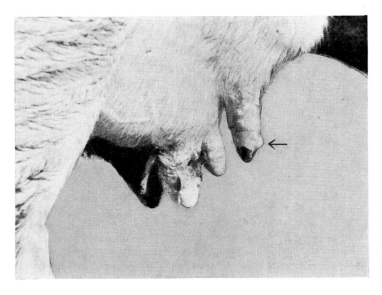

Fig. 54.   Foot and Mouth disease blisters on teats of a cow.
(Photo: Prof. H. Magnusson, Malmö)

References p. 440

Lesions resulting from ruptured blisters in the oral cavity where secondary infection is rare, heal within a few days. On the claws, however, severe inflammatory infections may often occur, causing panaritium, arthritis and phlegmones which may disable or even kill the animal.

In milk-cows the udder becomes inflamed by the virus at any stage, and secondary bacterial infection sets in, resulting in partial or total loss of the milk yield.

The damage caused by a FMD epizootic which is not amenable to vaccination of the non-infected cattle or to early methods of eradication, is strikingly extensive. Not uncommonly 40 to 60 % of the herds in a country are affected. According to the virulence of the virus, the death-rate may exceed 80% of the animals. Usually, however, it remains much lower, involving merely a small part of the herd.

The general condition of the animals seriously deteriorates, with the result that there is marked depreciation at slaughter. Because of the effects of the disease on the meat, it may be necessary to reject the entire carcass as unfit for human consumption. In addition to the direct loss of valuable foodstuffs during an epizootic of FMD, the economy of an affected country may suffer further serious losses owing to the imposition of regulations against importation by other countries to which cattle, beef and by-products would otherwise have been exported. Such restrictive regulations are not uncommonly extended to agricultural produce as well. When such a situation arises, the direct damage inflicted by a moderate epizootic in a cattle population of about 3 million head, may conservatively be assessed at 90 million dollars.

It was formerly believed that no animals other than ruminants and swine were susceptible to the natural infection. Later it was found that the guinea pig could be infected by intracutaneous injection of virus into the pads.

When this is done, within 24 hours a blister develops at the site of injection and this is followed by generalization of the infection after another 24 hours. In the guinea pig secondary blisters originate on the palms of the forefeet and on the mucous membranes of tongue and lips. Some time may elapse before the virus becomes adapted to the new cellular medium and a number of successive injections from guinea pig to guinea pig may be necessary to provoke the biphasic type of disease.

During the years following the discovery that the guinea pig is a useful laboratory animal for research on FMD, it has been found that many other animal species, such as rats, mice and hedgehogs, are susceptible to experimental infection. It has also been shown that the virus can develop in incubated fertile hen-eggs. Furthermore, Gillespie and Skinner independently discovered that day-old chickens could be successfully infected by injection of the virus into the tarsal vein. These animals showed inflammation of the gizzard and not uncommonly of the heart as well.

During epizootics among cattle one is repeatedly confronted with cases of stomatitis in humans which the patients themselves or the attending physicians suspect to be FMD. In most instances, however, the lesions do not resemble those found in cattle.

Human infections with FMD are exceptional, even during heavy epizootics involving millions of cattle. The low susceptibility of man to the virus is further evidenced by his direct and frequent association with cattle. Thus the hands of milking personnel would be excellent promoters of this viral infection should a higher susceptibility exist. In contrast to this, infections with cow pox on the hands and elsewhere, resulting from milking pox-infected cows, are a common occurrence.

Laboratory and stable personnel in FMD institutes have rarely shown infections. This has also been the author's experience over a period of 30 years, during which no human case was encountered in the State Institute for Veterinary Research in Amsterdam, although very large quantities of virus had been constantly grown and handled.

From all this it can well be understood why the susceptibility of humans has been doubted. Nevertheless, many cases of human infection have been described, most of them dating from a rather distant period, when accurate laboratory examination could not be carried out. Several cases were diagnosed merely on the strength of the clinical picture. The coincidence of stomatitis and a FMD epizootic was often sufficient reason for suspecting human infection or even to warrant it. Several people claim to have contracted FMD after drinking raw milk, even during a period when no cases of the disease were occurring in animals.

The following procedure is required in order to achieve a fool-proof diagnosis.

Either fresh material from blisters, or saliva containing the virus (a mixture of lymph from recently broken blisters and saliva), are sent to a specialized laboratory; or, if this is not feasible, bloodserum (about 20 ml of blood) is collected from a patient at a time when neutralizing antibodies are due to appear, *i.e.,* from 12 to 14 days after infection. Susceptible animals are inoculated with the suspected material. In guinea pigs the site of the intradermal inoculation should be their footpads. Several passages through the animals may be necessary before conclusive evidence of the presence of the virus is obtained. When, therefore, quick results are needed, a naturally susceptible animal such as a bovine, should be preferred. Such a bovine should of course not have suffered from the disease and should not have been vaccinated against it. Because guinea pigs are most often used for the examinations of human material, more cases would perhaps have been diagnosed if susceptible bovines had been used instead.

Also of importance for the diagnosis of FMD is the discovery made by Skinner, who found that unweaned mice are very susceptible to intraperitoneal injection of the virus. In positive cases suckling mice die within a few days, showing paralysis of the hindlegs and often also degeneration of the heart muscle.

Besides infection of experimental animals with material from blisters, a complement-fixation test can be done whenever a sufficient amount of the suspected material can be collected. It is then used as antigen and the serum of hyper-immunized guinea pigs is used as antibody.

It was formerly believed that a single and uniform virus is the cause of FMD. Since relapses were observed in bovines and swine which had just recovered from the illness, it was presumed that the immunity response was at fault. Vallée postulated that such relapses are due to differences in the quality of the virus rather than to inadequate immunity response. He discovered that similar clinical manifestations could be provoked by different types of FMD-virus. Infection with one type of virus either does not, or almost not, confer immunity to infection with an other type.

In addition to this, different variants can be encountered in one type which, although they are related in their immunogenical power, are most effective with the homologous one. From this it becomes apparent that accurate identification of the virus strains is rather complicated. In the Pirbright Virus Institute of Great Britain a reference laboratory for the purpose of exact differentiation of FMD-virus strains has been established.

A clear pattern of clinical symptoms will emerge only from human cases of foot and mouth disease which are based on demonstration of the aetiologic agent. According to Vetterlein, only 18 cases (to which the later published case of Garbe, Hussong and Pilz may be added) can so far be recognized as true instances. Additional infections would most probably have come to light had laboratory examinations been carried out more frequently in suspected cases.

In established cases the onset is characterized by headache, listlessness and sickness, after an incubation period of from 2 to 6 days. These symptoms vary in degree of severity and are sometimes associated with pharyngitis. Blisters are preceded by a sensation of tension, burning or itching. The appearance of blisters is not essential to the clinical picture, which may be restricted to the symptoms mentioned above. The disease in humans resembles that of susceptible animals in that its course is biphasic with formation of primary blisters followed by viraemia and secondary blisters. The latter are often seen on the palms of the hands (Fig. 55), on the volar surfaces of the fingers, the soles of the feet and the toes. Primary formation of blisters often occurs in the oral cavity. Sometimes these symptoms are localized there, the extremities remaining free. When they occur on the feet and hands, the blisters may vary in size from a pinpoint to the size of a sixpence. As a rule they barely protrude and are often surrounded by a red margin; the thicker the skin is, the flatter the blisters are. The same does not apply to the thinner membranes in the oral cavity, where the blisters are more prominent. Owing to their liquid contents they are tense at the outset, but dry up within 2 to 3 days. Though the liquid in them is usually clear and yellowish at first, it becomes turbid owing to the presence of leucocytes and fibrin. The aphthae may be elliptic or circular in shape and, when they are close together, they coalesce. After desiccation they slough off, leaving on the skin or mucous membrane a reddish surface which exudes serous fluid. Because the process does not involve

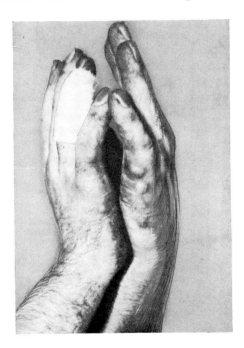

Fig. 55.   Foot and Mouth disease blisters on hands of a farmer.
(Photo: Dr. W. Pilz, Leverkusen, Cologne)

the entire skin or mucous membranes, and because the deeper layers of the epithelial covering remain intact, full regeneration soon ensues.

In cases of FMD uncomplicated by secondary infections, there is no formation of scars.

The nailbeds may also become painfully inflamed, sometimes showing vesicles that cause loss of the nails (Fig. 56). In the oral cavity and between the fingers and toes, the vesicles tend to rupture soon, recovery following 5 to 10 days thereafter. From experience gained so far it is known that secondary blisters may continue to appear for as long as 5 days.

Subjective discomfort is greatest whenever the oral mucous membrane is involved; eating, drinking and even talking become painful and there is an annoying increase of the salivary secretion. These symptoms, however, do not necessarily occur; they are absent when the extremities only are involved. Diarrhoea has been mentioned in one instance, by Gerlach, who

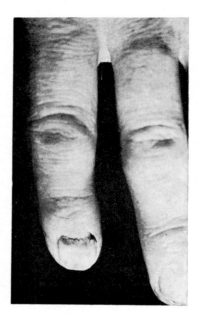

Fig. 56.   Loss of nail due to foot and mouth disease infection.
(Photo: Prof. H. Magnusson, Malmö)

described the case of his 5½ year-old daughter. It is, however, debatable in what measure the intestinal trouble could be attributed to direct influence of the virus.

Prior to the advent of vaccination, numerous cases of sudden death in young animals were observed during epizootics of the disease. Post mortem examinations revealed extended myocarditis showing a typical pathologic anatomical picture; the heart muscle presented localized white stripes which showed a tendency to quick calcification. This fatal form of the illness has also been observed in very young experimental animals of species that are usually little susceptible (guinea pig, rabbit, one-day old chicks, unweaned mice, etc.). In this connection it would be wise to issue a warning against the possible hazards to infants and young children during epizootics of foot and mouth disease from consumption of raw milk and from infected hands. Although no recorded case of sudden death among children is known, the possibility of serious results of infection should not be excluded. Gerlach believed that the heart involvement in the case mentioned above is an example of such relation.

It is likely that man can be infected in more ways than those recorded in established cases of the disease. Cases of accidental laboratory infections through wounds of the skin have been reported.

Cattle suffering from FMD are not the only potential hazard to humans. Cattle which have recovered from the infection or have been infected after vaccination, but show no outward symptoms of the illness, may also be sources of the infection. This can be explained by the long term production of small quantities of virus. It does not, however, alter the fact that man's susceptibility to the infection is very low. Up to the present no record of man-to-man infection exists. Nicolle and Bazolet, and others also, failed in their attempt to infect humans experimentally with foot and mouth disease. It is suggested that predisposing factors in the individual, rather than features of the virus, are important in bringing about the infection of human beings.

No systemic therapy for FMD is at present known. Treatment is symptomatic and is reduced to the topical application of drugs.

Many attempts have been made, to combat this dreadful epizootic disease. A hyperimmune serum prepared from bovines after repeated injections of virus was evolved by Loeffler and Frosch, the discoverers of the virus.

Because immune serum treatment alone will not control an epizootic, the destruction of diseased and exposed animals is advocated, in conjunction with other measures designed to halt the spread of the infection, *i.e.* disinfection of stables and confinement of animals from infected farms and adjoining areas. Where the geographical situation favours the application of such a programme, as, for example, in the United Kingdom, most outbreaks can be controlled by the so-called "stamping-out" system. In continental countries, however, this method, in order to be useful, would imply the sacrifice of most of the cattle population.

Many researches have been devoted to the problem of developing an effective method of vaccination. For the preparation of the first aluminium adsorbed formalized vaccine (Schmidt–Waldmann) the virus was propagated in susceptible bovines by means of multiple injections into the mucous membrane of the tongue.

Inactivation of the virus without impairing its antigenicity is achieved with formalin.

References p. 440

Another vaccine is prepared from FMD virus cultivated *in vitro* (Frenkel). Normal sheets of mucous membrane collected from the tongues immediately after slaughter of cattle are kept viable in a suitable medium. The elaboration of the virus culture into vaccine is essentially the same as the elaboration of the Schmidt–Waldmann vaccine.

Still other types of vaccine have been prepared, *e.g.* from cultures of the kidney cells either of calves or swine, or from suspended cell cultures, the virus being inactivated with formalin.

The discovery that FMD virus, after repeated injection into the tarsal vein of day-old chicks, loses its pathogenicity for cattle, but still retains its antigenicity, is due to the investigations of Gillespie, Zaharan, Delay and Fish. Kimron confirming their findings, claimed successful results with the use of a modified live virus vaccine in the management of an outbreak of FMD of the Asian type in Israel in 1959.

REFERENCES

ARKWRIGHT, J. A., *Lancet,* 214 (1928) 1191.
GARBE, H. G., H. J. HUSSONG and W. PILZ, *Vet. med. Nachr.,* 3 (1959) 1.
GERLACH, F., *Wien. klin. Wschr.,* 37 (1924) 210.
KANYO, B. and G. Z. OLAH, *Z. Immun. Forsch.,* 92 (1938) 20.
MAGNUSSON, H., *Berl. Münch. tierärztl. Wschr.,* 2 (1939) 421.
RINJARD, GRATIOLET and CHABROT, *Bull. Acad. vét. Fr.,* 12 (1938) 325.
SCHNEIDER, B., *Berl. Münch. tierärztl. Wschr.,* 25 (1951)
TRAUTWEIN, K., *Derm. Z.,* 57 (1929) 241.
WAHL, H., *Z. Tropenmed.,* 4 (1952) 1.

8

A. CH. RUYS

Cat scratch disease
(Maladie des griffes de chat, lymphoreticulosis benigna)

In 1950 Debré *et al.* and Mollaret *et al.* described a clinical entity in patients who suffered from a disease after they had been scratched by a cat. This disease had already been recognized in the U.S.A. by Foshay. It is characterized by a subacute, localized inflammation of lymph glands, which generally subsides without special treatment. As a rule, it becomes manifest in the regional lymph nodes draining a superficial wound. Although the abrasion may be caused by a variety of objects (thorns, wood or bone splinters), scratches or bites of cats are generally to blame.

The initial skin lesion usually persists for several weeks, appearing more or less inflamed, with or without small central necrosis and sometimes leaving a dark red scar. 2 to 3 weeks later, the regional lymph glands gradually become tender and enlarged. Some remain movable, others show signs of periadenitis, which often becomes suppurative. Sometimes additional groups of lymph nodes draining the site of the wound are involved, although lymphangitis and generalized adenopathy never occur. The spleen is not enlarged and the blood picture remains normal. The affected glands vary greatly in size, the larger ones sometimes becoming fluctuant or breaking down with a purulent discharge which is bacteriologically sterile.

Most of the patients have transient fever, with general symptoms which only exceptionally persist. A maculopapular, erythematous or fine papular rash of short duration may be observed. In rare cases the disease is complicated by encephalitis or other neurological symptoms (Paxson *et al.*, Debré *et al.*, Daniels *et al.*). When the primary lesion is on the eyelid or conjunctiva, the Parinaud syndrome may develop (Fig. 57). In some instances there is no recollection of an initial abrasion. In the oropharyngeal form of the disease, the portal of entry may be the mucosa. Pulmonary and mesenteric forms without any visible primary lesion are

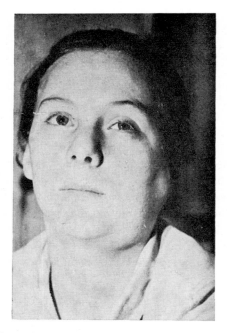

Fig. 57. Parinaud's conjunctivitis and purulent adenitis in cat scratch disease. (Courtesy: Dr. A. W. C. van Veelen and Dr. P. D. Stibbe, Utrecht).

also possible. After 3 weeks to 3 months the infection gradually subsides and is generally followed by an uneventful recovery.

The histological picture of the glands in the primary stage of the infection shows scattered localized inflammatory reactions of the reticular cells. In the subsequent stage micro-abscesses are formed with polynuclear leucocytes. Such abscesses may grow and may give rise to suppuration and sometimes they adopt a stellate form. The histological picture is non-specific and much resembles that found in tularaemia and lymphogranuloma inguinale (Nicolas–Favre). According to Hedinger the histological diagnosis is always uncertain; the more the reaction is reticular, the less probable it is that the condition is cat scratch disease. As Foshay (1932) suggested, the clinical diagnosis can be confirmed by an intradermal test with material taken from suppurative lymph nodes.

The antigen consists of pus collected aseptically, and diluted 5 times with normal saline solution and heated at 60° for 2 hours on 2 successive days. 3 to 4 days after intradermal injection of 0.1 ml of the antigen persons suffering from cat scratch disease react with a red, circumscribed papule, 6 to 10 mm in diameter, which is sometimes surrounded by a non-indurated red zone; in the centre a small vesicle may develop. The reaction subsides after 3 to 4 days. Not all antigens have the same potency. A positive skin test is of major diagnostic value, the reaction being highly specific. The Frei test in these patients is negative (Mollaret).

Up till now the causative agent of the disease has not been definitely determined. Contrary to Mollaret *et al.,* who claimed successful trans- mission to 1 out of 4 volunteers, as well as to monkeys, attempts by other investigators to infect a great variety of animals, including embryonated eggs, have so far failed. Moreover the presence of inclusion or elementary bodies has not been confirmed (Armstrong *et al.,* 1956).

It is generally believed that the infective agent of cat scratch disease is a virus, although no virus has been isolated. The assumption of Mollaret *et al.* that the virus belongs to the psittacosis–lymphogranuloma group is strongly doubted by others. Positive results in the complement-fixation test with an antigen prepared from lymphogranuloma venereum material (lygranum) were recorded by the French authors in most of their cat scratch disease patients. However, in other hands, this reaction gave results so variable that its diagnostic value was negligible (Prier, 1958).

The distribution of cat scratch disease is world wide and without seasonal preference. In most instances, there is a history of association with cats, with or without a scratch or a bite from this animal.

Cats as a rule show no evidence of illness and do not react to the skin test. On necropsy, cats suspected of having transmitted the disease did not show pathological changes. Inoculation of purulent material from patients does not result in any lesion. It has been suggested that cats transmit the disease mechanically. From epidemiological observations, it is assumed that cats carry the agent for only a short period, remaining infective for a few days, or at most for a few weeks. However, as long as the aetiological agent is not known, the epidemiological picture remains unclear.

No specific therapeutic measures are known to be of definite benefit, although chlortetracycline seems to shorten the febrile course. However, the drug is ineffective once suppuration has set in. Puncture of the suppurative lymph nodes may hasten recovery and in some cases their surgical removal is indicated.

REFERENCES

ARMSTRONG, CH., W. B. DANIELS, F. G. MACMURRAY and H. C. TURNER, *J. Amer. med. Ass.*, 161 (1956) 149.
DANIELS, W. B. and F. G. MACMURRAY, *J. Amer. med. Ass.*, 154 (1954) 1247.
DEBRÉ, R. and J. C. JOB, *Acta paediat. (Uppsala)*, 43 Suppl. (1954) 96.
DEBRÉ, R., M. LAMY, M. L. JAMMET, L. COSTIL and P. MOZZICONACCI, *Bull. Soc. Méd. Hôp. Paris*, 66 (1950) 76.
HEDINGER, C., *Schweiz. Z. allg. Path.*, 15 (1952) 622.
KALTER, S., J. E. PRIER and J. T. PRIOR, *Ann. intern. Med.*, 42 (1955) 562.
MOLLARET, P., J. REILLY, R. BASTIN and P. TOURNIER, *Bull. Soc. Méd. Hôp. Paris*, 66 (1950) 424; *Presse méd.*, 58 (1950) 1353; 59 (1951) 681; 701; 64 (1956) 1177.
PRIER, J. E., *Ann. N. Y. Acad. Sci.*, 70 (1958) 650.

9

N. GOLDBLUM

B virus infection

B virus infection in man is an acute encephalomyelitis which is usually fatal. Sabin and Wright (1934) first recorded a fatal case of B virus infection in man acquired through a bite of an apparently normal monkey. Within 3 days localized lesions developed at the site of the bite and were followed by regional lymphangitis and adenitis. A week later neurological signs ensued and an acute ascending myelitis developed. The patient died in respiratory failure. A filterable neurotropic agent was isolated from the brain, cord and spleen and was designated "B virus". A second fatal case, presumably infected by contamination of a wound with monkey saliva, was later reported by Sabin (1949). During the last few years several additional cases have been reported (Pierce *et al.*, 1958; Nagler and Klotz, 1958; Hummeler *et al.*, 1959). The only case on record, of recovery from what was presumably B virus aetiology, was reported from England (Breen *et al.*, 1958).

B virus *(Herpes virus simiae)* is 125 millimicrons in size. It is very susceptible to the action of formaldehyde, being inactivated in 48 hours at 36° by 4000 times diluted formaldehyde.

It is best preserved by freezing at −70°, or by lyophilization. B virus is closely related antigenically to the virus of herpes simplex *(Herpes virus hominis)* and to pseudorabies virus. It is highly pathogenic to rabbits by any route of inoculation; fatal paralysis follows 5 to 12 days after inoculation. A typical finding is the presence of eosinophilic intranuclear inclusion bodies in the nerve cells. Infant mice are also susceptible to infection. B virus grows readily and produces pocks on the chorioallantoic membrane of developing hen's egg. It grows in tissue cultures (rabbit kidney cells, monkey kidney cells and HeLa cells) causing typical balooning of the cells and the formation of giant cells.

The clinical features of B virus infection in man are those of an acute and fatal encephalomyelitis. The incubation period is between 10 to 21 days. The duration of illness prior to death has varied considerably, ranging from 1 day to 3 weeks. Pierce *et al.* have reported a fatal case in which there was no history of monkey bite 4 months prior to death. Death was sudden after an illness lasting less than 3 days. The clinical signs were more like those of a descending, than of an ascending, type. It is assumed that infection occurs through the nose, mouth or eye.

The main pathological findings in man are extensive changes and necrosis in the brain and spinal cord. Intranuclear inclusion bodies are occasionally found. Histologically diagnosis may be confused with herpes simplex encephalitis, owing to the similarity of the inclusions. Laboratory diagnosis is made by the isolation of the virus from the central nervous system.

Human infection is acquired through the bite of apparently "normal" monkeys or by contamination of wounds or mucous membranes by the saliva or tissues of monkeys. Melnick and Banker (1954) and Hull *et al.*, (1958) isolated B virus directly from the central nervous system of Rhesus monkeys. The disease in monkeys is probably inapparent or mild. Antibody studies indicate that both *Rhesus (Macaca mulatta)* and *Cynomolgus (Macaca irus)* monkeys are frequently infected by B virus. Antibody studies carried out in various monkey colonies showed that 20 to 80 % of monkeys have antibodies to B virus. Recently the danger of acquiring B virus infection has become greater, owing to the widespread use of monkeys and monkey kidney cell cultures for virus research and especially vaccine production. Wood and Shimada (1954) were the first to report the occurrence of B virus in monkey kidney cell cultures. Thus, protection of laboratory workers and individuals handling monkeys and monkey kidney tissue cultures has become a major problem. Control of B virus infection is based on the reduction of contact with monkeys, on the wearing of protective clothing and on the use of strictly aseptic techniques in the handling of monkey kidney tissue cultures.

REFERENCES

HULL, R. N. and J. C. NASH, *Amer. J. Hyg.*, 71 (1960) 15.
HUMMELER, K., W. L. DAVIDSON, W. HENLE, A. C. LABOCETTA and H. G. RUCH, *N. Engl. J. Med.*, 261 (1959) 64.
SABIN, A. B. and A. M. WRIGHT, *J. exp. Med.*, 59 (1934) 115.
WOOD, W. and F. T. SHIMADA, *Canad. J. publ. Hlth.*, 45 (1954) 509.

CHAPTER IV

FUNGAL DISEASES

A.   Superficial mycoses

B.   Deep mycoses

A. Superficial Mycoses

1

F. RAUBITSCHEK

Introduction

Pathogenic fungi responsible for the superficial or deep mycoses of man and animals are classified either according to the tissues they invade or according to accepted taxonomic rules. Those organisms which cause deep mycoses attack living cells and the lesions they produce in different structures are often pathognomonic for the causative species. The fungi which parasitize the horny tissues of the skin, are called dermatophytes, and they practically never attack living cells. The host–parasite relationship of the superficial mycoses is unique and is imperfectly understood; it does not necessarily conform to the usually accepted microbiological and pathogenetic conceptions.

2

Dermatophytes

Three genera of dermatophytes are recognized: *Trichophyton, Microsporum* and *Epidermophyton*. The last is exclusively anthropophilic, whereas the other two include both anthropophilic and zoophilic species. Epidemic spread in humans has occasionally been traced to direct or indirect contact with wild or domestic animals which were either diseased or acted as fungus carriers. The species of this group all have a peculiar preference for fully keratinized dead tissues. They live in the horny layer of the skin, or in the keratinized parts of nail, horn, hoof, hair and feather, in the form of branching hyphae.

Reproduction is by arthrospore formation. Microscopic examination of diseased tissue, cleared with KOH solution, usually reveals the fungus elements, but the identification of species is not possible in this "parasitic (life) phase". In the "saprophytic phase", on relatively simple culture media, characteristic colonies are produced. These contain various pigments and more or less complicated aerial fructification structures by which the species may be identified.

With the exception of one, or possibly two, organisms found in certain soils, the epidermal structures of man and animals just mentioned are the only known natural habitat of dermatophytes. These fungi are extremely resistant to adverse external influences and infected scales or hair kept in test tubes for periods of up to 18 months readily yield cultures when they are inoculated into suitable media.

The clinical lesions produced by dermatophytes are usually scaly, with very little inflammatory response. Certain organisms may, however, cause suppurative and granulomatous reactions. The mechanism leading to these reactions is not clearly understood. No actively secreted toxic or irritating substance, which might damage epidermal cells or diffuse through the unaltered epidermis, has yet been isolated. The primary clinical lesions of dermatophytosis (syn: epidermophytosis, tinea, ringworm) is a round, scaly patch, which spreads centrifugally and shows a tendency to central involution. Adjacent lesions may coalesce to form large polycyclic plaques. Sometimes small vesicles or pustules appear on the border or other parts of the lesion. The confluence and rupture of such vesicles may produce a denuded, moist or crusted surface. In hairy regions the fungi may invade the hair follicles and penetrate the hair shaft. The hair then quickly becomes filled with fungus elements, and in some types it is surrounded by a dense sheath of spores. Since the fungus extends downwards only into hair substance which is fully keratinized and does not invade the hair bulb or papilla, the hair continues to grow. When it is heavily parasitized, the hair loses its resilience and breaks off at, or somewhat above, the skin level. Most ringworm lesions therefore appear hairless, but on closer inspection many broken hairs can be seen projecting from the follicles or embedded in the scales or crusts. *T. schoenleini*, which causes favus in man and in some animals, is the only dermatophyte which may directly damage the hair papilla. After a certain period, due to an unknown mechanism, atrophy of the hair follicle and the surrounding skin occurs. The result is permanent baldness.

Hairs infected by some fungi fluoresce under specially filtered ultraviolet light (Wood's light), a fact which can assist in detecting early infections.

The susceptibility of the horny structures of man and animals to fungal attack is influenced by a variety of factors. Hair-bearing skin is affected mainly in young animals or humans, and in many cases the condition either clears up or ceases to spread when the host attains sexual maturity. On the other hand infection of certain other sites in humans seems to occur only at about puberty or during adult life. Hormonal influences may thus play an overall governing role. Nutritional factors may also affect the morbidity, as is suggested by the varying incidence of *tinea capitis* among children of different ethnic groups with different dietary habits. In animals the disappearance and reappearance of ringworm lesions has been induced by changing from a full to a deficient diet. The mechanism of such influences is unknown. When the fungus causes a more intense inflammatory reaction, sensitization of the skin of the whole body usually occurs. Concomitantly the skin shows a pronounced tendency to rid itself of materials containing the fungus, and infected hairs may then be spontaneously expelled from their follicles. This process sometimes leads to spontaneous cure. After healing, superficial lesions or hair infections which are only mildly inflammatory or are not inflamed at all leave no trace, whereas the more inflammatory granulomatous and kerion (abscess-like) types, in which deep tissue has been destroyed, heal with scar formation. In animals heavy itching sometimes occurs, which may, by interfering with normal feeding and sleeping habits, lead to considerable deterioration of the general health.

Infection takes place by the transmission of materials containing the fungus, such as scales or hairs. In view of the feeding and other habits of some animals, the localization of lesions about the face, on the hindquarters, or on the saddle area is understandable. Indirect transmission of infected materials by means of leather objects, chains, doorposts and fences, on which animals rub themselves either accidentally or in order to relieve itching, has been described. Infected material on the clothing of personnel handling animals can be transferred to other humans. Rats and mice may take part in the transfer of the infection by contaminating animal fodder and bedding straw, without themselves being infected. Some epidemics recurring in the same area after an interval of a few seasons have been traced to soil or to some inanimate object on which previously deposited fungi had remained viable for long periods of time.

In those animals in which spontaneous cure does not occur at sexual maturity the infection usually spreads. The deterioration of general health may necessitate the animal's destruction. Therapeutic measures are mainly directed towards stimulating the desquamation of the keratinous

layers of the skin, thus decimating the fungal population. Most compounds which have antimycotic activity against the saprophytic phase
on artificial media are less effective *in vivo*. They do not reach the fungi,
or they do not possess the same antifungal powers against the parasitic
life-phase, or they cannot be used in sufficient concentration, because
of their irritating and cytotoxic effects on the skin. An antibiotic recently
recommended and called "griseofulvin", is produced by several species
of *Penicillium* and it seems to have promising therapeutic effects when it is
given orally. Human ringworm infections contracted from cattle are
usually very suppurative, especially on the scalp and beard, and tend to
heal spontaneously. Some cases, however, still require X-ray epilation of
the affected area, followed by thorough mechanical epilation and the
prolonged local application of an antimycotic preparation.

Ringworm caused by Trichophyton species

T. mentagrophytes (syn.: *T. gypseum, T. interdigitale*) (Figs. 58, 59, 60 and 61)

This fungus mainly infects *cats* and *dogs; horses*, in which it causes
"girth itch", and *cattle* are occasionally affected. The fungus has been
recovered from lesions in guinea pigs, rabbits, chinchillas, muskrats,
oppossum, foxes, squirrels and even from a kangaroo. The lesions in these
animals vary from single or multiple scaly patches containing broken hairs,
to suppurative or granulomatous lesions. Microscopically the hairs are
seen to be invaded by hyphae and covered with small spores, which either
form chains or a dense layer. No fluorescence occurs under Wood's light.
In humans, however, at least in some geographic areas, the invasion of the
hair is of the *endothrix* type, and no fungal elements are seen on the
surface of the hair. The fungus has been occasionally isolated from soil in
caves and from animal dung, but it is very questionable whether it can
survive for long periods in these materials. The most important reservoir
of this dermatophyte is apparently in pet animals and wild and domestic
rodents, from which the fungus has been repeatedly isolated, even without
evidence of clinical disease. Human infections acquired from apparently
healthy laboratory animals have also been described. These animals very
often show no obvious hair invasion, although the fungus can be recovered by culturing from apparently healthy hairs. It must therefore be
assumed that a few dormant fungal elements carried on the hair, resume

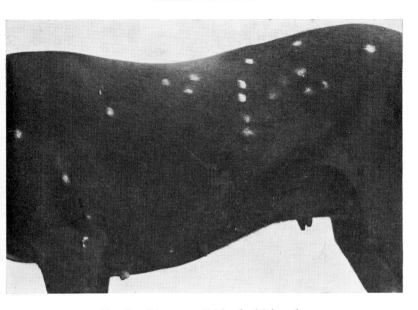

Fig. 58. Ringworm (trichophytia) in a dog.
(Photo: Department of Small Animal Diseases, Veterinary Faculty, State University, Utrecht)

their parasitic way of life when they are transferred to a suitable medium. Minute injury of the epidermis of the recipient is apparently necessary for the production of clinical infection. This, together with the tendency to spontaneous cure, explains the rarity of epidemics involving this organism. Only sporadic infections occur, even in families and close communities.

T. rubrum (syn.: T. purpureum)

In humans this organism produces ringworm of a chronic, very low grade inflammatory type, which is especially resistant to therapy. In cases with extensive skin lesions and involvement of several finger and toe nails, a history of the handling of animals is sometimes obtainable, but the first case of animal ringworm proved to be caused by this fungus in a dog was reported only recently. The owner of the animal suffered from long-standing tinea pedis and apparently infected the animal by scratching it with his bare feet. The organism has also been recovered from one other dog and from two cows. The hairs of the animals were not invaded and showed no fluorescence under Wood's light.

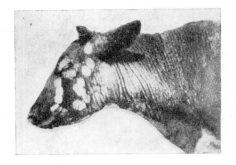

Fig. 59.   Ringworm (trichophytia) in a cow.
(Photo: Department of Internal Diseases, Veterinary Faculty, State University,
Utrecht)

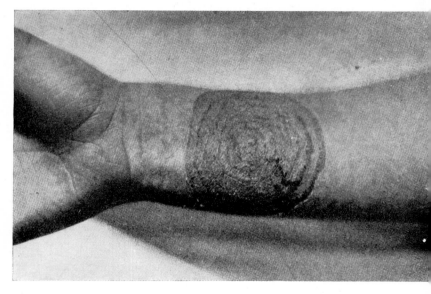

Fig. 60.   Ringworm (trichophytia superficialis) on arm of a farmer. (Photo: Department of Dermatology and Venerology, Medical Faculty, State University, Utrecht)

T. verrucosum (syn.: *T. faviforme discoides, T. album ochraceum*)

This *Trychophyton* species is the commonest cause of ringworm in *cattle*. *Horses, sheep, goats* and *donkeys* are also susceptible. The lesions in young animals of both sexes are mainly situated about the head and rump but

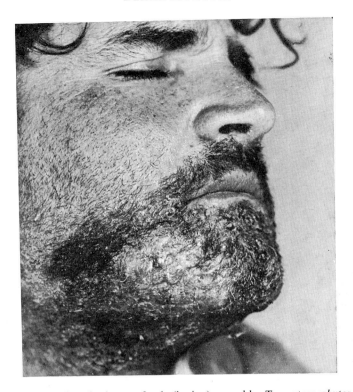

Fig. 61. Tinea barbae profunda (kerion) caused by *T. mentagrophytes*.
(Photo: Department of Dermatology and Venerology, Hadassah-University Hospital,
Jerusalem)

may appear on any part of the body. The lesions are at first round, boggy, hairless, covered with thick, grey scales and crusts and studded with the stumps of broken hairs. After removal of the crusts a red, granulating, moist surface is revealed. The oedema and inflammation later subside, the lesions becoming flat, scaly and hairless. Spontaneous healing often occurs when the animal reaches maturity. In *goats* and *sheep* (Fig. 62) the lesions are similar to those in larger animals, but sometimes the inflammatory reaction is minimal, with large areas of the body surface showing only scaliness and loss of hair. In sheep there are sometimes no distinct lesions, a very mild diffuse scaliness of the skin being the only evidence of infection. However handfuls of wool (hairs) may be easily pulled out and microscopical and cultural examination of these shows that they are heavily parasitized. Wool from such animals should prove inferior in textile manufacture.

Infection in *man* is usually suppurative. In children kerion lesions occur on the scalp, and in adults granulomatous *sycosis parasitaria profunda* may develop in the bearded area. The infection may be contracted as an occupational hazard by milkers who rest their heads on the flanks of infected animals. Infections of the glabrous skin are usually exudative.

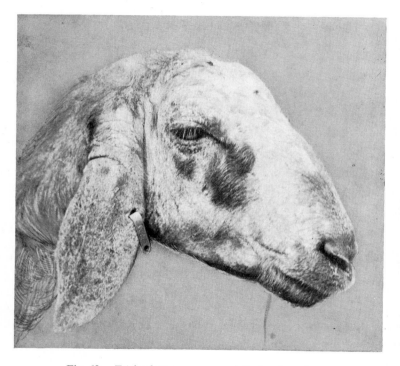

Fig. 62.   *Trichophyton verrucosum* infection in a sheep.
(Photo: Department of Dermatology and Venerology, Hadassah-University Hospital Jerusalem)

Indirect transmission from animal to man, by the various routes previously mentioned, has been described.

Microscopic examination of the infected hairs shows that they are invaded by hyphae and are covered by a sheath of spores. Cultures usually show the first signs of growth only after 2–3 weeks, *i.e.* much later than occurs with other dermatophytes. This fungus grows better at 30°–37° than at 26°, which is the temperature optimal for growth of most dermatophytes.

T. equinum

The organism is closely related to *T. mentagrophytes* and was, until recently, considered by most workers to be a variant of that species. However Georg showed that its different nutritional requirements and its *in vitro* behaviour towards equine and non-equine hair, warranted its classification as a separate species. It almost exclusively infects *equines,* but a dog is known to have been infected, probably by direct contact with diseased horses. The lesions are at first round, hairless, swollen and exudative, and become heavily crusted, dry and scaly when they are old. Intensive itching accompanies the lesions .They may be situated all over the body, head and extremities, but are usually most numerous in the saddle area, hence the name "girth itch" given to the infection. Direct transmission to *man* has occurred, mainly to personnel handling horses. There is no fluorescence of infected hairs under Wood's light. Hyphae and some arthrospores are seen inside the hair and varying amounts of spores, often arranged in longitudinal chains, are found on the hair surface. The cultural and microscopical appearances of the growth are very similar to those of *T. mentagrophytes.*

T. gallinae (syn.: *Achorion gallinae, Epidermophyton gallinae*) (Fig. 63)

T. gallinae causes the so-called favus of *fowls.* Chickens and turkeys are most commonly infected. The infection appears as thick, white crusts on the comb, wattles and cheeks, but it does not attack the feathers. It is mostly a benign disease and healing is spontaneous. The infection is said to be very common among wild birds in certain geographical regions. A dog in continual contact with infected fowls has contracted the disease. Only two cases of proved transmission to *human beings* are known, the best documented case being that of a child who contracted the disease from infected chicks. In this child a superficial type of scaly ringworm developed, with loss of hair on the scalp, but no invasion of the hair could be detected. In cultures the fungus produces a very characteristic red pigment which diffuses into the agar.

References p. 464

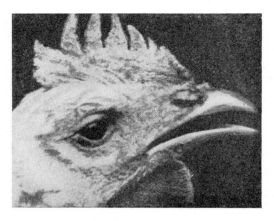

Fig. 63. "Favus" of chicken.
(Photo: Institute for Parasitic Diseases, Veterinary Faculty, State University, Utrecht)

T. schoenleini (syn.: *Achorion schoenleini*)

This dermatophyte is the cause of favus of *cats, dogs, rats* and *mice*. Infected animals usually show greyish, cup-like, dry crusts which adhere to the skin. These crusts are pierced by greyish, lustreless hairs, which can be easily pulled out. The skin beneath the crusts is inflamed and thin. If the disease persists, large areas of the skin become atrophic and scar-like, with loss of follicular pattern. In *children* the disease usually starts with scale patches on the scalp, which often develop pustules due to secondary bacterial infection. Saucer-shaped, sulphur-yellow, dry, adherent crusts, called "scutula", appear later (Fig. 64). Round, scaly, erythematous lesions of *tinea circinata* may develop on the glabrous skin. In severe and neglected cases the skin may become covered with very large scutula, there may be general adenopathy, and the glands may break down to form abscesses and fistulae. Deterioration of general health may then occur. Extensive skin involvement in humans usually occurs among people who live under low hygienic conditions, a circumstance which probably accounts for the contraction of the disease from cats and mice in some cases. However, transmission from animal to humans has not been proved. After successful treatment, bald, scar-like, hyper-pigmented and hypo-pigmented areas *(alopecia post-favosa)* may remain. The atrophic process is probably due to a toxic principle secreted by the fungus and first manifests itself by a loosening of infected hairs and later by progressive

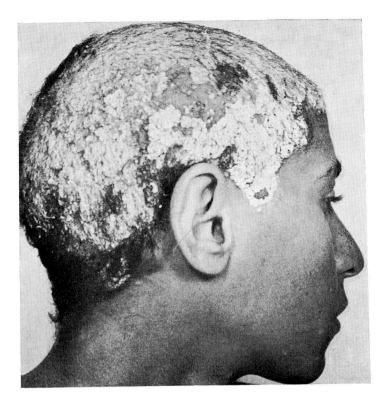

Fig. 64. Favus caused by *T. schoenleini* in a child.
(Photo: Department of Dermatology and Venerology, Hadassah-University Hospital, Jerusalem)

atrophy of the hair papillae and follicles. Since the crusts or "scutula" mainly consist of fungal elements, a similar mechanism presumably causes the atrophy of the underlying skin. The same principle may cause deterioration of the general health of the animal, sometimes terminating in its death. *T. schoenleini* thus behaves differently from other trichophyton organisms. There is, however, no experimental or other proof that it actually secretes a toxin.

On microscopic examination in KOH solution the infected hairs show *endothrix* invasion by fungal elements of various shapes which are, if the hair is examined immediately, usually surrounded by a mantle of gas. On standing, this gas disappears. The gas is probably CO_2 which is later absorbed by the alkali. Fungal elements are also found around the hair and in the horny lining of the follicle. The scutula consist of fungal growth intermingled with epidermal detritus and amorphous matter. Under Wood's light hairs infected with favus usually show a greenish-grey, dull fluorescence.

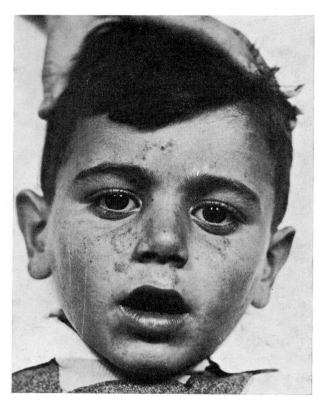

Fig. 65.   Tinea corporis caused by *T. megnini* in a child.
(Photo: Department of Dermatology and Venerology, Hadassah-University Hospital, Jerusalem)

T. megnini (syn.: *T. rosaceum, T. vinosum*)

This rare fungus is a cause of ringworm in *cattle* and *dogs*. The lesions in *man* (Fig. 65) and animals do not differ from those caused by other species of *Trichophyton*. Microscopically the hairs show an *ectothrix* type of invasion, with hyphae inside the hair and a dense sheath of rather large spores surrounding it. There is no fluorescence under Wood's light.

Ringworm caused by Microsporum organisms

M. audouini

Although in many countries this organism is the major cause of epidemics of *tinea capitis* amongst *children,* infection in animals has rarely been described. Some human cases have been traced to dogs and monkeys. In these animals, as in humans, the lesions are either scaly and hairless, or inflammatory and crusted. Broken hair stumps protrude from, or are embedded in, the scales or crusts. Under Wood's light the infected hairs show a bright bluish-green fluorescence. The fluorescent material can easily be extracted from the hair by hot water. Cultures of the fungus do not, however, fluoresce. Recent experiments have shown that a water soluble, mostly crystalline, fluorescent material can be extracted from keratinous structures of normal mammals, even though these tissues them-

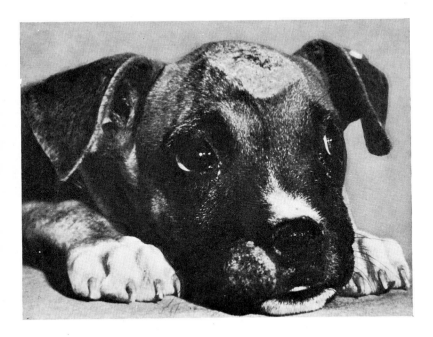

Fig. 66. *Microsporum canis* infection in a dog.
(Courtesy: U.S. Public Health Service, Communicable Diseases Center, Mycology Unit, Chamblee, Ga.)

References p. 464

selves do not fluoresce. The fluorescent effect may therefore be due to some chemical influence of the fungus upon the hair.

Microscopic examination shows that the infected hairs contain hyphae and are surrounded by a dense sheath of small spores, hence the generic name of the organism.

M. canis (syn.: *M. lanosum, M. felineum, M. equinum*) (Fig. 66)

This fungus is the commonest cause of ringworm of *cats, dogs* and other small animals, such as *monkeys* and *chinchillas,* and occasionally of *horses.* It has been observed in adult and young *lions* as a zoo-epidemic. Young animals are most susceptible to infection. The lesions may occur anywhere on the animal's body and are sometimes accompanied by severe itching. They appear as round, scaly, erythematous patches containing many broken hair stumps. Some lesions are more exudative, boggy, and covered with crusts. Infection in children tends to be of the more suppurative-kerion type. Under Wood's light infected hairs show a bright yellowish, green fluorescence. Microscopic examination reveals hyphae inside the hair and a surrounding dense mosaic-like sheath of small spores.

The fact that apparently healthy cats can be carriers of the fungus is of epidemiological importance. In some suspected animals, hairs that were normal by examination with the microscope and Wood's light have nevertheless yielded positive cultures.

M. gypseum (syn.: *M. fulvum, Achorion gypseum*) (Figs. 67, 68 and 69)

This organism causes ringworm in *cats, dogs, mice, rats, monkeys* and occasionally in *horses* and *humans.* The lesions are circular, scaly patches, which appear to be hairless because the hairs break off at skin level. Some lesions show a more acute reaction, with exudation and crusting, especially at the borders. In some cases the crusts resemble the scutula of favus lesions. Under Wood's light infected hairs usually show a slight greyish fluorescence or none at all. Microscopic examination reveals hyphae inside the hairs and a surrounding dense mosaic-like sheath of rather large spores. *M. gypseum* grows much more rapidly on culture than do other fungi belonging to the genus *Microsporum.* The fact that soil may be its normal habitat is of epidemiological importance. Tinea due to this organism is comparatively rare in humans. It appears probable that

463

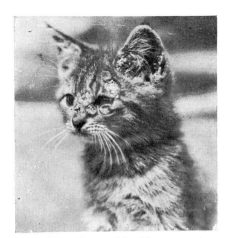

Fig. 67. "Favus" caused by *M. gypseum* in a cat.
(Photo: Department of Small Animal Diseases, Veterinary Faculty, State University, Utrecht)

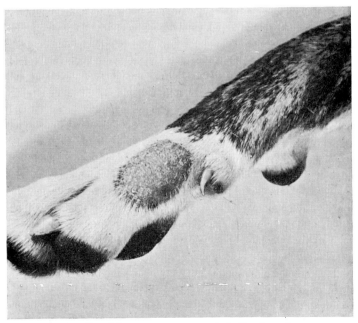

Fig. 68. *Microsporum gypseum* infection in a dog.
(Courtesy: U.S. Public Health Service, Communicable Diseases Center, Mycology Unit, Chamblee, Ga.)

References p. 464

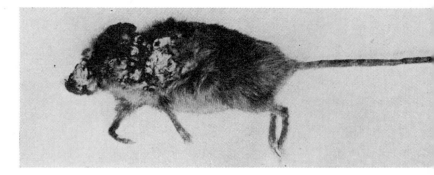

Fig. 69.   "Favus" caused by *Microsporum gypseum* in a mouse.
(Photo: Institute for Veterinary Pathology, State University, Utrecht)

animals become infected from contaminated soil and transfer the disease
to other animals, and occasionally to humans.

REFERENCES

BLANK, F., J. L. BYRNE, P. J. G. PLUMMER and R. J. AVERY, *Canad. J. comp. Med.*, 17 (1953) 396.
DUNCAN, J. T., *Brit. Med. J.*, II (1945) 715.
EMMONS, CH. W., *Trans. N.Y. Acad. Sci.*, 14 (1951) 51.
GENTLES, J. C. and J. G. O'SULLIVAN, *Brit. Med. J.*, II (1957) 678.
GEORG, L. K., *Trans. N.Y. Acad. Sci.*, 18 (1956) 639.
GEORG, L. K., *Vet. Med.*, 49 (1954) 157.
GEORG, L. K., W. KAPLAN and L. B. CAMP, *J. invest. Derm.*, 29 (1957) 27.
GORDON, M. A., *The Aub. Vet.*, (1951) 14.
KAPLAN, W. and R. H. GUMP, *Vet. Med.*, 53 (1958) 139.
LURIE, H. J. and M. WAY, *Mycologia*, 49 (1957) 178.
MENGES, R. W. and L. K. GEORG, *Publ. Hlth. Rep. (Wash.)*, 72 (1957) 503.
MUENDE, I. and P. WEBB, *Arch. Derm. Syph. (Chicago)*, 36 (1937) 987.
SCULLY, J. P. and M. M. KLIGMAN, *A.M.A. Arch. Derm. Syph.*, 64 (1951) 495.
THOMAS, B. A., M. LENNOX and J. T. DUNCAN, *Brit. Med. J.*, II (1945) 346.
TORRES, G. and L. K. GEORG, *A.M.A. Arch Derm. Syph.*, 74 (1956) 191.
VANBREUSEGHEM, R., *Trans. N.Y. Acad. Sci.*, 19 (1957) 622.
VILLANOVA, X. and M. CASANOVAS, *Presse Méd.*, 59 (1951) 1760.
WALKER, J., *Brit. Med. J.*, II (1955) 1430.
WILLIAMS, D. I., R. H. MARTEN and I. SARKANY, *Lancet*, ii (1958) 1212.

B. Deep mycoses

1

F. RAUBITSCHEK

Introduction

The deep mycoses are caused by a variety of fungi which are not taxonomically related. They occur in both animals and man, but direct transmission from one mammal species to another seems to be exceptional. In the last two decades much new knowledge has been gained of the epidemiological aspects of these diseases and of the biology and natural habitats of the organisms which cause them. Most of the fungi which cause deep mycoses are normally found in certain soils, or as saprophytes on vegetable matter. Disease in humans and in animals occurs by the introduction of the organism with dust through the respiratory tract or through injuries on the skin. The primary complex of the disease accordingly appears either in the lungs or the skin, and in the regional lymph nodes. In both humans and animals a generalization which is usually fatal may occur with involvement of all the internal organs.

Most of the deep mycoses occur in very restricted localities. It is not surprising to find that such wild animals as rodents living in these endemic areas are affected by asymptomatic or almost asymptomatic forms of the disease, but they nevertheless excrete large numbers of highly viable fungi into the soil. The virulence of the organism is thus maintained by repeated passages through animals.

The deep mycoses comprise *Coccidioidomycosis, Histoplasmosis, Blastomycosis* and *Sporotrichosis*. Further groups of fungous diseases affecting mammals are caused by yeast-like fungi and actinomycetes, and are hardly to be considered zoonoses. These organisms occur as normal saprophytes in the digestive, and sometimes the respiratory tract of a high percentage of healthy humans and animals. Severe local or general injury, serious disease or hormonal disturbance, may profoundly lower the resistance of the host and may favour the invasion of tissues by such saprophytes. The organisms may then become virulent parasites. Antibiotics, by suppressing antagonistic microorganisms and at the same time increasing the susceptibility of the host, may bring about a similar change in the behaviour of the fungus. Fungous diseases said to be due to common molds and occurring among certain professional handlers of pigeons and other animals have been insufficiently authenticated.

2

Coccidioidomycosis

In some areas of the U.S.A., *Coccidioides immitis* has been recovered from the soil, especially near the burrows of rodents. It was found that about 15 of the rodents trapped in one endemic area were suffering from a benign, asymptomatic form of the disease. The infection has often been traced to the inhalation of dust. Granulomatous lesions develop in the lungs and lymph nodes and sometimes undergo central necrosis. Rarely the disease may become generalized and prove fatal. Direct transmission between animals, or from animal to man, has not been reported.

REFERENCES

AJELLO, L., R. E. REED, K. T. MADDY, A. A. BUDURIN and J. C. MOORE, *J. Amer. Vet. Med. Ass.,* 129 (1956) 485.
ASHBURN, L. L. and C. W. EMMONS, *Arch. Path. (Chicago),* 34 (1942) 791.
EMMONS, CH. W., *Trans. N.Y. Acad. Sci.,* 14 (1951) 51.

3

F. RAUBITSCHEK

Histoplasmosis

Histoplasma capsulatum produces, in its saprophytic phase, characteristic tuberculate spores, which sometimes make its direct identification in soil samples possible. The fungus has been recovered from soils in the vicinity of abandoned chicken runs in the U.S.A., and in various parts of the world it has been found in caves containing heavy deposits of bird dung. In endemic regions skin sensitivity to histoplasmin has been revealed in a high percentage of apparently healthy humans and cattle. In these areas cattle, horses, dogs, cats and also wild rodents have been found infected. In many humans, as in these animals, the disease follows the inhalation of dust containing the spores. Primary granulomatous foci develop in the lungs and lymph nodes and these are sometimes accompanied by a moderate hyperpyrexia. In the majority of cases spontaneous healing occurs, with fibrosis and calcification of the lesions. Among animals, mainly dogs, and in a few humans, the disease subsequently generalizes and proves fatal. There is then involvement of all the internal organs and lymph nodes with a marked tendency towards involvement of the reticulo-endothelial system. The fever is usually remittent and often it is accompanied by cough, loss of appetite and weight. Epidemic outbreaks of a brief, acute condition, which is self-limited and produces symptoms of an infection of the upper respiratory tract, occurred among persons exploring caves, the floors of which were covered by the dung of wild birds ("Cave disease"). After recovery from this disease there remains a high sensitivity to histo-plasmin. Animals trapped in these areas were free from the disease. It is possible that birds may be carriers of the fungus, or that bird dung may provide a favourable medium for the organism present in soil and dust, keeping it viable for a considerable period of time. Experimental transmission of histoplasmosis from one dog to another has been reported, but the study was conducted in an endemic area and it is possible that the conditions of the experiment activated a latent infection. There is no report of human infection having been acquired directly from diseased animals.

REFERENCES

EDWARDS, P. QU. and J. HILLEBOE-KLAER, *Amer. J. trop. Med. Hyg.*, 5 (1956) 235.

EMMONS, CH. W., *Publ. Hlth Rep. (Wash.)*, 72 (1957) 981.

MENGES, R. W., M. F. FURCOLOLOW, H. W. LARSH and A. HINTON, *J. infect. Dis.*, 9€ (1952) 67.

MURRAY, J. F., H. J. LURIE, J. KAYE, C. KOMINS, R. BOROK and M. WAY, *S. Afr. med J.*, 31 (1957) 245.

RUHE, J. S. and P. D. CAZIER, *J. Amer. Vet. med. Ass.*, 115 (1949) 47.

ZEIDBERG, L. D., L. AJELLO, A. DILLON and L. C. RUNYON, *Amer. J. Publ. Hlth*, 4₂ (1952) 930.

4

F. RAUBITSCHEK

Sporotrichosis

Sporotrichum schencki occurs all over the world as a saprophyte on vegetable matter. It causes sporotrichosis in mules, donkeys and other animals. The disease may also occur as a localized asymptomatic infection in *dogs, cats, wild animals* and *birds*. The incidence of the disease among *humans* has diminished during recent decades, although it was once frequent in European countries, especially in France. Gardeners, florists and those engaged in vegetable processing or in packing objects in straw, are the most liable to the infection. The fungus usually enters the skin at the site of some minor injury and the primary lesions therefore occur mostly on the hands or upper parts of the body. An ulcerative infiltrated area, or sometimes a verrucous or acneiform lesion, develops at the site of entry. The infection spreads to the regional lymph nodes, producing the typical picture of gummatous sporotrichosis. In some animals, but rarely in man, the disease spreads to the lymph nodes, internal organs, periosteum and bones and eventually causes death. In man the disease is usually localized and takes a chronic, benign course. A few cases of transmission from animal to man have been reported. A veterinary surgeon, for example, contracted the disease from a mule on which he operated. Other cases have occurred after the bite of an infected parrot or rat.

REFERENCES

COLLINS, W. T., *Arch. Derm. Syph. (Chicago)*, 56 (1947) 523.
GOUGEROT, H., *Trans. N.Y. Acad. Sci.*, 50 (1950) 1348.
SILVA, M., *A.M.A. Arch. Derm. Syph.*, 65 (1952) 355.

5

F. RAUBITSCHEK

American Blastomycosis

Blastomyces dermatitidis, the causative organism of North American blastomycosis, has so far been found only in infected animal or human tissues. It causes granulomatous and abscess-like lesions in the lungs and thoracic lymph nodes, and occasionally in the viscera and skin, terminating in death. Blastomycosis occurs among horses and dogs. The mode of infection is unknown.

REFERENCES

LEE FOSHAY and A. G. MADDEN, *Am. J. trop. Med.,* 22 (1942) 565.
NEWVERNE, J. W., J. E. NEAL and M. K. HEATH, *J. Amer. vet. med. Ass.,* 127 (1953) 220.
SMITH, M., *J. Amer. med. Ass.,* 116 (1941) 200.

6

F. RAUBITSCHEK

Cryptococcosis - Moniliasis

Torula histolytica (cryptococcus neoformans) (a yeast-like fungus) causes torula meningitis in *man* and mastitis in *cattle*. *Candida albicans* causes moniliasis in *man* and *fowls*. Both organisms occur as normal saprophytes in humans and animals, and on plants. As has been already pointed out, the disease is probably endogenous and is not a true infection. However, an epidemic of moniliasis has been described among workers plucking geese which were contaminated with *Candida*. Maceration, caused by constant contact with water and the wet contaminated feathers, was considered to be a predisposing factor.

Recent clinical and laboratory observations seem to favour *pigeons* as vectors of human torulosis. *Torula histolytica (Cryptococcus neoformans)* has been frequently isolated from the nests and droppings of *pigeons*. It has been claimed that a primary respiratory infection may occur asymptomatically in humans who have had repeated close contact with pigeons. The organism subsequently remains quiescent, but it may resume activity with lymphatic or haematogenous spread, if the host's general resistance is lowered by some disease, such as malignant lymphogranuloma. This conception is supported by accounts of cases of asymptomatic torulomas of the lungs, which were incidentally detected during routine X-ray examination of persons who had been in contact with pigeons. The birds themselves do not develop the disease.

REFERENCES

HUEBSCHMANN, K. and P. FRAGNER, *Dermatologica (Basel)*, 114 (1957) 112.
LERNAU, CH., A. SHAPIRO and M. ASCHNER, *Vet. Med. (Israel)*, 4 (1947) 36.
LITTMAN, M. L. and S. SCHNEIERSON, *Amer. J. Hyg.*, 69 (1959) 49.
PERRUCHIO, P., R. BRUEL, C. LAGARDE and J. DELPY, *Presse méd.*, 67 (1959) 387.

CHAPTER V

PROTOZOAL DISEASES

1

O. THEODOR

Leishmaniases

The leishmaniases are a group of diseases caused by protozoa of the genus *Leishmania* of the family Trypanosomidae. Three main forms of leishmaniasis are generally recognized:

1. Visceral leishmaniasis or kala-azar, caused by *Leishmania donovani*.
2. Cutaneous leishmaniasis or Oriental sore, caused by *Leishmania tropica*.
3. American muco-cutaneous leishmaniasis (Uta, Espundia), caused by *Leishmania brasiliensis*.

While the three parasites are morphologically indistinguishable, their status as species is definitely established by serological and epidemiological evidence and by the characteristic clinical reactions they produce.

Agglutination and precipitin reactions, as well as complement fixation tests, have proved that the three species have both species-specific and common antigens, but that the species-specific antigens are predominant (Chang and Negherbon, 1947).

Visceral leishmaniasis includes a number of epidemiologically distinct forms of disease and it was, in the past, thought that some of them were caused by different species of *Leishmania*. Thus the Mediterranean form was thought to be caused by *L. infantum,* the disease in dogs by *L. canis* and the South American form by *L. chagasi*. All these strains of *Leishmania* are serologically indistinguishable from *L. donovani* and it is generally accepted today that they are, in spite of their epidemiological differences, identical with *L. donovani*.

The leishmaniases can be considered as zoonoses to a varying degree. The Mediterranean form of kala-azar is a zoonosis *par excellence*. It is mainly a disease of dogs, and human beings are infected only sporadically and to a much smaller percentage than are dogs. The Chinese, Central Asiatic and American forms resemble the Mediterranean form in most essential characters (age distribution, infection of dogs), but the disease in China shows, in some places, some resemblance to the Indian form. In the Indian form, however, an animal reservoir has not so far been demonstrated and the age distribution differs markedly from that of the Mediterranean form. The Sudanese form resembles the Indian form in some respects, but differs from it in others. Animal infection with Oriental sore has been demonstrated and it is particularly important and common in wild rodents in Central Asia. Animal infection with South American muco-cutaneous leishmaniasis has been found only rarely and no regular reservoir has so far been demonstrated. However, epidemiological evidence points to the existence of an animal reservoir in the Sudan and in South America, as the disease is contracted during travel through uninhabited areas, or while working in the forest.

The epidemiology of the leishmaniases has to be considered in conjunction with the biology of its vectors, which are various species of *Phlebotomus*.

Phlebotominae (sandflies) are small, hairy flies, 1.5–3 mm in length, which develop in soil, cracks in walls or rocks etc., wherever high humidity and decomposing organic matter create conditions favourable to them. Their development is relatively slow, requiring several weeks per generation in hot climates to several months in cooler climates, so that only a single generation per year appears in China, while several generations a year appear in tropical climates, where development may be practically continuous. Only the female sucks blood.

Their role as vectors has been definitely established by experimental transmissions by bite, and also by epidemiological evidence. No leishmaniasis is known to occur in the absence of *Phlebotomus*. Other theories of transmission which were held until recently, are today only of historical interest.

Adler and Ber (1941) experimentally transmitted Oriental sore to 5 human beings by the bite of *Phlebotomus papatasi*. 26 sandflies produced 28 lesions, of which 18 were produced on a single person by 9 sandflies.

Swaminath, Shortt and Anderson (1942) transmitted *Indian kala-azar* by the bite of *P. argentipes* to all of 5 persons on whom experiments were carried out. In China the disease has been transmitted to 8 out of 47 hamsters by the bite of *P. chinensis* which had been naturally infected on a dog (Chung *et al.*, 1950).

Each of the epidemiologically different forms of leishmaniasis is transmitted by one, or several, species of *Phlebotomus*, which are specifically adapted to the particular strain of *Leishmania* in the area, so that a high percentage of the sandflies become infected by biting and the leishmaniae undergo their specific biological cycle in them. Other species of *Phlebo-*

tomus, on the other hand, have a lower infection rate and the development of leishmaniae in them remains incomplete.

Leishmaniae are parasites of vertebrate animals, occurring in the body wherever cells of the reticulo-endothelial system are found (liver, spleen, lymph glands and bone marrow). They also appear in the peripheral blood in the monocytes and circulating macrophages, and in macrophages in the skin of certain animals (dogs, hamsters), in which they sometimes occur in great numbers.

In the vertebrate they occur in the form of the so-called Leishman-Donovan bodies, (L. D. bodies), which are elliptical cells, 3 to 4 μ long, with a nucleus and a kinetoplast, but without flagellum. In cultures and in the insect-host they assume leptomonad form, that is to say, they become elongated, with the kinetoplast at the anterior end and a long flagellum, but no undulating membrane.

Phlebotomus ingests macrophages containing L.D. bodies with its blood-meal or with tissue fluid. In its stomach the parasites grow flagella and assume leptomonad form. They multiply, move forward, attach themselves to the epithelium of the anterior part of the stomach near the oesophageal valve and later invade the pharynx and the mouth parts. The salivary glands are not involved. The anterior part of the stomach (cardia) often contains a dense mass of flagellates, which apparently fills the cardia completely, so that an analogy has been drawn to the "blocked flea" of plague (Smith *et al.,* 1940). This, however, is not correct. The dilator muscles of the pharynx and cibarium, and the elasticity of the epithelium of the stomach are capable of widening these organs sufficiently to allow the passage of blood, even when apparently completely blocked by parasites. Invasion of the tip of the mouth-parts seems to depend on chemical factors which influence the behaviour of the flagellates. Complete and accurate adjustment of these factors was apparently not obtained in transmission-experiments in the past, and this explains the many unsuccessful attempts to transmit the disease by bite.

During the second, infecting feed the parasites near the tip of the proboscis are passively deposited into the puncture wound. They are then taken up by the macrophages of the host, in which they begin to multiply.

In all leishmaniases diagnosis requires the demonstration of the parasite. In Indian kala-azar examination of blood smears with what Shortt called a "leucocyte edge", has given positive results in 70 to 80% of the cases. In the other forms of kala-azar parasites are too scanty in the blood for this method to be reliable. In these forms examination of the bone marrow by sternal puncture is today the method most commonly used. While spleen puncture is also used, it is less advisable, because of the danger of haemorrhage. Cultures of material obtained by spleen or bone marrow puncture from cases in which parasites are too scanty for direct microscopic demonstration, develop in about 1 week and cultures from peripheral blood in 2 to 3 weeks. The medium used is either N.N.N. or semi-solid blood agar. In Oriental sore material for culture should be taken with a glass capillary from the non-ulcerating edge of the lesion. In dogs either skin biopsy or excision of a small piece of spleen or examination of bone marrow should be carried out (iliac puncture). Examination of cutaneous ulcers of dogs infected with kala-azar is less reliable than examination of the apparently healthy skin. A number of serological tests (formol-gel test and others) have been used and are useful in many cases. They are, however, not specific and should not be relied upon alone.

1. *Visceral leishmaniasis or kala-azar*

This disease is characterized by irregular fever of long duration and by enlargement of the liver and spleen and it is fatal in the majority of untreated cases. It appears in various epidemiological forms in the different areas of its distribution. In most areas it is endemic or occurs sporadically, but in some areas it may from time to time lead to extensive epidemics.

It occurs chiefly in the Mediterranean region, India, China, Central Asia, East Africa and South America.

i. In the Mediterranean region, the disease primarily affects dogs and only occasionally human beings. It occurs throughout the entire region, mainly in the coastal areas, but is very rare in the Eastern parts of North Africa (Egypt). Southern Italy, Sicily, Malta, Greece and Crete are particularly heavily infected. The disease is endemic or sporadic; epidemics are unknown. Thus, the incidence in Catania (Sicily) is more or less static, involving approximately 250 cases per year in a population of over 250,000; about 90 cases per year occur in Malta in a population of 250,000.

Over 90% of the cases occur in children up to 5 years of age, and about 13% in children below one year. Parasites are rare in the peripheral blood, so that they cannot be demonstrated by the examination of blood smears, although they can be seen in blood cultures in the majority of cases. Thus in Italy and Palestine they could be cultivated from the blood in 33 out of 36 cases (91.7%) (Adler and Theodor, 1935).

The incubation period is difficult to determine, because of the usually slow and insidious onset of the disease. It has been shown to last only a few weeks in some cases, but in other cases it may have lasted several months. The main symptoms are an irregular, not very high fever, weakness, emaciation, enlargement of the spleen and liver, together with non-specific symptoms, such as diarrhoea and cough. In some cases there is an acute course with high fever. In a number of cases a dark pigmentation of the skin appears. The blood picture is characterized by leucopenia and anaemia. Progressive cachexia and loss of hair ensue. In the majority of cases, the untreated disease is fatal within several months or in one or two years. The Mediterranean form of the disease is difficult to treat and a marked drug resistance exists.

The main epidemiological feature of Mediterranean kala-azar is the infection in *dogs*, as first demonstrated by Nicolle in Tunis in 1908. Since then a large number of dogs have been found infected throughout the region.

A detailed table of infection rates in dogs in different localities has been given by Brumpt (1949). In most areas it varies between 5 and 10%. In Malta 11% of the dogs were found infected, with an estimated total of 1,500 infected dogs on the island. In a few places higher infection rates have been recorded, but in some localities this may have been due to the selection for examination of dogs with manifest signs of the disease. Infection in dogs is seasonal. The highest infection rates were found in the spring, before the onset of the sandfly season, and the lowest occurred in the winter. Thus in Algiers 7% of the dogs were found infected during the summer and 1% during the winter (Sergent, 1910), in Malta, 4% during the winter and 10% during the summer (Critien, 1911). This indicates that the animals become infected in the autumn and that the incubation period is 5 to 6 months (Adler and Theodor, 1932). The dogs either die off during the winter or some of them may recover spontaneously.

The infection rate in human beings at a given place is always much lower than that in dogs, as is shown by the figures given above for Malta. Infections both in dogs and in man often occur at the same focus of infection.

Thus, 90 dogs were examined in Canea (Crete). Of these 50, which came from parts of the town free from the disease, were found to be not infected. The other 40 came from an endemic focus of the disease, and 9 of them proved infected (Adler *et al.*, 1938).

Dogs may harbour leishmaniae in the bone marrow, liver and spleen without showing external signs of the disease for a protracted period of time. During this stage numerous macrophages containing leishmaniae are present in the apparently healthy skin of 40 to 50% of these dogs. This fact is of primary epidemiological importance, because 80 to 90% of the vector, *Phlebotomus perniciosus,* may become infected by feeding on such apparently healthy dogs. This is a specific phenomenon, since *P. papatasi,* for example, when it feeds on the same dog, becomes infected only at a rate of 6.7 to 20%. The infection rate in sandflies increases progressively as the skin infection becomes more intense. Thus, it increased in one dog, from 15% in May to 80% in October, and in another, from zero in June to 70% in October (Adler and Theodor, 1935).

The chief vector in the Western Mediterranean region is *Phlebotomus perniciosus,* but *P. major* is equally susceptible and gives even higher infection rates. Other vector species are *P. longicuspis* in Algeria, which was found naturally infected to a higher degree than *P. perniciosus* (13.5% in a kennel in which infected dogs were kept). *P. major, P. perniciosus tobbi* and *P. simici* are the vectors in the Eastern Mediterranean. *P. perniciosus* is particularly attracted to dogs and, while, in captivity, only 10% of the sandflies could be induced to feed on man, 50% or more fed readily on dogs (Adler and Theodor, 1935).

During the advanced stages of the disease visible dermal symptoms begin to appear, with emaciation, depilation, scaling of the skin, keratitis and seborrhoea (Figs 70, 71). Together with these symptoms anaemia develops

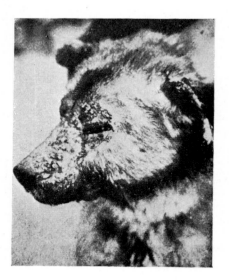

Fig. 70.   Kala-azar, skin lesions in a dog.
(Photo: Prof. I. Snapper; from G. Piekarski, Lehrbuch der Parasitologie, 1954; courtesy Springer Verlag, Berlin-Göttingen-Heidelberg)

ınd the disease is probably fatal in the majority of cases. The disease is
ıarticularly drug resistant in dogs (see below).

The pathological changes have been described in detail by Redaelli
1933) and by Adler and Theodor (1935). The histological changes in the
kin are mainly a selective infiltration of macrophages around hair follicles
ınd sebaceous glands.

In contrast to the high infection rates obtained by feeding sandflies on
logs, the infection rates in *P. perniciosus* fed on severe cases of kala-azar
n man are very low. Thus, only 3 out of 176 *P. perniciosus* (1.7%) and

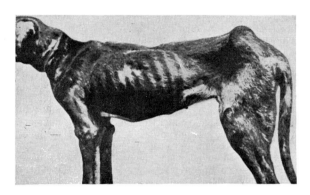

Fig. 71.   Leishmaniasis of a dog in Greece; extreme cachexia, alopecia and skin ulcers.
Photo: Dr. E. Papantonakis, Archiv für Schiffs und Tropen Hygiene, 1936; courtesy
Verlag Joh. Ambrosius Barth, Leipzig)

4 out of 64 (6.25%) became infected. (Adler and Theodor, 1931, 1935).
This may be explained by the fact that parasites are rare in the peripheral
blood and rare in, or absent from, the human skin.

ii. In India, the main endemic area is Assam and Bengal, with foci
along the Eastern coast of the peninsula and an isolated focus in Bombay.
The distribution of the disease closely corresponds to that of *Phlebotomus
argentipes,* as has been shown by Sinton (1925).

The age distribution differs markedly from that of the Mediterranean
form.

According to Napier (1946) only 12.4% of 387 cases occurred in children up to 5 years,
while 50% occurred in children and young adults of 5 to 15 years, and another 12% in
people of 15 to 20 years. McCombie Young (1924) gave a similar age distribution for

17,724 cases in Assam in 1922; 8.65 % of the cases were in children up to 5 years, 40.7 % in the age group of 5 to 15 years and 16% in people from 15 to 20 years.

Another feature peculiar to Indian kala-azar is the occurrence of large epidemics every 15 to 20 years. These outbreaks appeared in the endemic areas, but also invaded new regions. The last such epidemic occurred between 1917 and 1924. Thereafter its periodicity has been disturbed probably as a result of extensive campaigns of control with insecticides (Napier, 1946).

Transmission in India is by *P. argentipes*. Transmission experiments have been mentioned above. The success of these experiments is attributed to the fact that for their second meal the sandflies were fed on fruit juices which enhanced mass development of the flagellates and their tendency to invade the mouth parts.

Parasites are common in the peripheral blood in Indian kala-azar and can be demonstrated in 70 to 80% of the cases by the examination of blood smears. In consequence, infection rates in *P. argentipes* fed on human cases are much higher than those found in Mediterranean kala-azar and may reach 40 to 50%.

In Indian kala-azar areas no infection of dogs or other animals has been found. Thus 2,759 dogs examined in Madras were found to be negative (Patton, 1913). Similarly, 1,150 dogs in Madras (156 from an endemic focus of the disease) examined by Donovan, proved negative.

The common occurrence of parasites in the peripheral blood and the resulting high infection rates of *P. argentipes* fed on human cases suggest that in India man is the main source of infection for sandflies. Another possible source of infection of sandflies is the so-called *post kala-azar dermal leishmanoid*. This is a condition in which nodules containing parasites appear on the skin, generally 1 to 2 years after apparent recovery from the disease. Sandflies have been successfully infected by feeding on such lesions. Blood cultures are usually negative at this stage of the disease.

Indian kala-azar thus seems, as far as our knowledge goes, to be a purely human disease and it cannot be called a zoonosis.

iii. China. The disease is mainly endemic in East China in an area North of the Yangtse River, in part of Manchuria, and it also occurs in some scattered foci as far South as Canton. It is mainly found on the alluvial plains below 200 m altitude. In addition, endemic foci exist in Kansu province and in Sinkiang, forming a connection, however incomplete, with the Central Asiatic endemic area.

Some authors give an age distribution similar to that in India. Thus Young (1923) records 31.5 % of 762 cases in children under 10 years, and 40 % between 10 and 20 years. Patton and Hindle (1926) mentioned 32.2 % of 301 cases from Shantung in children up to 10 years, 32.5 % between 10 and 20 years and 22.8 % between 20 and 30 years. Only 3 children under 5 years were among the 301 cases. These statistics are based on hospital cases and the authors point out that "it is exceptional for Chinese country people to bring such small children for treatment". Wang and Wu (1959) recorded the following figures for Kiangsu province for 1951:

Age:	1–10	11–20	21–30	31–40	over 40 years
Percentage of cases:	33.9	28.9	17.4	11.7	8.1

On the other hand, Ho (1948) states that 95 % of 570 cases in North West China were children under 5 years and of these 89 were less than 1 year old. Chung (1953) records 63 % of 2,051 cases in North China in children under 10 years. Wang and Wu (1959) record 95.4 % of kala-azar cases in Kansu province, 89 % in Hopei in children under 10 years and 90 % of the cases in Shensi province in children under 5 years of age.

Dogs have been found infected mainly in North West China, but also in some areas in East China.

The infection rates recorded vary widely. Most authors give low numbers, particularly in recent investigations. Thus, out of 30,641 dogs examined in Shensi, 133 (0.43 %) were found infected (Li Chi Hsiao, 1957), in Kansu 90 out of 15,873 dogs (0.57 %), and in Tsinghai nearly 1 % of the dogs (Wang and Wu, 1959). The occurrence of human and canine cases in the same locality and sometimes in the same houses has been reported repeatedly, mainly in areas where the disease was prevalent in young children.

On the other hand, higher infection rates have been given for some localities. Thus, Koenigstein *et al.* (1950) record 59 dogs infected out of 100 examined in Hangchow in Chekiang province in 1949, but the authors point out that "the actual percentage will probably be much lower, as most of the dogs received were very emaciated. The better nourished were undoubtedly used for human consumption". This was confirmed by Wang and Wu (1959) who record the examination of 126 dogs in Hangchow in 1950 which all proved negative for kala-azar. The same authors report the examination of 14,109 dogs in Kiangsu province which all proved negative, and only a single dog among 10,368 examined in Anhwei province was found infected. In these provinces the age distribution resembles that of the Indian form.

The disease in dogs in China has a similar course as it has in the Mediterranean, with heavy infection of the skin and depilation and skin lesions in later stages. Parasites are present in the peripheral blood in higher numbers than in Mediterranean kala-azar. They were demonstrated in blood films by Wang (1937) in 9 out of 23 cases and, in a number of cases (Cash and Hu, 1927) in the skin. On the other hand, cases of dermal leishmanoid are very rare.

The transmitting sandfly is *Phlebotomus chinensis*, the distribution of which closely corresponds with that of the disease. Infection rates in *P. chinensis* fed on human beings are higher than they are in the Mediterranean. This is to be expected from the more common occurrence of parasites in the peripheral blood and in the skin. 7 to 19 % of *P. chinensis* became infected when they fed on human cases of kala-azar.

Infection rates in *P. chinensis* fed on dogs were much higher than in those fed on humans. Whereas 76.6 % of *P. chinensis* became infected by feeding on dogs, only 26.5 % of *P. mongolensis* were thus infected. Natural infections in *P. chinensis* have repeatedly been found, sometimes in a high percentage, particularly in the neighbourhood of kennels with infected dogs. Chinese authors have stressed the fact that *P. chinensis* is attracted by dogs, just as has been mentioned above for *P. perniciosus* in Malta. Thus, 1390 sandflies were caught in a dog-kennel during a single night. The fact that sandflies are attracted by dogs was also demonstrated by precipitin tests in which a considerable percentage of blood meals proved to be of canine origin.

Thus two different epidemiological forms of the disease seem to exist in China. Although these are not clearly separated geographically, the Mediterranean type seems to prevail in North-West China and in some parts of North China, while the Indian type is mainly found in Kiangsu, Anhwei and part of the Shantung province. The Mediterranean type of the disease in China is characterized by infection mainly in young children, though its incidence is low, and that it occurs in dogs. On the other hand, the majority of cases of the Indian type occur in older children and young adults, while dogs are not infected. The general incidence of the Indian type is much higher than that of the Mediterranean type.

Wang and Wu (1959) recorded an incidence of 32 % among the population in some villages in North Kiangsu, where cases of canine kala-azar were not found. Such an incidence approaches epidemic proportions, similar to those which are known only from kala-azar areas in India.

iv. In Central Asia the disease exists in an endemic area from Trans-Caucasia to Turkestan. There are large gaps in its recorded distribution

1ere. This may be due to the fact that large parts of the country are desert, 1teppe or mountainous and are either very sparsely inhabited or are unnhabited. Moreover, our knowledge of these areas is very incomplete. The disease is of the Mediterranean type.

According to Petrov (1939), over 90% of the cases are in children up to 6 years and 57% m children up to 3 years. Chodukin (1929) records 60% of the cases in Tashkent and 13% in Samarkand in children up to 3 years and 76 and 84% respectively in children up o 7 years.

In 1925 Chodukin examined 1,272 dogs in Tashkent and found 10.3% infected in May and 1% in November. This seasonal incidence thus closely resembles that in the Mediterranean (Chodukin, 1929, 1930). During 1926 to 1928, 27,092 dogs were examined in Tashkent of which 87 (0.32%) were found infected.

Latyshew *et al.* (1951) reported natural infection with kala-azar in *jackals* n the Vaksh valley in Tadjikistan, from which the settlers apparently icquired the disease.

The sandfly vector in West and Central Asia has not been definitely determined, but it is probably *P. perniciosus tobbi* in Transcaucasia and possibly a subspecies of *P. chinensis* in Turkestan. However, other species, belonging to the subgenus *Larroussius (P. keshishiani, P. smirnovi)* occur in the area, and may prove to be vectors of the disease.

It thus appears that the Mediterranean form of the disease, which is characterized by infection in dogs or jackals and young children, extends from the Mediterranean through the Caucasus and Turkestan into Central Asia and connects up with the Chinese endemic area through Kansu province. (See Map of World Distribution of Leishmaniasis, American Geographical Society, 1954).

v. East Africa. The disease is endemic in the Sudan and there are isolated foci in Kenya, mainly along the Tana River. It here closely resembles the Indian form, but resembles the Mediterranean form in some respects, for example in drug resistance and in the paucity of parasites in the blood. Leishmaniae have been demonstrated in the skin of 11 out of 94 cases examined and an initial lesion containing parasites has been found in some cases (Manson Bahr, 1959). The age distribution resembles that in India and dermal leishmanoid occurs. The disease is predominantly endemic, but small outbreaks of a few hundred to several thousand cases also occur (Kenya, Kitui district).

Several hundred dogs have been examined with negative results.

Isolated natural infections in a ground squirrel and in two gerbils have been recorded by Heisch (1957). Kirk (1956) concluded that no regular animal reservoir has been demonstrated, although a few animals (horses, monkeys) were found infected. He thinks, however, that on epidemiological grounds, such as the fact that people contract the disease while they are travelling through uninhabited areas, the existence of an animal reservoir cannot be excluded.

P. langeroni orientalis has been proved to be the vector in the Sudan with an infection rate of about 2% (Hoogstraal and Dietlein, 1963). *P. martini* has been found infected with *L. donovani* in Kenya (Minter and Wijers, 1963).

Isolated cases of human kala-azar and infection in dogs have been reported from Eritrea. 8 of 86 dogs examined in Asmara were found infected (Batelli *et al.*, 1944). It is thus possible that the Mediterranean form of the disease extends through Arabia into Eritrea.

Although the East African form of the disease resembles the Indian form in many respects, it will probably prove to be a separate epidemiological entity eventually.

vi. The *South American form* of the disease was originally described as being caused by a separate species, *L. chagasi*. Experimental work, however, proved that there is no difference between *L. chagasi* and *L. donovani* and these two forms are today considered to be identical (Cunha, 1938; Adler, 1940).

The disease is widely distributed throughout Brazil, as Penna (1934) proved by biopsies of the liver during a study of yellow fever. One of the important endemic centres is the province of Ceará, where the disease has been studied intensively by Deane and Deane for several years.

The age distribution resembles that of the Mediterranean form of the disease, but the percentage of cases in children under 5 years is lower. Thus, Alencar (1956) stated that 87% of the 231 cases in Ceará were in children up to 9 years and 67% in children under 5 years. Of the 41 cases reported by Penna, 25 were under 5 years, 4 up to 9 years, and 4 up to 15 years.

Infection in dogs has been demonstrated. Deane (1956) found 49 dogs infected out of 936 examined in Ceará (5.2%). Deane and Deane (1954) also found an animal reservoir in a wild canine, *Lycalopex vetulus*, in Ceará of which 4 out of 33 examined proved to be infected. 3 of the infected animals were among 10 caught in an endemic focus of kala-azar. Skin infection was found in 38 out of 49 infected dogs examined (77.5%) and in 3 out of 4 infected *Lycalopex;* skin infection was also established in 7 out of 43 human cases examined.

The sandfly vector in Brazil is *P. longipalpis.* 59 out of 238 *P. longipalpis* became infected when fed on dogs, and all 10 sandflies which fed on *Lycalopex* became infected. Parasites in the peripheral blood are apparently more numerous than they are in Mediterranean kala-azar. They were found by examination of blood films in 4 out of 43 human cases (9.3%). Accordingly, the infection rate in *P. longipalpis* fed on human cases proved to be much higher than it is in sandflies in the Mediterranean. 4 out of 14 human cases were infective for sandflies, and 14.8% of 81 sandflies fed on these persons became infected.

Two main epidemiological forms of kala-azar thus seem to exist:

(1) The Mediterranean form with infection predominantly in young children and dogs. This form is mainly endemic and extends from the Mediterranean through Central Asia into China and also exists in South America.

(2) The Indian form with the majority of the cases between 5 and 15 years, causing extensive epidemics in man but not infecting dogs. In East Africa the disease resembles the Indian form, but differs from it in a number of features.

2. *Cutaneous leishmaniasis or Oriental sore*

Oriental sore is widely distributed in the Mediterranean region and extends through the Middle East into Turkestan and North West India, where it is prevalent mainly in the dryer parts of the plains of the Indus and Ganges. It is found as far east as Delhi. There are isolated foci in Africa (Nigeria, Tchad) and isolated cases in East Asia.

In most areas Oriental sore and kala-azar have different distributions, due to the spread of their vector—sandflies. Thus in India the distribution of Oriental sore corresponds to that of *Phlebotomus sergenti*, and overlaps with the kala-azar area only to a slight extent. In other places where both diseases occur in the same area, close examination still reveals separate distributions. In Canea (Crete), Oriental sore is prevalent mainly in the old walled city, where *P. papatasi* and *P. sergenti* are common, while kala-azar is concentrated mainly in the suburb of Hagios Johannis, where *P. major* predominates (Adler *et al.*, 1938).

According to Deane (1956) the distribution of cutaneous leishmaniasis in Brazil is quite different from that of kala-azar.

Leishmania tropica causes purely local lesions which last for a year or two; it generally confers a persistent immunity and leaves characteristic scars. There are sometimes multiple infections, which are caused either by mechanical transmission, by spread through lymphatic channels or, in some cases, by multiple initial infection. The incubation period is often as short as 2 to 3 weeks, but it may be longer. A small papule first appears, which begins to ulcerate in the center and gradually enlarges (Fig. 72). Parasites are mainly found in the peripheral, non-ulcerating tissue. *P. papatasi* and *P. sergenti* have been shown to be its main vectors. Other species may also be able to transmit the disease (*P. perfiliewi* in Italy?).

Several species of animals have been found infected with Oriental sore (dogs, cats, a bear), but the number of infected animals in an area is always much smaller than that of infected human beings. The localization

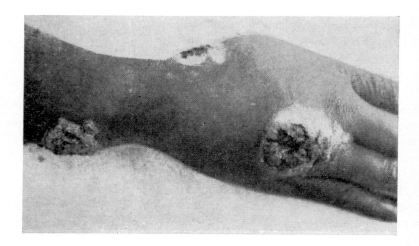

Fig. 72. Oriental sore.
(Photo: Dr. I. Katzenellenbogen, in Handbook of Tropical Dermatology, editor R. Simons, Elsevier, Amsterdam, 1952)

of the parasites in the human skin permits the infection of sandflies without requiring an animal reservoir. It may therefore be assumed that transmission is mainly from man to man.

A different situation apparently exists in Central Asia. Kojevnikov (1941) described two clinical forms of the disease, a rapidly ulcerating "moist" form with a short incubation period, and a non- or late ulcerating "dry" form with a long incubation period. He stated that lesions experimentally produced agreed in type with their parent lesions. It was also stated that the dry, chronic form occurred mainly in towns and the moist, acute form in rural areas. It has been shown that a rodent, *Rhombomys opimus*, acts as a reservoir for the moist form of the disease. 30% of the rodents examined were found to be infected. *P. papatasi* and *P. caucasicus* live in the rodent burrows and transmit the infection among rodents. *P. papatasi* occasionally transmits the disease to man. *P. caucasicus* in Turkestan apparently does not enter houses. 6 to 35% of the sandflies caught in the rodent burrows were found infected. In addition to *Rhombomys opimus*, rodents of some other species were found to be infected with sores on the ears, but less frequently than *Rhombomys*.

Oriental sore in some rural districts of Central Asia is thus definitely a zoonosis. Russian authors consider that the two forms of the disease are caused by different strains of *L. tropica* and state that one type of infection does not confer cross-immunity to the other, so that one strain might cause a zoonosis and the other not. On the other hand, Adler and Katzenellenbogen (1952) showed that the same strain of *L. tropica* (Jericho) can produce different forms of the disease, both ulcerating and "dry" forms, or even a subcutaneous nodule, and that experimental lesions may differ in type from their parent lesions, and also that there was no correlation between the type of the lesions and the length of the incubation period.

3. *South American muco-cutaneous leishmaniasis (Uta, Espundia)*

This disease is widely distributed throughout the South American continent from 30° lat. South to the Yucatan peninsula in Mexico in the North. Clinically it resembles Old World Oriental sore, but in a number of cases metastatic lesions appear in the mucosa of mouth and nose and may cause serious tissue destruction with fatal results (Figs. 73, 74).

Its causative organism, *Leishmania brasiliensis*, can be distinguished from *L. tropica* by serological methods.

References p. 492/493

Fig. 73.   Brazilian leishmaniasis showing noma. (Photo: Instituto O. Cruz, Rio de Janeiro; from Martin Mayer, Exotische Krankheiten, 1924; Courtesy: Julius Springer Verlag, Berlin-Göttingen-Heidelberg)

Fig. 73 ↓   Fig. 74 →

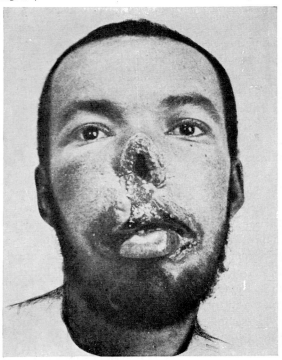

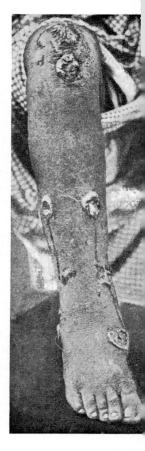

Fig. 74.   South American leishmaniasis.
(Photo: Piraja da Silva; from Martin Mayer, Exotische Krankheiten, 1924; Courtesy: Julius Springer Verlag, Berlin-Göttingen-Heidelberg)

Several species of *Phlebotomus* may be involved in the transmission of this form of leishmaniasis and some of them have been found infected in nature *(P. intermedius, P. migonei, P. pessoai, P. whitmani* and others). Deane (1956) called attention to the close correspondence of the distribution of the disease and that of *P. migonei* and *P. whitmani* in São Paulo and North East Brazil. Aragao (1922) infected a dog by the inoculation of *P. intermedius* previously fed on a lesion.

The fact that the infection is commonly contracted in forests is indicated by some of the vernacular names of the disease (Pian bois, chiclero ulcer). People often become infected when they are travelling through, or working in, the uninhabited forest. The existence of an animal reservoir is thus probable, but it has not so far been demonstrated. Dogs have been found infected, but, as in the Old World, not commonly enough to be considered as the regular reservoir. Other animals (aguti, paca) have been found infected occasionally, but, here also the evidence is not conclusive. There are apparently different strains of *L. brasiliensis*, which do not give cross-immunity against each other, as in the case of the different strains of Oriental sore in Central Asia. These strains also differ in the clinical aspect of the disease, and in the incidence of the lesions in the mucosa of the mouth and nose.

4. *Treatment and preventive measures*

The majority of cases of kala azar are fatal without treatment; Oriental sore disappears after some time without harmful effects except for the disfiguring scars; but South American cutaneous leishmaniasis may have fatal results in cases with serious destruction of tissue of nose and mouth.

This situation has been radically changed since the introduction of antimony therapy in 1915 by Di Christina and Caronia. Pentavalent antimony compounds are today the specific treatment for all forms of leishmaniasis. In addition, aromatic diamidines have recently been used. The majority of cases can be cured if treatment is begun early enough.

Strains of *Leishmania* differ markedly in their drug response. Indian kala-azar responds best to treatment, while Mediterranean and Sudanese strains of the disease require much higher dosages (Kirk and Sati, 1940).

Dogs are apparently highly resistant to treatment, both with pentavalent antimony compounds and with aromatic diamidines. Adler and Tchernomoretz (1946) failed to cure dogs with doses of up to 2 g of 4:4 diamidino–stilbene and up to 15 g of Neostibosan.

Preventive measures should be directed against adult sandflies. It is practically impossible to do anything against the early stages, because they breed deep in the soil, or in cracks in walls, rocks or other inaccessible places. The adult sandflies are, however, highly sensitive to modern insecticides and routine spraying of dwellings with DDT or BHC causes their rapid reduction or disappearance.

Since it is difficult, as has been stated above, to cure dogs, examination of all dogs in an endemic area, and not only of those showing external signs of the disease, is necessary. Infected dogs should be destroyed. Papantonakis (1939) reduced kala-azar in Crete to a few scattered cases by the systematic destruction of dogs.

Similarly, extermination of rodents by the use of chloropicrin in an endemic centre of Oriental sore in Turkestan all but eliminated the disease from the villages of the area.

REFERENCES

ADLER, S., *Mem. Inst. Osw. Cruz*, 35 (1940) 177.
ADLER, S. and M. BER, *Indian J. med. Res.*, 29 (1941) 803.
ADLER, S. and J. KATZENELLENBOGEN, *Ann. trop. Med. Parasit.*, 46 (1952) 25.
ADLER, S. and J. TSCHERNOMORETZ, *Ann. trop. Med. Parasit.*, 40 (1946) 320.
ADLER, S. and O. THEODOR, *Proc. roy. Soc. B.*, 108 (1931) 447; 110 (1932) 402; 116 (1935) 494.
ADLER, S., O. THEODOR and G. WITENBERG, *Proc. roy. Soc. B.*, 125 (1938) 491.
ALENCAR, J. E., *Apres XII Congr. Brazil. Belem. Para*, 1955.
ARAGAO, H. B., *Brasil Med.*, 36 (1922) 129.
BATELLI, C., A. COCEANI and M. ROSSI, *Boll. Soc. ital. Med. Hyg. Trop.*, 4 (1944) 497.
BRUMPT, E., *Précis de Parasitologie*, Vol. I, 1949, p. 270.
CASH, J. R. and C. H. HU, *J. Am. med. Ass.*, 89 (1927) 1576.
CHANG, S. L. and W. O. NEGHERBON, *J. infect. Dis.*, 81 (1947) 209.
CHODUKIN, N. J., *Med. Muisl. Uzbek. Turkm.*, *Suppl. Tashkent*, 1929; *Arch. Schiffs u. Tropenhyg.*, 34 (1930) 423.
CHUNG, H. L., *Chinese med. J.*, 71 (1953) 421.
CHUNG, H. L., L. C. FENG and S. L. FENG, *Peking Nat. Hist. Bull.*, 19 (1950) 301.
CRÈTIÈN, A., *Ann. trop. Med. Parasit.*, 5 (1911) 37.
CUNHA, A. M., *Mem. Inst. Osw. Cruz*, 33 (1938) 581.
DEANE, L. M., *Leishmaniose visceral no Brazil*, Rio de Janeiro, 1956.
DEANE, L. M. and M. P. DEANE, *O Hospital*, 45 (1954) 419.
HEISCH, R. E. *Afr. med. J.*, 34 (1957) 183.
HO, E. A., *Chinese med. J.* (Chinese Ed.), 34 (1948) 295.
HOOGSTRAAL, H. and D. R. DIETLEIN, *Amer. J. trop. Med. Hyg.*, 12 (1963) 165.
KIRK, R., *Trans. roy. Soc. trop. Med. Hyg.*, 50 (1956) 169.
KIRK, R. and M. H. SATI, *Ann. trop. Med. Parasit.*, 34 (1940) 83.
KOENIGSTEIN, R. P., Y. S. CHIU and K. C. TSAI, *Trans. roy. Soc. trop. Med. Hyg.*, 44 (1950) 347.
KOJEVNIKOV, P. V., *Trop. Dis. Bull.*, 41 (1944) 331.
LATYSHEV, N. I., A. P. KRYUKOVA and T. P. POVALISHINA, *Trop. Dis. Bull.*, 51 (1954) 37.
LI CHI HSIAO, *Chinese med. J.*, 75 (1957) 513.
MANSON BAHR, P. E. C., *Trans. roy. Soc. trop. Med. Hyg.*, 53 (1959) 123.
McCOMBIE YOUNG, *Kala Azar in Assam*, London, 1924.
MINTER, D. M. and D. J. B. WIJERS, *Ann. trop. Med. Parasit.*, 57 (1963) 24.

Napier, L. E., *Principles and Practice of Tropical Medicine*, New York, 1946.
Papantonakis, E., *Arch. Schiffs. u. Tropenhyg.*, 43 (1939) 273.
Patton, W. S., *Indian J. med. Res.*, 1 (1913) 1.
Patton, W. S. and E. Hindle, *Proc. Roy. Soc., London, B.*, 100 (1926) 379.
Penna, H. A., *Brasil Med.*, 46 (1934) 949.
Petrov, V. P., *Trop. Dis. Bull.*, 36 (1939) 794.
Redaelli, P., *Richerche sulla Leishmaniosi viscerali del Mediterraneo*, Catanea, 1933.
Sergent, Ed. and Et. Sergent, *Bull. Soc. Pathol. exot.*, 3 (1910) 510.
Sinton, J. A., *Indian J. med. Res.*, 12 (1925) 701.
Smith, R. O. A., K. C. Halder and J. Ahmed, *Indian J. med. Res.*, 28 (1940) 581.
Swaminath, C. S., H. E. Shortt and L. A. P. Anderson, *Indian J. med. Res.*, 30 (1942) 473.
Wang, C. W., *Chinese med. J.*, 52 (1937) 433.
Wang, Ch. Ts. and Ch. Ch. Wu, *Chinese med. J.*, 78 (1959) 55.
Young, C. W., *Chinese med. J.*, 37 (1923) 797.

2

P. H. VAN THIEL

Toxoplasmosis

In 1909 Nicolle and Manceaux described a micro-organism in a rodent, the gondi *(Ctenodactylus gondi)*, in Tunisia, designating it *Toxoplasma*. Splendore observed a similar organism in a rabbit in Brazil. It was only 30 years later that definite evidence was obtained of the role of *Toxoplasma* in human disease (toxoplasmosis). During the early period of observations many different organisms were called indiscriminately *Toxoplasma*, although they undoubtedly were other *Protozoa* or even *Histoplasma*, while others, which we now have ample reason to believe were *Toxoplasma*, had not been recognized as such, being designated by a variety of misnomers.

Jankú (1923) was perhaps the first to observe *Toxoplasma* in man, namely in the eye. The earliest evidence that *Toxoplasma* can infect human beings was offered by Wolf, Cowen and Paige in 1939, who described a case of encephalitis in a child. They demonstrated parasites with the typical morphology of *Toxoplasma* in the tissues and isolated the parasite from rabbits and mice that were injected with infected human brain material.

Morphologically the parasite appears in two forms (Fig. 75).

a. The proliferative form, which multiplies intracellularly in nearly all kinds of tissue cells, both those of the reticulo-endothelial system and those of the parenchyma of various organs, and also in muscle cells. This form is crescent-shaped or oval, with one sharp and one obtuse end, the nucleus being situated near the obtuse end. In the fresh state, these forms are from 4 to 7 microns long and about 2 to 4 microns wide. Reproduction occurs by repeated binary, longitudinary fission. When an affected cell is crowded with parasites ("pseudocyst"), it ruptures and releases parasites which then penetrate into noninfected cells.

b. The cyst form, which occurs only in the chronic phase of the infection; it consists of a resilient, thin membrane which encloses hundreds of *Toxoplasma* cells. The diameter of the cyst may reach 7 to about 60 microns.

Cysts have been observed in the central nervous system, the retina and in skeletal and cardiac muscle tissue. According to earlier beliefs, which led to the designation of these forms as "pseudocysts", the cysts were considerably enlarged tissue cells with walls which were merely the distended cell walls. Van der Waaij, however, argued that the wall of the cyst is of parasitic origin, so that it is more apposite to speak of cyst than of

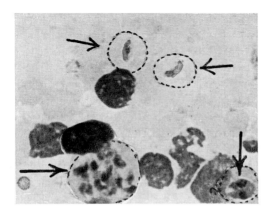

Fig. 75.   Various stages of reproduction of *Toxoplasma gondii* during the acute phase of toxoplasmosis in a mouse.

pseudocyst. He further concluded that possibly an interrelation exists between the encystment of *Toxoplasma* and the appearance in the host of specific defence against it.

Much controversy exists concerning the taxonomic status of *Toxoplasma*. So long as no more arguments are put forward, there is evidence in favour of its inclusion among the "unclassified *Sporozoa*" (van Thiel).

Next to man, a wide variety of animals, including primates, Artiodactyla, carnivores, rodents, marsupials, domestic birds, such as chickens, pigeons and ducks, and wild birds, such as pigeons and crows, may be infected. At first, the species occurring in man was called *Toxoplasma hominis* and those isolated from animals were named after the kind of host animal (*e.g. Toxoplasma canis* from the dog). Sabin established the morphological and immunological identity of *Toxoplasma* of human and animal origin. It then became evident that the causative organism of all forms of mammalian toxoplasmosis was represented by one and the same species, *Toxoplasma gondii*.

The absence of host-restriction in *Toxoplasma* led to a search for possible sources of human infection among lower animals, with the result that a significant correlation was revealed between the incidence of toxoplasmosis in man and its existence in some animals living in his immediate environment. Moreover, it has been shown that toxoplasmosis is enzootic among livestock. According to Hoare and many others, it is a typical zoonosis.

Next to the mouse, guinea pig, golden hamster and rabbit, the following animals have been experimentally infected: the dog and pig, certain rodents *(Mastomys coucha, Citellus citellus)* and the pigeon and canary. Monkeys and albino rats are relatively resistant, although Rhesus monkeys, when they are massively infected, may develop an acute and lethal toxoplasmosis (Mohr *et al.*). Experiments in the U.S.A. showed that a chronic infection can be induced in albino rats (Jacobs and Jones, 1950). However, with the exception of one strain, the author (1956) was unable to corroborate the American results with strains isolated in the Netherlands.

Three successive phases may be distinguished in the development of toxoplasmosis in man and essentially in animals as well (Frenkel and Jacobs): the acute, the subacute and the chronic phase. The rate of this progression varies in different hosts and according to the strain of *Toxoplasma* involved.

In the early *acute phase* proliferative forms of *Toxoplasma* multiply in a variety of the cells of most organs, causing cell destruction, necrosis and inflammatory reaction. Clinically, a febrile illness develops associated with encephalitis, myocarditis, interstitial pneumonitis, hepatitis, splenitis, lymphadenitis and, in man, a maculo-papular skin rash. In women who had given birth to clinically infected infants, no history of symptoms other than lymphadenopathy and fever – if at all – prior to parturition, could be evoked (Siim). This illustrates the difference in reaction to infection between adults and infants *in utero*, the latter frequently succumbing during the neonatal period.

Toxoplasmosis may cause abortion, stillbirth, immature and premature parturition (Makstenieks and Verlinde, 1957). Beverley and Watson (1961) isolated *Toxoplasma* from 15% of 39 aborted sheep foetuses, while no other pathogenic organism could be found.

In cases of asymptomatic infection in the mother, the disease can be diagnosed afterwards only by serological methods, *i.e.* by the complement-fixation test (Warren and Russ), in combination with the Sabin-Feldman dye test. The complement-fixation test becomes positive at a later stage than the dye test, the complement-fixing antibodies disappearing after 6–12 months. The dye test shows a titer which rapidly rises to a high value and falls slowly only in the course of years. A rising titer indicates acute toxoplasmosis. This cannot be achieved by the intracutaneous allergic test, described by Frenkel.

Laboratory animals, if they are infected with a strain virulent for their species, frequently die during the acute stage, pneumonia being the most common cause of death.

Final development of immunity is evidenced by subsidence of the parasitaemia and regression of the signs of infection. This is followed by a decline in the number of the parasites in the tissues and by remission of the lesions in the extraneural viscera.

In the *subacute phase,* however, despite this remission, progress of the infection occurs in the central nervous system, the eyes and occasionally elsewhere. The clinical form of this stage is most commonly encountered in infants infected *in utero,* occasionally in adults and in animals in which antibodies are demonstrable, although immunity is not strong enough to overcome infection of brain and eyes. In infants the disease is mainly characterized by meningoencephalitis, with symptoms of congenital toxoplasmosis which develop from a few days to many weeks after birth, *i.e.* the triad of symptoms: hydrocephaly, retinochorioiditis and cerebral calcifications. Sometimes microcephaly, psychomotor disorders, clonic and tonic spasms, strabismus, nystagmus and microphthalmus are associated with the symptoms just described.

Congenital toxoplasmosis usually pursues a progressive course, nearly always causing the death of the infant within a few weeks or months after birth. When the infant survives, residual effects may be observed in the fundus oculi, connected with visual disturbances, as well as convulsions, epileptiform seizures, hemiplegia, mental retardation, imbecility and debility.

The *chronic phase* is the state in which *Toxoplasma* continues to prevail predominantly in the cystic form. It appears to elicit little or no chemotactic response and may persist for lifetime.

According to Frenkel, cysts may rupture, and intense, necrotizing, inflammatory reaction may then occur. One would expect the number of cysts, their tendency to rupture, and their distribution according to organs

to have a bearing on the production of clinically apparent lesions. Van de
Waaij, however, showed that it is improbable that disintegration of the
cysts would be the cause of the release of toxoplasmas. In fact it may be
assumed that such releases are accomplished by single parasites, each of
which, when it escapes from the cyst, is in turn encysted. This process
would account for the increase in numbers of cysts localized in the mouse
brain and probably also in the brains of other animals as well as of man.

Dye tests are very frequently positive in apparently healthy human and animal popu
lations. Although there are solid grounds for concluding that the dye test is specific
(Mas Bakal, 1960), this does not imply that every positive reaction indicates clinical
toxoplasmosis. Especially low titers ($<$ 1/128), found on repeated examinations, do
not generally prove the existence of an active clinical process, except perhaps when the
eyes are affected. They may, however, indicate an earlier *Toxoplasma* infection.

With regard to the recording of positive dye tests in animals, one should take into
consideration the occurrence of a "*Toxoplasma*-hostile factor" (Jettmar) in the serum o.
sheep (Cathie and Cecil) and of cattle (Mas Bakal). This has not always been done
Consequently the diagnostic signification of positive dye tests may be questionable in
these, and possibly also in other, animals.

The sera of 33 % of 389 horses in Czechoslovakia, Bulgaria and Roumania showed
high titers by the complement-fixation test (Seeman, 1959).

Man, and most probably animals as well, may become infected with the
parasite at a very early age. Makstenieks and Verlinde found that 10 % of
infants in the first 3 months of life had titers caused by antibodies transmitted from the mother to the child through the placenta. After the first
year of life the percentage of children showing antibodies gradually increases, reaching about 15 % in 15-year old ones. This suggests a slow
increase in the frequency of infection with age. According to Van Soestbergen, in 388 soldiers in the Netherlands the titers were: in 36.9 % $<$ 1/4;
in 29.1 % 1/4; in 34 % $<$ 1/100 and in 5.4 % $>$ 1/100 (in 3 it was even
1/256, 1/512 and 1/2048 respectively). Since titers lower than 1/128 may
be found in a relatively high percentage of apparently healthy individuals,
their clinical interpretation in patients showing various signs of illness is
difficult.

Jacobs *et al.* (quoted by Hoare) have shown that, whereas young *dogs*
develop an acute disease of short duration (3 months), in adults the infection runs a symptomless or subclinical course. According to Frankhauser
there are two types of the disease in dogs: (a) the visceral form, characterized by fever, loss of condition, gastroenteritis with diarrhoea, and pneu-

monitis, death ensuing in 2 to 10 weeks; and (b) the nervous form, manifested by psychic disturbances and locomotor disorders. In the brain, lesions of meningoencephalitis are present, but there is no calcification. The parasites invade the intestinal wall, producing ulceration of the mucosa, whence they escape into the lumen of the intestine and may be discharged with the faeces.

The disease in *cats* is similar to that found in dogs (Olafson and Monlux).

In *cattle* the infection may pursue an acute course, with fever, dyspnoea and extreme weakness, as well as of central nervous disorders. The pathological changes include necrotic foci and calcifications (Sanger *et al.*).

Toxoplasmosis in *pigs* is of the same type as that found in cattle. In an epizootic outbreak with 50% mortality observed in the U.S.A. (Cole *et al.*, 1954), the disease was manifested by symptoms of debility, pneumonia, lack of coordination and enteritis with diarrhoea, but fever was absent.

According to Cole *et al.* the disease in *sheep* is characterized chiefly by symptoms referable to the respiratory and central nervous systems, with necrotic and granulomatous lesions in the corresponding organs.

Nothing is known of clinical manifestations in *horses*.

Toxoplasmosis occurs in wild *hares* as an acute, fatal systemic disease. Light or subclinical cases are seldom seen. The post-mortem picture is very characteristic; the lungs are oedematous and hyperaemic and there is a large amount of reddish serous fluid in the chest. The liver, spleen and mesenteric lymph nodes are enlarged and show necrotic foci (Christiansen and Siim in Denmark).

In *rabbits* the disease has an insidious onset, with emaciation, fever and sometimes subnormal temperatures, frequently with discharge from the eyes, muscular weakness, convulsions and probably encephalitis; in the liver necrotic foci have been found. The animals often die unobserved in their burrows. Latent inapparent infections may be most common (Lainson, 1955).

The most constantly observed lesions in *fowls* are those of pericarditis and myocarditis, encephalitis and ulcerating gastroenteritis (Erichsen and Harboe). Ratcliffe and Worth (1951) recorded the death of 13 mammals and 14 birds from toxoplasmosis in the Philadelphia Zoological Gardens over a period of 10 years.

Undoubtedly, more than one mode of transmission of the parasite exists. Because in animals and in man suffering from acute toxoplasmosis the parasites may be present not only in the internal organs and blood, but also in the faeces, urine, sputum, saliva and nasal and throat secretions. infection may be considered, theoretically at least, to be the result of close aerogenic or enterogenic contact with these excreta and secretions, or on the ingestion of food on which the latter have been deposited. Experimentally, however, it is difficult to transmit infection to a healthy animal, e.g. a mouse or rabbit, by bringing them into close contact for several months with animals suffering from acute or chronic toxoplasmosis, although von Kunert and Schmidtke (1954) succeeded in doing this by spraying peritoneal fluid containing proliferative toxoplasmas into cylinders holding mice or guinea pigs whose eyes had been protected.

The experiments of Wildführ (1956) and van der Waaij (1960) show that suspensions of free, proliferative, virulent toxoplasmas withstand desiccation poorly, namely, for only 8 hours at 18–19°; cysts, however tolerate drying at the same temperature for 26 hours.

Aerogenic transmission of toxoplasmas most probably occurs by short distance aspiration of infected sputum. It is hardly conceivable that aerogenic transmission of cysts should play a significant epidemiological role.

Because contact between the scarified skin of a test animal and free toxoplasmas leads to infection, animals and man may become infected through abraded or wounded skin or mucous membranes, or after they have been scratched, bitten or licked by animals excreting toxoplasmas (Makstenieks and Verlinde, 1957).

When dressing infected rabbits and hares, contamination of the hands and consequent conveyance of the parasites to the mouth is likely to take place.

Other routes of infection, such as the internasal (Roth) and conjunctival paths (Fialho), have also been suggested.

The parasites survive for long periods in a dead animal. If they are enclosed in cysts in rabbit carcasses, they will remain viable for as long as the rabbit is kept refrigerated or hanging at room temperature before it is eaten.

There is no consensus of opinion on the possibility of the oral infection of man and animals with *Toxoplasma*. This path does not lead easily to infection with free toxoplasmas, unless they penetrate into lesions of the mucosa of the mouth, throat or oesophagus, or eventually into the intact mucosa. The parasites are quickly destroyed by the hydrochloric acid

pepsin of the gastric juice at 37° (Holz and Bringmann, Schmidtke, Kozar
et al.). On the other hand, consumption of tissues containing cysts will
readily lead to the infection of laboratory animals. Cysts in meat and
other animal tissues may, therefore, be considered responsible for the oral
infection of man and animals.

In houses in which man, dog or cat alike suffer from toxoplasmosis,
these domestic animals will not always be the source of the human
disease; possibly all of them acquired the infection by eating undercooked
meat containing cysts (van Thiel and van der Waaij, 1955). De Roever-
Bonnet (1957) succeeded in cultivating Toxoplasma from the brains of 4
out of 31 sheep that had been declared fit for consumption. However, the
presence of toxoplasmas in the brain and lung does not by itself indicate
their prevalence in the skeletal muscles. Weinman and Chandler succeeded
in infecting pigs by feeding to them garbage from pigs or rats infected with
Toxoplasma. Jacobs (1957) infected mice by feeding the sediment from
the digested diaphragm muscles of 8 out of 50 pigs and of 4 out of 86
sheep.

High dye test titers in a group of vegetarians suggest a mechanism other
than by ingestion of meat, by which Toxoplasma infection may be
acquired (Jacobs).

In transmission experiments with maternal milk, young mice became
infected only after the mother had contracted an active generalized infection (Eichenwald), but when the mother mice were chronically infected,
no infection occurred (van der Waaij).

The transplacental transmission of Toxoplasma has been studied in
mice, and positive results were invariably obtained when the mother
animal had been contaminated during the first half of pregnancy; infection of the mother mouse during the second half of pregnancy never led to
infection of the foetuses. Piglets are congenitally infected only when the
sow is infected before the 84th day of pregnancy (Sanger et al.).

On the basis of experiments by van der Waaij, it may be assumed that
congenital infection in man and animals is likely to occur when infection
takes place during gestation, or when chronic toxoplasmosis has been
present before pregnancy, although in the latter instance only a few cysts
may have been formed. In such cases, the specific defense mechanism
will have declined to very low values and this will permit parasites which
have been released from their cysts, to reach the foetus by means of the
bloodstream. The presence of larger numbers of cysts reduces the likeli-

hood of foetal infection, because antibody production is stimulated as a result of the larger amount of steadily liberated *Toxoplasma* antigen.

Toxoplasmosis occurring enzootically in pigs has been observed by Farrell *et al.* in Ohio and by Momberg–Jörgensen in Denmark. Jacobs (1957) described cases in cattle. Epizootics have been recorded by Vivell and Buhn in rabbits and pigs, by Wiktor in tame rabbits and pigeons (80 % of the animals died), by Erichsen and Harboe in chickens and by Momberg-Jörgensen in mink, all of these animals living in captivity. Findley and Middleton and Elton *et al.,* recorded that 30 and 56 % of voles in nature carry the parasite.

Toxoplasma was recovered from 24.3 % of 140 Memphis cats (Jones *et al.*). In Copenhagen 10 out of 54 pet dogs gave significant positive dye test reactions; intestinal ulcers, lined with toxoplasma, were found at post-mortem examination (Siim, 1950). In hares toxoplasmosis has only been observed sporadically (in Denmark 9.4 % of 2,812). Enzootic infections were not found in any area with a large hare population (Christiansen and Siim).

Parasites were recovered from 7 out of 35 cats, from 2 out of 3 domestic ducks, from 3 out of 7 chickens, from 1 out of 16 pigeons and from 7 out of 121 mice *(Mus musculus)* in the immediate neighbourhood of a family in Memphis, which had been exposed to a common source of infection at a fairly recent date. No infections were found in wild sparrows (Gibson and Eyles).

Transmission from animals to man has yet to be substantiated, although many human infections were readily traced to a closely preceding infection of household pets (cat, dog), from which the parasite was isolated. In such cases, however, the possibility of simultaneous infection of man and animal should be borne in mind.

Makstenieks and Verlinde (1957) pointed out the fact that serological examinations yielded more positive results in household cats and dogs near to patients suffering from toxoplasmosis than in such animals chosen at random.

People in England who habitually handle rabbits showed a higher percentage of significant dye test titers than men in other occupational groups (Beverley *et al.*). Human infection by dogs or cats suffering from toxoplasmosis is promoted by man's tendency to close contact with the sick animals, while he is fondling them.

In view of the fact that the parasites persist for rather a long time in the hosts' blood-stream, the infection of blood sucking arthropods is not unlikely. In the intestinal tract of *Stomoxys calcitrans* the toxoplasmas remained viable for no longer than 22 hours at 25° at a relative humidity of 70%; in the bugs *Rhodnius* and *Triatoma* they remained viable for at least 6 days (Woke *et al.*) and in *Pediculus humanus corporis* 7 days. Transmission of *Toxoplasma* adhering to the proboscis is, epidemiologically, at most of incidental significance.

Non-bloodsucking flies may regurgitate toxoplasmas on to the food of man or animals for 2 hours after an infective meal. Toxoplasmas have not been found in the faeces of these flies. Another possible means of animal infection may be the ingestion of contaminated ectoparasites.

Intra-uterine infection from mother to foetus is rather frequent. Postnatal interhuman transmission of toxoplasmosis, however, has not been observed. There is no written evidence of transmission from man to animals.

Climatic conditions may influence aerogenic infection. Collected data suggest that toxoplasmosis is more prevalent in warm, moist areas than it is in cold or hot, dry regions (Jacobs, 1957). In Denmark and Sweden, however, the peak of incidence occurs in the cold season (Christiansen and Siim). We may assume that several as yet unknown ecological factors determine the epidemiology and epizootiology of toxoplasmosis.

Prevention of infection in man (especially in pregnant women) is only feasible by avoiding contact with suspected animals, especially dogs and cats. However, since the clinical picture is not distinct in the majority of cases, the aetiology of the disease will remain unrecognized. In regions where toxoplasmosis occurs in hares or rabbits, the dressing of freshly shot animals should be avoided. Only those animals which have been frozen at —30° and afterwards thawed can be dressed without danger (Christiansen and Siim). Physicians and nurses should be aware that the blood, secretions and excreta of man may be infectious; and the vet-erinarian should take a similar view of the blood, secretions and excretions of such animals.

Meat and offal should be duly cooked before it is eaten.

Neither vaccination, nor the administration of antisera have been tried to increase the specific resistance of animals and man. Congenital toxo-plasmosis is so rare that it does not warrant routine immunization of pregnant women and animals.

References p. 504

REFERENCES

BEVERLEY, J. K. A. and W. A. WATSON, *Vet. Rec.,* 73 (1961) 6.

CATHIE, J. A. B. and G. W. CECIL, *Lancet,* ii (1959) 229.

COLE, C. R., V. L. SANGER, R. L. FARRELL and J. D. KORNDER, *Proc. 15th. Int. Vet. Congr.,* 1954; *N. Amer. Vet.,* 35 (1954) 265.

FARRELL, R. L., F. L. DOCTON, D. M. CHAMBERLAIN and C. R. COLE, *Amer. J. vet. Research,* 13 (1952) 181.

FIALHO, S. A., *Wienn. klin. Wschr.,* 66 (1954) 817.

FRANKHAUSER, R., *Wien. tierärztl. Wschr.,* 38 (1952) 457.

FRENKEL, J. K. and L. JACOBS, *Arch. Ophthal. (Chicago),* 59 (1958) 260.

JACOBS, L., *Publ. Hlth Rep. (Wash.),* 72 (1957) 872.

JACOBS, L., J. S. REMINGTON and M. L. MELTON, *J. Parasit.,* 46 (1960) 23.

JETTMAR, H. M., *Arch. Hyg. (Berl.),* 139 (1955) 33.

JONES, F. E., D. E. EYLES and C. L. GIBSON, *Am. J. trop. Med. Hyg.,* 6 (1957) 820.

KUNERT, H. VON and L. SCHMIDTKE, *Z. Tropenmed. Parasit.,* 5 (1954) 324.

LAARMAN, J. J., *Docum. Med. geogr. trop. (Amst.),* 8 (1956) 293.

MAKSTENIEKS, O. and J. D. VERLINDE, *Docum. Med. geogr. trop. (Amst.),* 9 (1957) 213.

MAS BAKAL, P., *Thesis,* Leyden, 1960.

MOHR, W., H. WAHLE and A. STAMMLER, *Z. Tropenmed. Parasit.,* 6 (1955) 386.

MOMBERG-JÖRGENSEN, H. C., *Nord. Vet.-Med.,* 8 (1956) 227.

PIEKARSKI, G., *Z. Parasitenk.,* 14 (1950) 582.

ROEVER-BONNET, H. DE, *Docum. Med. geogr. trop. (Amst.),* 9 (1957) 336.

ROTH, W., *Schweiz. Z. allg. Path.,* 17 (1954) 502.

SCHMIDTKE, L., *Zbl. Bakt. I. Abt. Orig.,* 160 (1954) 470.

SEEMAN, J., *J. Hyg. Epidemiol., Microbiol. Immunol.,* 3 (1959) 229.

SIIM, J. C., *Proc.6th Int. Congr. Pediatrics,* 1950, p. 365; *J. Amer. med. Ass.,* 147 (1951) 1641.

SOESTBERGEN, A. A. V., *Trop. geogr. med.,* 11 (1959) 13.

THALHAMMER, O., *Toxoplasmosis bei Mensch und Tier,* Wien, 1957, 307 pp.

THIEL, P. H. V., *Acta Leidens,* 23 (1953) 121; *Antoni v. Leeuwenhoek,* 22 (1956) 243; 248.

THIEL, P. H. V. and D. V. D. WAAY, *Docum. Med. geogr. trop. (Amst.),* 8 (1955) 392.

WAAIJ, D. V. D., *Thesis,* Leyden, 1959; *Trop. geogr. med.* 11 (1959) 345; 12 (1960) 251.

WEINMAN, D. and A. H. CHANDLER, *J. Amer. med. Ass.,* 161 (1956) 229.

WILDFÜHR, G., *Z. Hyg. Infekt.-Kr.,* 143 (1956) 134.

3

J. VAN RIEL

Trypanosomiases*

1. African trypanosomiases (Sleeping sickness)

The vectors

African trypanosomiases belong to the rare diseases which are encountered solely in the intertropical zone. This geographical distribution is connected with strict life requirements of the blood-sucking *Diptera* belonging to the genus *Glossina*. The glossinae are also known as *tsetse flies* because of the peculiar noise produced by the flapping of their wings in flight. The diseases they transmit have, until lately, largely contributed to the isolation of Tropical Africa from the rest of the world and impeded its economic and social development. Human sleeping sickness is associated with high morbidity and mortality. Nagana, the African trypanosomiasis of animals, causes also heavy losses and virtually makes animal breeding difficult or impossible.

The consequent lack of food of animal origin partly results in the frequency of protein malnutrition or *kwashiorkor* which dominates most of the pathology of the Africans living in enzootic regions. Draught animals, like others, are severely affected, and their reduction or complete absence have forced the inhabitants of wide African areas to remain slaving labourers. By repercussion, areas free of tsetse flies became overpopulated and overstocked with subsequent soil erosion and poverty.

Fossile remains uncovered in miocene soils in Colorado do suggest that at one time *Glossina* may have had a wider area of distribution including the western hemisphere. Actually they are African flies. The absence of *Glossina* from the New World explains why, in spite of the transportation

* Original in French; translated by Dr. M. L. Levi.

to America of thousands of African slaves, among whom certainly many were infected with trypanosomes, there has never been created a focus of trypanosomiasis in that continent.

The glossinae require physical conditions such as are found in Africa in the zone corresponding to 15° latitude north and south on either side of the equator. Even in this vast zone of Africa their distribution is not uniform, the particular species of glossinae and their incidence being determined by the physical conditions of the environment and especially by the degree of humidity.

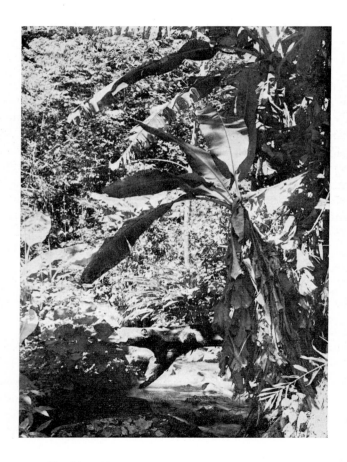

Fig. 76a.   Biotope of the tsetse fly, *Glossina palpalis*

Glossina palpalis needs shade, heat and a relative humidity grade of over 70%, condi- tions that are found on the banks of rivers and lakes bordered with high vegetation, shadowing dense bushes characteristic of much of the large equatorial forests in West Africa, in Congo and in the stretches of the Nile round the equator (Fig. 76a). This tsetse-fly is anthropophilic but feeds also on mammalian animals, birds and reptiles (crocodiles).

Glossina tachinoides thrives in areas of lesser humidity, such as clearer forests and bush around intermittent streams found in some areas of West Africa, where it re- places *Glossina palpalis*. It is also less anthropophilic and mainly attacks animals.

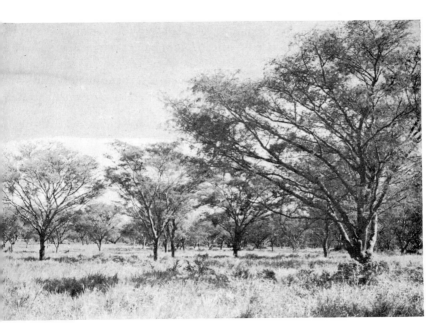

Fig. 76b.   Biotope of *Glossina morsitans*

Glossina morsitans seeks dryer areas with lower relative humidity, even less than 35%, in bushw here wild-life and game abound and it follows the latter's paths. (Fig. 76b). It feeds mainly on blood of wild and domestic animals although eagerly also biting humans inhabiting sparsely these semi-dry areas of East Africa, from the Sudan to Mozambique.

To the *morsitans* group belong *Glossina pallidipes* and *Gl. swynnertoni;* the latter is, however, more anthropophilic than *Gl. morsitans*.

The causal agents
The first species of pathogenic trypanosomes was discovered by Bruce in 1894 in bovines and equines suffering from nagana in Zululand, and it was called *Trypanosoma brucei.* Bruce confirmed the role of tsetse flies *(Gl. morsitans)* in 1897, that had already been suspected by Livingstone 40 years earlier. Dutton (1902), in Gambia, detected similar flagellates in the blood of a European suffering from irregular fever; he denominated the parasite *Trypanosoma gambiense.* Castellani (1903), in Uganda, observed the same parasite in the cerebrospinal fluid of patients with sleeping sickness. But it was Bruce again who clarified the aetiology of this dreadful disease by defining its causal agent *(T. gambiense)* and its vector *(Gl. palpalis).* Later on also *Gl. tachinoides* was recognized as a vector. In 1910, in North-East Rhodesia where *Gl. palpalis* is not found, Stephens and Langham isolated from man a trypanosome which they called *T. rhodesiense.* Its natural vectors are primarily *Gl. morsitans* and secondarily *Gl. swynnertoni* and *Gl. pallidipes.*

These 3 trypanosomes observed in the blood of man and animals, are morphologically similar. Their polymorphism, appearing more especially after passages in laboratory animals, is characterized mainly by variations in length (long, intermediate and short forms). In some of the latter the nucleus is displaced from the center of the cell towards the extreme end. The same evolution occurs within the insect vector; the ingested trypanosomes multiply in the midgut of the fly, giving rise to new, non-infective forms which reach up to the salivary glands and the proboscis where they multiply and yield infective forms termed metacyclic, to indicate that they finish the developmental cycle of the parasite.

The relationships between the three pathogenic trypanosomes are still under discussion. Should they, according to the unicist conception, be considered as strains of one and the same species, *T. brucei,* or are they, according to the pluralistic conception, 3 different species, *T. gambiense, T. rhodesiense* and *T. brucei?* Moreover, two dualistic theories have been developed, *viz.* (1) *T. gambiense* and *T. rhodesiense* are one and the same species proper to man, and (2) *T. rhodesiense* is identical with *T. brucei.* The controversy still continues, especially about the relationship of *T. brucei* and *T. rhodesiense* on the one hand and that of *T. gambiense* and *T. rhodesiense* on the other.

a. Relationship between T. brucei and T. rhodesiense. When *T. rhodesiense* was discovered, its identity with *T. brucei* was admitted because of morphological and biological similarity. Their polymorphism is more marked than that of *T. gambiense*, but today this feature has been shown to be a property dependent on the medium, and whatever differences exist in the ratio of eccentric position of the nucleus, this is merely quantitative. Their effects in laboratory animals are indistinguishable, both of them being more pathogenic than *T. gambiense*. Normal human serum, which is without effect on *T. gambiense*, is trypanocidal to the other two trypanosomes, though for *T. rhodesiense* only after laboratory passages. Both *T. brucei* and *T. rhodesiense* are transmitted by glossinae of the *morsitans* group.

Epidemiologically it is known that some nagana areas are sometimes free or nearly so of human trypanosomiases, although man and animals are bitten by the same fly-vectors. Moreover, all experimental inoculations to man of *T. brucei* have failed to infect him whether by injection of blood or by vector bite, even with a strain rendered resistant to the trypanocidal effect of human serum by mouse passage. (One exception has been recorded by Van Hoof (1947), where out of 7 volunteers bitten by *Glossina* carrying *T. brucei* he observed 3 weeks later the temporary presence of a few trypanosomes in the blood of one volunteer without any clinical symptoms). The unicist explanation of these failures is connected with the rarity of human receptivity for this trypanosome.

Infectivity may be considered to be a labile property; it was believed that *T. brucei* might, under certain conditions, become pathogenic to man, or that *T. rhodesiense* might lose its virulence. Long-term experiments in Tanganyika at Tinde have not, however, supported this view. Team work which was started as far back as 1936 by Corson and followed up by Fairbairn and Burtt, Willett and Fairbairn and by Ashcroft (1959) showed that transmission in *Gl. morsitans* of a strain of *T. rhodesiense* isolated from man and passed on sheep for 23 years had failed to affect its virulence for man. It persisted, only slightly diminished, for this long time, as shown by periodical tests on human volunteers. Similar passages on antelopes and on monkeys strengthen this conclusion. In these latter hosts the virulence to man was even exalted. From all this and from epidemiological evidence, Ashcroft concluded that *T. brucei* and *T. rhodesiense* are different species and that transformation of one type into the other, is to be considered very exceptional, if not impossible.

b. Relationship between T. gambiense and T. rhodesiense. Since the first descriptions of the latter species, emphasis was placed on the following features distinguishing it from *T. gambiense:* its greater polymorphism, the relative frequency of atypical forms with posterior nucleus, its greater virulence to laboratory animals and its resistance to human serum; all these characteristics are not absolute. The response of clinical cases of *T. rhodesiense* infection only to Suramin and Mel B rather than to the "ancient" arsenicals (like Tryparsamide which is very active against *T. gambiense*), has also been stressed.

It should be mentioned that in Nigeria, Lester (1938) isolated strains of *T. rhodesiense* intermediary in their characteristics (morphological, pathogenicity to laboratory animals, pharmacological). According to investigators at Tinde, the low virulence of a strain of *T. rhodesiense* which had repeatedly been passed through sheep, approached that of *T. gambiense*, whereas on the other hand, the pathogenicity of a strain which was propagated in monkeys and antelopes had been increased. They are more convinced now that human sleeping sickness is associated with one species of pathogenic trypanosome showing the characteristics of either *T. gambiense* or *T. rhodesiense* according to the main host in which they have lived and thrived. The differences possibly result from the fact that *T. gambiense* is exclusively a human parasite or nearly so, whilst *T. rhodesiense* ordinarily infects animals and less often man. British workers believe that *T. brucei* could be considered as the ancestral species which, by mutation, has given rise to a strain pathogenic also to man *(T. rhodesiense)*. By further adaptation to man in regions where he is the main host, this strain would have acquired the features of *T. gambiense.*

Animal trypanosomiasis or nagana

Following the recognition of *T. brucei* it became known that also monomorphic trypanosomes, such as *T. congolense* (Broden, 1904) and *T. vivax* (Zieman, 1905), could cause nagana in animals. Often these three trypanosomes were found associated in mixed infections. They are transmitted by glossinae of the *morsitans* group and respond to the same preventive measures.

The natural or experimental disease caused by *T. brucei* varies widely with the infecting strain and with the species of host animal. In equines, nagana usually assumes an acute course. After an incubation period of about 10 days there appear remittent fever, oedemata, anaemia, loss of hair, emaciation, and death usually ensues after 2 to 3 months. The disease is also serious in wild carnivores, camels, swine and dogs. Cattle, sheep and goats are definitely more resistant; the course of nagana in these species is usually chronic or even symptomless although some strains have been reported to cause severe mortality in cattle. Small laboratory animals are very susceptible to experimental inoculation.

The use of Antrycide made chemoprophylaxis of nagana possible. This should be associated with steps for the control of *Glossina*, such as bush-clearing, use of insecticides and destruction of game (though this latter measure must be carried out with discretion as otherwise it may be harmful).

Nagana – as has been mentioned above – indirectly constitutes a serious problem to human welfare by affecting resources of food.

Sleeping sickness associated with Trypanosoma gambiense

The zone of incidence parallels that of the vectors: *Gl. palpalis* and *Gl. tachinoides*. At the end of the 19th and the beginning of the 20th century, the disease was localized in small foci, but later, due to human shift and colonization, it has widely spread in the vast zone occupied by the trans-mitting vectors without, however, being present in all of the area. It is usually endemic, but sometimes severe epidemics increase still more the grave social significance of this plague. Whilst laboratory transmission of the disease can succeed with *Gl. morsitans*, this fly does not transmit it in nature.

The development of the disease in man comprises two stages. The early stage – both parasitaemic and haemolymphatic – is characterized by fever, very much varying in type and intensity, an erythematic skin rash (trypanides), tachycardia, and adenopathia, usually detected by palpation of the deep cervical chain. A later stage is ruled by nervous localizations: meningo-encephalitis with pronounced changes in the cerebrospinal fluid, changes in sensibility, and motor and psychic disturbances especially affecting sleep and consciousness. The course is generally prolonged, possibly 2 to 4 years, and ends in a most impressive state of emaciation (Fig. 77). Cases with slight or no symptoms do occur.

Laboratory diagnosis is direct, when detecting the causal agent in lymph (usually acquired by puncture of a cervical node) or in thick blood-drops, or indirectly by the complement-fixation test, using a group-specific antigen prepared from *T. equiperdum*. Changes in the cerebrospinal fluid can help in assessing the stage of the disease and its prognosis in individual cases.

Animal reservoirs of *T. gambiense* probably could be found in monkeys and antelopes which have experimentally been shown to be susceptible

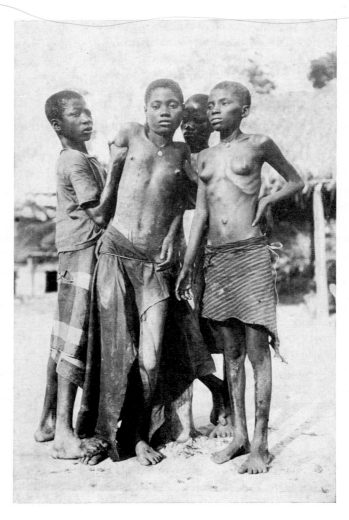

Fig. 77.   Emaciation caused by African trypanosomiasis (Sleeping sickness).
Photo: Broden, 1905

Certain species of antelopes *(Tragelaphus spekei)* do carry a trypanosoma morphologically identical with *T. gambiense*. Among domestic animals, the dog was found naturally infected and, experimentally, both the pig and the goat were infected during numerous passages of the parasite, although by these passages the index of transmissibility to man progressively decreased (Van Hoof *et al.*). These results are not as clear as those obtained at Tinde with *T. rhodesiense,* the latter being much more strict and demonstrative. However, the above mentioned animals can hardly be considered to form natural reservoirs of *T. gambiense,* nor should trypanosomiasis caused by this parasite be ranged among the zoonoses. The minor role of the animal reservoir is corroborated by the following facts: the human disease occurs in densely populated areas with little or no game; it is spread along the paths of communication on the African continent; prophylactic measures based solely on treatment of the human reservoir have been remarkably successful.

Systematic detection of human cases, as shown by Belgian physicians in Central Africa, forms the basis of prevention. Mobile medical teams track cases and treat them with trypanocidal drugs (Tryparsamide, Suramine, Pentamidine, Mel B). Large-scale application of these measures of chemotherapy have, in the former Belgian Congo, reduced the index of new infections from 1.2% in 1926 to 0.25% in 1940. Chemoprophylaxis, using Suramine first and later Pentamidine, have reduced this index to 0.025% in 1957, *i.e.* in an endemic area with 6,000,000 inhabitants 120 new cases in 10,000 inhabitants would have appeared in Congo in 1926, and only 2 in 1957. Notwithstanding the possibility of the advent of chemo-resistant strains of trypanosomes, similar results recorded by British, French and Portugese services confirm the soundness of this approach.

Eradication measures should logically be completed by controlling *Glossina.* When populations had been moved to areas free of flies, the disease could have been controlled, but in practice, transfer of population meets with considerable resistance. Clearing bush is helpful in that it forces the flies to move elsewhere for denser, shadier and wetter surroundings. However, the high cost of labour involved is prohibitive. This factor more and more encouraged the use of insecticide sprays (DDT or Dieldrin) on trees, foliage and riverside vegetation.

It should be remembered also that, where, according to Scott (1959), in some remote areas of northern Ghana, an animal reservoir of *T. gambiense* seems to be responsible for the low endemicity of sleeping sickness in man, prevention should include measures directed against such animal source of infection.

References p. 521

Sleeping sickness associated with Trypanosoma rhodesiense
The distribution of *Glossina* flies of the *morsitans* group which serve as vectors of *T. rhodesiense*, is much wider than the foci of sleeping sickness of this type. Contrary to what obtains with *T. gambiense*, which is very widespread in West and Central Africa, the *rhodesiense* type appears sporadically in sparsely populated zones of East Africa. Whereas *Gl. palpalis* is capable of transmitting *T. rhodesiense* under laboratory conditions, *Gl. morsitans* is nearly exclusively the vector in nature; *Gl. pallidipes* and *Gl. swynnertoni* have been incriminated as accessory vectors. However, recently Southon and Robertson (1961) reported that out of 21 strains of pleomorphic trypanosomes which they had isolated from *Gl. palpalis*, one strain seemed to be *T. rhodesiense* (as classified by virulence to laboratory animals, resistance to Tryparsamide and infectivity to man).

The clinical picture resembles that described above for *T. gambiense* although there are some quantitative differences. The course is more acute, the parasitaemia more intense, the hyperthermia more constant, the lymphatic reaction less so. Whilst invasion of the nervous system appears early, the nervous symptoms are less prominent, possibly because the patient dies from sepsis or myocarditis before neurologic symptoms get set. The duration of the disease averages one year. This rather rapid course, however, is not without exception, as is also the case with the chronicity of *T. gambiense*. In both infections cases do vary in gravity and duration. The methods of laboratory diagnosis are identical.

The epidemiology of the two human trypanosomiases differs markedly. The strictly localized foci of *T. rhodesiense* in bush, dense with game and flies, and the sporadicity of cases, made it plausible that apart from the human reservoir responsible for the cycle man–fly–man, demonstrable in certain foci, an animal reservoir might also play a role and possibly be the more important source of infection. The incidence and course of sleeping sickness due to *T. rhodesiense* in Tanganyika led Fairbairn in 1948 to believe that the infection could be introduced by human cases into free areas where it would owe its low endemicity to persistence in wild animals. At Tinde, experiments proved the susceptibility of antelopes to *T. rhodesiense* and the persistence in them of its virulence to man. Wild animals in endemic areas were examined to see if they harboured a polymorphic trypanosome pathogenic to man. Thus, Ashcroft (1959) inoculated blood from 74 wild animals to rats in two foci in Tanganyika.

One strain of trypanosome, obtained from an antelope, *Alcelaphus cokei*, proved non-pathogenic to two volunteers and, therefore, was considered to be *T. brucei*. Heish *et al.* (1958) in Kenya in a zone where *T. rhodesiense* is endemic in man and where this trypanosome was encountered in the local vector *(Gl. pallidipes)*, succeeded in isolating a polymorphic trypanosome by direct inoculation of blood from an antelope *(Tragelaphus scriptus)* to the rat. 0.25 ml of blood of this animal rich in trypanosomes, some of which showing nucleoposterior stages, were inoculated to a human volunteer; trypanosomes developed at the locally inflamed site and appeared in the blood in small number by the 8th day. The hyperthermia of 106.9° F. (41.6° C) and the gravity of the symptoms by the 9th day made treatment with Suramin imperative. Rapid and uneventful recovery followed. This was the first successful transmission of an animal trypanosome to man; the pathogenic character together with its proven resistance to Tryparsamide and its susceptibility to Mel B justified considering it as *T. rhodesiense*. In addition to the earlier mentioned arguments, this experience contributes to the conviction, expressed by several authors, that Rhodesian trypanosomiasis should be included among the zoonoses.

Prophylactic approach to Rhodesian trypanosomiasis is quite different from that applied to sleeping sickness due to *T. gambiense*. Mass prophylactic treatment, found so efficient in control of the latter, gave only palliative results in areas affected by *T. rhodesiense*. Regrouping of the scattered human population, thereby compelling game, and consequently also *Gl. morsitans*, to move off, has been especially recommended. The method of "discriminative clearing" of bush, which is based on the knowledge of the ecology of *Glossina*, consists in destroying the type of vegetation in which these flies tend to concentrate. Insecticidal sprays may perhaps be helpful where *Gl. pallidipes* is the vector. Their use in the vast fly belts of *Gl. morsitans* and *Gl. swynnertoni*, however, appears to be impracticable.

In essence, African trypanosomiasis of man presents two epidemiological aspects: one of a zoonosis observed in areas where the animal is an important reservoir of the parasite and where zoophilic glossinae are the vectors; the other where the transmitting flies live in closer contact with man who is there practically the sole reservoir of the trypanosome. Their adaptation to vertebrate hosts is reflected by two forms of the disease: the one acute, where the animal is the important reservoir, the other less acute, where man is the main host.

2. Chagas' disease or American trypanosomiasis

The causal agent, *Trypanosoma cruzi,* was discovered by Carlos Chagas (1909) and found in the intestine of the reduviid bug, *Panstrongylus megistus.* The vertebrate host, man or animal, shows the trypanosome under two morphological forms: (a) the *Leishmania*-like form, non-motile, without flagellum and undulating membrane, localized inside reticulo-endothelial cells or muscular fibres of the heart- and voluntary muscles, where they multiply and develop to trypanosomes, and (b) a form which invades the blood stream. There, in their adult stage, they measure about 20 μ in length, and are characterized by a thickish body, a large terminal blepharoblast and an undulating slightly curled membrane.

Biting reduviid bugs belonging to the order *Hemipterae* or *Rhyngota* constitute the vectors of Chagas' disease. In them the ingested *T. cruzi* undergo a developmental cycle including first *Leishmania*-like forms in the stomach; then *crithidia* forms appear in the midgut with a free flagellum and a short undulating membrane, and finally mature adult meta-cyclic trypanosome forms occur in the hindgut; the latter are incapable of further division but they are infective. It is reckoned that for complete maturation and elimination of the metacyclic forms through the anus, 20 days are required.

T. cruzi, excreted with the faeces of the biting bugs is capable of pene-trating the intact skin or mucous membranes of the vertebrate host, and more easily in scratch wounds, or through the local allergic area of reac-tion that follows the bite. They spread through the lymphatic system. Experimentally, the biting bug was shown to be capable, in rare cases, to transmit the disease directly through its bite but this is unusual, the common vehicle being the faeces. Infection of the vectors through cannibalism or/and coprophagy is possible so that the vertebrate host is not indispensable for infection of the bug. The latter mechanisms, how-ever, have no importance from an epidemiological point of view.

T. cruzi grows easily on artificial media, much more so than other pathogenic trypanosomes. On culture they undergo a cycle similar to that occurring in the guts of the bug. Cultures are infective only when they contain metacyclic forms.

The blood-sucking bugs transmitting the disease belong to the families *Triatoma, Rhodnius* and *Panstrongylus*. The species *Triatoma infestans* is most common in northern Argentina; both *Panstrongylus megistus* and *Rhodnius prolixus* are abundant in northern South America. Some forest bugs maintain and perpetuate the infection in wild hosts but do not practically infect man. The main sources of human infection are reduviid bugs living near or in human habitations. Primitive houses with roofs of mud or palm leaves afford excellent sites for the bugs. They bite preferably at night. Round human endemic foci the role of reservoir host is played by domestic animals, namely dogs, cats and pigs (Hoare, 1960), and the percentage of infected bugs varies from 2 to 60. Cases of transmission via the placenta or milk of nursing mothers to their babies or through blood-transfusion, although reported, are exceptional.

Chagas' disease is rightly classified amongst the zoonoses. The reduviid bugs infect themselves when sucking blood from man or animals. By serum-precipitation tests carried out on the intestinal contents of these bugs the animal species on which they parasitize has been determined.

Trypanosomes apparently indistinguishable from *T. cruzi* have been found in *man* and various animals such as *armadillo, marsupialia (opossum), rodents, canids, raccoons* and *mustelidae*. In many cases, however, exact determination of these parasites was lacking.

Everything points to the fact that the wild-life reservoir in Chagas' disease is of secondary epidemiological importance as compared with domestic animals living in the near neighbourhood of man, and especially *dogs, cats* and, in some countries, also *guinea pigs*. This situation, however, may considerably vary with the area. Thus in zones where the vector is *Triatoma infestans*, a bug that lives close to man (in northern and southern Brazil for example), Chagas' disease appears like a domestic zoonosis. A survey based on xenodiagnosis * that was carried out by De Freitas showed an incidence of 30% *T. cruzi* infections in dogs, 20% in cats as against 6% in the human population. In a personal communication Deane reports that in the Amazon Valley, with dense forests in the north of Brazil, free of domestic blood-sucking reduviid bugs, no human trypanosomiasis has ever been detected; no cats and only two dogs were

* In this method of survey, laboratory-bred bugs *(Triatoma)* are directly fed on the skin of suspected cases or on their blood through an artificial membrane. Positive results are those in which trypanosomes in their crithidia stage are recovered from the faeces of the bugs about 30 days after the infective meal.

proven infected, whilst the incidence in species of wild animals carrying trypanosomes indistinguishable from *T. cruzi*, was high, especially in *opossums, armadillos* and *ferrets*, but less so in *squirrel-monkey, anteaters* and wild *rats*. Numerous species of *bats* also carry "*T. cruzi*-like" trypanosomes, but, although many of these are closely related with *T. cruzi*, they are not identical with it.

Factors that directly or indirectly bring man to closer contact with the vector, such as bad hygiene, poor housing and poverty, tend to increase the endemicity of the disease. The infection occurs mainly in rural areas, with seasonal fluctuations of the climate, and especially during the hot summer months when the bugs are most active. Children are more prone to contract the disease as they are more exposed to the risk of infection. In them, as well as in adults freshly entering endemic areas, the course of the disease is usually most severe.

A study group on Chagas' disease that met in Washington in 1960, under the auspices of the American Bureau of Hygiene (functioning as an Office of the W.H.O. for the Americas) estimated that 35,000,000 individuals are exposed, of which about 7,000,000 are actually infected by *T. cruzi*. The mortality due to American trypanosomiasis is known to be high and the invalidity accompanying the chronic forms has serious economic consequences. The infection in man and in animals has been found in all countries of North and South America, with the exception of Canada and possibly Cuba. Its incidence is greatest in Brazil and northern Argentina, whilst in other South American countries (Venezuela, Bolivia), it appears to be on the increase.

The symptoms of Chagas' disease are varied. Several authors believe that the majority of human infections are asymptomatic. The initial symptom is a painless oedematous swelling of the eyelids (Romaña's sign), often limited to one eye only and accompanied with hyperaemia and conjunctivitis. This symptom was considered to be indicative of infection with *T. cruzi* although it might also be an allergic reaction to the saliva of the bug. The frequency of the facial portal of entry has been explained by the attraction that increased CO_2 concentration of the air has on the insect vector. The fever is of the remittent type with evening peaks reaching 39–40° C and it is associated with symptoms of general infection. The lymph nodes are enlarged, especially the axillary and inguinal glands. The liver and spleen are slightly increased in size; there is an accelerated pulse rate and hypotension. The electrocardiogram is variable, and its changes are sometimes very marked, though mostly transient in character. In young children death may be the result of cardiac insufficiency or due to a fulminating infection with meningo-encephalitis. In this acute stage the mortality is about 10%. In many cases the patient recovers. When the chronic form sets in, the disease is dominated by cardiovascular symptoms varying in severity from slight changes of the electrocardiogram with little or no visible signs to severe cardiac insufficiency and death. The damage to the heart results from its invasion by the trypanosomes causing minute ischaemic infarcts with often hypertrophy and dilatation of the right heart. In some endemic areas about 10% of the inhabitants have been known to show serious heart trouble caused by Chagas' disease. The parasites tend also to invade the muscularis of oesophagus and stomach resulting sometimes in dilatation and atony of these organs. In severe acute cases, especially in children, diffuse meningo-encephalitis is observed (Noetzal et al., 1958), associated with nodular disseminated foci in the central nervous system. The severity of the lesions appears to depend on the area, on the resistance of the host, his nutritional status, as well as on the virulence of the strain of T. cruzi involved. It is known that in Brazil the disease is usually more severe than elsewhere. Complications such as megaoesophagus, megacolon and chronic neurological disorders have been ascribed to infection with T. cruzi. Mortality rates of chronic forms are difficult to assess.

Early in the course of the disease diagnosis is based on the demonstration of the parasite in blood smears, and especially by the thick drop method. Later, in the chronic stages, parasites being scanty, they can be revealed by haemoculture (in about 16% of cases) or by animal inoculation, especially in puppies (12% efficiency), but the methods of choice are that of xenodiagnosis as mentioned above (70–80% efficiency when repeated at intervals), and of the complement-fixation test, which is both specific and reliable.

Medical treatment of Chagas' disease is symptomatic, as clinically active remedies are still lacking. In experimental animals some antibiotics and drugs of the nitrofuranes and 8-aminoquinolines groups have given encouraging results.

Emphasis should be placed on prophylaxis based on the improvement of hygienic conditions, better housing, and on education of the masses. In the poor areas all this presupposes social and economic reform of great magnitude. Insecticidal sprays, especially chlorine derivatives of hydrocarbons, have been used in emulsions or watery suspensions. Dieldrine and HCH are used in preference to DDT. Two of 3 applications at 30 to 180 days' interval have been found necessary when dealing with reduviid bugs. The former should be used with great care because of its toxicity to man and animals; HCH is less toxic but its efficiency requires further study. Organic compounds of phosphorus have also been tried. Acquired resistance to antiparasitic sprays has not been observed.

3. Other trypanosomiases

T. rangeli (syn. *T. guatemalensis*) is transmitted by reduviid bugs *(Rhodnius prolixus)*, often in association with *T. cruzi*. Morphologically it is distinguished by its punctiform blepharoplast, situated at a distance from the caudal end and by the large size and curliness of its undulating membrane. Surveys based on examination of fresh unstained smears from the intestinal contents of reduviid bugs have often caused confusion. The complement-fixation test with *T. cruzi* as antigen is negative in infections caused by *T. rangeli*. In South and Central America, where it is found in wild and domestic animals and in man (800 cases detected in Venezuela), its pathogenicity is still unproven.

Reduviid bugs are known to carry still other trypanosomes, which are more easily distinguishable from *T. cruzi: T. diasi, T. conorrhini* and *T. myrmecophagae.*

TRYPANOSOMIASES   521

REFERENCES

ASHCROFT, M. T., *Trans. Roy. Soc. Trop. Med. Hyg.*, 52 (1958) 1307; *Ann. Trop. Med. Parasit.*, 53 (1959) 137; *Trop. Dis. Bull.*, 56 (1959) 1073.
DAVEY, D. G., *J. Trop. Med. Hyg.*, 7 (1958) 546.
DEANE, L. M., *Rev. Inst. Med. Trop. S. Paulo*, 3 (1961) 15.
ETHES, Y. and F. PICK, Trypanosomiase américaine, in VAUCEL (Ed.), *Médecine Tropicale*, Paris, 1952. Mise à jour, 1957.
FAIRBAIRN, *Trop. Dis. Bull.* 45 (1948) 1.
FREITAS, J. L. P. DE, *Bol. Ofic. sanit. panamer.*, 49 (1960) 552.
GILLET, J., *J. Inst. Roy. Coll. Belge, Bull. des Séances*, 25 (1954) 326.
HEISCH, R. B., J. P. MAHON and P. E. C. MANSON-BAHR, *Brit. med. J.*, (1958) 1203.
HOARE, C. A., *Zool. Zh.* (Russ.), 39 (1960) 801.
LESTER, H. M. O., *Ann. trop. Med. Parasit.*, 27 (1933) 361.
LUMBRERAS, H., W. FLORES and A. ESCALLON, *Z. Tropenmed. Parasit.*, 10 (1959) 6.
NASH, T. A. M., *Trop. Dis. Bull.*, 57 (1960) 973.
NOETZAL, H., P. ELEJALDO and E. DIAS, *Z. Tropenmed. Parasit.*, 9 (1958) 27.
PHILIPS, N. R., *Ann. trop. Med. Parasit.*, 54 (1960) 397.
PIFANO, C. F., *Bol. Ofic. sanit. panamer.*, 49 (1960) 563.
SCOTT, D., *W. Afr. med. J.*, 8 (1959) 165.
SOUTHON, H. A. W. and D. H. H. ROBERTSON, *Nature*, 189 (1961) 411.
VAN HOOF, L., *Trans. roy. Soc. trop. Med. Hyg.*, 40 (1947) 728.
WILCOCKS, C., *Trop. Dis. Bull.*, 57 (1960) 433; 58 (1961) 549.
WOODRUFF, A. W., African Trypanosomiasis, Chagas' Disease, in FAIRLY, WOODRUFF and WALTERS (Eds.), *Recent Advances in Tropical Medicine*, London, 1961, p. 480.
World Health Organization, Tech. Rept. Ser. No. 202 (1960), *Chagas' Disease*, Washington D.C., March 1960, Geneva, p. 21.

4

J. VAN DER HOEDEN

Simian Malaria

It was, until recently, generally assumed that the sole mammalian host of the malaria parasites of man is man himself.

Although man must be considered to be by far the largest reservoir of the plasmodia which cause human malaria, in certain regions of the world apes and monkeys form an independent potential source of human infection, this situation being comparable with that of jungle yellow fever.

Human malaria is caused by four species of the protozoan genus *Plasmodium*. These species are: *P. vivax, P. falciparum, P. malariae* and *P. ovale*, which cause tertian, tropical, quartan and *ovale* tertian malaria respectively. Malaria in the lower *Primates* is caused by *P. inui, P. cynomolgi, P. knowlesi, P. kochi, P. brasilianum* and other species. Some of these have been differentiated into subspecies or varieties. Several are identical with, or are very closely related to the malarial parasites of man.

P. rodhaini found in the chimpanzee, and *P. brasilianum* found in monkeys of the New World, are similar to *P. malariae; P. reichenovi* found in anthropoid apes is indistinguishable from *P. falciparum; P. schwetzi* in the gorilla and chimpanzee and also *P. cynomolgi* closely resemble *P. vivax*.

In principle the pathology of simian malaria is much like that of malaria in man.

In 1932, Knowles and Das Gupta successfully transmitted *P. knowlesi* from naturally infected monkeys found in the Malayan jungle, to man and produced, as a result, typical attacks of malaria which had a daily periodicity.

Injection of the blood of African baboons suffering from a heavy form of malaria due to *P. inui* into other baboons, *Macacus rhesus* and man, gave rise to severe attacks of malaria with a schizogonic cycle and large numbers of parasites in the blood. This condition promptly disappeared on treatment with quinolysine.

Inverse infection with the blood of the volunteers infected with *P. inui* brought about a malignant form of malaria in the monkeys (Ionescu–Mihaiesti *et al.*, 1934).

In the African forests, plasmodia of the *malariae* type are transmitted by anopheline mosquitoes both to man and chimpanzees.

Transmission experiments with *P. vivax*, *P. falciparum* and *P. ovale* of human origin through anopheline vectors was successful on anthropoid apes.

According to Garnham (1958), *vivax*-type infections in man in the Amazon region of South America have been held to be of simian origin.

Experimental, as well as accidental, laboratory infections of man with *vivax*-parasites of *Macacus* monkeys have been recorded from America (Eyles *et al.*, 1960).

During large scale experiments with *Rhesus*-monkeys in the National Institutes of Health, using the *bastianellii* strain of *P. cynomolgi* (originating from *Macara irus* in Malaya), two workers spontaneously developed tertian malaria, *vivax*-type plasmodia similar to those of the *bastianelli* strain being found in the blood of both of them. Similar attacks with numerous *P. cynomolgi* in the blood, occurred in two volunteers, as well as in *Rhesus* monkeys, after the injection of the blood of the laboratory workers first infected. The disease was promptly cured by treatment with chloroquine. Two other volunteers underwent similar attacks after they had been bitten by *Anopheles freeborni* carrying *P. cynomolgi bastianellii* acquired from *Macaca rhesus*. The results of cross-immunity investigations with the infected individuals and monkeys supported the view that reciprocal transmission between monkeys and man may occur under natural conditions.

In addition to these highly suggestive data, Eyles *et al.* cited a report by L. Schmidt of a spontaneous attack of malaria in a member of the staff of the Cincinnati hospital, who had been working with the *bastianellii*-strain of *P. cynomolgi*. Injection of the blood of this person into a *Rhesus* monkey produced a characteristic *cynomolgi*-like form of malaria.

The *bastianelii* strain of *P. cynomolgi* (fairly recently isolated from a monkey) established parasitaemia in 12 of 13 volunteers who had been bitten by infected *A. freeborni* or *A. quadrimaculatus*. The M-strain of

P. cynomolgi (maintained via blood passages for more than 25 years) was much less readily transmitted between monkey and man, but its transmissibility markedly increased after few serial passages through man, by which the intensity of parasitaemia and the heights of fever quickly rose (Schmidt *et al.*, 1961; Coatney *et al.*, 1961; Contacos *et al.*, 1962). There was no clear difference between monkey → mosquito → man, and man → mosquito → man transmissions.

In comparison with the extremely extensive reservoir of malaria parasites present in human populations, transmission of simian malaria to man at the present time is no more than an epidemiological curiosity. It may represent a hazard to laboratory investigators and persons living in territories in which monkeys and anthropophilous mosquitoes are carrying malaria plasmodia which can infect both man and monkeys. This risk may be present especially in the jungle, where control by insecticides is not practicable.

In regions from which human malaria has been eradicated, the hazard connected with simian malaria will depend largely on environmental factors.

REFERENCES

BEYE, H. K., M. E. GETZ, G. R. COATNEY, H. A. ELDER and D. E. EYLES, *Amer. J. Trop. Med. Hyg.*, 10 (1961) 311.

COATNEY, G. R., H. A. ELDER, P. G. CONTACOS, M. E. GETZ, R. GREENLAND, R. N. ROSSAN and L. H. SCHMIDT, *Amer. J. Trop. Med. Hyg.*, 10 (1961) 311.

CONTACOS, P. G., H. A. ELDER, G. R. COATNEY and C. S. GENTHER, *Amer. J. Trop. Med. Hyg.*, 11 (1962) 186.

EYLES, D. E., G. R. COATNEY and M. E. GETZ, *Science*, 131 (1960) 1812.

GARNHAM, P. C. C., *J. trop. Med. Hyg.*, 61 (1958) 92.

IONESCU–MIHAIESTI, C., G. ZOTTA and E. RADACOVICI, *C. R. Soc. Biol. (Paris)*, 115 (1934) 1311.

KNOWLES, R. and B. M. DAS GUPTA, *Indian med. Gaz.*, 67 (1932) 301.

SCHMIDT, L. H., R. GREENLAND and C. S. GENTHER, *Amer. J. Trop. Med. Hyg.*, 10 (1961) 679.

5

J. VAN DER HOEDEN

Balantidiasis

Balantidium coli is a large egg-shaped *Ciliate* (length: about 50–200 microns, width: 40–80 microns). It has a cosmopolitan distribution in pigs and man. Most commonly it is found in domestic hogs and often in monkeys. It has also been recorded in various other wild animals (wild boars, rats). Man is a relatively rare host to *Balantidium*. There is a locally different incidence in pigs. In New Guinea the infection rate in swine mounted to 100 %; in Belfast it was found to be 74 % and in other places the parasite was rare or absent. In certain regions of New Guinea *Balantidium* cysts were found in 28 % of the Papuan population (Couvée and Rijpstra, 1961).

It is generally admitted that *Bal. coli* is a commensal in the intestinal lumen of swine. On the contrary, in monkeys it penetrates into the wall of the large bowels, sometimes causing extensive tissue destruction with fatal outcome. Similar processes develop in man, the lesions and clinical symptoms closely resembling those produced by *Entamoeba histolytica*. In a number of cases there is no obvious damage to the tissues. The acute course of human balantidiasis is characterised by multiple or diffuse ulceration and gangrene with perforation of the intestinal wall. Sometimes the appendix is involved. Chronic infection follows a course similar to amoebic dysentery with heavy profuse diarrhoea.

The incidence of *Bal. coli* in man often correlates with that in domestic pigs in the same area. Appasov (1958), who studied the distribution of *Bal. coli* among wild and domestic animals in Kazakhstan (U.S.S.R.), pointed out that persons having close occupational association with pigs, run the greatest risk of becoming infected. On the other hand attention has been drawn to the transmission from man to man without an intermediate animal carrier.

This occurs especially in population groups living in a crowded insanitary environment. Ferri (1943) recorded 20 cases of which 7 terminated fatally, in a mental hospital in Tomsk (Siberia); many of the patients worked in a pig farm attached to the hospital. Six cases of balantidial dysentery and 5 symptomless *Balantidium* carriers were observed among the children of a ward in the same hospital. These children had no association with hogs and the author believed that the unhygienic habits of the mentally disturbed inmates facilitated interhuman faecal infection. McCarrey (1952) recovered 87 human cases of balantidiasis within 10 months in South Persia, among the Muslims who had no contact with swine.

Improvement of hygienic conditions, especially where man is employed in pig breeding and slaughter, is of major importance in the prevention of balantidiasis. In endemic areas manure of the sties should not be used for dunging of kitchen gardens.

Treatment with Carbasone, Acetarsol, Stovarsol, aureomycin or terramycin has yielded favourable results.

REFERENCES

APPASOV, R. N., *Trudy Inst. Zool. Acad. Sci. Kazakh.*, 9 (1858) 198.
COUVÉE, L. M. J. AND A. C. RIJPSTRA, *Trop. geogr. Med.*, 13 (1961) 284.
FERRI, L. V., *Med. Parazit. (Mosk.)*, 11 (1942) 108; Ref.: *Trop. Dis. Bull.* 40 (1943) 459.
MCCARREY, A. G., *Brit. med. J.*, (1952 I) 629.

CHAPTER VI

ZOOPARASITIC DISEASES

A. Helminthozoonoses

B. Diseases caused by arthropod parasites

A. Helminthozoonoses

1

Nematodiases

a. Trichinelliasis

Trichinelliasis is caused by *Trichinella spiralis,* a nematode of minute dimensions (female, up to 4 mm, male, up to 2 mm long). Among the nematodiases this is the most serious, because it frequently endangers the life of the host.

The parasite was first recognised by Owen in 1835, who called it *Trichina spiralis.* When Raillet, in 1896, discovered that the generic name *Trichina* had already been used by Meigen in 1830 to denominate a genus of flies the Rules of Zoological Nomenclature made it necessary to alter the name of the worm. The correct name of the parasite at present is *Trichinella spiralis.* However, the old name *Trichina* is firmly anchored in common language, and the term trichinosis or trichiniasis instead of trichinelliasis is widely used in medical literature. In the following account the parasite will be referred to as *Trichinella,* for short.

Human trichinelliasis occurred in early epochs of European civilisation without its nature being realised. Epidemics were apparently common in the Middle Ages, and it is presumed that many a case of witch-burning or persecutions of Jews accused of poisoning wells were based on mis-interpretation of outbreaks of trichinelliasis.

Trichinella lives in the lower part of the small intestine and in the upper part of the large intestine. The adult worm is not very injurious. Symptoms occurring during the infection are connected with the multi-plication of the parasite and its life cycle within the same host.

Trichinella has a unique life cycle, which was elucidated in the middle of the last century mainly by Leuckart, Virchow and Zenker, working independently. It is remarkable for its lack of host-specificity, since it may live in almost any mammal, including man, and, under certain conditions in some species of birds.

The host (either man or animal) becomes infected by ingesting meat containing encysted viable larvae. Such meat needs not be raw; many kinds of meat-dishes and sausages are insufficiently heated to ensure the death of the trichinella larvae they contain.

The meat fibers and the capsules enclosing the larvae are digested within a few hours, sometimes while they are still in the stomach. It should be noted that the acid reaction of the contents of the mammalian stomach does not impair the vitality of trichinella larvae. According to Ritterson (1959) trichinella cysts readily dissolve in a solution of collagenase, but are unaffected by trypsin, pancreatin and hyaluronidase.

In the intestine the liberated larvae creep between the villi, moult several times and rapidly develop into adults. However, not all ingested larvae develop to the adult stage; a number of them are eliminated, mostly during the first 24 hours (McCoy, 1938; Zimmermann et al., 1959). Animals already previously infected eliminate a higher percentage of larvae than those infected for the first time. Even after this initial elimina tion a part of the developing larvae subsequently die and are passed out of the body (Gursch, 1949). The young worms reach maturity and copulate after less than 2 days. The female penetrates through the mucosa up to about half the length of its body in cluding the vulva. Anchored in the tissue it continues to grow and develops ova, which hatch *in utero*. The young larvae escape from the worm's vulva and directly enter the lymph spaces of the intestinal wall of the host.

Shedding of the larvae continues for several days or weeks, until the adult trichinella dies. There are indications that the immunity which develops during the initial period of infection is the cause of the death and elimination of the adult worms. In cases of heavy infection, the host may die before the lifespan of the parasite has expired.

The degree of infection, the longevity of the adult *Trichinella*, and the intensity of the pathological reaction depend mainly on the sensitivity of the host species, but also on the number of invading parasites, and on the age and constitution of the particular host. Apparently not all age-groups are equally susceptible to trichinella infection. Nolf and Zaiman (1941) demonstrated that, in rats, the younger the animal the lower is the infec tion rate, while the contrary was observed by Matoff (1937) in the dog.

Usually, the larger the number of infecting larvae the higher is the degree of infection. Heavy infection interferes with the development of immunity and thus increases the longevity of the parasites.

In man the adult trichinellae usually begin to die out during the fourth week after the onset of the disease. However, in individual cases they have still been found alive many weeks later. Carter (1949) observed gravid females in the mucosa of the duodenum and jejunum at post mortem examination 115 days after the appearance of clinical symptoms. In experimentally infected animals the longevity of the parasite varied in different host species. In the guinea pig, which is regarded as being the most susceptible laboratory animal, the adult trichinellae may live for 30–37 days in the small intestine and up to 55 days in the caecum. In dogs the trichinellae usually die out during the second week (Roth, 1938). The longest life span of adult trichinellae (up to 13 weeks) was observed in gophers (a small wild rodent, *Citillus richardsoni;* Offutt and McCoy, 1941).

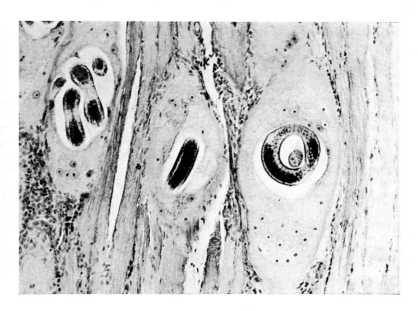

Fig. 76.   Trichinella spiralis. Section of muscle with cysts in early stage of formation.
(Original photo)

Adult trichinellae begin to produce larvae between the fourth and sixth day after infection. During the period of their sexual activity trichinella presumably produces on the average of 1 larva every half hour.

The larvae, laid in the tissue of the villi, at once reach the central lacteals. From there they are carried by the lymph through the mesenteric glands to the thoracic duct, vena cava, heart and lungs, and eventually they enter the arterial circulation. The microscopic dimensions of the larvae (80–120 microns long and 6–12 microns in diameter) facilitate their passage through capillaries. Yet, on their way through the lungs, the larvae damage the capillaries and this apparently causes the extensive haemorrhages and pneumonic lesions, which are often associated with heavy infections. Transported through the blood system, some of the larvae reach tissues in which they cannot develop. Here they are immobilized by leucocytes, killed and dissolved by them.

In general, only the larvae which reach the skeletal muscles can develop further. In cases of heavy infection they may also settle in other tissues. The larvae enter the muscle fibers through the sarcolemma. They appear in the muscles on the sixth to seventh day after infection, their number increasing every day for as long as the females living in the intestinal mucosa continue their production. After the larva has settled in a muscle fiber, the affected part of the fiber at once shows signs of degeneration; it loses its striation, widens, the sarcoplasm becomes granular, the nuclei grow larger and become rounded. Cellular infiltration sets in around the affected spot about a fortnight after the infection and eventually an increasing number of fibroblasts appear. In the meantime, the place where the larva rests becomes swollen and filled with detritus and degenerated nuclei (Fig. 76). Two weeks later the larva has reached ten times its initial size. It now rolls itself into the characteristic spiral and a capsule is gradually formed out of the surrounding fibroblasts. On the nineteenth or twentieth day after infection the infiltration diminishes and the larva has by then reached about 1 mm in length. A few days later the capsule loses its filamentous character and becomes homogeneous; it measures 0.3–0.4 mm in length. Detritus and some fat globules derived from the breakdown of the muscle fiber are visible at its poles and a delicate net of capillaries appears around the capsule. The larva then acquires its final form and remains unchanged and motionless for variable periods. It absorbs food and oxygen from the capillaries surrounding its capsule and metabolises actively all the time. In experiments carried out by McCoy *et al.*, in which infected rats were fed with radioactive phosphorus, the latter was detected in the trichinella larvae as early as 2 hours after feeding. There are reports (McCoy *et al.*, 1941) stating that trichinella larvae may, although rarely, be alive in human muscle as long as 30 years after the disease presumably had been contracted.

In cases of slight infection it may be necessary to examine several grams of muscle to find a single larva. In heavy human infections hundreds of larvae and in very susceptible animals thousands of encapsuled larvae may be counted in 1 gram of muscle (Roth, 1935). As *Trichinellae* live longer in the guinea pig than in any other laboratory animal, in this host a worm produces a very large number of larvae (up to 2,400) during its total life span.

After a quiescent period of variable duration, the larva dies and calcification sets in. The process of calcification is not uniform; sometimes it may start in the capsule while the larva is still alive and infective. In mice and rats the first signs of calcification become visible at the poles, 14 to 16 months after the infection took place. Sometimes the dead larva calcifies first, and this is followed by calcification of the rest of the content of the capsule. Fully calcified capsules may be seen 2 years after infection. According to Nevinny (1927) the process of total calcification of the trichinella cyst in man takes from 14 to 40 years.

The young larvae become infective on about the 17th day, that is to say, before full development of the capsule. In this condition they can, when they are swallowed by a suitable host, start a new life cycle.

Although the larvae can settle in any skeletal muscle, they show a distinct predilection. Thus, the diap' ragm and the intercostal muscles, the muscles of the larynx, eye, and tongue, are invaded by far greater numbers of larvae than the other muscles. It is accepted that in man the diaphragm is the muscle most heavily infected. Zebrowska (1960) found that, in cats, the intercostal muscles are the ones that are most intensely infected. In the guinea pig the masseters, the muscles of the neck and anterior extremities are the sites of preference (Jensen and Roth, 1938).

Trichinelliasis occurs in two epidemiological phases: it may be either *sylvatic, i.e.* in wild animals, without any connection to man or domestic animals, or *synantropic* *, *i.e.,* connected with animals living in close association with man.

It is often assumed that trichinelliasis is mainly linked with man and swine, the latter being the usual source of human infection. Although it is true that the pig is the main vector of human trichinelliasis, man serves only as an occasional host and is a blind alley for the trichinella.

Recent investigations show that trichinelliasis is spread along a variable and ramified net of interchangeable parasite-hosts in which not infrequently wild animals play the only part. Trichinella prevails not only in regions in which human infections occur, but also in areas in which these are unknown.

It should be borne in mind that trichinella is not restricted with respect to its hosts; it can thrive in practically every mammal. In nature it may occasionally occur even in animals which do not eat meat, such as, for instance, shrews or whales. In experimental infections all mammals, among them the laboratory animals, including bats, sheep and others and, under special conditions, even young birds, are susceptible. The natural hosts of trichinella are wild carnivorous and omnivorous mammals which constitute the reservoir from which the infection spreads to synantropic and domestic animals and eventually to man. Trichinelliasis of wild animals is especially prevalent in temperate and Arctic regions and is maintained mainly in predatory animals. In some instances an astonishingly large percentage of various local mammalian species is infected. For instance, according to Hovorka (1957), in Czechoslovakia the following animals were found infected in nature: lynx *(Lynx lynx)* in 66%, wild cat *(Felis sylvestris)* in 15%, wolf *(Canis lupus)* in 33%, and

---

* The term "synantropic animals" was introduced by E. J. Pavlovsky, to denote animals for which proximity to human habitation constitutes their natural biotope.

fox *(Vulpes vulpes)* in 30%. Tretiakova (1953) found in Bashkiria (South Ural) trichinelliasis in 85.7% of wolves, 80% of badgers, 94.7% of foxes and 60% of weasels. Mielnikova (1960) records 8.4% infection with trichinella in the wild boar in Tadjikistan (North of Persia), while Dubinin (1952) found 24% of these animals infected in the Volga delta. In comparatively thinly populated regions, such as Central Russia and Latvia, the wolf is the animal most infected, with an incidence of up to 100% (Bobrov, 1955). In central Europe the fox takes over this role (Hovorka, 1957, in Czechoslovakia; Kozar and Warda, 1960, in Poland). This animal was found infected in Italy (Leinati and Marazza, 1957), in Sweden (Hermansson, 1943), in Switserland (Joorg and Britschgi, 1944), and also in Dagestan (East Caucasus, by Nikitin, 1960), where human trichinelliasis is unknown. Zimmermann *et al.* (1960), observed trichinellas in 13 species of wild animals in Iowa.

A strikingly high frequency of infection is found in all species of bears, especially in the Arctic. For years, it was supposed that bears acquired infection only when they are kept in zoological gardens, but recent investigations have shown that they are infected in nature as well. Natural infection of bears was recorded in the American and Asiatic Arctic, in the Southern Urals, in Caucasus and in other regions (Schultz and Kastorskii, 1949, Tretiakova, 1953).

Our knowledge of the prevalence of trichinelliasis among wild animals is still fragmentary. Often, observations made in the same region by different investigators have shown marked discrepancies. For instance the data published by Kazlauskas (1958) and Mustekaite and Prusaite (1959) in Lithuania fluctuated in wolves between 0–100% and in foxes between 22–50%. Even repeated investigation in the same region may produce varying results (Zimmerman *et al.,* 1959).

The ways in which trichinelliasis spreads among wild animals are not sufficiently clear, but certainly there are many. Undoubtedly the large predators become infected by preying on small ones, and all of them by eating the dead bodies of infected animals, including those of their own species. Even animals which are not usually carnivorous may under certain circumstances acquire trichinella infection. For instance, Nosik *et al.* (1948) found 2 out of 17 field mice infected with trichinellae in a haystack near to which the body of an infected wolf had been deposited. Cannibalism, which is common among certain mammals, notably rodents, plays a significant role in the maintenance of trichinella infection in nature. The latter fact used to be taken as the basis for the presumption that rodents are the principal animal group in which trichinelliasis is maintained in nature and that they serve as its main transmitters to other animals, in particular to swine and eventually to man. This argument has lost strength since recent surveys (Bielayeva, 1957; Kozar and Warda, 1956; Mustekaite and Prusaite, 1959; Lukashenko, 1960) have shown that rodents may be free from trichinella in regions in which the infection is common in large predators and also occurs in man.

Merkushev (1950) and Bielayeva (1958) showed that some carrion insects may retain viable trichinella larvae in their digestive tracts, thus temporarily serving as passive vectors.

Some authors have stressed the hazard caused by indiscriminate discarding of animal carcasses by hunters. In regions in which hunting is common, this source of infection can be an important factor in the dissemination of trichinelliasis in nature.

The fresh faeces of recently infected mammals may in some instances serve as sources of infection for other mammals, by soiling their food. According to Merkushev (1955) the faeces of carrion eating birds may also contain viable larvae of trichinella.

However attractive the observations on animal trichinelliasis may seem to be for the elucidation of the epidemiology of human infection, one should consider this factor with some reserve. Comparative investigations show that the interconnection between human and animal epidemiology, and the transmission of infection between domestic and wild animals are both variable and unpredictable.

As has been mentioned, it has been known for about 100 years that man becomes infected by eating pork. In general the incidence of trichinelliasis in swine in endemic localities is low, being mostly no more than a fraction of 1%. Only in exceptional circumstances, as for instance, in the outbreak in the Lebanon to be quoted below, was the incidence found to be high. Yet, the importance of swine as the source of human infection is great, considering that one pig may supply a hundred or more infective meals. It is especially great in localities in which people are used to consuming meat products (sausages) made of insufficiently heated pork.

The suitability of the pig as a vector of trichinella is accentuated by its degree of tolerance to the infection. In adult pigs only severe infections cause symptoms of disease and even death. According to Schwartz (1938) no clinical signs are observed in swine which, at autopsy, show less than 800 larvae per gram of diaphragm muscle.

The problem of how trichinellae reach the pig has been the object of much controversy. According to an early hypothesis advanced by Leuckart (1860), swine mainly acquire the infection by eating dead rats. The rat is an omnivorous animal and can easily become infected by eating the flesh of dead animals (scrap from slaughterhouses, domestic refuse, the discarded corpses of hunted animals, etc.) or as a result of cannibalism. Ill or weak members of a rat colony, or those which die in the nest, are devoured, and thus an infection, once it has reached a rat colony, is constantly maintained. It should also be noted that the rat is very susceptible to trichinelliasis, 2 larvae being sufficient to produce infection (while a guinea pig requires at least 10 larvae). Slight infection is well tolerated by rats and symptoms comparable to those in other host animals do not appear (Hall and Wigdor, 1918).

Before the advent of modern meat hygiene, trichinelliasis of man and domestic animals occurred much more frequently than it does at present. When slaughter-houses were merely slaughter-sites, open to scavenging animals, the local rats were heavily infected. Billings (1893) found infection in almost 100% of the rats in the slaughter-house of Boston, and Fessler (1878) found it in 50% in Bromberg (Germany). However, the infected rat is not necessarily the only, or even the main, vector of trichinella, to pigs. It appears that under ordinary conditions the occurrence of trichinelliasis in swine and rats, as well as in other animals, does not coincide. Examples of an unusually high incidence of trichinelliasis in rats in the vicinity of slaughter-houses in contrast with an insignificant incidence in other parts of the same town may indicate rather that, conversely, the infection of the rats originated from swine (Bierezhanzev, 1960). In some instances the rat serves only as an additional factor, which creates the vicious circle: rat – swine – rat. It should also be noted that domestic mice may also be infected: in more than 3% of mice in Odessa, South Russia (Lukashenko, 1953) and in more than 2% in West Russia (Bielayeva, 1954) trichinellae were found. Thus mice may occasionally represent a source of the infection of swine.

Mark, as long ago as 1888, concluded that trichinelliasis of pigs results from the ingestion of infected meat offal. Nowadays it is generally accepted that, in countries in which swine are raised on an industrial scale, feeding with waste from slaughter-houses and dead animals forms the main mode of spread. A striking example of the propagation of trichinelliasis by scrap feeding was given by Pigury (1943), who recorded epidemics in Beirut (Syria) in which 15% of the pigs were infected in an isolated piggery in which the pigs had been fed with the scrap of animals raised in the same place.

In discussing the ways in which domestic and synantropic animals become infected the unorthodox ways of spread for which man is responsible should not be ignored. Domestic scrap may introduce trichinelliasis into a farm in a locality where no local sources of infection exist. The peculiar habit of feeding swine with the carcasses of skinned animals reared on farms or with hunted fur animals has been pointed out by several observers (Rochman, 1950, *et al.*).

Various other explanations of the spread of trichinelliasis have been suggested. Some authors have advanced the theory that transmission of trichinella is possible by the ingestion of the fresh faeces of recently infected animals which are eliminating viable larvae or adult worms. However, other investigators (Lintz, 1916; Hall, 1937; Gould *et al.*, 1943) assert that this mode of transmission is rare and is in reality insignificant. Moreover, Robinson and Olson (1960) believe that infection through faeces is unlikely, because the eliminated larvae do not survive longer than 2 hours in a dry environment and about 4 hours under moist conditions.

Katz (1960) and Matov (1957, 1960) found that not only larvae, but also young female worms (except those 24–28 hours old) ingested by experimental animals (mice) would produce infection. This means that even animals harbouring only the intestinal stage of trichinella may serve as a source of infection to carrion feeders and, among them, swine.

Trichinelliasis in rats and swine is apparently responsible for a high incidence of trichinelliasis among domestic carnivores, *e.g.*, cats and dogs.

The following examples of heavy infection may quoted:
Incidence in cats: in Warsaw (Poland), 20% (Gronek, 1948); in Riazan (Centr. Russia), 28% (Merkushev, 1939); in Norway, 18% (Aaser, 1941); in Mexico (Mexico), 25% (Nunez and Mazzotti, 1948); in U.S.A., 5–21% (Zimmermann and Schwartz, 1958). *Incidence in dogs:* in Poland, 9.3% (Kozar and Warda, 1960); in Roumania, 8.3% (Talos, 1935; Oprescu *et al.,* 1956); in Bielorussia, 20% (Koriazhnov, 1957); in Manchuria, 26–61% (Wan Gei-Chai, 1960); in Norway, 18% (Aaser, 1941); in U.S.A., 1–17% (Zimmermann and Schwartz, 1958). Ohbayashi and Sato recorded in 1957 trichinelliasis in a dog in Japan, where this infection had been, until then, unknown. It should be pointed out that these figures represent only incidentally collected data which do not show the average rate of infection, but merely the extent to which the

incidence may rise. Though dogs and cats sometimes show very high infection rates, this usually occurs in very limited areas, mostly in the vicinity of improperly constructed slaughter-houses to which local dogs and cats have access.

In early experiments it has not always been possible to infect dogs. It was, therefore, supposed that the dog is a unsuitable host-animal. Later, it appeared that the intensity of infection in the dog depends on its age. Young animals are more susceptible and the infection produces more severe symptoms like anorexia, diarrhoea, weakness and elevated temperature.

As has been explained above, domestic and synantropic animals are susceptible to trichinelliasis and doubtless suffer damage to their health. However, as an animal disease, trichinelliasis is not regarded as being a cause of significant economic loss. Illness of domesticated animals due to trichinella is almost unknown. Cases have been recorded in the pig, for example, which showed as many as 1,500 cysts per gram of muscle tissue, although these hosts never seemed to be ill (Ruprecht, 1864). However, although animals become sick, and even die in experimental infections, this is very rare under farm conditions.

The only instance in which animal trichinelliasis is regarded being a direct economic hazard is when it affects farm reared fur animals. On some farms on which the food contains garbage from slaughter-houses or the carcasses of the skinned fur animals, large numbers of the breeding stock may succumb to trichinelliasis (Aaser, 1941).

Special conditions for the maintenance of trichinella infection exist in the arctic regions, where the greater part of the fauna consists of carnivorous animals and hunting is a prevalent occupation of the population. The flesh of the animals is widely used for human consumption, while the offal, as well as the carcasses of inedible animals, are fed to sledge dogs or thrown away. This situation results in a high incidence of trichinelliasis in man and animals (over 45 % of dogs on the average and even 92 % in some localities, with up to 1000 cysts per gram of muscle).

According to Rausch et al. (1956), 11.7% of mammals comprising 23 different species are infected in Alaska. Most frequently infected are polar foxes (up to 80%), 3 species of bears (in 52% of the white bears) and other carnivores which habitually not only feed on prey, but also eat the bodies of dead animals, including those of their own species.

On examination of the muscles of animals in Greenland, Roth (1950) found the following infection rates: in dogs, 66.5 %; in polar bears, 27.7 %; in walruses, 0.9 % and in seal, 1.9 %. Kuitunen (1954) found that 4.8 % of walruses on the northern shores of Canada were infected. Other authors (Vibe, 1950) acknowledged the infection of walruses, seals and whales.

The route of infection of walruses, which normally feed on molluscs, and of seals, which mainly eat fish, is not completely understood. It was observed, however, that these animals sometimes feed on the bodies of land animals, for instance dogs, which have been swept into the sea. Vibe (1950) suggested an other explanation. He pointed out that in polar waters the bodies of dead animals are disintegrated by swarms of amphipods (crustaceans), in which trichinella larvae may live long enough to enable infection of seals, which eat the amphipods.

Some authors suppose that certain species of polar birds which feed on dead animals may disseminate the infection. The birds do not digest the trichinella larvae, but eliminate them with their excreta, in which the larvae may remain alive and infective for some time. In some instances birds themselves probably become infected, as has been observed by Rausch et al. (1956), who found trichinella-like larvae in the muscles of a bird (Stercorarius pomarinus).

However, even in polar surroundings depleted of fauna, the rat may be a predominant element in the epidemiology of trichinelliasis. One such example is given by Schiller (1952), in which 12 % of the rats living on a refuse dump in the isolated Aleutian island of Adak, were found to be infected.

Other wild rodents apparently play an insignificant part in the spread of trichinelliasis in arctic regions. Söntgen (1931) investigated 521 field voles from a region in which infection in foxes was frequent, with negative results.

Although there are allusions to trichinelliasis in the early records of the civilised world, the proof that the disease actually occurred was obtained only when it became possible to identify the causative agent under the microscope. Doubtless trichinelliasis was widespread in Europe before the middle of the last century. At present human trichinelliasis occurs in varying degrees of frequency in many temperate regions, i.e., in Central and North Europe and in North and South America, but it is unknown in Australia, as well as in some Asiatic countries in which the population does not eat pork. It is also not propagated in tropical countries, including the whole of Africa and the Pacific Islands. Recently, however, trichinelliasis has been observed in Kenya (Nelson and Forrester, 1962) and, according to Holtz (1962) the infection was found in dogs and pigs in Sumatra.

It might be expected that, with the development of meat hygiene during the last century, especially in the more advanced countries, the incidence of trichinelliasis would have greatly decreased or even disappeared completely. However, a number of recent severe outbreaks show that the time for complacency has not yet arrived. As a matter of fact, trichinelliasis still exists in many civilised countries, prevailing either as a widespread but unnoticed infection, or in the form of serious though rare sporadic outbreaks.

The following recent outbreaks may be quoted as examples: in Beirut (Lebanon) in 1939, over 500 cases (Saad, 1940; Pigoury, 1943); in Oslo (Norway) in 1940, 687 cases (Aaser, 1941); in Wolverhampton (England) in 1941, about 500 cases (Jolly, 1943); in Santiago (Chile) in 1947, 422 cases (Neghme, 1949); in Westfalen (Germany) in 1950, 436 cases (Petrasch and Gaaze, 1952); in Bydgoszcz (Poland) in 1958, 308 cases (Gancarz and Dymek, 1960); in the region of Debrecen (Hungary) 6 outbreaks involving 71 persons (with 3 deaths) recorded during the last 10 years (Nemeseri and Szabo, 1960).

In addition to epidemic outbreaks, individual cases diagnosed on the basis of clinical manifestations occur with varying frequency in most endemic countries. One of the most serious examples is Bielorussia where 709 sporadic cases of trichinelliasis were recorded in 1955 (Leikina, 1957). Sometimes cases occur in places in which the disease was hitherto unknown. Thus, Berni and Mazzi (1957) recorded an outbreak in Italy, in which 9 persons were involved. However, neither the recorded outbreaks nor the individual cases reflect the true incidence, because the majority of infections are symptomless or subclinical and therefore escape from the statistics. Even severe cases are frequently not recognised as such and are not recorded. Epidemiological evaluation of occult trichinelliasis based on sensitive serological tests or the artificial digestion of muscle samples taken at random from routine human necropsies, recently disclosed a hitherto unsuspected high degree of prevalence.

Wright, Jacobs and Walton (1944) recorded 15–28% infections in several localities of the United States; Walker (1948) discovered an incidence of 36.3% in Alabama; Mazzotti (1944) 7.6% in Mexico City; Neghme (1944) 12.5% in Santiago (Chile); Diaz *et al.* (1960) as many as 57% in a small village in the Andes mountains in Chile;

Young (1947) 10.8% in England; Kozar *et al.* (1950) and Piusinski (1960) 4 and 15% in Bialystock and Warsaw (Poland) respectively. High, although not exactly evaluated incidences are recorded from several regions of the Soviet Union, *e.g.* Bielorussia, Litva, parts of Ukraine, Kasakhstan etc. (Bezsonov, 1960).

This high prevalence in man is due to the consumption of insufficiently cooked pork or pork products. Although, in most civilised countries, legislation provides for either the microscopical inspection of slaughtered pigs and the boiling of scrap which is to be used as food for swine, practice shows that universal enforcement of these measures is difficult. Moreover, many infections originate from uninspected animals slaughtered on small farms.

The value of the statistics quoted above is rather limited. With the improvement of sanitary measures the results may be drastically changed. The example of Beard (1951) is instructive to this point: during the years 1949/50 post-mortem examinations in San-Francisco showed an incidence of 8% as contrasted with 24% reported by McNaught and Anderson in 1936. This change has been attributed to the more stringent enforcement of meat hygiene measures and the diminished use of garbage as pig-food.

Occasionally other animals providing human food have been the sources of infection, for instance, the *wild boar* in Palestine (Wortabet, 1881; 1883) and in the Caucasus (Marmashvili, 1955); the *badger* in Kazakhstan (Chun-Syun, 1958), the Caucasus and Russia (Simionova, 1947); the *beaver rat* (*Myocastor coypus*) in Switzerland (Rubli, 1936). *Bear* meat has been the cause of several serious cases of human trichinelliasis.

The earliest recorded outbreak of this kind occurred when a ham made of bear meat was consumed in Germany in 1888 (von Bockum-Dollfs). Later, polar bear meat caused illness in München in 1913 (Boehm). Subsequently a number of similar infections were recorded, some of them recently *e.g.* in Stuttgart (Germany) in 1930, when 100 people fell ill and 13 died after eating insufficiently cooked meat of a polar-bear served in a restaurant (quoted from Roth, 1950). Several outbreaks in the Soviet Union have been described recently.

A few decades ago dogs were used as food in some German towns. According to Gould (1945) the slaughter of dogs for this purpose was practised in three German cities (Breslau, München and Chemnitz), and between 1904 and 1924 examinations of more than 42,000 dogs showed that 1.18% of them were infected. Seifert (1874) described an epidemic which originated from the flesh of dogs.

Arctic regions offer particularly favourable conditions for the spread of human trichinelliasis. Certain customs of the aborigines especially facilitate it. Thus the Eskimos depend on the flesh of sea mammals for their food. Polar-bear, walrus and seal are the main animals used. In spite of the fact that Eskimos usually cook their meat, outbreaks of trichinelliasis occur. According to a "Review of the National Research Council" (Ottawa, 1954), trichinelliasis was recorded in some tribes of Eskimos at a rate as high as 95%. The epidemic in Disco Bay (Greenland) in 1947, described by Thorborg *et al.* (1948), involved over 300 cases with 23 deaths. It is supposed (Parnell, 1934; Roth, 1950) that the frequent outbreaks of "meat-poisoning" among Eskimos are in fact outbreaks of trichinelliasis.

As has been mentioned earlier, there is no distinct correlation between the prevalence of trichinelliasis in wild animals and in man. The parasite may exist in a certain region without involving man in its life cycle. The relationship between trichinelliasis of man and that of swine is often inverse. In spite of the common occult infections of man, swine are usually only lightly infected.

In regions in which customs, religion or sanitary measures prevent man from eating raw pork, infection may exist in nature while decades may pass without a single human case. In Israel, for instance, under natural conditions, the dog, cat, lynx, fox *(Vulpes nilotica)*, jackal *(Canis aureus)*, mongoose *(Herpestes ichneumon)* and wild boar *(Sus scrofa)* have been found infected, while no human case of trichinelliasis has been recorded for over 80 years.

The clinical course of trichinelliasis in man is markedly irregular. Slight infections may be symptomless. Intensive infections, however, produce several clinical signs, of which only two are characteristic, namely the very high eosinophilia (up to 80%), and the oedema of the face, which is mainly suborbital. In most lightly infected cases these symptoms are not pronounced. Other signs, such as an unstable temperature, general malaise, myalgia, pain in the joints and coughing occur but are not pathognomonic, and therefore most of the cases which do not occur during an epidemic are not correctly diagnosed. Most often they are confused with rheumatic fever (Terry and Work, 1940).

The incubation period varies, even in individuals during the same outbreak. It is generally more than 4 days and rarely exceeds 20 days.

The symptoms of trichinelliasis may be classified in three stages: (1) the period during which the adult worms develop in the intestine

(2–3 days); (2) the period of muscle invasion (approximately 2 weeks); (3) the period of gradual recovery (approximately 2–3 months).

The first signs appear 24–72 hours after the ingestion of infected food. The patients show symptoms of gastro-intestinal disturbances, nausea and vomiting, with a rise of temperature, sometimes above 38°. The picture often suggests typhoid or paratyphoid fever. About 3 days after the onset of the disease, headache, muscular pains and oedema of the face appear, their intensity corresponding to the intensity of infection. At the same time eosinophilia becomes pronounced. Generally it increases, although rarely, even in fatal cases, it may be low (Terry and Work, 1940). Excruciating pain is especially felt in the muscles of the extremities, the intercostals and the eyeballs. Breathing becomes difficult, and a painful cough may be very disturbing. In grave cases haemorrhages occur in the retina. In intensive infections cerebral symptoms, and in cases which end fatally a non purulent meningitis and encephalitis are common. According to Sheldon (1941) involvement of the central nervous system occurs in 10–17% of the cases. Sometimes somnolence and delirium are pronounced. On rare occasions a rash appears. These symptoms grow in intensity for about 2 weeks, while eosinophilia reaches its peak. The absence of eosinophilia often has a grave prognostic significance. At this time the patient either dies in coma or the symptoms gradually subside.

It is generally accepted that when, some 2 or 3 weeks after the start of the disease, immunity develops, the clinical symptoms gradually disappear. The nature of the immunity and its curative effect are not completely understood.

The picture of trichinelliasis is variable even in the same epidemic outbreak. The diagnosis of sporadic cases especially that of light infections may be very difficult, because in these cases the symptoms are common to many familiar diseases.

The most serious damage is done to the cardiovascular and central nervous systems. Myocarditis may be the predominant pathological process and in isolated cases it may be mistaken for rheumatic fever (Terry and Work, 1940).

The immediate cause of the symptoms which develop in the course of trichinelliasis is not sufficiently understood. Some authors assert that the clinical symptoms express the reaction of the host to invasion by the parasite rather than the direct effect of the parasite on the host tissues (Philipson and Kershaw, 1960; Rachon and Januszkiewicz, 1960). Rostafinska (1960) showed that the serum of persons infected with trichinella does not possess the histamine-binding property in the Parrot and Laborde test, and she concluded that the pathogenesis of trichinelliasis is allergic in character.

The course of light infections may be confined to 2 or 3 weeks, after which time the patient can gradually return to his normal regime, but in intensive infections, which do not end fatally, the complications mentioned above, as well as general malaise may continue for months. A fall of temperature and the return of sleep are favourable signs. Vomiting and delirium at the end of the third week indicate a dangerous condition. Pneumonia or oedema caused by heart failure, and also a rapid decrease of the eosinophilia, denote an unfavourable outcome. Death usually occurs in stupor or coma in the fourth or fifth week of disease.

The mortality from trichinelliasis varies greatly, depending on the intensity of the infection. Epidemics with mortality rates up to 16% of the infected persons have been recorded. On the other hand, there are outbreaks without any fatalities. Death depends on two factors, *i.e.* the number of larvae invading the muscles and the natural resistance of the host. Neither factor is predictable. The immunity is complex and it is not absolute. Immunity which acts against the adult stage of the parasite living in the intestine develops independently from that directed against the larvae migrating in the tissues. There is apparently no immunological process which acts on the encysted larvae.

Immunity against trichinella infection is manifested in various ways. McCoy (1940) showed that immune rats eliminate a large proportion of the young worms through violent peristalsis during the first 24 hours. Rappaport and Wells (1949) observed reduction in the size of the adult trichinellae and reduction in the number of new-born larvae in immunised mice. Efforts to produce artificial immunisation of animals have not led to practical methods.

The most interesting attempt to produce immunity was by means of irradiated larvae. It was found by several authors (Tyzzer and Noneij, 1917; Schwartz, 1921; Semrad, 1937; Levin and Evans, 1942; Evans, Levin and Sulkin, 1941; Alicata, 1951; Gould *et al.* 1953, and others) that X-ray irradiation is injurious to trichinella larvae and that the injury is proportionate to the dosage of the radiation. A large dosage kills them, but under appropriate low dosage (10,000 R) they are sterilised, although they retain vitality and develop in the intestine of the host to their full size, just as non-irradiated larvae do. They do not cause clinical symptoms, but their presence may produce the desired immunity against subsebuent infection with normal cysts (Hendriks, 1952; Sadun *et al.* 1957; Kim, 1957). It has been proposed that this phenomenon might be used for the immunization of pigs, but it has not yet been accepted for practical application.

Attempts have been made to produce passive immunity by the injection of convalescent serum (Trawinski, 1935; Culbertson and Kaplan, 1937, 1938; Culbertson, 1942; Oliver Gonzalez, 1941; McCoy and Bond, 1941; Dorin, 1946, and others). The results, however, were conflicting and their application has not been sufficiently corroborated in practice.

Several serological tests have been devised for diagnostic purposes, among which are the intradermal, precipitin, complement-fixation, flocculation, circum-larval precipitation, micro- and macro-haemagglutination-, larval immobilisation and the fluorescent antibody tests. Some of these tests are used in routine diagnosis; others are still in the experimental stage.

Serological diagnostic methods are important, not only in human infections, but also in animals, particularly in swine, in which the presence of encapsulated trichinella larvae cannot usually be established clinically and cannot always be detected by quick microscopic examination. Various methods have been proposed for diagnosing trichinelliasis in swine prior to slaughtering; among them are an intracutaneous allergic test (made on the ear) and a precipitation test.

Both clinical and laboratory methods may sometimes fail to provide decisive results. Certain symptoms, mainly the swelling around the eyes and the eosinophilia, are suggestive of trichinelliasis. In such cases examination of a small piece of skeletal muscle, the size of a match-head, pressed between two pieces of thick glass, may reveal the infection. The presence of trichinella larvae is a definite proof of infection, while their absence does not necessarily exclude it, because they may be scanty or absent from the particular sample of muscle tissue biopsied.

Various muscles may be chosen (for instance *M. gastrocnemius*), but examination of the intercostal muscles is the most promising. It should also be kept in mind that, besides the inconvenience biopsy causes to a patient with high fever and tender muscles, it carries the risk of causing phlegmonous inflammation. Kathe and Poters (1943), who recorded two such cases, presume that trichinelliasis might predispose the wound to septic infection. It should be pointed out that encysted and distinctly spirally coiled larvae may not be observed in man before 3 weeks after the onset of the disease.

In cases of heavy infection the larvae may occasionally be discovered in the circulating blood. For this purpose 10 ml of venous blood is laked in 100 ml of 3% acetic acid, centrifuged and the sediment examined (Stäubli's method). The larvae can be recognized as they show, at about the middle of their bodies, a characteristic unstainable area, the genital primordium (Stäubli, 1909). This method is, however, unreliable. Similarly unreliable is the search for the young trichinellae which are sometimes eliminated with faeces in the early days of the infection.

References p. 548/549

Despite intensive search during the last 120 years for an effective remedy against trichinelliasis, no specific treatment has as yet been found It should be borne in mind that, in choosing a therapeutic agent against trichinelliasis, 3 different stages of the causative agent must be considered first, the adult worm, which is partly embedded in the intestinal mucous membrane, secondly, the young larva present in the blood and migrating through the tissues, and thirdly the larva embedded in the muscles. While it may be possible to affect the female and the migrating larva, the larva in the muscle fibers is securely protected by its capsule and is inaccessible to therapeutic agents. Many drugs have been tried with variable, but mostly doubtful, effects.

Recent observations show that corticosteroid therapy may greatly, and sometimes dramatically, alleviate the subjective symptoms. In cases of successful treatment the temperature falls, the oedema and myalgia disappear, and the patient feels better. However, these hormones are not harmful to the worms and do not alter the course of the disease. On the contrary, it is believed that cortisone increases the longevity of the adult trichinellae (*i.e.* the number of larvae) and suppresses the degree of acquired immunity. Some authors (Lord, 1958) advocate, therefore, abstention from the use of cortisone in the treatment of trichinelliasis. There are indications that Dithiazanine reduces the number of adult worms and larvae (Kuzmicki, 1962).

In spite of the lack of specific therapy, symptomatic treatment may bring relief to the patient. Sedatives, given by the mouth or injected, are indicated in almost all cases.

Since the most important epidemiological factor in the spread of trichinelliasis is the consumption of insufficiently cooked or otherwise heated pork, it should be remembered that a single hog may provide many meat meals, and that even in cases of inapparent infection of this animal, each meal may constitute a most serious hazard to the consumers. In many countries the danger of eating infective pork is reflected in legislative measures, which forbade the slaughter of hogs, except in licensed slaughter-houses in which the meat is inspected by competent personnel and infected carcasses are either destroyed or sterilized.

The inspector collects several samples of muscle weighing about 1 gram and then divides them into smaller pieces which are squeezed between two thick glassplates (compressor).

Examination is done either through a low power microscope or by the use of a specially constructed lantern, in which the compressor serves as a lantern slide, the picture being projected on to a screen. It is customary to choose for examination a piece of the diaphragm, such in view of the particular predilection of trichinella larvae to this organ. Next in attractiveness to the larvae are the masseters and the muscles of the pharynx (Luengo and Rodriquez, 1954). This routine inspection will reveal only grossly infected meat and some of the more lightly infected cases may pass unnoticed. In view of the high costs of the method it has not been made obligatory in every country in which trichinelliasis of hogs is likely to occur.

Serological methods have also been tried for the diagnosis of trichinella infection in animals. The precipitin test, advocated by Trawinski (1934), Nelson (1939) and others, gives 5–15% of false reactions and cannot, therefore, be relied upon.

Soulsby (1960) showed that a precipitation test in which an aqueous trichinella extract is used as antigen, may yield positive results in infections with other nematodes.

Trichinous meat should not be consumed until the larvae have been destroyed. Heating until a temperature of 60° has been reached throughout the meat will render it innocuous. Keeping the meat for at least 20 days at a temperature of −15° or lower, will also make it non-infective. It should be noted, however, that such processing methods generally affect the quality of the meat. Salting for at least 45 days in 10% brine kills the larvae.

According to Gould et al. (1954–'55) irradiation with gamma rays at 30,000 R makes infected pork innocuous and does not reduce its palatability; however, the high cost of the installation makes this method impracticable.

The following rules have been laid down by the Federal Meat Inspection Regulations in the U.S.A. for pork which is to be eaten without cooking: Pieces not exceeding 15 cm in thickness or stored in containers not more than 6 inches in depth, should be frozen for 20 days at −15°, for 10 days at −23°, or for 6 days at −29°. Larger pieces must be kept at low temperatures for longer times (Wright, 1954).

Objection has been raised (Thompsen, 1956) against the sterilization of lightly infected pork, because this action deprives the population living in an endemic region of the comparatively harmless natural immunization which results from the consumption of small numbers of larvae in their food. This argument cannot be considered without serious criticism.

Feeding pigs on raw slaughter-house scrap is one of the most important factors in the spread of trichinelliasis among these animals. When this fact became evident some countries issued legislation which made it obligatory to cook scrap destined to be swine food. The beneficial effect of this measure is evident if the situations in Canada, where it is properly enforced, and the U.S.A. where it has been issued only in some of the

References p. 548/549

States are compared. According to Cameron (1940, 1943) garbage-fed hogs in Canada are infected at the rate of 0.2%, while in the U.S.A. the infection rate amounts to 5%. At the same time the incidence of the infection, according to the examinations of human corpses, is 1.5% in Canada, and about 17% in the U.S.A.

Proper construction of slaughter-houses is one of the prerequisites of trichinelliasis control. An establishment which is not isolated from its surroundings by a suitable fence, and is accessible to dogs, cats and rats, cannot be regarded as being fully safeguarded; on the contrary, it sometimes constitutes a serious source for the spread of trichinelliasis.

Proper disposal of home refuse should supplement preventive measures. Gaugusch (1949) has shown that encysted trichinella larvae can survive at a temperature of 18–25° for up to 260 days, even when the surrounding muscle has completely decomposed. Unattended rat-infested refuse dumps may become foci from which trichinelliasis is spread (Schiller, 1952).

It is obvious that many measures, if they are properly applied, can reduce the spread and incidence of trichinelliasis in man and domestic animals. There is, as yet, no hope that the infection can be totally eradicated. Sylvatic trichinelliasis lurking in places inaccessible to human interference will always be liable to encroach on human surroundings.

REFERENCES

BABERO, B. B., R. V. RAUSCH and E. L. SCHILLER, J. Parasit., 42 (1956) 259.
BIELAYEVA, M. YA., Zool. Ž., 33 (1954) 714.
CAGNOLATI, G. C. and B. MERIGHI, Parassitologia, 1 (1959) 78.
GOULD, S. E., Trichinosis (Springfield), 8 (1945) 356.
GOULD, S. E., H. J. GOMBERG and F. H. BETHELL, J. Amer. med. Ass., 154 (1954) 653.
HOVORKA, J., Wiad. Parazyt., 3 (1957) 231.
KAGAN, I. G., J. infectious Dis., 107 (1960) 65.
KOO, S. Y., Lingnan Sci. J., 21 (1945) 39.
KUITUNEN-EKBAUM and Z. W. FLEMING, Canad. J. publ. Hlth, 40 (1949) 514.
LEHMENSICK, R., in BORCHERT (Ed.), Probleme der Parasitologie 1956, p. 148.
LEINATI, L. and V. MARAZZA, Chinese Vet., 82 (1959) 1.
NEGHME, A., G. F. RIVERA and M. ALVAREZ, Bol. chil. Parasit., 10 (1955) 73.
NELSON, G. S. and A. T. T. FORRESTER, Wiad. Parazyt., 8 (1962) 17.
OHBAYASHI, M. and H. SATO, Japan J. vet. Res., 5 (1957) 39.
OLSEN, O. W., J. Parasit., Suppl., 46 (1960) 22.
REINHARD, E. G., Exp. Parasit., 7 (1958) 108.
RITTERSON, A. L., J. Parasit., Suppl., 45 (1959) 36.
ROTH, H., Acta med. scand., 126 (1946) 17; Bull. Off. int. Epiz., 34 (1950) 197.
WITENBERG, G., Arch. Schiffs-u. Tropenhyg., 37 (1933) 37.
WRIGHT, W. H., L. JACOBS and A. C. WALTON, Publ. Hlth Rep. (Wash.), 59 (1944) 669.

ZAIMAN, H., G. OMI and L. GAPINSKI, *Amer. J. Hyg.*, 57 (1953) 306.
ZAIMAN, H., J. M. STONEY and N. C. HEADLEY, *Amer. J. Hyg.*, 61 (1955) 15.
ZIMMERMANN, W. J., E. D. HUBBARD, L. H. SCHWARTE and H. E. BIESTER, *Proc. Iowa Acad. Sci.*, 67 (1960) 578.

b. Dracontiasis

Dracontiasis or *dranunculiasis* is a disease caused by the nematode worm *Dranunculus medinensis*, the correct name of which is *Füllebornius medinensis*, and in vernacular terminology the Guinea worm or rishta (in

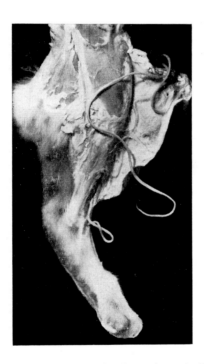

Fig. 77. *Dranunculus medinensis* in leg of a domestic cat in Israel (original photo).

Asian parts of the Soviet Union). This very long nematode (which may be 1.20 m long, but is only about 2 mm wide) lives in the connective tissues, slowly but continuously moving along a tortuous path in all parts of the body.

The Guinea worm was one of the earliest of the human parasites to be

recognized and was already known to the ancient Egyptians, Arabs and Indians. Apart from man, it occurs in numerous wild and domestic animals, including the dog, cat (Fig.77), horse and monkey. A similar species is found in North America in the raccoon, fox, mink and other animals, but there is no general agreement as to whether it is an identical or related species.

The infection results from drinking water containing the infected inter- mediate host, which is an almost microscopic copepod of the genus *Cyclops*.

The worm found in human infections is usually a female. The males, which are much smaller, copulate early and disappear soon afterwards. The growing female produces numerous eggs which hatch while still in the uterus. The genital opening of the female worm is closed and the larvae are therefore not laid, but remain inside the female, accumulating there for about 1 year, the female meanwhile becoming distended with her progeny. When filled with larvae the female worm approaches the surface of the skin of any part of the host's body, and there causes a blister which finally bursts and allows the anterior end of the female worm to protrude from the opening. Usually the blister is formed on a part of the skin which comes into frequent contact with water, *e.g.* the back or the bare feet of water carriers. The open sore thus produced often becomes infected with bacteria and then develops into an ulcer. The process of blister formation destroys the cuticle over the anterior end of the worm and the adjoining part of the uterus contained therein, thus providing an outlet for the larvae. When the ulcer comes in contact with water, the worm contracts and ejects a drop of whitish fluid containing myriads of larvae which actively swim away. If these are swallowed by a *Cyclops*, the larvae enter the body cavity of this crustacean and there develop during the next 2–4 weeks into spirally-coiled infective larvae. Further development requires that the infected *Cyclops* shall be swallowed by the final host, in which the freed larvae enter the connective tissues, thus completing the life cycle of the parasite.

During the process of liberation of the larvae, which continues for a number of days or weeks, the worm is slowly pushed out of the opening in the ulcer until the loose remnant can easily be removed (Fig. 78). This process is accompanied by local inflammation, sometimes of considerable extent, which incapacitates the patient. When the entire worm has left the wound, the inflammation usually subsides quickly and the lesion heals. Occasionally, however, especially when the anterior part of the worm has been torn away and the remaining portion is not capable of emerging, bacterial infection sets in and, this, if it is not suitably treated, may cause phlegmone, gangrene, septicaemia, synovitis or other serious conditions.

Not infrequently the mature worm does not find its way to the in- tegument. In this case it dies in the tissues without discharging its accumu-

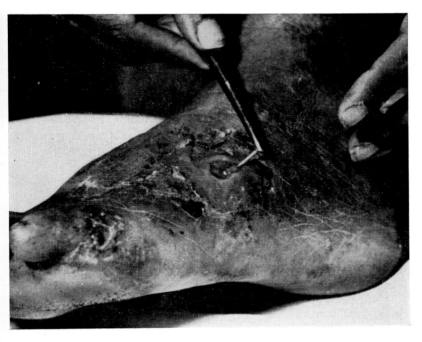

Fig. 78. Dracontiasis; ulcer with emerging worm on the foot of a Yemenite Jew (courtesy Dr. I. Pfeiffer, Pardess Katz Hospital of Infectious Diseases, Israel).

lated progeny. Part of the worm becomes phagocytised; the rest calcifies without provoking any subjective symptoms. Such calcified remains of dead Guinea worms may show up in X-ray pictures of various parts of the body. In endemic localities they are a common accidental finding. Occasionally scores of such "mummies" of Guinea worms are dispersed all over the body (Fig. 79).

In many cases one single worm settles in the human body, but several worms may appear in succession, forming new ulcers. The presence of the parasite does not produce immunity; in endemic localities superinfections and reinfections are quite common. Botreau-Roussel (1928) reported a case of dracontiasis in Senegal in which more than 100 Guinea worms were removed from one man.

Often infected individuals do not realize that they harbour the parasite, the period of worm-migration usually being clinically symptomless. Sometimes, however, allergic signs appear in the form of patchy erythema, urticaria, nausea and diarrhoea. As soon as the ulcer has been formed these symptoms disappear, and may be replaced by other toxic manifestations. Although eosinophilia has been recorded, it is not pathognomonic in dracontiasis.

According to the estimate of Stoll (1947) about 48 million people suffer from dracontiasis. It is prevalent over the whole continent of Africa and in southern Asia, as well as in China and Korea. In certain areas of Africa over 80% of the population are carriers of Guinea worms. Its

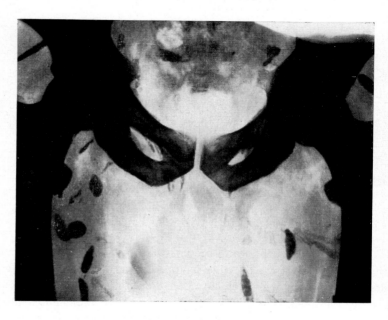

Fig. 79.   Dracontiasis. Röntgenograph of the pelvic region of an immigrant from Yemen showing calcified remains of 24 guinea worms (courtesy Dr. Breslau, Hadassah Hospital, Jerusalem, 1956).

incidence is greatest in arid, rural regions where the population is dependent, for drinking purpose, on water which has been stored in open cisterns or pools. These sources of potable water are often grossly polluted and develop rich plankton among which several species of *Cyclops* abound.

Besides its wide human distribution, dracontiasis may occur as a purely animal infection. Chun-Siun (1958), for instance, found over 11% of stray dogs infected in Kizylordy (Soviet Kazakhstan), where no human infection was known. In the majority of cases, however, under unhygienic conditions, both people and animals are infected, and it is difficult to decide which source is the more important for the dissemination of the Guinea worm.

In principle, control of dracontiasis is comparatively easy if adequate sanitary measures can be enforced. Potable water must be stored in basins inaccessible to pollution by man or animals, and it must be periodically cleansed of vegetation which gives shelter to crustaceans. The water can be cleared of *Cyclops* by means of insecticides, among which Gammexane is effective and cheap. The introduction of *Gambusia* or other insectivorous fish may by itself be sufficient to keep the water-cisterns free from crustaceans.

The town of Bokhara in Tadjikistan (U.S.S.R.) may be cited as an example of successful control of dracontiasis. About 30 years ago this locality was hyperendemic, hardly a person escaping recurrent infection. Potable water was drawn from open cisterns and distributed by water-carriers who entered the water barefoot to fill the skin-sacks. All

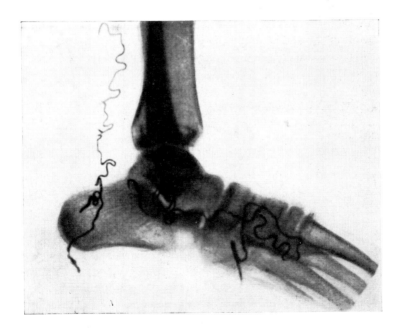

Fig. 80. Dracontiasis. X-ray photo of two lipiodol-injected guinea worms in human foot (from: Botreau-Roussel, in Bull. Soc. Pathol. exotique, 1928).

References p. 554

these water-carriers were infected at one time or another with Guinea worms. Under these circumstances the abundant *Cyclops* were constantly exposed to the larvae. After proper sanitation of the general water supply had been carried out, dracontiasis was eradicated and did not reappear.

The best method of extraction of the worm, after it has appeared in the ulcer, is the aboriginal one, practised in endemic regions by witch-doctors. The head-end of the parasite is fastened by a thread to a wooden stick and is covered with a water-compress for 1 or 2 days. Every day a piece of the worm emerges from the wound and is rolled onto the stick. After approximately a fortnight, the whole parasite has been removed and the wound then closes without complications. Considering the tortuous shape of the worm in the tissues (Fig. 80), it is clear that the removal cannot be accomplished by forcible traction; the pulling must be done gently and gradually, for, if rupture occurs,the remaining part becomes a focus of secondary bacterial infection.

When multiple infection is suspected or diagnosed, drug treatment should be applied. The most effective of the numerous drugs which have been used is tartar emetic, given intravenously. Elliot (1942) recommends infiltration of the site in which the worm is located with an emulsion of phenothiazine in oil.

REFERENCES

BOTREAU-ROUSSEL, P., *Bull. Soc. Path. exot.*, 21 (1928) 103.
FAIRLEY, N. H., *Indian J. med. Res.*, 12 (1924) 351; 369.
KATZENELLENBOGEN, I., *Dermatologica (Basel)*, 108 (1954) 129.
LINDBERG, K., *Bull. Soc. Path. exot.*, 39 (1946) 318.
MCCONNELL, R. L., *J. trop. Med. Hyg.*, 17 (1914) 337.
SCOTT, D., *Ann. trop. Med. Parasit.*, 54 (1960) 32.

c. *Strongyloidiasis*

Strongyloidiasis is caused by very small nematode worms belonging to the genus *Strongyloides,* a genus which includes numerous species parasitic in various vertebrates (mammals, birds, reptiles and amphibians). Two of these species, *S. stercoralis* and *S. fülleborni* appear as parasites of man. Human strongyloidiasis is common in the tropics, but less so in the sub-tropics, while isolated cases are reported also from temperate zones *e.g.* in NorthAmerica and Central Europe.

One of the peculiarities of spacies of the genus *Strongyloides* is the heterogenic life cycle, during which a parasitic generation alternates with a free living one, the former being represented by parthenogenetic females.

Strongyloides stercoralis is the more important of the two species mentioned.

The parasitic female is about 2.5 mm long and lives in the mucosa and sub-mucosa of the small intestine, mainly of the duodenum. In heavy infections the worms spread along the whole of the small intestine and eventually invade the pancreatic and biliary ducts. The eggs are laid within the tissues where they hatch. The emerging rhabditiform larvae* escape into the lumen of the intestine and are voided with the faeces. Subsequently these larvae, which are about 0.5 mm long. live in the soil, feed on organic matter, and moult twice within a few days. Either of two different developmental stages may result from the second moult, signifying a direct or an indirect life-cycle.

In the *direct life cycle* the larva retains the skin cast of at the last moult and, after 2 to 3 days, becomes the "filariform" infective stage, which has a long oesophagus, devoid of a bulb. This form continues life in the soil for up to 50 days and it can penetrate the intact human skin. Naturally barefoot people are most exposed. Once under the skin the larva works its way to the lymphatic or venous system and is carried, by way of the heart, to the lungs. When it arrives in the capillaries of the lung, the larva breaks through the endothelium into the alveoli and undergoes an additional moult. It then enters the bronchioles and is carried by the ciliated epithelium to the larynx-pharynx, from which it is swallowed. By this complex route the larva reaches the duodenum, where it penetrates into the mucosa and is transformed into a parthenogenetic female within 4 or 5 days. This female proceeds to deposit eggs between or under the epithelial cells; two days later rhabditiform larvae appear in the faeces and the life cycle starts anew.

When the worm develops by the *indirect cycle*, the rhabditiform larva is transformed, within one day, into a free-living adult male or female (morphologically distinct from the parthenogenetic parasitic female), which lives in the soil as a saprozoic organism. When the free-living female is about 1 mm long, it begins to lay eggs, and this continues for several days, after which the female dies. A new generation develops from the eggs she has laid. These larvae undergo two moults within 2 or 3 days and then become filariform larvae identical with those produced during the direct cycle, and these are very infective. In rare instances the rhabditoid larvae of the free-living generation may again become free living adults.

There are strains of *S. stercoralis* which preferably follow the direct mode of development and others which tend to follow the indirect one. In accordance with changing environmental conditions some, however, may alternate between these two modes

---

* The rhabditiform or rhabditoid larva is distinguished by an oesophagus provided with a globular posterior extremity, the "bulb",

(Galliard, 1951). After several passages through dogs, any strain of human *Strongyloides* changes into a predominantly indirectly developing strain. Temporary cooling of the larvae or changing of the medium produces alterations in the ratio of direct-indirect strains (Beach, 1936; Faust, 1937; Galliard, 1951; Premwati, 1958).

There is apparently no correlation between the intensity of the infection and the form of the life-cycle of the strain concerned, although in most cases of severe infection a directly developing strain is involved.

Strongyloidiasis in *man* may be almost symptomless, but frequently it manifests itself from the moment the larva penetrates the skin. At first there may be intense itching, followed by the formation of a small papule, and by spreading oedema and painful lymph-nodes. This reaction may last up to a week. Passage of larvae through the lungs may be accompanied by urticaria, asthmatoid respiration and eosinophilia (de Langen, 1928). Strong bowel movement accompanied by pain in the epigastrium is the commonest sign of intestinal invasion. Sometimes the disease appears with a sudden attack of diarrhoea, which may subside and recur intermittently. If the disease persists, it may cause debility and loss of body-weight.

The presence of the parasite in the intestinal mucosa does not necessarily give rise to perceptible lesions or even to cellular reactions. Sometimes, however, extensive ulceration of the epithelial tissue may be observed. Eosinophilia always appears, but its intensity varies.

There is no age-predilection for strongyloidiasis, though it mostly affects adults. Camain *et al.* (1955) described an acute fatal case in a child 2 years old, in Dakar.

The longevity of the parasitic female is not definitely known, but is presumably short. In some cases human strongyloidiasis disappears spontaneously after a short duration. Occasionally, however, the infection may last, if left untreated, as long as 30 years (Kyle *et al.*, 1948), and this may happen even in localities in which the possibility of reinfection can reasonably be excluded.

Fülleborn and other investigators presumed that, in cases of persistent infection, re-infection is affected by filariform larvae which develop in faecal material adhering to the anal region and invade the host on the spot, thus constantly replenishing the parasite load. Faust (1937) offered a different explanation, namely, that in some instances filariform larvae (of a so-called "dwarfed" type) develop in the intestine, enter the tissues and follow the usual migration without leaving the host (hyperinfection), a view also shared by Harz (1946, 1954) and Galliard (1949, 1951).

In many instances, for reasons unknown, autoinfection persists continuously, and in some mild cases this may be evidenced by the frequent appearance of pulmonary infiltrations, renal haemorrhages and the presence of larvae in the sputum or urine. When hyperinfection is abundant, it may cause a fulminating course of the disease terminating fatally. In such cases the numerous larvae incessantly invading the body of the host gain entrance into the major blood circulation and can be found in every part of the body, including the kidneys, liver and brain (Askanazy, 1900).

While resistance to reinfection has been observed in animals, recovered from a *Strongyloides stercoralis-infection*, such increased resistance is presumably absent from man.

The highest incidence of strongyloidiasis has been reported in the Rio Doce area (Brazil) and in the city of Inquitos (Peru) where 58 % and 60 % of the population respectively were found infected (Gomes de Moraes, 1948; Gonzalez-Ungaburu, 1955). Faust (1931) recorded that 20 % of the village population of Panama were infected; Coutinho *et al.* (1951) observed the larvae of *Stercoralis* in 12 % of the children in Sao Paulo (Brasil); Buckley (1946) detected the infection frequently in some Rhodesian villages; Sadun and Vajrasthira (1952)–in North Thailand– and Fan (1959) in some communities in Formosa, recorded an incidence of 18 %. Human strongyloidiasis becomes rarer the farther one moves away from the tropics.

An odd feature in the spread of strongyloidiasis is its comparative rarity. Because the direct type of the life history of *Strongyloides* is very similar to that of the hookworm, it would seem that the prevalence of both species of parasites should be equal. In fact, however, strongyloidiasis is everywhere much less frequent than hookworm disease. This is the more puzzling since *Strongyloides* is often more prolific thanks to the exogenous reproduction of its free-living generation. The less extensive spread of *Strongyloides,* as compared with that of the hookworm, may perhaps partly be explained by the shorter longevity of the filariform larvae of the former species.

Clinical symptoms cannot alone be relied upon to establish the diagnosis. Peptic ulcer is the commonest misleading differential diagnosis (Hinman, 1938).

The only exact basis for diagnosis is provided by the recovery of *Strongyloides* larvae from the excreta (faeces, intestinal contents, sputum). The number of larvae excreted in the stool does not indicate the severity of the infection. In some cases in which the infection may be quite intensive, only a few or no larvae appear. In such cases the larvae may be more easily discovered in cultures then by direct examination of the faeces. Deschiens (1925), Jones (1950) and others, consider that microscopy of fluid aspirated from the duodenum is much more efficient than examination of the faeces.

Fülleborn (1926) proposed a cutaneous test, in which powdered *Strongyloides* larvae are used as antigen. Brannon and Faust (1949) demonstrated the presence of specific antibodies in a precipitin test. However, neither of these tests has gained popularity.

There is no universal treatment of strongyloidiasis in man. The best drug, which frequently gives satisfactory results, is medicinal gentian violet, orally administered in gelatine capsules. In some cases the infection is refractory to this treatment (Fisher, 1946) and repeated administration of the drug is necessary to get rid of the parasite. Some authors attribute efficacy to Hetrazan, chenopodium oil, hexylresorcinol and Dithiazanine, but the merits of these drugs have yet to be substantiated.

Strongyloides stercoralis is predominantly a human parasite, but it also causes spontaneous infection in the *dog*, the *cat, orang-utan, chimpanzee, gibbon (Hylobates concolor)*, and *coati (Nasua narica)*. In monkeys the eggs, rather than the larvae, are eliminated with the faeces (Desportes, 1945). In spite of proven susceptibility of these animals to *S. stercoralis* the part they play as reservoirs of human infection is not clear. However, the dog must be regarded as a potential source of human infection On numerous occasions dogs have been infected experimentally with human strains and in several instances also experimental infection of human volunteers with the canine strain of the parasite has been successful. Yet the dog is rarely found to be spontaneously infected, even in localities in which infection is common in man. It should be noted that susceptibility of dogs to *Strongyloides* infection varies according to the strain of the worm and size of the inoculum. Galliard (1951) showed that dogs in Tonkin are easily infected with the local strain of *Strongyloides*, but not with strains imported from Africa or the Antilles.

The pathological picture of strongyloidiasis in the dog is similar to that in man. In most cases, the disease in canines is mild and lasts only for weeks or months, as contrasted with the years of infection in man. Hawkins and Dunlap (1947), however, recorded a fatal case of natural canine infection in Michigan (where human cases are extremely rare); the infected dog passed loose, bloody stools. Only in a few instances has a high incidence been recorded, as for example in a publication of Burrows and Lillis (1960) who found that 16% of puppies in kennels n New Jersey were infected. Chandler, in an intensive study of helminth nfections in India, found an incidence of *Strongyloides* in approximately 50% of some human population groups, but no dogs were infected personal communication, quoted by Augustine, 1940). The course of the infection in dogs differs significantly in individuals and in age groups. Galliard (1939) was able to provoke a massive experimental infection which killed young dogs within 10 or 12 days, whereas adult dogs developed only symptomless infections.

In view of the difference in the pathogenicity of strongyloidiasis in man and the dog, some authors (Brumpt, 1936; Augustine and Davey, 1939) expressed the opinion that the strains which invade man are distinct from those which infect dogs. This view might justify the proposal made by Brumpt (1922) that the parasites of the dog should be regarded as belonging to a separate species, *Strongyloides canis*. This view, however, has not been sufficiently corroborated.

To sum up the varying and sometimes contradictory observations, it may be concluded that *Strongyloides stercoralis* is represented by numerous strains which show different degrees of adaptation to the dog.

As in man, diagnosis of infection in the dog may be made by demonstration of the larvae in the faeces. Their number does not indicate the intensity of the infection. Galliard (1939, 1951) observed that *Strongyloides* larvae frequently become scarce or totally disappear from the faeces of the dog, even during an intensive infection. This is presumably due to the strongly proteolytic action of intestinal ferments, which destroy the larvae before they reach the anus.

It should also be noted that fresh dog faeces may contain the larvae of other nematodes, mainly those of *Ancylostoma* or *Uncinaria* living in the intestine, or of *Filaroides osleri* and *Aelurostrongylus obstrusus,* which live in the lungs, as well as *Rhabditis macrocerca* and *Rh. clavopapillata,* which may be present in the perianal area.

Not much is known about the treatment of strongyloidiasis of dogs. Gentian-violet may be useful but, as in human infection, it is not always effective. Other therapeutic means are: repeated saline purgation, oil of chenopodium given by the mouth (Galliard, 1950) and the administration of Soluseptazine, hexylresorcinol, Anthiomaline and several organic compounds (chlorophenyl-phosphorothionate, according to Levine *et al.,* 1959).

The part played by the domestic cat in spreading the infection is not clear. Cats are rarely found infected with *Strongyloides*. However, a high incidence has been recorded in a few cases (Chandler found 20% of cats

infected in Calcutta, while Calero recorded 51 % infection in Panama city)
Experimental inoculation undertaken by several authors showed
contradictory results. Sandosham (1952) could not infect either of two
cats with material collected from one human patient, but a heavy infection
was caused with material from another man. Sandground observed that
in Java, where *Strongyloides* infection is common in both man and cats
larvae obtained from feline faeces failed to penetrate the human skin
Similarly, in the experience of Galliard in Tonkin, the cat proved re
fractory to infection with the human strain.

Next in importance as a reservoir of *Strongyloides stercoralis* are
certain monkeys, notably the chimpanzee. Desportes (1945) showed that
this host is liable to acquire a spontaneous infection which could ex
perimentally be transferred to other hosts. Spontaneous infection in the
chimpanzee and the gibbon proved lethal to these hosts, while experi
mental infections produced with the larvae excreted lasted 3 months in a
human volunteer, 3 weeks in a dog and was fatal to a cat.

Several species of the genus *Strongyloides,* in addition to *S. stercoralis*
have been reported from primates. The best known is *S. fülleborni,* which
commonly lives in Old-World monkeys (the relevant records have been
summarized by Premvati, 1958), and rarely in man.

Strongyloides fülleborni is morphologically similar to *S. stercoralis* but
may be distinguished from it by a peculiar post-vulvar constriction in the
free-living female. It develops just as the human species does, but some
times, not only in animals but also in man, eggs instead of larvae are
eliminated with the faeces.

S. fülleborni causes spontaneous infection in the orang-utan, baboon
and in several other Old-World monkeys, but apparently it canno
establish itself in New-World monkeys or in the cat.

Chandler (1925) found that practically all Rhesus monkeys in the
Calcutta Zoo which died from various causes, were harbouring *S. fülle*
borni without showing symptoms of that infection. However, other cases
have been recorded in which this species was highly pathogenic.

Man and the *dog* may acquire only a transitory infection with *S*
fülleborni. According to Buckley (1946), *Strongyloides fülleborni* is wide
spread among the inhabitants of Rhodesian villages, the incidence reach
ing 30%. Wallace *et al.* (1948) reported a case of spontaneous human

nfection with *S. fülleborni* contracted in the Philippines. The infection persisted for at least 1 year and 7 months. A case of experimental infecion in a human volunteer, recorded by Tomita (1941), lasted 11 months.

The numerous Old-World monkeys which are nowadays being imported into Europe and North America for experimental purposes and or the production of vaccines should be regarded as potential disseminators of this parasite.

REFERENCES

ASKANAZY, M., *Zbl. Bakt.*, 27 (1900) 569.
AUGUSTINE, D. L. and D. G. DAVEY, *J. Parasit.*, 25 (1939) 117.
BLACKLOCK, B. and S. ADLER, *Ann. trop. Med. Parasit.*, 16 (1922) 283.
BUCKLEY, J. J. C., *J. Helminth.*, 21 (1946) 111.
CHANDLER, A. C., *Indian J. med. Res.*, 13 (1925) 213; *Parasitology*, 17 (1925) 426.
CHITWOOD, B. G. and G. L. GRAHAM, *J. Parasit.*, 26 (1940) 183.
CRAIG, C. F. and E. C. FAUST, *Clinical Parasitology*, 5th ed., Philadelphia, 1951, 1032 pp.
DESCHENS, R. E. A. and O. TAILLANDIER, *Bull. Soc. Path. exot.*, 18 (1925) 525.
DESPORTES, C., *Ann. Parasit. hum. comp.*, 20 (1945) 160.
FAUST, E. C., *Proc. Soc. exp. Biol. (N.Y.)*, 28 (1931) 919; *J. Amer. med. Ass.*, 98 (1932) 2276.
FAUST, E. C. and A. DE GROAT, *Amer. J. trop. Med.*, 20 (1940) 359.
FUELLEBORN, F., *Arch. Schiffs- u. Tropenhyg.*, 18 (1914) 26; 30 (1926) 721.
GALLIARD, H., *C. R. Soc. Biol. (Paris)*, 128 (1938) 572; *Ann. Parasit. hum. comp.*, 25 (1950) 441; 26 (1951) 67.
HARTZ, P. H., *Arch. Path.*, 41 (1946) 601.
HINMAN, E. N., *Rev. Gastroent.*, 5 (1938) 24.
KYLE, L. H. and D. G. MACKAY, *Ann. intern. Med.*, 29 (1948) 1014.
PALMER, E. D., *Amer. J. trop. Med.*, 30 (1950) 91.
PREMVATI, *Canad. J. Zool.*, 36 (1958) 36, 185, 447.
SANDGROUND, J. H., *J. Parasit.*, 12 (1925) 59; *Amer. J. Hyg.*, 6 (1926) 337.

d. Trichostrongyliasis

Trichostrongyliasis is caused by species of nematodes belonging to the family *Trichostrongylidae*. Mostly these are hair-like worms, about 1 cm long, which often are reddish when they are alive. Primarily they inhabit the stomach, and small intestine of domestic ruminants, but some species may also establish themselves in man and in a variety of other mammals. Apart from man and domestic ruminants they have been found in the following animal species: bison, buffalo, mountain sheep, wild goat,

chamois, deer, rendeer, elk, antelope, gazelle, roebuck, horse, pig, rabbit
hare, ground squirrel, nutria, opossum, porcupine, and others.

A large number of *Trichostrongylidae* have been differentiated. The life cycle of all thes
species is similar. The development is direct, *i.e.* they do not use an intermediate host. I
the eggs, which are eliminated with the faeces, a first-stage larva develops and hatche
within a few days. In the soil or on pastures the larva undergoes two moults and i
finally transformed in a resistant infective stage capable of maturing on being swal
lowed by a suitable host. The infective stage of most of the species climbs up grasse
or other pasture plants and is ingested by herbivore animals. The young worms settl
in the digestive tract (the abomasum or small intestine), where they develop into adult
in about 4 weeks. The immature stages of some species of the genius *Ostertagia* tem
porarily burrow in the submucosa where they pass through a so-called histotropi
phase, then return to the lumen of the intestine where they matureinto adult worms

Trichostrongylids, also called stomach worms, are wide-spread all ove
the world, and they are so common in cattle and sheep that hardly an
of these animals is free from them.

Trichostrongylids when in small numbers, may be almost harmless
but large numbers of them may cause serious disease and even death
Heavy infection of livestock constitutes a most important economic
problem. Great losses occur either through death or unthriftiness of the
afflicted animals.

The various species of trichostrongylids differ in their pathogenicity to
the domestic animals. In human pathology these differences are insufficiently known, and it is therefore customary not to distinguish between
the various species of trichostrongylid worms.

Until a quarter of a century ago, it was thought that trichostrongyliasi
was fairly rare in man, but later it appeared that, apart from sporadic infections, there exist in several regions of the world localities in which the
disease is a common endemic human infection. Man is most frequently
affected in rural surroundings where contamination of the soil with
animal excrements creates an abundance of infective larvae and many
opportunities for ingestion exist. Yet, in endemic regions high incidence
has been found among the urban population as well.

Endemic areas are found in Africa, and are dispersed throughout the
whole of South Asia, from the Mediterranean to the Pacific. Kalantariar
(1927) recorded a 15% incidence in Armenia, where 6 species of trichostrongylids were identified as human parasites. Biocca (1959) found 6

species in 46 % of the population in certain communities in Persia, where people keep cattle in their dwellings. Watson (1953) found infection with *T. colubriformis* in up to 25 % of the population in some localities of Iraq. Abdel Malik (1937) recorded an 11.5 % incidence of trichostrongyliasis in children in Cairo, while Lawless *et al.* (1956) found that 70 % of the adult population of an Egyptian village were infected. Endemic foci have also been recorded in Pakistan, India, Japan, and other countries. Sporadic infection occurs in most cattle-raising countries, including the United States.

The pathology of trichostrongyliasis in man is not fully known. The worms are mostly lodged in the mucosa of the small intestine, occasionally invading the gall-bladder. The infection may last several years. When the number of parasites is small, the infection may be symptomless. In cases of massive infection, however, the clinical picture may be disturbing, with nausea, abdominal pain, anaemia and general weakness.

The diagnosis may be made by demonstration of the characteristic eggs in the stool. However, differentiation of the particular species cannot be established in this way because the eggs of the majority of species in this group are similar in shape and size. The species can be determined by examination of the infective larvae obtained in stool-cultures. The eggs of the trichostrongylids resemble those of hookworms, and are often confused with these by inexperienced laboratory personnel.

No specifically effective treatment is known. Tetrachlorethylene or Ascaridol, which are effective in the treatment of other nematode infections, fail to cure trichostrongyliasis. Kalantarian (1934) and other Soviet investigators recommended the use of a thymol suspension administered through a duodenal tube.

Control of trichostrongyliasis consists of improvement of personal hygiene together with treatment of infected cattle with appropriate drugs (nicotine sulphate, phenothiazine).

The infective larvae survive dryness for many months.

REFERENCES

BIOCCA, E., *Parassitologia,* 1 (1959) 21.
BIOCCA, E., I. PAGGI and P. ORECCIA, *Parassitologia,* 2 (1960) 345.
HARTSTON, W., *Brit. med. J.,* 2 (1950) 526.
HEYDON, G. M. and A. K. GREEN, *Med. J. Aust.,* 1 (1931) 619.

HUNTER, G. W., L. S. RITCHIE and others, *J. Parasit.*, Suppl. 34 (1948) 34.
KALANTARIAN, H., *Arch. Schiffs- u. Tropenhyg.*, 38 (1934) 41.
LAWLESS, D. K., R. E. KUNTZ and C. P. A. STRONE, *Amer. J. trop. Med. Hyg.*, 5 (1956) 1010.
LIE KIANG JOE, *J. Parasit.*, 33 (1947) 359.
WATSON, J. M., *Parasitology*, 43 (1933) 102.

e. Larval nematode infections

i. Larva migrans

α. *Introduction.* Apart from the larvae of parasitic worms, which are specific to man and must in the course of their life cycle migrate through human tissues in order to reach a predestined site where they develop to maturity, man may be invaded by the larvae of several different parasites which are specific to animals, but only accidentally infect the human body. Such larvae may be of various origin: insects, pentastomids, worms or other animals; but they all have one common property *i.e.* they wander indiscriminately among the tissues in a vain search for a suitable site and do not develop to maturity, as they would in a proper host.

The term *larva migrans* was coined by Croker (1893) for such accidental parasites, which, as he observed, migrate under the skin. As observations on such larvae accumulated it appeared that they vary, not only in their identity, but also in their mode of behaviour in the human body, each species producing a peculiar syndrome. For this reason the infections produced by these larvae have been primarily classified, according to the manner in which the larvae move in the human body. Beaver *et al.* (1952) showed that the larva of the dog ascarid *(Toxocara canis)* can enter the internal organs of man, and they formulated a new concept of infection by the larvae of non-specific parasitic worms. They suggested a differentiation between *visceral larva migrans,* a term which denotes any helminth larva which enters deep tissues, and *cutaneous larva migrans, a* term which is applied to larvae confined to the sub-cutaneous tissues which cause the condition called *creeping eruption.*

These terms are often used to indicate, not the larva itself, but the syndrome it produces.

In their wanderings through the tissues the larvae bring about pathological reactions, which are often serious. The parasite itself is rarely found, and therefore can seldom be determined specifically. When the larva can be identified, its name is included in the diagnosis, which otherwise simply stands as *larva migrans.*

The syndromes produced by different species of worms may show slight biological and pathological variations. Thus, in some infections the clinical picture indicates the probable aetiological factor. In these cases the infections are usually treated under separate headings. Several such syndromes will be described separately in the chapters on fascioliasis, cercarial dermatitis, sparganosis, gnathostomiasis, strongyloidiasis and tropical eosinophilia. As a result of the separation of these infections, the terms *cutaneous larva migrans* and *visceral larva migrans* are retained chiefly to denote syndromes constituting the bulk of diseases caused by nematode larvae which normally develop in domestic carnivores.

β. Cutaneous larva migrans. The now widely-used term *cutaneous larva migrans* is applied to several conditions known also as *dermatitis linearis migrans* (Looss, 1911), *creeping eruption* (Kirby-Smith *et al.*, 1926), *ground itch*, etc. This syndrome arises when larvae of a nematode parasite of an animal penetrate the skin of man and move around in the sub-cutaneous tissue.

Usually this condition is ascribed to the larvae of several species of animal hookworms *(Ancylostoma caninum, A. brasiliense, A. ceylanicum, A. tubaeforme, and Uncinaria stenocephala)*, but other, even unrelated species may occasionally provoke similar symptoms. The hookworms mentioned are common parasites of *dogs* and *cats*, though they also live in various wild carnivores. The latter animals serve only under exceptional circumstances as disseminators of human infection.

Not only the larvae of other hookworm species, but also those of other nematodes (human hookworms, *Strongyloides stercoralis, Gnathostoma spinigerum*) have been found to cause creeping eruption. On rare occasions the larva of the cattle hookworm *(Bunostomum phlebotomum)*, or an undertermined species of *Capillaria* have been identified as the causative agents. Although there is no unanimity of opinion as to the identity of the larvae responsible for creeping eruption, it is generally accepted that most cases are due to infection with larvae of the cat hook-worm, *Ancylostoma brasiliense*.

The adult form of species whose larvae are involved in creeping eruption can easily be identified. The larvae, however, are so similar that identification is rarely possible. In most cases, therefore, creeping eruption is diagnosed only by its clinical appearances. Clinically there is little difference between the eruptions produced by the various species of nematodes.

In spite of the multiplicity of species involved in producing *larva migrans,* their life cycle in the normal host is similar. Worm eggs are evacuated with the faeces of the infected animals. In each egg a non-infective larva develops within 2 or 3 days. When the temperature and humidity are suitable, the larvae hatch out in the soil, and after another 3 or 4 days the infective stage is reached which is capable of entering the normal definitive host, either through the skin or through the mouth. Skin infection occurs by direct contact. After migration in the bloodstream, the larvae arrive in the lungs where they emerge from the blood capillaries and enter the air-passages. They then migrate to the pharynx, are swallowed and thus arrive in the intestine in which they settle and mature. When infection occurs through the mouth, the complicated migration just described is apparently not necessary; the larvae are simply swallowed and develop directly in the intestine.

Under favourable conditions these same larvae may penetrate the human skin, but then the migratory instinct of the infective larvae fails. They wander under the skin, following a tortuous path along which arises an inflammatory, erythematous or vesicular reaction, called *creeping eruption* (Fig. 81). The parasite is located between the *stratum germinativum* and *stratum corneum* of the skin, at some distance from the visible end of the burrow. Movements of the larvae are followed by extension of the linear inflammation, and are accompanied by intense itching. In cases of infection with the larva of *Strongyloides stercoralis* the process spreads very rapidly (Beaver, 1956). Frequently, secondary contamination with bacteria occurs, and the resulting inflammation gives rise to pustules and abscesses. Sometimes, especially in cases of multiple infection, constitutional symptoms appear.

The condition is never fatal, but causes much discomfort, varying with the intensity of infection. In man the life span of the larvae of animal hookworms is usually short. When the parasite dies, the lesions heal.

It should be noted that larvae of the *human* hookworm and those of *Strongyloides stercoralis* normally enter the human body through the skin and sometimes cause a characteristic papular or pustular reaction, called *ground itch, miner's itch* or *sand itch.* This condition closely resembles creeping eruption, but lasts only a short time; the larvae eventually behave like those of animal hookworms in their natural hosts, *i.e.* they enter the lymphatics or blood and proceed on their way to the lungs and intestine.

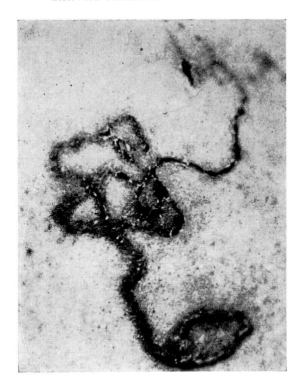

Fig. 81. Creeping eruption in skin of a man, caused by nematode larva (courtesy, Kirby-Smith et al., Arch. Dermatol. and Syphil., 1926).

Creeping eruption occurs mostly in warm and damp climates in localities with sandy soil, in which the ecological conditions are favourable for the survival of the larva in the soil until it encounters a suitable host. Barefoot and lightly clothed people in hot climates are more exposed to the infection. Some regions are notorious for the high incidence of creeping eruption. For instance, Kirby-Smith (1925) reported 2,500 cases in Florida during a period of 14 years. The same author (1929) recorded 179 admissions within 20 days only. Homes (1953) recorded 200 cases in Maracaibo (Venezuela), and Knox (1953) stated that 1 out of every 2,000 persons in the Mississippi Gulf coast shows the infection.

Creeping eruption commonly occurs in children who play in places polluted by the excrements of dogs and cats. Sand boxes used as playgrounds are especially attractive to cats for depositing their faeces. The localisation of the lesions in children is mainly on the buttocks, feet and hands.

Another aspect of creeping eruption is its character as an occupational disease of workers whose profession brings them in contact with the soil, e.g., gardeners and plumbers. In South Asian countries creeping eruption is most prevalent among sweet-potato growers, ricefield workers, tea-picking labourers and other people who cannot avoid contact with grossly contaminated soil. In this group the lesions appear most frequently on the legs and hands.

Some of the invading larvae of *Ancylostoma brasiliense* and *A. caninum* may occasionally reach the human intestine and settle there as true parasites (Beaver, 1950, Witenberg, 1951: *A. caninum;* Ciso, 1930: *A. brasiliense*).

The larvae, while passing through the lungs, may provoke an eosino-philic reaction (Löffler's syndrome). In endemic areas the simultaneous occurrence of two syndromes has been noticed (Wright and Gold, 1946).

The prognosis of creeping eruption is favourable. A large proportion of the persons affected recover spontaneously. When, however, untreated lesions are contaminated by scratching, healing may be delayed for weeks or even months.

There is no known specific treatment for creeping eruption. Kirby-Smith (1926) recommended refrigeration of the site of maximal itch by spraying it with ethylchloride, or by treating it with carbon dioxide snow (dry ice) or crushed ice mixed with salt. Repetition of this treatment is sometimes necessary. Hevia (1958) claimed cure of creeping eruption by treatment with diethyl-carbamazine (Hetrazan) administered *per os.*

Under primitive conditions, when the soil is grossly polluted with the excrements of dogs and cats, it is difficult to prevent infection. In endemic localities parents should be advised to get rid of sand boxes, or at least to keep them closed to cats. Strong salt solution, or the frequent application of borax, would presumably kill the larvae in the ground.

y. Visceral larva migrans. The sporadic occurrence of nematode larvae in human tissues is well known to pathologists. Beaver *et al.* (1952) were the first to interpret this finding as an infection with errant larvae of canine or feline ascarids and they proposed the term *visceral larva migrans* for the syndrome caused by this infection. Subsequently the attention of numerous investigators was focussed on the role played by non-specific nematode larvae in the human body in various regions of the world.

The species of nematode usually reponsible for this condition is *Toxocara canis*, which normally lives in the intestine of the *dog*, rarely in that of other carnivores. It has been proved experimentally on animals (Brill, *et al.*, 1953; Dent and Carrera, 1953) that it can settle in non-specific hosts including man (Smith and Beaver, 1953). Man becomes infected by ingesting eggs in which the larvae have already developed. It has been recognised that this may occur, although to a lesser extent, with the eggs of some other nematode species too.

The eggs of *T. canis* eliminated from the dog with the faeces contain only an ovum. Under favourable external conditions of temperature, humidity and shade, about 20 days are required for the development of an infective larva. In a suitable environment eggs containing infective larvae may remain viable for several months. When swallowed by a dog, the eggs hatch in the intestine and the larvae, after burrowing into the intestinal wall, enter the blood circulation. After a few days they pass through the liver and reach the lungs. From this point onwards, depending on the age of the host, the behaviour of the larvae differs.

Toxocara canis is essentially a parasite of young *dogs* (Noda, 1938, 1961); in older dogs it behaves as it does in an unsuitable host. In puppies up to 40 days old the larva follows the normal migration along the liver-lung route. From the lung, by way of the trachea and oesophagus, it reaches the small intestine, in which it develops to maturity. In puppies 40–70 days old some of the larvae which pass through the lung-capillaries enter the general circulation and are carried to various tissues. When they settle in muscles or organs they may become encapsulated; this occurs rather frequently in the liver, kidneys and brain. In adult dogs practically all the *Toxocara* larvae are thus distributed in the tissues. Either encapsulated or free, the larvae may survive for up to 2 years without undergoing growth or development.

If infective eggs of *T. canis* are accidentally swallowed by *man*, the larvae apparently behave as in the adult dog. However, they are not so readily inactivated and encapsulated as in the canine host and they wander about erratically and indiscriminately in various organs and tissues. Some of the larvae become entangled in foci of inflammatory reaction, giving rise to granulomata, which are characteristic of the infection. There is evidence that some of the larvae remain active for a year or longer, causing chronic or intermittent pathological reactions in the tissues, in which they actively bore. Their pathogenicity to man is greater than it is to dogs. In some instances tissue damage is so great that it causes generalized reactions. Exceptionally the infection may terminate fatally, especially when vital organs like the brain or liver are involved (Van Thiel, 1960).

The destructive action of *Toxocara* larvae may be mainly mechanical because of the considerable size of the parasite (*ca.* 0.4 mm in length and 0.02 mm in width). Yet, some observers also attach importance to the concomitant influence of sensitization developed during previously undetected, similar infections.

The principal symptoms provoked by the migrating *Toxocara* larvae are chronic extreme eosinophilia and hepatomegaly, sometimes accompanied by other signs which vary in severity, such as pneumonitis and allergic phenomena. Granulomata in the liver are characteristic lesions.

The appearance of these various symptoms depends on the number of the invading larvae and on the tissues involved. In some instances the wandering parasites do not produce any localised reaction, but cause pronounced systemic manifestations, such as eosinopilia; the latter alone is suggestive of the diagnosis.

In addition to the generalized reaction, certain peculiar phenomena have been related to *visceral larva migrans*. Nematode larvae were found in about half of the eyes enucleated from patients suspected of pseudogliomata, which were investigated histologically by Wilder (1950) in the U.S.A.; in the remaining cases examined by him, a tissue reaction characteristic of nematode endophthalmitis was observed. Originally these parasites had been identified as larvae of the human hookworm but Nichols (1956), on reexamination of 5 cases of Wilder's material, identified the larvae as those of *Toxocara canis*. 4 similar cases have been described by Ashton (1960) in England.

T. canis is common in all parts of the world and in some localities it affects as many as 80% of dogs. The potential exposure of man to infection with this parasite is therefore considerable. The much higher incidence of infection in the young has been related to the unhygienic habits of small children and their occasional geophagy (Beaver *et al.*, 1952).

It has been found that not only the larvae of *T. canis*, but also those of other ascarids of domestic carnivores may produce the syndrome of *visceral larva migrans,* namely *Toxocara mystax* (= *T. cati*) of the cat, and *Toxocaris leonina,* the primary host of which is the dog. The degree to which these species are involved is not exactly known.

It should be noted that in some cases, *visceral larva migrans* follows *cutaneous larva migrans,* both being produced by the same parasite (usually a larval hookworm) (Wright and Gold, 1946; Wilder, 1950). In cases of larval gnathostomiasis these two syndromes often replace one another. The larva of *Ascaris lumbricoides* of man may further confuse the diagnosis. Ordinarily, this larva migrates in the human body just as the larva of *T. canis* does in puppies. Occasionally, while it is passing through the lungs of sensitized persons, it provokes a severe eosinophilic pulmonary reaction (Löffler's syndrome) which resembles to a certain degree the syndrome caused by *visceral larva migrans.* In fact, Löffler's syndrome and any form of *larva migrans* involve similar processes, *i.e.,* a response of the sensitised organism to the presence of an unspecific tissue parasite. Each of these is caused by different species of larvae and the course of the reaction usually shows certain specific peculiarities.

There are no clear-cut clinical signs which alone could assure the diagnosis of *visceral larva migrans.* The only certain proof is the demonstration of the larvae in the tissues by biopsy. However, this method is not always successful; even when fragments of the parasite are available, identification in microtome sections is often impossible. Exact determination of the larvae has not infrequently been made in material obtained at post mortem examination; in these cases the parasite was found most abundantly in the liver, brain and lungs. Peptic digestion of a large sample of tissue considerably facilitates their detection.

The larvae of human and animal ascarids are very similar and their structure differs in accordance with their age and the method of fixation. More recent publications present detailed descriptions of the anatomy of the larvae of ascarid species likely to infect man, namely *Toxocara canis, T. mystax, Toxascaris leonina* and *Ascaris lumbricoides* (Wright, 1935; Sprent, 1956; Nichols, 1956; Sacher, 1957).

No reliable serological test for the diagnosis has as yet been devised, because the majority of the reacting antigens are not specific. Sadun *et al.* (1957) obtained encouraging results with the bentonite flocculation reaction using the purified acid-soluble protein fraction of *T. canis* as antigen. Kagan *et al.* (1959) proposed an improved haemagglutination test, for which they claim specificity at high titer.

There is no specific treatment for *visceral larva migrans.* Hetrazan or cortisone, tried by several investigators, give only slight temporary improvement.

REFERENCES

AUGUSTINE, D. L., *J. Parasit.*, 13 (1927) 256.
ASTRUP, A., *Acta derm.-venereol. (Stockh.)*, 25 (1945) 389.
BEAVER, P. C., *Amer. J. trop. Med. Hyg.*, 15 (1956) 737; *Publ. Hlth Rep. (Wash.)*, 74 (1959) 328.
BURROWS, R. B. and W. G. LILLIS, *N.Y. St. J. Med.*, 60 (1960) 3239.
DOVE, W. E., *Amer. J. Hyg.*, 15 (1932) 664.
HOMEZ, C. J., *Rev. Med.-quir.*, 28 (1954) 43.
KAGAN, I. C., L. E. NORMAN and D. S. ALLAIN, *J. Immunol.*, 83 (1959) 297.
KIRBY-SMITH, J. L., W. E. DOVE and G. F. WHITE, *Arch. Derm. Syph. (Chic.)*, 13 (1926) 137; *Amer. J. trop. Med.*, 9 (1929) 179.
LIE, K. J. and G. J. BRAS, *Documenta neerl. indones. Morb. trop.*, 2 (1950) 288.
MAPLESTONE, P. A., *Nid. med. Gaz.*, 68 (1933) 175.
MERCER, R. D., H. Z. LUND, R. A. BLOOMFIELD and F. E. CALDWELL, 80 (1950) 46.
NICHOLS, R. L., *J. Parasit.*, 42 (1956) 363.
SANDGROUND, J. H., *Geneesk. T. Ned.-Ind.*, 79 (1939) 805.
SANDOSHAM, A. A., *J. Helminth.*, 26 (1952) 1.
SMITH, M. H. O. and P. C. BEAVER, *Pediatrics*, 12 (1953) 491.
WRIGHT, D. O. and E. M. GOLD, *Arch. intern. Med.*, 78 (1946) 303.

ii. Gnathostomiasis

Gnathostomiasis in man is caused by the nematode *Gnathostoma spinigerum*. Although several other species of the same genus have been incriminated in cases of human infection, later work on the morphology and bionomics of this genus suggest that they are synonymous with *G. spinigerum* (Miyazaki, 1960). Man harbours only the larvae of the parasite, and his infection is accidental. The normal final hosts of *G. spinigerum* are *cats* and *dogs* living with or near to humans and, in nature the tiger, leopard, lynx and possibly other wild *Felidae*. In these hosts the adult worms reach about 2 cm in length. They live half imbedded in large nodes which are produced in the wall of the stomach. This parasite is common in the Far East (Bengal, Thailand, China, Ceylon, the Philippines and Japan). In the endemic area of Kiushu up to 35% of cats and 4% of dogs were found infected. Up to 50 adult worms have been found in a single cat.

The life history of *G. spinigerum* is complicated, since it requires two obligatory intermediate hosts, while additional facultative hosts are often involved. The freshly laid eggs are in a one or two-cell stage and they can develop further only if they reach fresh water, in which the larva hatches out after 7 or more days. When the larva is swallowed by a *Cyclops* (a small copepod crustacean) it enters the body cavity and develops into the next stage in the course of about 10 days. The *Cyclops* must now be eaten by a second intermediate host, usually a fish; the larva burrows into the muscles and becomes encysted. It is subsequently transformed into the *infective* stage. During the ensuing month it reaches maturity if it is swallowed by a suitable final host.

The larva of *Gnathostoma spinigerum* is not particular with respect to its second intermediate host. Many cold blooded animals may serve this purpose *e.g.* fish, crabs and crayfish, frogs and snakes. In each endemic area certain species of fish are the predominant hosts of the *Gnathostoma* larvae. In Japan *Ophiocephalus argus* and *O. tadianus* are the most infected fishes, up to 99% of them being infected in endemic areas, while over 300 larvae may be lodged in a single fish. In the fish the infective larva is enclosed in a cyst. It reaches a length of up the 4 mm, is covered by thick rows of sharp spines and is provided with a head-bulb armed with 4 rows of strong hooks. When swallowed by a suitable final host, the larva pierces the stomach wall and enters the liver, in which it wanders for about 3 months. At the end of this period it reaches its full size and returns to the stomach, piercing now its wall from the outside, and attaching itself to the mucosa by means of its strong spiny head-bulb. Hyperplasia of the surrounding tissue ensues at the site of the anterior part of the worm, the other part hanging in the lumen of the stomach. If, however, the infective larva is swallowed by an animal unsuitable as a final host (a bird or mammal, including man) it grows only slightly in the liver, and soon leaves this organ without finding its way back to the stomach. Now the parasite begins to migrate indiscriminately through various tissues, as if it were looking in vain for a suitable site for settlement. When they are enclosed in food, such larvae may be transferred to another unsuitable host in which they continue to wander. During these movements through the tissues of such a facultative host, the larvae may cause severe damage with their hooks and spines. In endemic regions many fish-eating animals, such as snakes or herons, may serve as facultative hosts and become heavily infected with the larvae of *G. spinigerum.*

Man shares the role of facultative host and in him these larvae may cause serious disease. In most cases only a single larva develops and is responsible for the resulting clinical symptoms. Multiple invasions are rare. Toumanoff and Phung (1947) quoted a case in which 7 larvae were removed from the breast of a patient.

In the human tissues the infective larva grows very slowly, often reaching 10 mm in length; only in rare instances does it develop to maturity.

Epidemic human gnathostomiasis occurs in localities in which the population customarily eats dishes made of raw fish, snakes or chicken. Numerous highly endemic foci are known in Thailand and Japan, while less important ones occur all over the Far East. Before the second world war, little attention had been paid to human gnathostomiasis and no

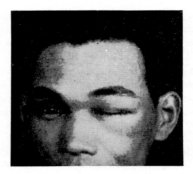

Fig. 82.   (a) Oedematous form of gnathostomiasis.

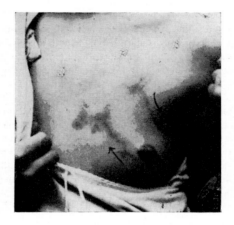

Fig. 82.   (b) Creeping eruption form of gnathostomiasis. (acc. to Miyazaki; Courtesy
Kyushu Mem. Med. Sci., 1954).

reliable statistics of its incidence were available. Since the discovery
of the endemicity of the syndrome, hundreds of patients harbouring the
parasite have been recognized every year. For example, Doi, in 1950
(quoted by Miyazaki, 1960) reported on 1264 cases in his practice
in Japan. Sporadic cases have been recorded in Australia and Israel, a
fact which indicates that the infection has a wide distribution.

The syndrome is caused by the combined action of mechanical injury
due to the movement of the armed larva in the tissues, and inflam-

matory, toxic and allergic reactions elicited by the parasite's excretions and secretions. Eosinophilia occurs in practically all cases. The most conspicuous clinical symptom is a migrating intermittent oedema which develops around the site of the larva (Fig. 82a). The larva may move 1 cm per day, and the location of the oedema moves together with it. Since the larva wanders indiscriminately through all tissues, every organ of the human body may be involved (Fig. 82b). The path of the larva is unpredictable, and so are the symptoms. Cases have been described in which it migrated in the viscera, passed to the head and the cranium and emerged through the orbit. Sometimes the larva migrates under the skin, causing a typical picture of creeping eruption (see below). The erratic movement of the *Gnathostoma* larva in the human body may last for years (16 years in the case of Toumanoff and Phung, 1947) or it may end with an abscess (on the tip of a finger, in the throat, or in other places), through which the larva is eliminated. Sometimes, during the movement of the larva, the symptoms disappear temporarily, but they reappear violently when vital organs are invaded. The most alarming symptoms develop when the larva enters the brain and the eye (Witenberg *et al.*, 1950). The damage done to the liver or lungs may also be very serious. In addition to extensive mechanical damage, the wandering larva may cause serological phenomena, which have been investigated by Yamanako (1958).

A saline extract injected intravenously into a guinea pig, which had been sensitized 24 hours previously by subcutaneous injection of the same antigen, produces the Schwarzmann phenomenon (haemorrhagic necrosis). The same antigen repeatedly injected subdermally produces the Arthus phenomenon. The serum of persons showing an intradermal reaction positive to *Gnathostoma* antigen, elicits a Prausnitz-Küstner reaction in noninfected persons.

In endemic localities symptoms which indicate the presence of wandering *Gnathostoma* larvae are often observed, whereas in fact the larva is rarely seen.

The diagnosis may be supported by a simple skin test. Miyazaki (*loc. cit.*) stated that a 1/50,000 saline extract of the worm (adult or larval) provokes a reaction which reliably indicates the infection. The reaction is of the immediate type.

There is no effective medication for human gnathostomiasis. In some cases surgical removal of the parasite is indicated.

REFERENCES

MIYAZAKI, I., *Exp. Parasit.*, 9 (1960) 338.
PROMMAS, C. and S. DAENGSVANG, *Indian med. Gaz.*, 49 (1934) 207.
TOUMANOFF, C. and LE-VAN-PHUNG, *Bull. Soc. Path. exot.*, 40 (1947) 168.
YAMANAKA, T., *Igaku Kenkyu*, 28 (1958) 2043.
WITENBERG, G., J. JACOBI and S. STECKELMACHER, *Opthalmologica*, 119 (1950) 114.

f. Zoonotic filariases

The term *filariasis* denotes an infection with any species of filariid worms.
About 10 species of this Nematode family may be parasitic in man, each
of them producing a specific syndrome. These nematodes live in the
tissues or in the lymph glands and are viviparous. Their larvae, the microfilariae, are, according to species, either dispersed in the connective tissue,
or they swarm in the blood. Microfilariae of some species show the
remarkable phenomenon of periodicity, *i.e.*, they appear in the circulating
blood and disappear periodically either during the day or during the night.
When these microfilariae are ingested by specific blood sucking insects,
they develop into the infective stage, and can then be transmitted to the
final host by bite.

Until recently it was thought that the species of filariae occurring in
man were strictly specific but recent research has shown that in West
Africa and East Asia at least 3 species occurring in man may develop in
animals, *i.e.* in reservoir hosts. These are: *Brugia malayi*, *Loa loa* and
Acanthocheilonema streptocerca. The syndromes provoked by these parasites are called respectively: filariasis malayi, loaiasis and streptocerciasis.
In addition, a species as yet undefined, presumably causes a syndrome
called tropical eosinophilia. Apart from the species of filariidae which are
specific to man, some species specific to animals may occasionally invade
man and induce pathological changes. To these belong species of the
genus *Dirofilaria* known under the group name *Filaria conjunctivae* and
an as yet insufficiently investigated species, *Wuchereria vauceli*, described
by Galliard (1955) in Madagascar.

i. Filariasis malayi

Filariasis malayi denotes filariasis which is associated with the so-called *malayi* type of microfilariae *(Microfilaria malayi)*. It is found in the blood of the inhabitants of an extensive geographic area, comprising a large part of south-eastern Asia, as far as Korea, Indonesia and some of the Pacific Islands.

This type of microfilaria is characterised by a swelling in the tail which contains a prominent nucleus. It was discovered by Brug in Sumatra (1927), who differentiated the worm from *Microfilaria bancrofti*. Rao and Maplestone (1940) were the first to describe the adult filaria and assign it together with the latter species to the genus *Wuchereria*. Recently, Buckley (1960) proposed a separate genus for this species, *Brugia*. For a long time, *B. malayi* was regarded as being strictly specific for man, until Poynton and Hodgkins (1938) found a "malayi" type of microfilaria in the Kramonkey in Malaya. Subsequent investigations showed that morphologically indistinguishable species of filariae occur in a number of domestic and wild animals (cat, tiger, pangolin, moon-rat, monkeys).

Intensive study showed that some of these microfilariae are larvae of *Brugia malayi*, while others belong to *Brugia pahangi*.

Wilson *et al.* (1958) pointed out that *Brugia malayi* (then called *Wuchereria malayi*) is, in fact, represented by two separate strains which, in spite of the morphological similarity of the adults and microfilariae, differ distinctly in their specificity for different vectors, their infectivity to the cat, their geographical distribution and their different periodicity. In subsequent papers these investigators distinguished between the strictly *periodic form*, with markedly nocturnal periodicity, and the *semi-periodic* form, which shows some nocturnal rise in the microfilaraemia, but the microfilariae are readily found at all times. The geographical distribution of these "forms" in man is imperfectly known for most of the endemic localities, but it has been defined in Malaya. Both occur in rural areas, are absent from towns and cause the same syndrome.

The *periodic* form of *B. malayi* is predominant in man in all the endemic regions. It occurs in the coastal rice-fields of the north-western part of Malaya, centering on Penang Island. Although it may be transferred experimentally to animals, the latter are not specific hosts. In the cat the microfilariae are always scanty and it is, therefore, believed that this animal is not an important source of human infection. However, Rhesus monkeys *(Macaca mulatta)* and the leaf-monkey *(Presbytis obscurus)* are suitable hosts for this strain.

The *semi-periodic* form of *B. malayi* mainly prevails in the central and eastern districts of Malaya in fresh-water swamp forests (along the Perak and Pahang rivers). It is readily transmissible to a variety of animals, and cats are particularly good hosts. Microfilariae appear in cats as early as $2\frac{1}{2}$ months after inoculation and persist in large numbers for long periods thereafter. They have been found in 76% of dusky-leaf monkeys, and it is considered that this species forms an important reservoir from which man can be infected. The parasite can be successfully transmitted to hamsters white rats and dogs.

The main vectors of *M. malayi* are mosquitoes of the genus *Mansonia* the larvae of which live attached by their siphons to the air cushions o floating water plants. Certain species of the genera *Anopheles* and *Armigeres* may also act as vectors.

In Malaya, where *filariasis malayi* has been extensively investigated children are found infected very early in life. The infection rate rises with age, reaching a peak of over 56% at the age of 4 to 10 years (Edeson 1961). The relatively limited prevalence in highly endemic localities i explained by the biting habits of the vectors, which feed chiefly on cattle and comparatively rarely on man.

Edeson and Duckley (1959) studied the development of *B. malayi* in the cat. The micro filaria is about 200 microns long and 5 microns wide. In mosquitoes it develops in the thoracic muscles to the infective stage. The infective larvae settle in the lymphatics o the definitive host, usually close to the site of the inoculation, but some of them ma migrate to distant parts of the lymphatic system. Generally the final location is reached in less than 24 hours. Microfilariae appear in the peripheral blood between 75 and 140 days after infection. The male worm reaches its maximum size at maturation in approximately 70 days, while the female continues to grow after maturation for abou 300 days.

The onset and development of the disease varies greatly from case to case In many instances few clinical signs are observed, despite the presence of microfilariae in the blood. The most common symptoms are: enlargement of the lymph glands, eosinophilia and pulmonitis. Adeno-lymphangitis often accompanied by swelling of a limb, fever and sterile abscess appear at irregular intervals ("episodic" attacks); the frequency of these attack varies with the individual infected and usually they last a few days. Presumably these attacks are allergic in nature. A certain percentage of case develops elephantiasis several years after infection. Whereas up to 20% of people between the ages of 20 and 60 years may develop elephantiasis usually no more than 10% of the total population do so. Elephantiasis occurring in filariasis malayi is mainly confined to the legs below the knees; it may be debilitating and may, for this reason, present a considerable health problem. Scrotal elephantiasis, common in Bancroftian filariasis, is almost unknown in filariasis malayi.

No treatment is known for the elimination of the adult filariae. *Suramin* (given intravenously) is considered to be the most effective drug.

but its relative toxicity makes its application unsuitable for wide use. On the other hand microfilaraemia can be successfully suppressed by diethylcarbamazine (Hetrazan, Notezine, Banocide, Caricide, etc.). When this is properly given to the total population, it may within several years drastically reduce the incidence of any filariasis, including that of the *malayi* type (Beaver, 1961).

It is difficult to achieve full control of filariasis malayi under natural conditions. Control of the mosquito vectors is a complex problem and depends on the bionomics of the local species. It should be supported by removal of floating vegetation by hand or by the use of herbicides.

REFERENCES

BEAVER, P., *Wld Hlth Org. Monogr. Ser., Helminth.*, 2, 1960, 54 pp.
BUCKLEY, J. C. C., *Ann. trop. Med. Parasit.*, 54 (1960) 75.
CHOW, C. Y., Bull., *Wld Hlth Org.*, 9 (1953) 571.
DISSANAIKE, A. S. and D. C. PARAMANATHAN, *Trans. roy. Soc. trop. Med. Hyg.*, 55 (1961) 299.
EDESON, J. F. B., *Wld Hlth Org., Monogr. Ser., Fil.* 28, 1961, 24 pp.
EDESON, J. F. B. and R. H. WHARTON, *Ann. trop. Med. Parasit.*, 52 (1958) 87.
GALLIARD, H., *Ann. Parasit. hum. comp.*, 32 (1957) 271.
LAING, A. B. G., J. F. B. EDESON and R. H. WHARTON, *Ann. trop. Med. Parasit.*, 54 (1960) 92.
POYNTON, J. O. and E. P. HODGKIN, *Bull. Inst. med. Res. Malaya*, 1 (1938) 25.
TURNER, L. H., *Trans. roy. Soc. trop. Med. Hyg.*, 53 (1959) 154.
WILSON, T., *Trans. roy. Soc. trop. Med. Hyg.*, 55 (1961) 107.

ii. Loaiasis

Loaiasis is caused by the filarial species, *Loa loa*, which is a parasite in man in the rain forest belt of West Africa and in the Equatorial Sudan. The adult female is 5–7 cm and the male 2–3 cm long. The worm lives in the connective tissues in which it constantly migrates, often appearing under the skin and mucous membranes, including the conjunctiva, hence the popular name "eye-worm". It is remarkable that this migration does not provoke any mechanical trauma or tissue reaction. Usually several specimens of the worm are involved in every infection; up to 40 worms have been recorded from a single individual (Gordon *et al.*, 1950).

The epidemiology of loaiasis has not yet been elucidated completely. It has long been assumed that *Loa loa* is specific to man only. Sandground (1936), summarizing the observations of Treadgold (1920), Vogel (1927) and also his own, showed that the species of *Loa* found in some African and American monkeys are morphologically similar to the species found in man, so much so that they may all be regarded as representing one single species. However, Duke *et al.* (1958, 1960) and Gordon *et al.* (1949, 1958) demonstrated that the microfilariae of the strain of *Loa* occurring in monkeys in West Africa show a nocturnal periodicity in the blood, which contrasts with diurnal periodicity of the human strain. They also expressed the opinion that, although experimental cross infection between man and monkeys is possible, the monkey probably plays no part in the epidemiology of human loaiasis, because, under natural conditions, the monkey strain is transmitted by a tabanid species *(Chrysops langi* and *Chr. centurionis)* which live in the forest canopy and do not bite man. On the other hand, Woodman and Bokhari (1941) described a human strain of *Loa loa* from the Sudan, which showed irregular or nocturnal periodicity.

The significance of the above data for the epidemiology of human loaiasis is still under consideration. It is impossible to correlate them until additional knowledge is available. On the other hand, the life history of the parasite has been fairly well studied in monkeys.

The adult worm releases vast numbers of microfilariae, which initially concentrate in the internal organs; they regularly appear in the blood during day time, but almost disappear from it during the night.

Duke (1960), experimenting with monkeys, demonstrated that microfilariae of both the diurnal and the nocturnal strains accumulate in the lungs before they periodically invade the peripheral blood. From this reservoir in the lungs, which is maintained throughout the infection, only a part of the microfilariae are released into the circulating blood. After 3–5 months the number of microfilariae in the blood stream becomes static. It is thought that the mechanism which regulates the release of microfilariae into the circulating blood is situated in the spleen. The microfilariae do not change while they remain in the human body, but they develop into the infective stage in the fat-body of blood-sucking tabanid flies (mainly *Chrysops siliacea* or *C. dimidiata*). After about 12 days they concentrate in the proboscis of the fly, from which they enter the human body during the subsequent act of biting. In man, the parasite matures in about a year.

The tabanid flies mentioned above breed in stagnant waters and need a blood meal for the production of their eggs. They attack man during the hours of daylight, mostly in forest clearings surrounding the villages.

The reaction of the human host to the presence of these parasites varies from case to case. Eosinophilia appears invariably and may reach over 70%. Years may pass before serious symptoms are noticed, but sooner or later transient oedemas on various parts of the body set in, often on the face or scalp (Calabar swelling). Such oedemas reappear at short intervals, usually in different locations and although they may cause serious inconvenience, they never suppurate. In rare instances cerebral or cardial disturbances may aggravate the conditions. All these symptoms are believed to be allergic in origin. "Calabar swellings" make their first appearance at very variable periods after initial infection; Coutelen (1935) noted a variation of between 2 months to 6 years. Microfilariae may be absent from the peripheral blood, despite the presence of adult worms under the conjunctiva.

It has been stated that the adult *Loa loa* may live in man for 4–15 years, but it is known that some individuals who have been reinfected have suffered continuously from these worms for as long as 24 years.

Human loaiasis may be completely cured with Hetrazan or similar compounds, which kill both the microfilariae and the adult worms. This treatment may, however, cause an allergic reaction, which is sometimes severe. It is accompanied by oedema, itching, a brief transient rise of temperature, malaise, nausea, joint pains and rarely by encephalopathy. These conditions may be relieved by antihistaminics.

REFERENCES

COUTELEN, F., *Bull. Soc. Path. exot.*, 28 (1935) 126.
DUKE, B. O. L., *Nature*, 179 (1957) 1357; *Ann. trop. Med. Parasit.*, 54 (1960) 15.
DUKE, B. O. L., and D. J. B. WIJERS, *Ann. trop. Med. Parasit.*, 52 (1958) 158.
GORDON, R. M., L. J. CHWATT and C. M. JONES, *Trans. roy. Soc. trop. Med. Hyg.*, 42 (1949) 315.
GORDON, R. M. *et al.*, *Trans. roy. Soc. trop. Med. Hyg.*, 14 (1950) 11.
JANSSEN, P. G., *Bull. soc. Path. exot.*, 51 (1958) 632.
KENNEY, M. and R. HEWITT, *Amer. J. trop. Med.*, 30 (1950) 895.
SANDGROUND, J. H., *Ann. Soc. belge Med. trop.*, 16 (1936) 1.
WOODRUFF, A. W., *Trans. roy. Soc. trop. Med. Hyg.*, 44 (1951) 479.

iii. Streptocerciasis

Streptocerciasis is due to a filarial species *Acanthocheilonema strepto-cerca* (= *Dicheilonema streptocerca*) which occurs in man and chimpan-zees in limited regions of West and Central Africa. This type of filariasis has as yet been insufficiently studied and it is even not known whether the parasite is better adapted to man or to the ape. In some localities up to

100% of the aborigines are infected (Van den Berghe and Chardome, 1952). Its pathogenicity is apparently low, although annoying papular eruptions have been described by Duke (1957).

The adult worm has not been recovered from man, but presumably it lives in the subcutaneous and connective tissues, as it does in the chimpanzee. The microfilariae are found in the skin, and are freqeuntly associated with the microfilariae of *Onchocerca volvulus*. *A. streptocerca* is transmitted by a small gnat, *Culicoides grahami,* which is abundant in endemic localities. The worm is very susceptible to diethylcarbamazine, which rapidly clears the skin of microfilariae. Some authors presume that, contrary to what happens in other filariases, in streptocerciasis the secondary reactions (itching, headache, nausea, oedema, etc.) do not appear after this treatment.

REFERENCES

DUKE, B. O. L., *Ann. trop. Med. Parasit.,* 51 (1957) 364.
PEEL, E. and M. CHARDOME, *Ann. Soc. belge Med. trop.,* 26 (1946) 117.
VAN DEN BERGHE, L. and M. CHARDOME, *Trans. roy. Soc. trop. Med. Hyg.,* 46 (1952) 99

iv. Tropical eosinophilia

In some tropical regions, notably in India and Indo-China, there appears a peculiar pathological condition in man, known as tropical eosinophilia (also called Meyers and Kouwenaar's syndrome (1939), Frimodt-Moeller disease (1940) or Weingarten's eosinophilia (1943). It is characterized by the following symptoms, of which the first occurs always and is the most significant:

(1) marked eosinophilia (up to 85%) and leucocythaemia;
(2) asthmatoid attacks of cough, often associated with slight rise of temperature and general malaise;
(3) multiple mottled shadows on the radiogram of both lungs, sometimes accompanied by increased hilar shadows;
(4) occasional swelling of the lymph nodes and spleen; and
(5) a chronic course of the disease if not treated.

Pathological changes are observed mainly in the bronchi and include macrocytic and eosinophilic infiltration associated with necrosis of the bronchioles and deformation of the local vascular system. In advanced cases the process is irreversible and may end fatally.

The aetiology of this syndrome has baffled many investigators. The observation made by Weingarten and others that the disease readily responds to treatment with antifilarial drugs (arsenicals, Hetrazan, anthiomaline, etc.) suggested that possibly filarial worms are responsible for it. Although microfilariae usually are not found in the blood of the affected persons, they have been observed in their lymph nodes. This seems to be an additional indication of tropical eosinophilia being the result of filarial infection. These filariae apparently are not fully adapted to man. They can invade him accidentally, but fail to produce microfilariae which they usually do in their natural hosts. On the other hand, in man, their activity may elicit serologic and allergic responses, which result in systemic and pulmonary eosinophilia. This view has been supported by several records.

Microfilariae have been observed in serial sections of excised tissues of persons suffering from tropical eosinophilia in various parts of the world (Meyers and Kouwenaar (1939), Bras and Lie Kiang Joe (1951) and Riesel and Groen (1951) in Indonesia; Friess et al. (1953) in Tonkin; van der Saar and Hartz (1945) in Dutch Guiana). Furthermore, Danaraj and Schacher (1951) demonstrated that in Malaya all of 69 cases of tropical eosinophilia showed positive complement-fixation reactions with an antigen made from the dog-filaria, *Dirofilaria immitis,* which gives a group-reaction to filarial antibodies.

Galliard and Mallarmé (1955) observed microfilariae of the *malayi* type in a lymph-node punctate obtained from a case of tropical eosinophilia of 4 years standing. The most suggestive evidence as to the identity of the causative agent of the disease has been provided by Buckley (1958), who produced the syndrome experimentally by inoculating 2 volunteers with larvae of filariae *(Brugia)* which normally live in the cat and monkey.

In this context it is noteworthy that the species which has long been regarded as *Wuchereria malayi* in the Malayan Peninsula, is in fact a complex of at least 3 different filarial species of the genus *Brugia,* of which only 1 (a periodic strain of *Brugia malayi*) is specific for man, while the other 2 (*Brugia pahangi* and the semiperiodic strain of *B. malayi*) are parasites of cats and monkeys. Experimental inoculation of these animal-filariae into man was followed by development to the adult stage, but for some unknown reason their microfilariae did not appear in the peripheral blood.

The fact that tropical eosinophilia has been observed, not only in the Asian tropics (India, Ceylon, the East Indies, Japan, the Philippines), but also in Central and South Africa and the West Indies, where species of

Brugia do not occur, strongly suggests that other filarial species may also provoke the syndrome of that disease.

It should be emphasized that the symptoms characteristic of tropical eosinophilia indicate a state of general hypersensitivity to some unknown agent rather than a specific disease. Hence, this process may appear, not only in infections with various specific and non-specific parasitic helminths, but also in cases in which other parasites, for instance mites, are involved.

Suspected cases of tropical eosinophilia must be differentiated from other syndromes in which eosinophilia is pronounced, *i.e.* asthma, Hodgkin's disease, infectious mononucleosis, and primarily from Löffler's syndrome, which is caused by larvae of the human strain of *Ascaris lumbricoides* during their habitual migration through the lung. Tropical eosinophilia must also be differentiated from *visceral larva migrans* brought about by the larvae of canine ascarids (see pages 569–571, and Table XXXI).

TABLE XXXI

DISTINGUISHING FEATURES OF THREE SYNDROMES
IN WHICH EOSINOPHILIA IS CONNECTED WITH HELMINTHIC INFECTION

	Tropical eosinophilia	*Visceral larva migrans*	*Löffler's syndrome*
Course of infection	chronic (long duration)	chronic (short duration)	acute (transitory)
Response to anti-filarials	mostly prompt	none	none
Occurrence	in the tropics	universal	predominantly in temperate regions
Rise of temperature	slight but chronic, with transitory exacerbations	variable	transitory, of short duration
Hepatomegaly	in about half of the cases	always pronounced	transitory
Splenomegaly	frequent in inacute phase	inapparent	inapparent
X-ray shadowing	chronic, mottled	transitory, atypical	variable in type, quickly resolving
Lymphadenitis	common	infrequently	none
Asthma, Urticaria	common, chronic	rare, transitory	of short duration, if present

The diagnosis of tropical eosinophilia is based on clinical and haematological examinations. Serological tests with filarial antigen are of little value in areas in which filariasis is endemic because they are group-specific. In cases in which the diagnosis has been established, treatment with diethylcarbamazine (Hetrazan) produces improvement or even cure (Baker *et al.*, 1959).

REFERENCES

APLEY, J. and G. H. GRANT, *Lancet*, i (1944) 308.
BAKER, S. J., K. T. RAJAN and S. DEVADATTA, *Lancet*, 1 (1959) 144.
BALL, J. D., *Trans. roy. Soc. trop. Med. Hyg.*, 44 (1950) 237.
BUCKLEY, J. C., *Trans. roy. Soc. trop. Med. Hyg.*, 52 (1958) 336.
DANARAJ, I. J., L. S. DA SILVA and J. F. SCHACHER, *Amer. J. trop. Med. Hyg.*, 8 (1959) 151.
FRIESS, J., N. PIERRON and J. SEGALEN, *Bull. Soc. Path. exot.*, 46 (1953) 1037.
FRIMODT-MOELLER, C. and R. M. BARTON, *Indian med. Gaz.*, 75, (1940) 607.
GALLIARD, H., *Riv. Parassit.*, 15 (1954) 403.
GALLIARD, H. and J. MALLARMÉ, *Sang*, 26 (1955) 520.
RIESEL, J. H. and J. GROEN, *Docum. néerl. indones. Morb. trop.*, 3 (1951) 320.
WEBB, J. K. G., *Indian J. Pediat.*, 27 (1960) 147.
WEINGARTEN, R. J., *Lancet*, i (1943) 103.
WINTER, H., *Z. Tropen med. Parasit.*, 6 (1955) 99.

v. Human infections with other animal filariae

In addition to 10 species of filariae of which man is the specific host, other filariae, which are usually parasitic in animals, may occasionally establish themselves in the human body. As a rule, however, they cannot reach maturity in this uncommon host and they either become encapsuled, or die, or are eliminated through a suppurative process. Cases of parasitism of this kind have been summarized by Desportes (1939) and Faust (1957). Although in most of them the parasites have been extracted and studied, their descriptions have usually been inadequate for their exact taxonomic determination.

This is understandable when the difficulty of classifying the immature stages of nematodes is remembered. Moreover, in the majority of cases immature females were obtained, whereas it is the male characteristics which are usually decisive in the determination of species or even of the genus of nematodes. Another difficulty is due to the fact that these parasites have been described under more than a dozen names. The commonest of these names are: *Filaria oculi humani* Nordman, 1832; *F. lacrimalis* Dubini, 1850; *F. lentis* Diesing, 1851; *F. palpebralis* Pace, 1866; and *F. conjunctivae* Adario, 1885.

On only few occasions have extracted worms been described in detail by competent helminthologists and, according to Faust (1957), practically all of these bear great resemblance to the genus *Dirofilaria*, which includes numerous species, all parasites of mammals. In 4 instances it was possible to establish the species exactly, *viz.*: *Dirofilaria magalhaesi* from the heart of a child in Brazil (Blanchard, 1895), *Dirofilaria repens* from the eye-lid of a person in Russia (Skrjabin, *et al.*, 1930), *Dirofilaria luisianensis* from the heart of a patient in U.S.A. (Faust, *et al.*, 1941), and *Dirofilaria spectans* from the finger of a man in Brazil (Texeira de Freytas *et al.*, 1953).

By analogy with these findings, and considering certain morphological characteristics of the recovered worms, modern investigators have similarly attributed the remaining records to the genus *Dirofilaria*. In his review Desportes *(loc. cit.)* designated all the undefined parasites recorded in the literature by the collective name *Dirofilaria conjunctivae*, although the correctness of this name remains problematic.

Faust (1937) divided the genus *Dirofilaria* into 2 subgenera: *Dirofilaria*, characterised by a smooth cuticle, and *Nochtiella*, showing longitudinal rows of small bosses on the cuticle. In his review of 1957 this author suggested that two canine parasites belonging to the subgenera just mentioned are possibly the main culprits: *D. (D.) immitis*, which is normally parasitic in the heart of the *dog* and *fox* and *D. (N.) repens*, which is parasitic in the subcutaneous tissue of dog and *cat*. *Man* serves as an accidental host of both these two species. In spite of the very high prevalence of these parasites in their normal hosts, human infections are comparatively rare. Faust presented a list of 31 cases of infection with *Dirofilaria conjunctivae* in man, but at least a similar number should be added to complete the list of published records. The latter cases occurred chiefly in Europe, Africa, North and South America, southern Asia and Ceylon.

The life histories of only a few species belonging to the genus *Dirofilaria* are known; for all of them blood sucking insects, mostly mosquitoes, serve as intermediate hosts which transmit the larvae to the final host by bite.

The tissue reaction produced by *D. conjunctivae* in man is usually slight; it is evidenced by mild inflammation and itching, which are frequently accompanied by nodule formation around the growing worm. In a few instances migratory movement of the larva has been observed.

Dirofilaria immitis has extraordinary biological characteristics. It may live in the dog for up to 7 years (Fülleborn, 1929), and may remain all this time in the right ventricle of the heart or in the pulmonary artery, being obviously not disturbed by the relentlessly strong stream of blood. Usually a bundle consisting of a number of males and females (the latter up to 30 cm long) may live together. Dogs harbouring a few *D. immitis* suffer little so long as the parasites are alive, but when the worms die, they are carried by the blood into the lung vessels, where they produce an infarct which often causes the sudden death of the host. The presence of numerous worms provokes endocarditis, ascites, loss of vitality and other pathological conditions. In localities in which the parasite is endemic (for instance South China) most dogs die as a result of this infection.

Dirofilaria repens is half as large as the species just mentioned and lives under the skin of the dog, cat and some other mammals. A great number of these worms may be dispersed all over the body of the animals without causing pathological manifestations.

The presence in animals of the filariae mentioned above can easily be diagnosed by examination of the blood, in which the microfilarial larvae of these worms can be found. The microfilariae of *D. immitis* appear in the peripheral blood during all the 24 hours of the day, but they are most numerous during the night. In *D. repens* this periodicity is less pronounced.

If the number of worms is small, infected dogs may be cured by injections of Antimosan or Fuadin. Treatment with Hetrazan kills the microfilariae and, thus, renders the affected animals non-infective, without killing the adult worms.

REFERENCES

DASHIELL, G. F., *Amer. J. trop. Med. Hyg.*, 10 (1961) 37.
DESPORTES, C., *Ann. Parasit. hum. comp.*, 17 (1939–'40) 380.
FAUST, E. C., *Z. Tropenmed. Parasit.*, 8 (1957) 59.
FAUST, E. C., E. P. THOMAS and J. JONES, *J. Parasit.*, 27 (1941) 115.
FORBES, J. G., *Trans. roy. Soc. trop. Med. Hyg.*, 12 (1918) 11.
SKRIABIN, K., *Med. Parazit. (Mosk.)*, 9 (1940) 119.

g. Rare human nematodiases

i. Capillaria infections

α. *Capillaria hepatica infection.* Several species of the nematode genus *Capillaria* affect man. The commonest and best known is *Capillaria hepatica,* also called *Hepaticola hepatica.*

References p. 591

For 30 years this species remained on the list of specific parasites of the rat and some other mammals. However, in 1924 MacArthur found its ova in the liver of a British soldier in India who died with the symptoms of "pyaemia". Since then 3 more human infections have been recorded, all diagnosed post mortem. Meanwhile the elucidation of the life history of this nematode has provided an explanation of the epidemiological aspects of the infection.

Capillaria hepatica is a small and very thin worm, the female measuring about 20 mm in length and *ca.* 0.1 mm in width, the male being about half as long. As a matter of fact, nobody has yet succeeded in securing an undamaged whole worm, for it is so fragile that only fragments can be removed from the tissues. The anterior extremity tapers gradually, the posterior end is blunt. It lives in the liver, winding sinuously through the parenchyma. The female lays eggs in the liver tissue, where they accumulate in large masses forming characteristic whitish spots which are macroscopically visible under the surface. The eggs (51–68 microns long and 27–35 microns wide) resemble those of *Trichuris, i.e.,* they are oval and thick-shelled, and have plugs at both poles. They differ from the eggs of Trichuris in being larger (Trichuris eggs are 49–54 microns long) and in that their surface is pitted, while that of the eggs of *Trichuris* is smooth; the plugs of the eggs of *U. hepatica* are moreover flat and do not protrude.

The eggs, containing at most 8 metameres, are not passed out of the host, but remain unchanged in the liver as long as the host lives. After the death of the host they are liberated on the ground, either after the carcass has disintegrated, or when the infected host body has been eaten by an other animal, often an animal of the same species; this second host disseminates the undigested eggs with its faeces. In the presence of sufficient oxygen, larvae develop in the liberated eggs within 1 to 2 months. When these infective eggs are ingested by a suitable mammal, or by man, the larvae hatch in its intestine, migrate to the liver and, after another month, develop to the adult stage (Wright, 1931; Shorb, 1931; Luttermoser, 1938). The larvae are either carried to the liver by the blood of the portal system or they penetrate actively through the wall of the caecum into the body cavity and from this enter directly through the surface of the liver. Larvae may sometimes be carried to the lungs or other organs, but in these locations they do not mature and soon die.

It is now evident that, as a rule, the infected host does not eliminate the eggs of the parasite; consequently infection can be diagnosed only by dissection or biopsy. Yet eggs of *Capillaria hepatica* have been found on numerous occasions in the faeces of man. These eggs were in transit through the digestive tract of persons who had eaten the liver of an infected animal. Such eggs are not yet embryonated and they do not hatch, even if they are alive and are not digested. In a village in Panama Wright (1938) found eggs of *Capillaria hepatica* in over 8 % of examined people. Later Foster (1932) and Johnston (1939) explained that these cases were due to ingestion of the livers of the peccaries (a small pig-like forest animal, *Tayassu peccari spiradens*) and monkeys *(Ateles geoffroyi* and

Cebus capucinus immitator). Isolated cases of such spurious infections have been observed in various parts of the world (McQuown, 1950, in Louisiana; Skrjabin *et al.*, 1929, at lower Amur River; Dinulescu, 1957, in Roumania).

Capillaria hepatica has been found in all continents (including Alaska, New Guinea, Japan, Australia and Europe). It is apparently not particular with respect to its host, because it has been found in more than 40 species of mammals: rodents, carnivores, ungulates, primates and man. The animal most frequently infected is the house *rat*. Tubangui (1931), for instance, found the infection in 90% of the rats in the Philippines; Luttermoser (1936) found 86% of the rats infected in Baltimore; Gupta and Randhawa (1960) 50% in Delhi. This frequency in rats is explained by the cannibalistic habits of rodents in general and particularly of the domestic rat. In certain regions other wild rodents are also often infected (Cochrane, 1957, in Africa). Among domestic animals *C. hepatica* occurs in the *pig*, *cat* and *dog*. The pathology of *Capillaria hepatica* infection in these hosts is insufficiently known. Small animals probably soon die of atrophy of the liver. Smit (1960), in South Africa, found indications of long-standing infection in the dog.

As has been explained above, the eggs of *Capillaria hepatica* are not eliminated from the parasitised animal. It is assumed that the same occurs in human infection. This probably explains why, in some localities in which a high prevalence of infection was found among rats, only a few fatal infections were observed in human beings. Presumably slight human infections are not rare in regions in which *Capillaria hepatica* is prevalent among the small rodents and where low hygienic conditions enable the dispersed eggs of the parasite to reach man (Lubinsky, 1956), These infections are not revealed by characteristic symptoms and remain undiagnosed.

In cases of heavy human infection, or in those complicated by concomitant diseases, the outcome is usually fatal. It is, however, impossible to judge from the total of fatal cases recorded, to what extent *Capillaria* contributed to the lethal outcome. The clinical picture shows extreme weakness, anaemia, leucocytosis and eosinophilia up to 80%. The infection provokes serious disruption of the histological structure and physiological function of the liver. The organ is mostly enlarged and shows a variable number of whitish specks on its surface, consisting of egg-masses. In microscopic sections multiple granulomata with necrotic center, formed around separated or massed eggs, are visible in varying density; cirrhosis is mostly pronounced. Solitary, tubercular-like foci also appear in the lungs and kidneys. The unaffected liver parenchyma, blood vessels and bile capillaries often retain their normal appearance, a fact which indicates a considerable degree of adaptation between the parasite and the host. However, the relentless progressing cirrhosis finally leads to liver failure. In one case death followed as lately as 2 years after the onset of the disease (Otto *et al.*, 1954).

The above mentioned clinical picture of *Capillaria hepatica* infection bears some resemblance to *visceral larva migrans*. Indeed, in certain instances the syndromes are indistinguishable, and it may, therefore, be presumed that the former is more common than is now apparent (Beaver, 1956).

No effective treatment of the condition has yet been found. Control of rats is the main preventive measure to be recommended. Dead rats must not be left to be eaten by swine (see also the chapter on *trichinelliasis*) or to disintegrate in the soil. It should be remembered that Momma (1930) and Shorb (1931) have shown that flies can disseminate the eggs of *Capillaria hepatica*, which, according to Luttermoser (1938), remain viable under external conditions for about half a year.

β. Thominxiasis. Thominx aerophila (also known as *Capillaria aerophila*) is a common parasite of carnivores (*cat, dog, fox, wolf*, etc., in the Old and New World), in which it is located in the nasal cavity, trachea and bronchi.

Burrows and Lillis (1960) found 7% of *dogs* and 10% of *cats* infected with this parasite in the vicinity of New York. *Thominx aerophila* sometimes causes high mortality in reared fur-animals.

It has been found 6 times in the Soviet Union (Podyapolskaya, 1958) in *man* in whom it caused serious disease.

Although this species is rather long (the female measuring up to 20 mm), the worm is hardly visible, because it is only 0.06–0.07 mm wide. According to Romanov, 1958, the worms developing in wild animals are much larger than those in man. The body is thickest at its posterior extremity and becomes gradually thinner in the anterior half of the body. The ova which are 59–80 microns long, have two polar plugs, resembling those of *Trichuris*, from which they can be distinguished chiefly by the peculiar network pattern on their surfaces.

There is a controversy about the life history of this parasite. While Christenson (1938) asserts that the development is direct, Podyapolskaya (1958) thinks that earthworms serve as intermediate hosts. The known cases in the Soviet Union occurred in garden

workers, who had presumably swallowed infected earthworms with soiled fresh vegetables.

In man the infection is accompanied by acute bronchitis or broncho-
pneumonia, and sometimes asthmatic attacks. Cough with copious purulent and sometimes bloody excretion cannot be influenced by ordinary
treatment. The recovery is slow, while asthma-like attacks may persist for
years. It has been claimed that the instillation of very dilute solution of
iodine gives good therapeutic results.

REFERENCES

COCHRANE, J. C., L. SAGORIN and M. G. WILCOCKS, *S. Afr. med. J.*, 31 (1957) 751.
CHRISTENSON, R. O., *Libro Jubilare L. Travassos*, Rio de Janeiro, 1938, 119.
FAUST, E. C. and W. H. MARTINER, *J. Parasit.*, 21 (1935) 322.
FOSTER, A. I. and C. M. JOHNSON, *Proc. roy. Soc. trop. Med. Hyg.*, 32 (1939) 639.
LUBINSKY, G., *Canad. J. comp. Med.*, 20 (1956) 457.
LUTTERMOSER, G. W., *Amer. J. Hyg.*, 27 (1938) 321.
OTTO, G. F., M. BERTHRONG, R. E. APPLEBY, J. C. RAWLINS and O. WILBUR, *Bull. Johns Hopk. Hosp.*, 94 (1954) 319.
PODYAPOLSKAYA, V. P. and V. F. KAPUSTIN, *Helminthic Diseases of Man*, Moscow, 1958.

ii. Physaloptera infection

The nematode *Physaloptera caucasica* (male 1.5–5 cm, female 2.5–10 cm
long) is a specific parasite of African monkeys. It lives in the stomach,
firmly attached to the mucosa by a pair of lips. It also has been found in
the orang-utan, *Macaca sylvana* (Indo-Malayan apes) and in a *Capybara*
kept in zoological parks in the U.S.A. The latter infections were probably
acquired in captivity by the ingestion of cockroaches or beetles which are
considered to be intermediate hosts of this nematode (Petter, 1960). It has
been stated that this species is common in man in certain parts of Africa
(Leiper, 1911) and it has been found once in Brazil (Soriano-Lleras, 1955)
and in India (Sing and Rao, 1954). A record from Israel (Witenberg,
1951), diagnosed on eggs discharged in human faeces, may be regarded as
doubtful.

The pathological action of *Physaloptera caucasica* in man is insufficiently known. Curiously enough, this species was originally described as a
parasite of man in the Caucasus as early as 1902 (Linstow), although
there are in this area no monkeys which could serve as a reservoir of
infection.

REFERENCES

FAUST, E. C. and C. F. GRAIG, *Clinical Parasitology*, 1951, pp. 398.
LEIPER, R. T., *J. trop. Med. Hyg.*, 14 (1911) 209.
SCHULZ, R. S., *Ann. Parasit. hum. comp.*, 4 (1926) 74.
WITENBERG, G., *Harefuah*, 41 (1951) 180.

iii. Human infections with animal ascarids (Butcher's dermatitis)

Many domestic dogs and cats harbour in their intestines specific ascarids, the species found in dogs being *Toxascaris leonina* and *Toxocara canis* while the species found in the cat is *Toxocara mystax*. These species occasionally also develop to maturity in a variety of related wild carnivores and in man. Except for specific hosts most of the larvae do not settle in the intestines but wander through the tissues and are eventually encapsulated. The same may occur in man when he ingests the fully developed eggs of these worms. The migrating larvae may cause substantial harm, which is manifested in the syndrome called *visceral larva migrans* (*vide* p. 568).

Mendheim *et al.* (1952), summarizing the literature on various ascarids specific to animals, found 19 records of *Toxocara mystax* in man, 1 of *T. canis,* whereas the other canine species *(T. leonina)* apparently has never been recorded as a human parasite. *Lagochilascaris minor,* a parasite probably restricted to wild Felidae, has been observed in abscesses in 4 human cases, 3 of which situated in the subcutaneous tissues. On the other hand, the species of *Ascaris* specific to man *(A. lumbricoides)* has been only rarely observed as a parasite of other animals, namely in the orang-utan, the dog, cat, sheep, musk-rat *(Ondatra zibethica),* and squirrels *(Sciurus indicus; S. pygerythrus)*. Considering the ubiquity of human ascariasis and its rarity in animals, no epidemiological importance can be ascribed to the infections of the animals just mentioned. Further, it should be noted that eggs of *A. lumbricoides* are frequently seen in the excreta of dogs; these are cases of pseudoparasitism, due to the ingestion of human faeces by dogs.

Ascarids of animals can be indirectly responsible for human suffering, namely by causing so-called *butcher's dermatitis, swine itch* or *cattle itch* (Schwartz, 1931). This is a skin affliction, which primarily affects the hands, occurring in persons who handle the organs of freshly slaughtered animals. It is found especially among the personnel of meat-packing plants. Its aetiology is believed to be connected with sensitisation of these persons against ascaris-antigen occurring as a result of infection with *A. lumbricoides*, and occupational contact with the antigen which is present on the entrails of pigs and cattle which harbour related ascarids *(A. suum* and *Neoascaris vitulorum* respectively) and have antigenic components in common with the *Ascaris* of man. The dermatitis appears several days after such contact and may last from a few days up to several weeks. It is characterized by erythema, vesicles the size of a pinhead, and an eruption, and is accompanied by intense itching. The lesions may spread over adjacent areas. The process occurs in varying degrees of severity and is sometimes recurrent. In some individuals it persists for several years.

REFERENCES

SCHWARTZ, B., *J. industr. Hyg.,* 13 (1931) 233.
MENDHEIM, H., G. SCHEID and J. SCHMIDT, *Z. tropenmed. Parasit.,* 3 (1952) 368.

iv. Human infections with animal hookworms

Apart from the specific hookworms of man *(Ancylostoma duodenale* and *Necator americanus)*, several species of hookworms specific to animals have been recorded as accidental parasites of man, namely: *A. caninum, A. brasiliense* and *A. ceylanicum.* The larvae of these species invade man in the way in which they invade their specific hosts, *i.e.* domesticated and wild carnivores. In the majority of human infections they wander in the tissues without reaching the intestine. Occasionally, however, the larvae succeed in arriving there, and develop to maturity as intestinal parasites. During their migrations through the tissues they cause *creeping eruption or visceral larva migrans* (vide: p. 563).

There are only a few records of human infection by adult *A. caninum* (Witenberg, 1951). On the other hand, numerous cases of infection with *A. brasiliense* and *A. ceylanicum* have been recorded, but the identification of the parasites seems now questionable. Most authors (*e.g.* Lane, Faust, Chandler) regarded the 2 last-mentioned species as synonymous and grouped them together under the name *A. brasiliense.* However, Boicca (1951) reexamining 36 specimens described by Gordon (1922) in Brazil as *A. brasiliense,* found that, in fact, 35 were *A. ceylanicum* and only one was *A. brasiliense.* Consequently Biocca (1952) reinstated both species as valid and doubted whether man is susceptible to infection with *A. brasiliense.*

Summing up recent observations, the conclusion may be drawn tha'
A. ceylanicum is third in importance as a hookworm-species pathogeni(
to man. This species is common in cats and dogs in tropical countries o'
both the Old and the New World. According to Chandler (1957) it ac
counts for about 4% of the cases of adult hookworm infection in man ii
India. Additional hosts of it are wild cats (Felis bengalensis, F. temmincki)
civet cats (Viverra mallaccensis), squirrels (Callosciurus caniceps, C. no
tatus) in South East Asia and the civet cats (Viverra civetta and V. genetta,
in Africa.

On the other hand it should be noted that specific human hookworm:
are occasionally found as parasites of animals. Although, under exceptional circumstances, animals may serve as reservoirs of human hookworms, little epidemiological importance should be ascribed to thes(
findings. Among animals which may thus act as reservoirs of Necato/
americanus are the gorilla, the rhinoceros, anteaters (Manis) and severa'
species of monkeys, whilst the gorilla, the orang-utan, the chimpanzee,
species of gibbon, and the pig, may be reservoirs of Ancylostoma duodenale.

Clatham (1942) regards Necator suillus, a parasite of pigs, as a strain o'
the human hookworm, N. americanus, which has become specifically
adapted to the pig. Buckley (1933) demonstrated, by successfull infection
of a volunteer, that the porcine parasite must be regarded a potential
human parasite.

REFERENCES

ADLER, S., Ann. trop. Med. Parasit., 16 (1922) 293.
BIOCCA, E., J. Helminth., 25 (1951) 1.
BUCKLEY, J. J., Brit. med. J., I (1933) 699.
CHANDLER, A. C., Amer. J. trop. Med. Hyg., 6 (1957) 438.
GORDON, R. M., Ann. trop. Med. Parasit., 16 (1922) 223.
WITENBERG, G., Harefuah, 41 (1951) 180.

v. Human infections with animal Trichuris species

It is generally accepted that Trichuris trichiura (often called Trichocephalus
or whipworm) is the only species of this genus which is parasitic in man.
However, recent observations indicate that one, or possibly two, other
species may settle in the human body, namely the swine whipworm (T.
suis) and the dog whipworm (T. vulpis).

Species of Trichuris inhabit the large intestine, rarely the ileum. The adults are a few cm long and consist of two parts: a long, thin anterior part and a shorter, wider posterior part. The parasite is firmly attached by the anterior part of its body to the tips of the intestinal villi. The mode of feeding of whipworms is not adequately known; traces of blood have been found in the worms, a fact which suggests that blood constitutes at least a part of the food of these worms (Glikina, 1958). Other investigators presume that the food is absorbed through the outer integument of the worm.

Small numbers of whipworms are harmless, but in intensive infection they may cause severe intoxication and even death.

All the species of *Trichuris* are morphologically much alike and the specific identity of some of them is still *sub judice*. Species which are indistinguishable in shape from those which occur in man are frequently harboured by pigs, monkeys and apes. Most authorities regard the Trichurids found in *primates* as being identical with those observed in *man*, but opinions are divided concerning the porcine species. Cameron (1958) favours the opinion that the human and porcine species are identical, and he consequently thinks that the pig is a reservoir of human infection. On the other hand, Dinnik (1938), Tukolevsky (1940) and others claim to have demonstrated by unsuccessful experimental cross-infection, as well as by the results of detailed morphological examination, that the species of man and swine are distinct, and they call the latter *Trichuris suis*. At all events, even if the possibility of human infection with porcine or monkey strains (or species) were admitted, this has no real significance for the epidemiology of trichuriasis in man, because *T. trichiura* of man is ubiquitously distributed, even in regions from which pigs and monkeys are absent.

Apart from "*T. suis*", another species of the genus present in animals should be considered a potential human parasite, namely *T. vulpis,* which is normally parasitic in dogs and foxes. Human infection with this species is, however, rare. As an example may be cited a case, described by Hall and Sonneberg (1956), of a 4-year old child in Maryland. Dinulescu (1958) has recorded a high incidence of this infection among the employees of dog-kennels in Bucharest.

REFERENCES

BEZUBIK, B. and S. FURMAGA, *Acta parasit. pol.,* 7 (1959) 591.
CAMERON, T. W. M., *Ann. N.Y. Acad. Sci.,* 70 (1958) 564.

DINULESCU, G., et al., Trop. Dis. Bull., 55 (1958) 902.
DINNIK, N. N., Med. Parazit. (Mosk.), 7 (1938) 907.
PAVLOVSKY, E. N. and V. A. SONDAK, Parazit. Sbornik. 13 (1951) 35.
SCHWARTZ, B., J. Parasit., 13 (1926) 83.
SKRYABIN, K. J., N. P. SHIKHOBALOVA and I. V. ORLOV, Osnovy Nematodologii, 6
  (1957) 126.

vi. Gongylonema infection

The genus *Gongylonema* is represented by some 30 species of which one, *G. pulchrum*, may appear as an accidental parasite of man. The worm has a threadlike shape. The female measures up to 15 cm long and is about 0.5 mm wide, the male being half that size. The worms live under the mucosa of the oesophagus of *swine, cattle, sheep* and other mammals, mainly ruminants, all over the world. Accidental hosts in addition to man, are *hares, bears* and several species of *monkeys*. Although in the proper hosts the worms sometimes appear in great numbers, they exert little pathogenic effect.

In the Ukraine, according to Chebotariov *et al.* (1959), up to 94% of cattle, 95% of sheep and 37% of pigs are infected with *G. pulchrum,* the number of these animals varying from one to several hundreds. A similar high incidence of infection in cattle has been observed in other regions.

The adult *G. pulchrum* either moves slowly along a characteristic zigzag path under the mucosa, or it lies spirally rolled in a 5 to 10 mm wide papule. The eggs are extruded into the oesophageal lumen and are passed out with the faeces of the host. The life cycle of the parasite requires an insect intermediate host. Numerous beetles, among them domestic cockroaches, may play this role. The definitive host becomes infected by ingestion of an insect which contains the fully developed encysted infective larva.

Infection of man rarely occurs. About 20 cases have been recorded in the literature, chiefly in Europe, the U.S.A., China, Ceylon and New Zealand. In most cases immature worms were extracted from the mucosae of the mouth. Rarely the almost mature worm has been found in a specific organ, the oesophagus (Feng *et al.,* 1955). Kamalov (1953) described a case, observed in the Caucasus, in which 6 adult specimens of *G. pulchrum* were extracted in the course of 10 months from under the buccal mucosa of a man. Faust and Martinez (1935) mentioned a case presumable of pseudo-parasitism, in which eggs of *Gongylonema* were found in human stools.

The worms cause disturbing local symptoms in man, but no serious consequences have ever been noted.

All the reported cases of *Gongylonema* infection of man have been attributed to *G. pulchrum*. In most of these cases, however, the determination of the species was based upon examination of the immature worms, so that the validity of the determination is only approximate and other common species of the genus cannot definitely be excluded (*e.g. G. neoplasticum*, which is ordinarily a parasite of rats). As a matter of fact, the various species differ little from each other; they show major differences only in the anatomical topography of the mature male.

REFERENCES

BAYLIS, H. A., *J. trop. Med. Hyg.*, 28 (1925) 71.
CHEBOTARIOV, R. S., *Acta parasitol. pol.*, 7 (1959) 23.
KAMALOV, N. G., *Skrjabin Anniv. Vol.*, 1953, p. 273.
LEIPER, R. T., *Brit. med. J.*, (1926) 504.
SAMBON, L. W., *J. trop. Med. Hyg.*, 28 (1925) 39.
THOMAS, L. J., *Proc. helminth. Soc., Wash.*, 19 (1925) 124.

vii. Oesophagostomum infection

The nematode-genus *Oesophagostomum* includes numerous species which are parasitic in various domesticated and wild animals. Eight of these species are parasites of apes and monkeys and 3 of them have also been found in man on several occasions *(O. stephanostomum* in Africa and South America, *O. bifurcum* in Africa and Asia, and *O. aculeatum* in Asia).

Oesophagostomes are small worms (1–2 cm long), living in the large intestine. The life-histories of most of the species just mentioned have not yet been adequately studied, but they seem to be similar to that of related species in sheep, or to *Ternidens deminutus* (vide p. 599). Oesophagostomes are common parasites of *monkeys*, the incidence sometimes exceeding 50 % (Bebuzik and Furmaga, 1959). They cause severe dysenteric attacks, which may be fatal when the worms are present in large numbers. Human infections have been only rarely recorded. Except for the 4 % incidence among African prisoners in Nigeria, as reported by Leiper (1913), all records indicate only occasional infections produced by a few worms. One should, however, take into account that, in the light of recent systematics, the identification of the parasites recorded by Leiper is not certain. The fact that on 2 occasions (Chabaud and Larivière, 1958; Lothe, 1958) immature worms have caused subcutaneous nodules, indicates that man is an unsuitable host and that human infection therefore should be regarded an accidental occurrence.

REFERENCES

BAYLE, R. J. and R. J. PAILLET, *Bull. Soc. Path. exot.,* 52 (1959) 32.
BEZUBIK, B. and S. FURMAGA, *Acta parasit. pol.,* 7 (1959) 591.
CHABAUD, A. G. and M. LARIVIÈRE, *Bull. Soc. Path. exot.,* 51 (1958) 384.
LEIPER, R. T., *Trans. roy. Soc. trop. Med. Hyg.,* 6 (1913) 265.
SIANG, T. K. and L. K. JOE, *Docum. Med. geogr. trop. (Amst.),* 5 (1953) 123.
SWELLENGREBEL, N. H. and M. M. STERMAN, *Animal Parasites in Man,* Princeton, N. J., 1961, 652 pp.
TRAVASSOS, L. and E. VOGELSANG, *Mem. Inst. Osw. Cruz,* 26 (1932) 251.

viii. Syngamiasis

Syngamiasis is caused by *Syngamus laryngeus**, a nematod eliving in the upper respiratory tract of cattle and other ruminants, without provoking obvious harm. Its geographic distribution includes localities in India, Malaya, the Philippines, Central Africa, the West-Indies and Brazil. In the Island of Trinidad more than half of the sheep and 15% of the cattle were found to be infected; over 75 pairs of worms were counted in one sheep (Buckley, 1934). Man is infected accidentally. Amaral (quoted by Pessoa, 1958) summarized 22 cases of human infection, of which 7 were from Brazil.

The generic name of the worm denotes its characteristic biological feature, namely, the fact that the male is firmly attached to the female *in copula* for the whole of its life, the pair thus showing the form of a Y. In the living state *Syngamus* has a blood-red colour. Both the male and the female are fixed to the mucosa by a strong buccal sucking capsule. The female reaches 20 mm, the male 6 mm in length. The life history is still obscure.

In man the parasite causes paroxysms of cough, asthmatic attacks, dyspnoea, haemoptysis and irritation in the throat and nasopharynx. In one

---

* According to the latest nomenclature, *S. laryngeus* belongs to the genus *Mammomonogamus,* but the traditional name *Syngamus* is used here for convenience.

of 3 cases described by Saint Prix (1950) in Martinique, the symptoms lasted for 6 months. The disease usually terminates when the worms are expelled by coughing.

REFERENCES

BUCKLEY, J. J. C., *J. Helminth.*, 12 (1934) 47.
FONT, J. H., *Bol. Asoc. méd. P. Rico*, 35 (1934) 331.
HOFFMAN, W. A., *Bol. Asoc. méd. P. Rico*, 24 (1932) 703.
PASSOS, W. and C. BARBOSA, *Rev. Brasil. Med.*, 5 (1948) 340.
RYZHIKOV, K. M., *Osnovy Nematologii*, 1 (1949), Acad. Sci. U.S.S.R.

ix. Ternidens infection

Ternidens deminutus is a small nematode (female 8–16 mm long, male somewhat smaller) living in man and various Old-World primates, including the gorilla and chimpanzee, in scattered areas of the southern half of Africa (including Mauritius) and in the tropical regions of South-East Asia (including Indonesia). It is not certain whether *man* or other animals are the main host of this species. An incidence as high as 65% has been recorded in the population of some African localities (Sandground, 1931) while infection of 21% of the *monkeys* imported from China was established by Bezubik and Furmaga (1959).

Present knowledge of the life-history and geographical distribution of *Ternidens* is still fragmentary. Morphologically, the worm and its eggs resemble the much more common hookworms, and it may be presumed that confusion between these species has sometimes obscured the identification of *Ternidens*.

The adult worms live in the large bowel, attached to the mucosa by a strong goblet-shaped sucking capsule. They feed on blood. The eggs (80 microns in length) are passed with the host's faeces; the larvae hatch in the soil. After 2 molts they become infective. Further development requires ingestion by a suitable host. The larvae then burrow into the intestinal submucosa, causing the formation of a nodule, inside which the pre-adult stage is formed. At this stage they eventually break through into the intestinal lumen and develop there into the adult worm.

The pathological significance of *Ternidens* infection in man has not been fully clarified.

References p. 600

REFERENCES

AMBERSON, J. M. and E. SCHWARZ, *Ann. trop. Med. Parasit.*, 44 (1952) 227.
BEZUBIK, B. and S. FURMAGA, *Acta parasit. Pol.*, 7 (1959) 591.
CRAIG, C. F. and E. C. FAUST, 5th ed., Philadelphia, 1951, 1032 pp.
SANDGROUND, J. H., *Ann. trop. Med. Parasit.*, 25 (1931) 147.

x. Thelazia infections

There are several species of nematodes of the genus *Thelazia*, all of them parasites of the conjunctiva or lacrimal sacs of mammals or birds. Some of these species constitute a serious hazard to domestic animals since they may cause blindness. Most common is this parasite in China, Siberia and Czechoslovakia. All species of *Thelazia* need arthropods as intermediate hosts which are swallowed by the final hosts. Human infection occurs accidentally and rarely; they are mostly acribed to *T. callipaeda* which mainly parasites in *dogs*. In some cases it may be assumed that other species of the same genus can also produce human infection.

In *man Thelazia* causes constant irritation and scarification of the conjunctiva and cornea, ensuing abundant lacrimation. The infection may be easily terminated by removal of the thread-like worm by pincers, after instillation of cocaine solution.

REFERENCES

CRAIG, C. F. and E. C. FAUST, *Clinical Parasitology*, 5th ed., Philadelphia, 1961, pp. 1078.
HOVORKA, J., *Wiadom. Paraz. (Poland)*, 5 (1959) 379.

xi. Anisakiasis

A peculiar syndrome, observed in several persons in Rotterdam and neighbouring places, was caused by nematode larvae (Straub, 1955). Van Thiel *et al.* (1960) identified the parasite as a larva of *Anisakis* sp. of the family *Heterocheilidae* which usually inhabits the viscera of small fish (herring, mackerel, cod, etc.) that serve as intermediate hosts. The adult worm is found in aquatic predators (shark, ray, seals).

Healthy people are suddenly attacked with violent abdominal colic and fever, often indicating urgent surgical treatment. At laparotomy the nematode larva is found in the intestinal and stomach wall, causing phlegmonous eosinophilic infiltration and ileus. In few cases the course was fatal.

Human infection with "herring-worm disease" is due to the habit of swallowing fresh or insufficiently salted fish (especially the so-called "green herring") containing *Anisakis* larvae. It is presumed that ingestion of these larvae for the first time does not bring about clinical symptoms but sensitises the intestinal wall locally against repeated contact with the larvae (Kampelmacher and Kuipers). Consequently, subsequent swallowing of similar larvae may cause severe local allergic reaction creating the above mentioned syndrome.

If the herring is gutted immediately at sea, the larvae are removed with the intestine. However, if the fish is kept for some time and gutted ashore, the larvae have meanwhile migrated from the viscera to the muscles in which they reach the human intestine. Therefore, gutting and curing should be done soon after the catch, and distribution of "green herring" should be prohibited.

Strong brine (1 : 12 for 7 days), high temperature (55 C°) and freezing to — 20° C for 24 hours kill the larvae.

REFERENCES

KAMPELMACHER, E. H. AND F. C. KUIPERS, in the press.
VAN THIEL, P. H., F. C. KUIPERS AND R. TH. ROSKAM, *Trop. geogr. Med.*, 12 (1960) 97.
VAN THIEL, P. H., *Parasitology*, 52 (1962) 16.

2

G. G. WITENBERG

Trematodiases

Introduction

Trematodiases, often called *distomatoses*, are infections caused by trematodes. This term, although still frequently used is an anachronism, derived from the old name *Distoma* which embraced most digenetic trematodes until the beginning of the current century. In the progress of classification, however, the trematode species were distributed between numerous separate genera while the genus *Distoma* was disqualified as a taxonomic unit.

Several species of the trematodes are parasites both of man and animals, and because each of them causes a different syndrome and also differs in the sense of epidemiology and control, it is desirable to call every infection by a name derived from that of its specific causative agent.

a. Fascioliasis

Fascioliasis is a systemic disease caused by liver-flukes of the genus *Fasciola*, which are among the largest of the trematodes. These worms are common parasites of sheep and cattle all over the world and live in the bile ducts of the liver. In animals, *Fasciola* causes thickening and dilatation of the bile ducts and toxic degeneration of the adjacent liver tissue. Slight infections are generally quite well tolerated, but heavy infections cause serious disease and high mortality.

In endemic localities up to 60% of infected livers may be condemned for human consumption and losses of millions of dollars are thus caused. In some regions the breeding of sheep and cattle becomes unprofitable and even has to be abandoned because of the ravages caused by *Fasciola*.

The parasite occurs mainly in swampy regions or in the vicinity of flooded pastures, because it requires a fresh-water snail (species of the genus *Lymnaea*) as intermediate hosts. There are two species of the genus *Fasciola*. *F. hepatica* occurs in many temperate regions of all continents; in tropical regions it is replaced by a larger species, *F. gigantica*.

F. hepatica is leaf-shaped and may be up to 4 cm long. Its eggs (approx. 150 microns in length) are passed out of the host in its faeces. They must reach fresh water for further development. Within a few weeks (much longer during the cold season), they mature and the larvae (miracidia) hatch out and invade a snail. Inside the snail many generations of cercariae come into being through asexual multiplication. The cercariae escape from the snail and attach themselves to plants, on which they become encysted metacercariae. These metacercariae are resistent to exposure to the air when the water recedes. According to Taylor (1952) they remain in the shade infective for a period of up to 6 months. Animals acquire infection by eating infected plants or by drinking water containing cysts washed off the vegetation. When the metacercariae arrive in the intestine, they escape from the cysts and migrate through the intestinal wall to the liver in which they settle down.

In ordinary circumstances, human infection rarely occurs. Outbreaks are most frequently recorded in countries in which people are accustomed to eat watercress. However, this is not the only factor which promotes the infection in man. Infection may also occur by drinking water containing freely floating metacercariae.

The geographical distribution of human fascioliasis is not adequately known. According to Coudert and Triozon (1958) the most serious infections have been recorded in France, where about 500 persons were involved in several outbreaks during the years 1956–1957. Among other countries in which sporadic outbreaks have been observed, the following may be quoted; in Hawaii, at least 19 recognised outbreaks have been recorded in the past (Alicata and Bonnet, 1956); in Mexico, 13 outbreaks were summarised by Hernandez-Chinas *et al.* (1959); in Chile, 68 cases have been reviewed by Faiguenbaum (1958); in Cuba, 85 cases were reported during the period 1931–1939 (Kouri and Basnuevo, 1939). Sporadic cases have been observed in Central Europe, the Soviet Union, Britain (Facey and Mardsen, 1960) and other countries.

In man, as in animals, infection of the liver is often not confined to the bile ducts, but spreads to the surrounding parenchyma, giving rise to inflammatory and degenerative sequelae.

The onset of the disease is usually abrupt. The often very disturbing acute symptoms of hepatic colic, high fever and urticarial eruption of the Quincke type, last for about 3 months. Cough often occurs in the initial period. Usually enlargement of the liver and spleen, eosinophilia (up to 65%) and jaundice develop. In severe cases appendicular, peritoneal, nervous and psychic symptoms may complicate the picture. When the disease takes a chronic course of slow evolution the patients may lose weight and become invalids. The intensity of the syndrome depends on the number of parasites. If these are few, the infection may be symptomless, or the symptoms may be slight at the beginning, but at a later date (sometimes in the course of several years) digestive and hepato-biliary troubles (e.g. cirrhosis, obstruction by calculi, secondary infections) complicated by acute febrile crises, may set in. Cholelithiasis is a common after-effect of the infection. Complications next in frequency are: obstructive icterus and hepatic cirrhosis. Rarely empyema of the gall-bladder is observed (Coudert and Triozon, 1958; Facey and Mardsen, 1960).

During the course of fascioliasis, anaemia often develops. This is generally attributed to a haemolytic toxin produced by the parasite. There are, however, indications that the anaemia of fascioliasis is caused by chronic haemorrhages (Jennings et al., 1956), which is feasible, considering that Fasciola hepatica mainly feeds on blood (Hsu, 1939: Stephenson, 1947).

The parasite is not as well adapted to man as it is to animals. Human infections differ from those in animals in that in man, Fasciola does not always develop in the liver. Thus, in man it often behaves as a larva migrans, wandering in the tissues as if it were searching in vain for a suitable site for settling down. The young worm, migrating erratically through various organs, may grow to a size of 1 cm, causing damage to the tissues and sometimes giving rise to abscesses, from which it can be eliminated with pus. This event has even been observed in such unusual sites as the larynx. Migrating Fasciola larvae may be found simultaneously with adult worms in the bile ducts and may then cause additional symptoms which are liable to confuse the clinical picture. Wandering larvae may also cause unpredictable complications. For instance, Cattan et al., (1953), quoted by Gallais et al. (1955), recorded a case of transient hemiplegia in a 36-year old man, who passed eggs of F. hepatica in his faeces.

The diagnosis can most reliably be made by demonstration of the characteristic eggs of the worm in the faeces. However, as long as the parasites are still young (up to 4 months), or are living in organs other than the liver, the eggs may be absent. In such cases the illness can easily be confused with other pathological processes, and sero-logical diagnosis may be helpful. Coudert (1955) recommended an intradermal test with a lyophilised antigen as superior to other tests. Minning and Fuhrman (1955) found that an alcoholic extract from *Fasciola* is specific and most valuable in the complement-fixation test. A very sensitive agglutination test with antigen adsorbed on collodion has been proposed by Coudert and Coly (1956).

It should be noted that in localities in which people are accustomed to eat the livers of infected sheep or cattle, undigested ova of *F. hepatica,* the so called transit eggs, may appear in fair numbers in the faeces. Such eggs may lead to a false diagnosis. In order to find out whether the excretion of eggs denotes a true or a spurious infection, the patient must be put on a meatless diet for a week. During this time all the remnants of both the ingested liver and the parasites are eliminated and examination of the faeces can be repeated. The absence of eggs may be then interpreted as proof that those previously found were transit eggs. If, however, eggs reappear, it proves that a true infection is present. Alternatively, duodenal sounding may quickly reveal the presence of ova when a true infection is present.

Most cases of human fascioliasis have been attributed to *F. hepatica,* only a few to *F. gigantica.* It is not known whether this is due to a particular affinity of the former species for man or whether other factors are responsible.

The control of fascioliasis in cattle or sheep should be approached from two angles. First, the animals must be treated with carbon-tetrachloride (sheep) or hexachlorethane (cattle) given by mouth, which kill and eliminate the parasites. This treatment must be applied systematically to the whole herd. On the other hand, destruction of the snail-carriers should be undertaken. Dusting the banks of infected ponds and swampy areas with copper-sulphate, pentachlorophenate or some other mollusci-cide is practicable and may reduce the incidence to a tolerable degree.

Elimination of the parasite from cattle does not always free the endemic region from *Fasciola hepatica,* because this species also infects other domesticated animals, such as pigs and horses. It also thrives in some wild herbivorous animals, such as deer and chamois, and notably in rabbits and hares, which are also important as reservoirs of the parasite in the vicinity of human habitations. Olsen (1948) for instance, recorded 32% infection among jack-rabbits in Texas.

Laboratory animals are also susceptible to infection with *Fasciola* and

can acquire infection through ingesting green food. How easy the spread
of infection may be has been shown by Trofimov and Alyabova (1959),
who lost over half of their experimental guinea pigs in a sudden outbreak
caused by contaminated grass. Unexpected epidemics may occur in other
experimental animals. Bezubik and Furmaga (1959) recorded infection
of 5% of monkeys *(Macacus rhesus)* brought from China, which were
carrying one to 14 specimens of *F. hepatica.*

For the treatment of human infection daily intramuscular injections of
emetine hydrochloride for 10 consecutive days are effective in eliminating
the parasite from most patients. Because outbreaks of fascioliasis often
have a familiar character, it is advisable whenever a clinically evident
sporadic case occurs, to examine the whole family.

Control of the cultivation of watercress (which in France, for instance,
amounts to tens of tons yearly) is another important measure. Human
consumption of watercress should only be permitted where no animal
manure has been used for the cultivation of the cress, and where proper
precautions have been taken to avoid soiling the ponds with animal ex-
crement. Watercress growing wild should be regarded as being unfit for
human consumption.

REFERENCES

ALICATA, J. E., *Hawaii med. J.,* 12 (1953) 196.
COUDERT, J. and M. COLY, *Ann. Parasit. hum. comp.,* 31 (1956) 489.
COUDERT, J. and F. TRIZAN, *Presse méd.,* 65 (1957) 1586.
FAIGUENBAUM, J., *Bol. chil. Parasit.,* 13 (1958) 29.
HSU, H. F., *Chin. med. J.,* 56 (1939) 122.
JENNING, F. W., W. MULLIGAN and G. M. URQUHART, *Exp. Parasit.,* 5 (1956) 458.
STEPHENSON, W., *Parasitology,* 38 (1947) 123.

b. Plant-borne intestinal trematode infections

At least 2 species of trematodes transmitted by the consumption of
aquatic plants cause human intestinal infections in the Far East, namely
Fasciolopsis buski and *Gastrodiscoides hominis.* Though these two species
are taxonomically unrelated, they have the same geographical distribution
and probably have similar life histories, while both are propagated by
animal hosts. By their pathological action they create both medical and
veterinary public health problems.

i. Fasciolopsiasis

Fasciolopsiasis is caused by *Fasciolopsis buski,* one of the largest trematodes, which is related to the liver flukes of the genus *Fasciola.* The genus *Fasciolopsis* differs from *Fasciola* in anatomical details and in that its representatives do not live in the liver, but in the intestine, of man and the pig.

Fasciolopsis buski is a leaf-shaped, flat, elongated worm reaching 5 cm in maximum length and 2 cm in width. It feeds on blood. The worms are very profilic, every female laying many thousands of eggs daily (according to Barlow, 1925: up to 15,000; according to Stoll and Kwei, 1927; up to 25,000). The eggs, which pass out of the final host in its faeces, are usually oval, but they vary in shape and size (100–180 microns). The life cycle is similar to that of *Fasciola, i.e.* it requires a fresh-water mollusc as the only intermediate host. However, the snail must be a species of the genus *Planorbis* (*Hippeutis*) or *Segmentina.* The cercariae emerging from the snail encyst on water plants, often edible ones, which may be ingested by the final host. The adult worm matures within about 5 weeks.

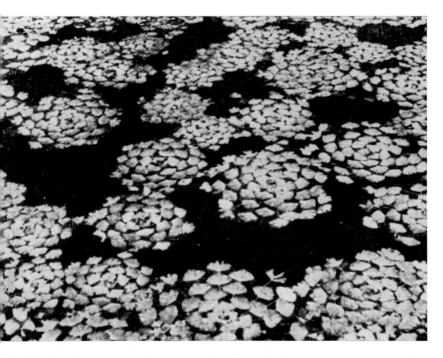

Fig. 83.   Pond surface showing growth of cultivated caltrop, the main vector of *Fasciolopsis buski* (courtesy Prof. H. Vogel, Arch. Schiffs Tropenhyg., 1936).

Fasciolopsis buski is commonest in the south-eastern part of continental Asia. Some areas are highly endemic foci; they are mainly found in the Yang-Tse Valley (Chekiang Province, China) where, in some villages, up to 80% of children are infected (Hung Sie Lü, 1933; Vogel, 1936), in Assam (Buckley, 1939), Formosa (Hsieh, 1960), and the vicinity of Canton and Hong Kong. They also occur in certain localities in Bengal, the Philippines and Indonesia.

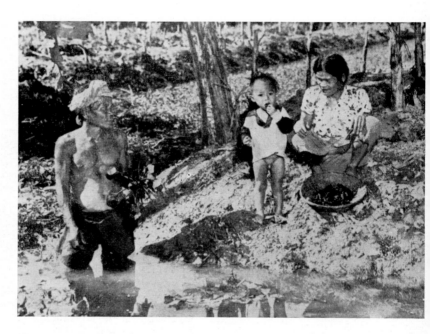

Fig. 84. Child eating water caltrop harvested by his parents in Thailand (courtesy Sadun and Maiphoom, Amer. J. trop. med. Hyg., 1953).

The most important factor in the spread of human fasciolopsiasis is the water-nut or water caltrop *(Trapa natans)* (Fig. 83). This plant grows wild or is cultivated for its nuts in basins of stagnant water or irrigation channels. The nuts are enclosed in a fleshy angular shell, which is usually peeled with the teeth so that the nut can be eaten raw (Fig. 84). This plant is favoured by the snails which transmit *Fasciolopsis*. The metacercariae of *Fasciolopsis buski* often settle on the nut shell and are swept into the mouth of persons peeling the nuts. Other plants which play a similar role, but to a lesser degree, are *Eliocharis tuberosa* (the tubers of which are eaten) and water-cress *(Nasturtium aquaticum)*. Children are usually fond of caltrop nuts and accordingly are as a rule, more intensively infected than adults.

There is a perplexing point in the epidemiology of fasciolopsiasis. Several investigators have noted that the incidence of this infection in man does not coincide with the incidence in domesticated animals. For instance, Barlow (1925) found no infection in pigs in China, in localities in which it was common in people. Mathis and Leger (1911) observed the opposite in Tonkin, where 6% of the pigs were infected as contrasted with very rare cases in man. There are also localities in which man and animals are infected to an equal degree.

It seems probable, that, as happens with some other parasitic worms, there may be local strains of *F. buski* which are better adapted either to man or to animals. Galliard and Ngu (1947), think that there is only one common species of *Fasciolopsis,* which affects both man and the pig, and that the dissimilar infections of these two hosts and the differences in the geographical distribution can be explained by other factors. They consider for example that the scarcity of *F. buski* in man in Tonkin noted by Mathis and Leger *(loc. cit.)* is probably due to the fact that in that country the plants carrying the metacercariae serve mainly as animal food and that man always cooks them before they are eaten.

Fasciolopsis infection is an important cause of disease and debilitation in endemic areas. Its incidence rises during abundant rains, which facilitate the multiplication and spread of the snail-carriers. The severity of fasciolopsiasis depends on the number of parasites present. In people in whom a few parasites have developed, the symptoms may be mild, while, in heavy infections, intestinal disorders of varying severity appear a month after the ingestion of the metacercariae; these are manifested by emaciation, colicky pain and intermittent diarrhoea. In advanced infections oedema of the face, ascites (Fig. 85) and anasarca may develop (Sadun and Maiphoom, 1953), while many (*e.g.* 500) worms may cause death (Sadun, 1957).

Microscopical examination of the stools reveals the peculiar eggs of *Fasciolopsis,* and this is decisive for the diagnosis.

The infection may be eradicated comparatively easily by anthelmintics,

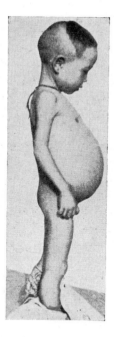

Fig. 85. Ascites caused by heavy fasciolopsiasis (Chekiang, China) (courtesy, Prof.
H. Vogel, Arch. Schiffs-u. Tropenhyg., 1936).

among which hexylresorcinol, thymol, or tetrachlorethylene are the most effective. In man the parasite has a comparatively short life span and in the absence of reinfection it disappears spontaneously after approximately 6 months.

For control of the infection, public education, aiming mainly at abstention from drinking unfiltered water and eating raw caltrop nuts or other water plants is most important. Measures should be taken to protect pigs, which may serve as reservoirs and spread the infection. The control of snail-carriers, though it is theoretically possible, is not feasible in localities which are periodically flooded during every rainy season, or in those in which the caltrop is artificially cultivated in ponds and is fertilized with human sewage.

ii. Gastrodiscoides infection

Gastrodiscoides hominis is a relatively small trematode (approx. 1 cm long) belonging to the paramphistomid group. It is characterised by a peculiar

:xpansion of the posterior part of the body, which serves as a dispropor-
ionally large sucker and firmly fastens the parasite to the mucosa of
he large intestine in which the parasite lives.

The name *hominis* has been given to this parasite because it was first
ound in man. Yet man is probably a secondary host, the primary host
)eing the hog, which, in many localities, is infected to a high degree.
Gastrodiscoides has also been recorded in monkeys, a mouse-deer
(Tragulus napu) and a field rat *(Rattus rattus brevicaudatus)* in Java
Sandground, 1940).

The geographical distribution of *G. hominis* is chiefly limited to south-
:astern Asia (Malaya, Assam, India), but a record in a wild boar in the
Soviet Kasakhstan (Badanin, 1929) indicates that its range of distribution
nay be wide. Human infections vary in intensity and frequency. In an
Assam village, investigated by Buckley (1939), an incidence of 40%
vas recorded.

The life history of *G. hominis* is not exactly known; it is supposed that
t is similar to that of *Fasciolopsis buski,* both species being frequently
ound in common infections. The average length of the ova of *Gastro-
liscoides* is 160 microns.

Although the pathology associated with *Gastrodiscoides* has not been
nvestigated in detail, it is known that the disease is mild, the main symp-
oms being intestinal discomfort and diarrhoea.

Gastrodiscoides hominis readily responds to treatment with conventional anthelminthics, among which thymol is the most efficacious. A soap-
aline enema alone may expel a number of parasites lodged in the
)osterior part of the colon.

REFERENCES

BARLOW, C. H., *Amer. J. Hyg., Monogr. Ser.,* 4 (1925) pp. 98.
BUCKLEY, J. J., *J. Helminth.,* 17 (1939) 1.
GALLIARD, H. and D. V. NGU, *Ann. Parasit. hum. comp.,* 22 (1947) 16.
HSIEH, H. C., *Formosan Sci.,* 14 (1960) 95.
HSU, H. F. and S. Y. Li, *Thapar Commem. Vol.,* Lucknow, 1953, 133 pp.
SADUN, E. H. and CH. MAIPHOOM, *Amer. J. trop. Med. Hyg.,* 2 (1953) 1070.
VOGEL, U., *Arch. Schiffs- u. Tropenhyg.,* 40 (1936) 181.

c. Dicrocoeliasis

The trematode *Dicrocoelium dendriticum* (known also under the name
D. lanceolatum or "small liver fluke") is a parasite of sheep and cattle.

However, it is not specific to these hosts and can live in more than 50 species of mammals and in man. Hares, rabbits, deer and numerous small rodents are frequently infected and serve as a natural reservoir. The worm is elongated and flattened, measuring up to 12 mm in length. This very injurious parasite lives in the small bile ducts and produces thickening of their walls, extreme hyperplasia of the epithelial layer and fibrosis of the liver. In cases of slight infection the symptoms may not be apparent, but in intensive infections mass mortality of animals may occur. In many a locality sheep breeding had to be discontinued because of the ravages caused by *Dicrocoelium*. In man, who usually harbours only a few specimens, it causes incapacitating chronic cholangitis and hepatitis.

Dicrocoelium dendriticum is commonly found all over Central and Southern Europe, in the central belt of Asia and in some localities of South and North America.

In spite of the fact that the parasite was described by Rudolphi as early as 1803, its life history has only recently been unfolded, and even at the present time it has not been completely elucidated. Noller (1928, 1929) and Vogel (1929) first indicated that *Cercaria vitrina,* which was discovered by Linstow in 1879 and develops in land snails, may be the larva of *Dicrocoelium.* This was experimentally proved by several observers (Neuhaus, 1939; Vogel, 1954; Krull, 1958; Svadzhian, 1956), but the final mode of infection of the definitive host is still the subject of controversy. It is certain that the eggs, which already contain developed larvae (miracidia) when laid, are eliminated with the faeces and disseminated on the pasture, where they can be ingested by land snails. The miracidia hatch in the intestine of the snails and migrate to their internal organs, where they develop two generations of rediae and eventually long-tailed cercariae. The latter emerge from the snail tissues into its breathing chamber and collect there in small masses, glued together by thick slime. These slime-balls of cercariae fall out of the breathing chambers of the snails and stick to the grasses on which the snails are living. Their further fate is variously explained. According to Neuhaus and others, experimenting in Europe, animals become infected by ingesting these cercariae. However, according to the opinion of Krull and Mapes (1952), who conducted experiments in North America, the slime-balls have to be taken in by certain species of ants, which carry them to their nests and feed them to their larvae, in which the cercariae develop into metacercariae. When these larvae subsequently develop into adult ants, they may be swallowed by grazing animals, in which the metacercariae hatch, migrate to the liver and develop to maturity. It seems probable that development of *Dicrocoelium* is possible in both these ways, each of which depends on circumstances still unknown.

While dicrocoeliasis of live-stock is widespread in endemic localities, it is rare in *man*. The presence of the eggs of the parasite in human faeces is not necessarily a proof of infection of man. In endemic localities, so called *transit eggs* of *Dicrocoelium* appear frequently in human faeces. When man has eaten the liver of an infested animal, he digests the organ tissue and the parasites it contains, but the eggs are only partially digested; the undigested eggs may then appear in great numbers in the faeces. In order to ascertain whether the infection is real or spurious the patient must abstain from eating meat (liver) during several days and a second stool examination must be done. In cases of real infection, the eggs of the parasite will persist after the procedure mentioned.

No reliable remedy is known against dicrocoeliasis in live-stock. In man, according to some authors (Signier, 1952), emetin and antimonials may be helpful, although some authors (Pasternak, 1958), claim that this therapy is not effective.

REFERENCES

KRULL, W. M., *Cornell Vet.*, 48 (1958) 17.
KRULL, W. M. and C. MAPES, *Cornell Vet.*, 42 (1952) 603.
NOELLER, W., *Tierärztl. Umsch.*, 38 (1932) 190.
NEUHAUS, W., *Z. Parasitenk.*, 10 (1938) 476.
SCHEID, G. and H. MENDHEIM, *Z. Tropenmed. Parasitol.*, 2 (1950) 142.
SVADZHIAN, P. K., *Izv. Akad. Nauk Armenian S.S.R.*, 9 (1956) 89.
VOGEL, H. and J. FALCAO, *Z. Tropenmed. Parasitol.*, 5 (1954) 275.

d. Fish-borne trematode infections of the liver

Apart from fish-borne trematode infections of the intestine, there are numerous similar infections of the liver. They are common in piscivorous mammals and birds, while some occur also in man. Human hepatic trematode infections are widespread in endemic regions and constitute a serious public health problem. They are mainly caused by the species: *Clonorchis sinensis, Opisthorchis felineus* and *O. viverrini.* The life history and pathogenicity of these species are similar, the differences being quantitative rather than qualitative and attributable mainly to the different size of the respective worm species. Each of these parasite species is associated with a particular geographical region.

i. Clonorchiasis

Clonorchiasis is caused by *Clonorchis sinensis* *, a lancet-shaped trematode, 1 to 2.5 cn long. This trematode lives in the biliary ducts of man and some carnivorous and omni vorous mammals, such as dogs, cats and pigs. The eggs are 26–34 microns long and they are eliminated with the faeces. The subsequent life history is similar to that of the heterophyids to which clonorchis is related, *i.e.,* the ova must reach fresh water, in which they are ingested by mud-eating snails of the genus *Bithynia* or related genera The cercariae which develop in the snail escape into the water and attack fish, in the muscles of which they encyst as metacercariae. The final host becomes infected by ingesting the raw fish. The metacercariae are lodged mainly in the muscles, especially those near the skin, and are often absent from the fins or scales. The number of meta cercariae in one fish varies from one to several hundreds; young fishes are usually more heavily infected than old ones.

The metacercariae are liberated in the intestine of the final host and enter the biliary system, either through the portal vein system, or by creeping directly through the bile ducts. Rarely, *Clonorchis* is found in the pancreatic duct (Kobayashi, 1920). The maturation of the worms takes 4–5 weeks.

Only a small proportion of the metacercariae reach their destination, so that usually but a few of them develop. In exceptional cases up to 10,000 worms have been counted in one individual (Blanchard, 1891). Apart from *man, dogs* and *cats* are commonly also infected in endemic localities; exceptionally *wild carnivores* (such as the Korean otter, the marten or the badger) are infected in nature, while rabbits and guinea pigs can be infected artificially. In man *Clonorchis* is long-lived, the longest recorded longevity being 25 years (D. Moore, 1924); in the dog the life span of the parasite does not exceed $2\frac{1}{2}$ years (Brumpt, 1927). The cat is apparently a more suitable host than the dog (Faust and Khaw, 1926).

Clonorchis feeds chiefly on the epithelium of the bile ducts, but it also swallows the epithelial secretions and occasionally blood (Hsu, 1940). The parasite provokes a characteristic reaction of the surrounding tissues: hyperplasia of the epithelium in the form of spongy adenoid growth which obstructs the lumen of the ducts, thickening of the duct wall proper, and finally progressive cirrhosis of the liver tissue (Fig. 86).

Light infections may remain symptomless for years. In multiple in-

---

* Some investigators are of the opinion that there is no justification for retaining the genus *Clonorchis* which they regard as synonymous with *Opisthorchis*. However, owing to long-standing tradition, the name *Clonorchis* and *Clonorchiasis* is generally accepted.

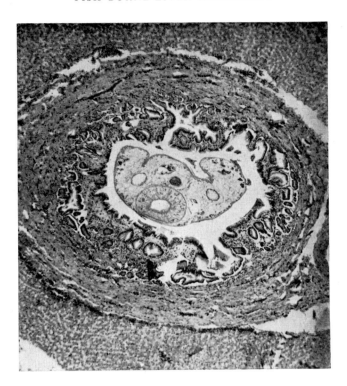

Fig. 86. Section of liver showing *Clonorchis* in a bile duct; hyperplasia of the duct wall and epithelial layer (original photo).

fections these changes lower the vital power of the organism and may result in cachexia or even death. The following symptoms appear soon and slowly grow in intensity: intestinal discomfort, icterus, intermittent fever, bradycardia; and later, colicky attacks resembling those caused by lithiasis and sometimes vomiting of bile containing material.

When bacterial infection aggravates the process, the condition usually becomes serious, holiangiohepatitis being the most common sequela (Fung, 1961). Malignant change in the adenomatous tissue of the bile-ducts is one of the most serious consequences of clonorchiasis. It is believed that primary carcinoma of the liver, which is rather common in Canton (China), is related to the endemicity of clonorchiasis in this region (Hou, 1955, 1956).

In 1947 Stoll estimated that there were some 19 million people infected with clonorchiasis. The distribution of the infection is geographically limited mainly to the South-Eastern part of Asia. China is the country most heavily infected, with Japan as second. The principal endemic area of clonorchiasis in China is the Kwantung province, with the town of Canton as its center (Hsu and Chow, 1937).

The incidence of infection in the population, the prevalent fish-eating habits, the variety of local fish species that serve as intermediate hosts and the intensity of infection in the latter, all combine to maintain the endemicity. The usual methods of processing fish are also a factor defining the spread of clonorchiasis. Wykoff (1959) showed that the metacercariae of *Clonochis* survive when they are kept for 40 days at 3–6° C and 50% of them remain viable for 60 days.

It has been estimated that in the provincial localities the incidence varies between 3 and 100%. In Canton Hospital, over 11% of patients have eggs of *Clonorchis* in their stools, while some selected groups show a much higher rate (beggars: 80%). *Clonorchis* is encountered in all classes of the population, and occasional visitors who cannot refrain from tasting the dainty local fish-dishes often become infected. Out of about 40 fish species known to be carriers of clonorchis-metacercariae 24 are found in China, with *Ctenopharyngodon idellus* (Fig. 87) and *Mylopharyngodon aetiops* the most heavily infected.

Artificial fish breeding is one of the factors which contribute to spread of clonorchiasis in Kwantung Province. It is an important branch of the

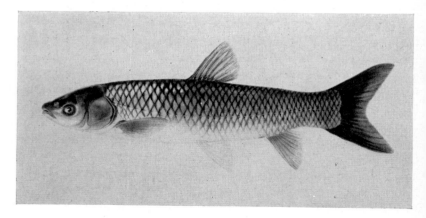

Fig. 87. Ctenopharyngodon idellus, the main vector of the metacercariae of Clonorchis sinensis in the Canton area (China). (Photo Prof. H. Vogel).

local agriculture and the most suitable carriers of *Clonorchis* are bred intensively. The system of breeding favours their infection. The fish are not cultivated from the spawn, but the fry are caught in the rivers and are used as the initial breeding material. Usually they are already infected when introduced into the ponds. In addition, the use of nightsoil to encourage the growth of the plankton or to serve directly as food for the fish is widely practised, and the sewage is systematically discharged into the ponds. Often especially attractive latrines are built over the ponds to supply the valuable faecal material (Fig. 88). Fishponds are favourable environments for the multiplication of snails, which serve as the first intermediate hosts of *Clonorchis*.

Both man and animals are responsible for the dissemination of clonorchiasis. Dogs and cats, to which the fish offal is accessible, are usually more heavily infected than is man; hence they serve as important disseminators of *Clonorchis* eggs. In some localities of the northern part of China, where the consumption of raw fish is not customary and human infection is therefore rare, the incidence of infection in dogs and cats is high (Hsu and Khaw, 1936).

In the Tonkin Delta clonorchiasis is very common, while along the upper reaches of the river the incidence amounts to only 4–9% (Gaillard, 1939).

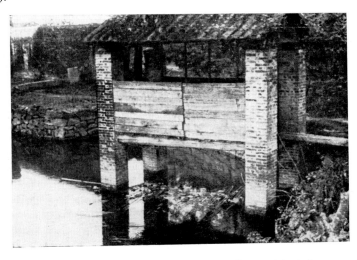

Fig. 88.   Latrine built over a fish pond near Canton for provision of manure to the plankton (courtesy Prof. H. Vogel, Hamburg, 1937).

According to Kobayashi (1934), in some heavily infected districts in
Japan, *Pseudospora parva* is the most important carrier of metacercariae
of *Clonorchis*, while other fish-species are infected to a much lesser degree.
Human clonorchiasis is prevalent in most parts of Korea, where it sometimes affects over 40% of the population (Kobayashi, 1924). Here it was
found that the local otter *(Lutreola sibirica)* was heavily infected and
served as an important reservoir host. Skrjabin *et.al.* (1929) reported the
occurrence of clonorchiasis among the aboriginal tribes living along the
Amur River, where dogs and cats and some wild carnivores are also
infected. Kadenazi (1940) recorded the infection of pigs in the region of
Khabarovsk. Clonorchiasis in Hawaii has been attributed to fish imported from endemic regions.

Clinical findings known in endemic localities are suggestive of the
diagnosis. Stool examination detects most infections but it may fail in
cases of new or light infection and in these instances duodenal sounding
may be helpful.

It should be borne in mind that the diagnosis of clonorchiasis made by stool examination may, under certain circumstances, be erroneous, because the eggs of two species of
Opisthorchis and one species of *Metorchis* (which may also occur in man in some
localities where clonorchiasis occurs) are very similar to those of *Clonorchis* and
morphological differentiation is difficult. However, from a medical point of view, this is
of little importance because the pathology and treatment in both instances is similar.

There is no simple or sure treatment of clonorchiasis. Chloroquin is the
most effective drug, but the prolonged administration schedule and high
dosage required, often cause undesirable toxic side effects. Weng (1959)
proposed the combination of chloroquin with emetine, which gives
reasonably satisfactory cure rates. Side effects are observed and the
author, therefore, recommends this treatment only when other methods
have failed.

Faust *et al.* (1926) showed that gentian violet is highly toxic to *Clonorchis* in cats and they assumed that this drug will also be useful for the
treatment of human infection. Podyapolskaya (1958) recommended
hexachlorethane.

Prevention of clonorchiasis depends mainly on successful public health
education, aimed towards the dissemination of knowledge on the life
history of the parasite. The primary measure, namely, abstention from
eating raw fish, is sufficient to prevent spread of the infection.

REFERENCES

CHOU, P. C., *J. Path. Bact.*, 70 (1955) 53.
CHU, S. H., *Chin. med. J.*, 75 (1957) 473.
FAUST, E. C., YAO KE-FANG, O. K. KHAW and C. YUNG-AN, *Proc. Soc. exp. Biol. (N.Y.)*, 23 (1926) 607.
FAUST, E. C. and O. K. KHAW, *Amer. J. Hyg., Monogr. Ser. No. 8* (1927) 283.
HOEPPLI, R., *Chin. med. J.*, 47 (1933) 1125.
HSU, H. F. and C. Y. CHOW, *Chin. med. J.*, 51 (1937) 341.
KAN, H. C. and H. VOGEL, *Festschrift Bernhard Nocht*, 1937, pp. 225.
KOBAYASHI, H., *Mitt. med. Hochsch. Keijo*, 7 (1924) 1.
PODYAPOLSKAYA, V. P. and V. F. KAPUSTIN, *Moscow, Medgiz. Publ.*, 1958, 663 pp.
SADUN, E. H., B. C. WALTON, A. A. BUCK and B. K. LEE, *J. Parasit.*, 45 (1959) 129.
WENG, H. C. *et al.*, *Chinese J. int. Med.*, 7 (1959) 1175.

ii. Opisthorchiasis

Opisthorchis felineus is second in importance among parasites of the human liver. Its anatomy is similar to that of *Clonorchis sinensis*, but it measures only up to 12 mm in length. The fluke was discovered by Rivolta in 1884 in cats and dogs in Italy and has subsequently been found in many regions of Europe and Soviet Asia in *man*, the *dog*, the *cat*, the *fox* and the *ermine*.

It has essentially the same life cycle as *Clonorchis sinensis*. Its first intermediate host in all known foci is the small fresh-water snail, *Bithynia leachi*, which lives in semi-stagnant waters and swamps and may be extremely abundant. In one instance cited in Siberia, nearly 6,000 specimens of this snail were counted per one square meter of bottom; over 20% of the snails were infected and shed cercariae (Plotnikov, 1959). According to Vogel (1934), the eggs of *Opisthorchis* remain infective for 3 months at 8°. At the optimum temperature, cercariae begin to leave the snail approximately by the end of the second month. At lower temperatures, the formation of cercariae may require 10–12 months (Goriachev, 1953). Numerous species of cyprinoid fish serve as second intermediate hosts and harbour the encysted metacercariae of the fluke in their muscles. At 18–20°, the metacercariae develop to the infective stage in about 6 weeks. Development of the adult worm in the final host requires some 4 weeks. A minimum of 4½ months is required for *O. felineus* to complete its life cycle.

In endemic foci up to 100% of susceptible species of fish may be infected and the number of metacercariae in them is occasionally very great. The metacercariae can well withstand the low temperature at which the fishes hibernate, so that the latter remain infected all the year round.

The main host of *Opisthorchis felineus* is the cat, in which the parasite develops to its maximal size. Cats and dogs are always more heavily in-

TREMATODIASES

fected than is man; however, the presence of *Opisthorchis* in local cats does not necessarily correspond with its occurrence in man. Vishnievskaya (1959) found that 85% of the cats in a South Russian region were infected, but not a single case was observed among the 2½ million human inhabitants of that region. In some localities in Central Siberia up to 22% of the foxes are infected (Bruskin, 1954). Lissitskaya (1958) recorded that 5% of the water voles *(Arvicola amphibius)* in South-East Russia were infected.

Human infection with *Opisthorchis felineus* is one of the major clinical and public health problems in extensive regions of Central Siberia and to a lesser degree in other foci in Asia and Europe. Stoll (1947) estimated that 1,700,000 people were infected with *Opisthorchis*. At that time "East-Prussia" constituted the important endemic region, but this focus has since then, almost disappeared (Gerwel, 1957). The main contemporary foci of human opisthorchiasis are in the Soviet Union. Plotnikov (1959) who drew a vivid picture of its endemicity in this country, distinguished four main endemic regions: the basins of the rivers Ob and Irtish in Central Siberia, those of the river Kama, west of the Ural Mountains, that of the Lower Dniepr in the Ukraine, and Kazakhstan (Central Asia). Sporadic cases of human opisthorchiasis occur in numerous other localities, for instance in Caucasus.

In Siberia not only the nomad aborigines, who feed mainly on fish, but also the city dwellers are heavily infected. Over 83% of the population in the town of Tobolsk (1948) were found infected, while the incidence in the children of the town was more than 36%. At the same time the incidence in cats was 100% and in dogs 90%. In an other survey, carried out in the same town, the worm burden in 18% of the infected livers was as high as 1000–1500. In individual cats as many as 6,000 worms have been counted. In some places in western Siberia the total human population and all domestic carnivores are heavily infected. The aboriginal tribes are most affected. Skrjabin (1950) recorded a case in which 25,000 worms were counted at post-mortem examination.

In Kazakhstan a considerable number of human, canine and feline infections have been recorded, and 100% of certain species of fish carry metacercariae (Ssidorov, 1960). Opisthorchiasis in the Ukraine is mainly restricted to the settlements of fishermen along the Dniepr, where the incidence may exceed 50% in isolated localities (Schulmann et al., 1955). There is but scanty information on the epidemiology of opisthorchiasis in the Urals, where in some regions, according to Mulmienko (1959), up to 64% of men and 100% of cats are infected.

The clinical and pathological picture of opisthorchiasis resembles that of clonorchiasis. The symptoms vary and depend on the number of worms and the duration of the infection. Subjective symptoms are: asthenia, weakness, headache, nausea and pain in the liver. Clinical signs suggest cholecystitis and cholangitis. Indications of the infection are: slight jaundice, ascites, loss of weight, the presence of the worm eggs of this fluke in the faeces and a lowered liver function-test. The blood picture often remains normal (Kondratiev, 1932). According to Ozieretskovskaya (1957) in 1–3% of patients the infection is associated with interstitial hepatitis and cirrhosis of the liver. Ashkanazy (1900), Rindfleisch (1910) and others maintain that in some cases this process gives rise to primary cancer of the liver and Boyko (1957) found that this had occurred in over 7% of persons who died of opisthorchiasis.

The longevity of *Opisthorchis felineus* is as yet not conclusively established. Plotnikov and Zierchaninov (1932) maintained that the parasite does not live for longer than 3 years. Batiusheva (1957) presented records of 2 fatal cases of longstanding opisthorchiasis in which the duration of the disease was 15 and 18 years. In these cases, the main pathological change was widespread cirrhosis of the liver accompanied by ascites.

The custom of consuming uncooked, slightly salted or frozen fish, the promiscuous pollution of water with excrements, and the abundance of dogs and cats that feed mainly on fish offal, all help to maintain opisthorchiasis in its endemic form.

It is presumed that man is the chief agent in the spread of infection with *Opisthorchis* and that he does this by indiscriminate dissemination of his excreta containing the eggs of the fluke. Domestic animals, cats, dogs, and, to some extent, wild carnivores, such as foxes, although some of them are heavily infected, play only a secondary part in the spread of the parasite, because they pollute the snail inhabited waters to a lesser degree than man.

No satisfactory treatment of human opisthorchiasis has hitherto been developed. Gentian violet was advocated by Faust and Yao (1926) but Erhard (1935) found that it is not effective; he regarded Fuadin (Neoantimosan) as being partially effective. In experiments of Pantiukhin (1957) chloroquine diphosphate (Aralen) and hexachlorethane have proved partly successful. Emetine and tartar emetic have some effect (Kondratiev, 1932), but, in view of the damage to liver tissue, their application involves a risk.

There is insufficient experience of the treatment of dogs and cats. Plotnikov and Zierchaninov (1932) found that for these animals the subcutaneous administration of carbon tetrachloride was very effective.

References p. 624

Khamidullin (1960) found that hexachlorethane emulsified in bentonite was effective for dogs.

The control of all forms of opisthorchiasis might be easy, when one considers that abolition of the habit of consuming insufficiently cooked fish would suffice. Public health education is the proper means towards this end. Unfortunately this, although feasible in urban areas, is not readily applicable in the vast, undeveloped rural regions in which primitive ways of life and age-old culinary habits are not easily changed. Snail control and the prevention of river pollution is impracticable in rural Asia, but proper handling of town-sewage may diminish the prevalence of the disease.

Another control measure is the proper storage of fish. According to Plotnikov and Zierchaninov (1932) all metacercariae die within 3 days in a 15% saline and within 10 days in a 5–10% saline solution. It is presumed that the commercial method of salting fish, as practised in the fisheries, kills the metacercariae if it is continued for 10 days or longer. Freezing up to −10° must be maintained for at least 5 days in order to kill the metacercariae.

The diagnosis of human opisthorchiasis may be ascertained by demonstrating the characteristic eggs of the parasite in the stool.

iii. Far-East opisthorchiasis

Apart from *Opisthorchis felineus* which is, as has been explained above, endemic in several foci within the temperate zone of Europe and Asia, there is a large region of endemic opisthorchiasis in the south-eastern corner of Asia: North-East Thailand (Mekong Valley) and Laos, which is due to a different species, *Opisthorchis viverrini*. This species closely resembles *O. felineus* morphologically and in its life cycle, but differs from it by slight anatomical details and by adaptation to particular local snails of the genera *Bithynia* and *Vivipara*.

Opisthorchiasis viverrini has been recently studied by Sadun *et al.* (1953–1958) and by Harinasuta and Vajrasthira (1960). It was revealed that the endemicity affects about 2,000,000 people and constitutes a highly important public health problem. An average of some 25% of the population is infected; in one community an incidence of 80% was observed. Cats and dogs share the infection, even in localities in which human infection is scanty. In nature the parasite occurs n piscivorous animals, notably in the civet cat *(Felis viverrina)*. Like other fish-borne infections, Far-East opisthorchiasis is due mainly o the habit of eating raw fish and to the pollution of fishing grounds. The ole of reservoir hosts may be significant, but is secondary in importance.

Harinasuta and Vajrasthira *(loc. cit.)* recognise three degrees of in-ensity of the disease caused by *O. viverrini*. When less than 1,000 eggs of the parasite are found per ml of faeces, symptoms are mild or absent. n cases of moderate infection (1000–30,000 parasite eggs eliminated per nl of stool) the course has a chronic character, showing diarrhoea, with no relation to meals, dyspeptic flatulence, aggravated by fatty food (to vhich patients consequently become averse), recurrent pain over the hepatic region lasting for a few days, moderate jaundice, mild fever 37.5–38.5°) continuing for several days and a moderately enlarged liver, with or without oedema.

Heavy, long-standing infection frequently terminates fatally, showing widespread hepatic cirrhosis, with cachexia, ascites, oedema of the legs or of a large part of the body, prominent superficial abdominal veins and, in are instances, carcinoma. Eggs of the parasite have not necessarily to appear in the faeces.

Several drugs have been tried (Fuadin, tartar emetic, gentian violet, gold salts) with little success. Lately Sadun *et al.* (1955)have recommended hloroquine, which seems to be rather effective.

Control of *Opisthorchiasis viverrini* is similar to that of northern Clonorchiasis and it is equally difficult to carry it out, because of the poor hygiene and the faulty culinary traditions of the inhabitants in endemic regions.

v. Rare opisthorchid infections

Apart from the 3 species of opisthorchids which constitute serious public health problems, several other species of the same family *(Opisthorchidae)*, which are normally parasitic in fish-eating animals, may accidentaly in-ect man and cause harm to him. These are *Amphimerus norverea, Metorchis conjunctus* and *Pseudamphistomum truncatum*. All three are parasites of the bile ducts or gall bladder and their pathogenicity is similar to that of the opisthorchids mentioned above. Those species can be correctly identified only by examination of adult worms expelled by anthelmintic treatment or obtained post-mortem. Because it is often difficult to collect such material, the number of diagnosed cases is very limited. It may therefore be presumed that the actual incidence of human infections is much higher than the existing records would suggest.

REFERENCES

ASHKANAZY, M., *Dtsch. med. Wschr.*, 30 (1904) 689.
GORITSKAYA, V. V., *Med. Parazit. (Mosk.)*, 26 (1957) 65 (Suppl.).
HARINASUTA, H. and S. VAJRASTHIRA, *Ann. trop. Med. Parasit.*, 54 (1960) 100.
LISSITSKAYA, L. S., *Med. Parazit. (Mosk.)*, 27 (1958) 109.
OZIERETSKOVSKAYA *et al.*, *Med. Parazit. (Mosk.)*, 26 (1957) 439.
PANTIUKHOV, A. M., *Med. Parazit. (Mosk.)*, 26 (1957) 298.
PLOTNIKOV, N. N., *Trudy Sovieshch. po Bolesn. Ryb. (Ac. Sci. U.S.S.R.)*, 9 (1959) 208.
PODLESNOY, A. V., *Med. Parazit. (Mosk.)*, 28 (1959) 235.
SADUN, E. H., *Amer. J. Hyg.*, 62 (1955) 81.
SADUN, E. H., *Amer. J. trop. Med. Hyg.*, 6 (1957) 416.
SADUN, E. H. and C. CHARMNARNKIT, *Amer. J. trop. Med. Hyg.*, 4 (1955) 1080.
SKRJABIN, K. I. and A. M. PETROV, *Trematody Zhiv. Chelovieka*, 4 (1950) 81.
VOGEL, H., *Zoologica*, 33, 86 (1934) 103.

e. Other fish-borne trematode infections

There is a large group of diverse, usually very small, trematodes causing intestinal infections in man and animals as a result of consumption of raw fish containing metacercariae of the parasites. These trematodes belong chiefly to the family *Heterophyidae*. Rarely representatives of other families cause similar infections in man, *e.g. Nanophyetus salmincola, Echinochasmus perfoliatus, Clinostomum complanatum* and *Prohemistomum vivax*. The differentiation of the species of these trematodes is simple when the adult worms are available, but it is usually impossible to differentiate their eggs, which are very similar in related species and genera. From the point of view of public health group-determination is sufficient, because the life histories, modes of infection and control of all these species are alike.

i. Heterophyiasis

Heterophyiasis is caused by any one of the numerous species and genera of the trematode family *Heterophyidae*. These are small, oval flatworms living in the intestine of carnivorous and piscivorous mammals and birds. Some of the species are also parasites of man. They have peculiar morphological characteristics (*i.e.*, a common male and female genital duct and no copulatory organs), as well as a similar life cycle which requires two intermediate hosts: a mollusc and a fish.

About 10 species belonging to 6 genera have been found parasitic in man, mainly in the Far East and eastern Mediterranean regions.

The heterophyid species recorded as human parasites are listed in the following table:

Name of parasite	Records of human incidence	Records of animal incidence
Heterophyes heterophyes	Mediterranean and Far East	Mediterranean and Far East
H. dispar	Egypt (?)	Egypt
H. equalis	Egypt (?)	Egypt
Stellanthasmus falcatus	Philippines	Eastern Mediterranean and Far East
Metagonimus yokogawai	Japan, Rumania, Spain, Indonesia	Rumania, Central and South-East Europe, Spain, Far East
Haplorchis calderoni	Philippines	Philippines
H. taichui	Philippines, Formosa	Egypt, Far East
H. yokogawai	Far East, Indonesia	Far East
H. vanissima	Philippines	Philippines
Stamnosoma armatum	Japan	Egypt
Tocotrema lingua	Greenland	Europe, North America

As far as may be judged from contemporary observations, the pathological changes in the intestine caused by different species of the parasite are similar. They are grouped here under the common heading *heterophyiasis*. The worms, living in the middle of the small intestine, penetrate between the villi, sometimes reaching the Lieberkühn's crypts. Small numbers of the flukes produce mild irritation of the mucosa, accompanied by pain and mucous diarrhoea. In most cases the course of human infection is benign. Massive invasion may, however, cause a troublesome enteritis with serious complications.

The diagnosis is based on demonstration of the characteristic eggs or the parasites in the faeces. The ova of all heterophyids, are, however, similar in shape and size. Their presence, therefore, in faeces cannot help in the identification of particular species.

The incidence of heterophyiasis is always higher in carnivorous animals than it is in man. Human infection is common in regions in which the consumption of raw or insufficiently cooked fish is customary.

Animal hosts which have access to open water which they may pollute with their excreta are important agents in the dissemination of heterophyiasis. For this reason the sanitary disposal of sewage and the exclusion of raw fish from the diets of both man and domestic carnivores are important in the prevention of heterophyiasis.

α. *Heterophyes infection.* A typical and most common species infecting man is *Heterophyes heterophyes.* The worm measures about 2 mm. Its eggs, which are 20 to 25 microns long, contain a miracidium. They must reach brackish water to be eaten by an appropriate snail (*Pirenella conica* in Egypt; *Cerithidium singula* in Japan). In the snail's intestine the miracidia hatch, penetrate into their organs and there produce cercariae which escape back to the water, invade a fish and encyst, mainly in its muscles, as metacercariae. The final hosts, among them man, become infected by eating fresh or insufficiently cooked fish carrying the metacercariae.

The parasite is specific to the molluscan intermediate host, but not to either the fish or final host. Numerous species of fish can act as second intermediate hosts, but the mullet is most abundantly infected.

In the Near East, apart from man, *dogs* and *cats* are the primary hosts. These animals are mainly responsible for the dissemination of the eggs of this species. Other hosts are the *jackal, black rat, fox, wildcat,* and among birds, the *pelican, hawk* and *black kite.*

In some localities peculiar geographical and demographical conditions favour the maintenance of the infection. Thus, the great brackish lagoons of the Nile Delta in Egypt, which serve as basins for the semi-artificial breeding of mullet, contain countless *Pirenella* snails on the bottom, Usually all the mullets carry the metacercariae of *Heterophyes,* often in considerable numbers. Every surrounding village participates in the fishing trade and the population habitually eat raw fish, while sanitary facilities are practically absent. Moreover, almost all the local cats and dogs are infected, so that the life-cycle of the parasite is ensured in this environment. The fish are sold all over the country and are also exported.

Khalil (1928) estimated that 65% of the schoolchildren in the town of Matarieh were infected.

H. heterophyes has also been recorded in Spain, Greece, Morocco and Turkey. Possibly the whole Mediterranean basin is an endemic region.

β. Metagonimus infection. *Metagonimus yokogawai* is the next most frequent representative of the heterophyids occurring in man. This is a small, pyriform trematode, 1–2.5 mm long, characterised by an asymmetrical arrangement of some of its genital organs. It inhabits the small intestine and occurs in *man, dogs, cats, pigs* and *foxes.* It is prevalent in the Far East (China, the Delta of the Amur River, Korea, Japan, the Philippines), Central Europe (Czechoslovakia, Rumania, Southern Russia) and in Spain. As a human parasite it is of some importance only in the Far East; in Europe it occurs mainly in carnivorous mammals. In some localities in Japan half the population are infected (Joyeux, 1944). The infection is also common among the aborigines of the Soviet Far Eastern provinces.

The life history of this species and its pathogenicity are similar to those of *Heterophyes.* Ciurea (1933) found metacercariae of *Metagonimus* mainly under the scales of 5 different species of cyprinoid fish in the Danube Delta.

γ. Extra-intestinal heterophyiasis. Peculiar sequelae of heterophyiasis have been brought to light in the Philippines by Africa and associates (1935–1940). Here the consumption of dishes containing fish is widespread while heterophyid metacercariae were found in 14 species of fishes.

In this area several heterophyids are common in man; the species most frequently encountered is *Haplorchis yokogawai.* It appears that the local heterophyid species do not always confine themselves to the intestinal lumen, but may bore through the mucous membrane and deposit their eggs in the tissues. These eggs enter the circulation and are carried with the bloodstream to various parts of the body, where they eventually clog the capillaries, causing small thromboses, haemorrhages and granulomas. Serious consequences may arise when vital organs, such as the myocardium or the cerebro-spinal complex, are invaded. The situation may be still more aggravated when the whole worm enters the blood vessels and is carried to vital organs to settle. This process has been observed in both man and animals.

Over 11% of 297 autopsies carried out in the Philippines showed intestinal infection with some kind of heterophyid, and in approximately one third of these cases extra-intestinal lesions were present. Africa *et al.* (1940) tend to explain fatal cases by the pathological changes, among which are acute cardiac dilatation, right ventricular endocarditis and chronic passive congestion of the liver, spleen or kidney. The syndrome resembles "cardiac beriberi". The spread of infection in endemic localities is facilitated by the manner in which fish-food is prepared. Dishes are customarily made of raw fish, with the addition of sauces and spices, and the mild salting of these dishes keeps the metacercariae alive for several days. The metacercariae are killed by heating the fish to at least 60° for 3 minutes, or by pickling in a 10% salt solution for 4 days, or in a saturated solution in 2 days.

The life span of the parasite in the body is brief, presumably only a few months. When their expulsion is desired, the worms can be readily eliminated by tetra-chlorethylene, hexylresorcinol, thymol or other anthelminthics.

The eradication of the snails in endemic regions is not a practical measure for the control of heterophyids. Treatment of human infections may possibly reduce the spread of the parasites, but it cannot eliminate them as long as animals continue to disseminate the eggs of the parasite. Public education, aimed at eliminating the habit of eating raw fish is the most effective preventive measure. Kitchen refuse should be properly handled and fish offal should be made inaccessible to domesticated carnivores.

ii. Nanophyetiasis

Nanophyetus salmincola, a trematode which is less than 1 mm long, was formerly included among the heterophyids, but now it is assigned to the family *Troglotrematidae.* It was first described in the *dogs, coyotes* and *foxes,* living in a belt along the Pacific Coast of the United States. The infection develops in the host after ingestion of raw salmonid fish and is accompanied by severe symptoms of disease, which is called "salmon poisoning". Cordy *et al.* (1950) and Philip (1955) proved that the disease is not caused by *Nanophyetus* itself, but by a micro-organism, *Neorickettsia helminthoeca,* which is carried by the trematode parasite and is transmitted to its progeny through the eggs. In the dog it multiplies in the cells of the reticulo-endothelial system.

Subsequently it was found that the same trematode (regarded as a distinct species, *N. schikhobalovi*) is a parasite of the aborigines of the Soviet Far East, including Sakhalin. Thousands of this small worm may be found in one individual (Ssinovitch, 1959), and in some localities almost the entire population is infected. No human case of nanophyetiasis has as yet been recorded in America.

Infected people suffer from discomfort, abdominal pain and transient diarrhoea or constipation. These symptoms are provoked by *Nanophyetus*, but not by the *Neorickettsiae*, to which man is naturally resistant.

The eggs of the *salmincola* are 62–72 microns long. They must reach fresh water, in which, usually after several weeks, the miracidium develops inside the egg. It hatches out and penetrates into an appropriate snail. The short-tailed cercariae eventually leave the snail and invade salmonid fishes; in these they encyst as metacercariae in the muscles and internal organs. In endemic foci up to 100% of these fishes may be infected. The final hosts become infected by eating insufficiently cooked fish. The worms mature and begin to lay eggs after 5–8 days. Their life span does not exceed a few months, but man is susceptible to reinfection.

Canines, primarily the dog, are the most susceptible animals. The accompanying neorickettsial infection is characterized by severe symptoms of general intoxication, to which the hosts usually succumb within 2 weeks. Other animals, such as cats, minks, martens and badgers are susceptible to *Nanophyetus* infection, but they are not affected by the neorickettsiae.

The diagnosis is made by coproscopical examination. In Far Eastern countries confusion may arise by mistaking the eggs of *Nanophyetus* for those of *Paragonimus*.

Treatment with male-fern extract, acridin derivatives or thymol is usually successful in human cases. Dogs may be freed of the parasites with the aid of arecoline while sulphonamides and antibiotics control the rickettsiae within 24 hours.

iii. *Rare fish-borne trematode infections*

Echinochasmus perfoliatus, a trematode about 2 mm long, is a common parasite of *dogs* and *cats* in some parts of Europe and Asia. It has also been found on several occasions in man in the Far East. Kobayashi (1934) mentioned 12 species of fishes belonging to several families, which may be intermediate hosts of this species. The metacercariae are located mainly in the gills.

Prohemistomum vivax occurs in North Africa, Israel and Rumania in the *kite (Milvus migrans)* and in domestic carnivores. It has been recorded once in *man*, in Egypt, the infection being a heavy one.

Clinostomum complanatum is a large species, reaching 1.5 cm in length. Normally it lives in the throat of the *heron* and the *pelican*. Its metacercariae are found mainly under the skin of fishes. A few cases of accidental human infection have been described. Witenberg (1944) believes that the infection of inhabitants of the Lebanon known as "halzoun", which has been ascribed to *Fasciola hepatica*, is partly due to *Clinostomum complanatum* (and partly to the local leech). (*vide* page 604).

Chandler (1928) discovered, that the trematode, *Isoparorchis hypselobarbi*, is fairly common in man in the Manipur Valley (India). It causes gastro-intestinal disturbances and is apparently acquired by the ingestion of adult worms which normally live in the air bladders of certain siluroid fishes.

REFERENCES

Heterophyiasis

AFRICA, C. M., W. DE LEON and E. Y. GARCIA, *Acta Med. Philippina, Monogr. Ser. No. 1*, 1940, 132 pp.
COLLOMB, H., R. DESCHIENS and J. DEMARCHI, *Bull. Soc. Path. exot.*, 53 (1960) 144.
HUNTER, G. W., L. S. RITCHIE and C. PAN, *J. Parasit., Suppl.*, 37 (1951) 17.
LIE KIAN JOE and TAN KOK SIANG, *Amer. J. trop. Med. Hyg.*, 8 (1959) 518.
PODYAPOLSKAYA, V. P. and Y. F. KAPUSTIN, *Helminthic Diseases of Man*, Moscow, Medyidz. Publ., 1958, 663 pp.
WELLS, W. H. and W. BLAGG, *Amer. J. trop. Med.*, 5 (1956) 266.

Nanophyetiasis

BENNINGTON, E. and I. PRATT, *J. Parasit.*, 46 (1960) 91.
BOMBELO, I. A., *Abstr. Address. All Sov. Un. Helminthol. Soc.*, 1960, pp. 18.
CORDY, D. R. and J. R. GORHAM, *Amer. J. Path.*, 26 (1950) 617.
DOWHAM, C. R., B. T. SIMMS and F. W. MILLER, *J. Amer. vet. med. Ass.*, 68 (1926) 701.
PHILIP, C. B., *J. Parasit.*, 41 (1955) 125.
SKRYABIN, K. J. and V. P. PODYAPOLSKAYA, *Zbl. Bakt., I. Abt. Orig.*, 119 (1931) 294,

f. Invertebrate-borne trematode infections

Invertebrate animals serve as basic food for a great part of the verte-brates, but exceptionally for man. In such rare instances the ingestion of invertebrate carriers of parasites specific for animals may incidentally transmit the infection to man. In some localities where people are used to eat crustaceans, mollusks or insects, these infections may even occur in endemic form. The main trematode species connected with this kind of human infections are *Paragonimus westermani, Spelotrema brevicaecum* and *Euparyphium ilocanum*, while other species invade man merely occasionally.

i. Paragonimiasis

Paragonimiasis is caused by a trematode parasite, *Paragonimus westermani*, which lives primarily in the lung, but also in the brain and visceral organs of man and various carnivorous mammals.

The living parasite is ovoid or almost globular, flattened on one side, 7 to 12 mm long and reddish-brown. It is lodged in cyst-like cavities in the lung, which are connected with the bronchi by a small opening through which the excreta of the worm and its eggs are discharged. Usually every cyst contains one pair of worms. The eggs which escape from the cysts are oval and measure 80 to 118 microns in length. They reach the pharynx with the bronchial mucus and are then swallowed and passed out in the faeces. Hatching takes about 3 weeks. The miracidium develops in fresh water and needs a suitable snail (of the genera *Semisulcospira, Tarebia, Assimenia*) for its multipli-cation and development of the cercariae. The cercariae are liberated during a prolonged period into the surrounding water. They have almost no tail, but they nevertheless move actively and attack crustaceans which serve as obligatory second intermediate hosts. These crustaceans may be species of fresh-water crabs of various genera (*Erio-cheir, Potamon, Paratelephusa*, and others) or crayfishes. Over 20 species of crustacean vectors have been recorded. Some of the cercariae encyst on the carapace or on the extremities of the crustaceans, but mostly they enter through the softer parts of the exoskeleton and reach the gills, muscles or internal organs, in which they encyst and become metacercariae. In some regions it was found that 100% of the crabs were carrying metacercariae of *Paragonimus*.

Infection of the final host comes about by ingestion of raw or insufficiently cooked crabs or crayfish containing the encysted metacercariae of the parasite. These are set free in the duodenum, where they burrow through the intestinal wall. Reaching the peritoneal cavity, they penetrate through the diaphragm to the lung and settle in the small bronchioles. As they grow and develop into adult worms, the bronchiole expands. forming a cavity about the size of a pea, which is lined with a thick, fibrous layer. Such cysts usually are found in the deeper tissues and are inhabited by two, or sometimes by several, worms. The parasite feeds on blood and mucus. Its excretions often contain blood and are discharged into the bronchi in a rusty slime. Some worms may be lodged in the viscera, including the liver, mesenteric lymphnodes, muscles or brain. In these sites the parasite causes the formation of large granulomas or abscesses containing pus, numerous ova and necrotic material. Maturity is reached and eggs are produced within about 6–10 weeks. The adult worms may live in the lung for up to 20 years.

Paragonimus westermani is not specific with respect to its final hosts; it develops in many domestic and wild mammals which feed on the crustacean intermediate hosts. The infection is often sylvatic. The parasite has been found (even in areas in which human infection is unknown) in the tiger, leopard, civet cat, mongoose, monkey, and other animals. Human infection is endemic in some regions in which the dog, cat, rat and pig may be also involved, these species serving as reservoirs of the infection (Tang, 1940; Chen, 1936).

In endemic localities man spreads the infection through lack of hygiene (indiscriminate spitting and dispersal of faeces) and the habit of eating raw crabs. Where crabs are taken boiled, human infection is attributed to contamination of the fingers with the metacercariae derived from crabs. Rarely metacercariae encyst in the water and reach the host while he drinks (Ameel, 1934; Rock *et al.,* 1953). Local customs explain the frequency of human paragonimiasis in some areas. Thus in Korea the ingestion of raw crabs is regarded as a remedy against fever, diarrhoea, whooping-cough and other illnesses.

In addition to *Paragonimus westermani,* several other species of the same genus are known as parasites of mammals in localities in which human paragonimiasis is unknown. In Japan 4 species are found (Miyazaki, 1959); of these *P. westermani* is the commonest. *P. ohirai,* which is normally parasitic in dogs and some wild carnivores has been recently incriminated as a cause of human infection (Norio So, 1959; Araki, 1959). *P. kellicotti* occurs in North America in the cat, mink, dog, muskrat, opossum and other animals. A single human infection by this species has been recorded.

Human paragonimiasis of the lung has an acute onset associated with a rise of temperature and eosinophilia, but the clinical aspect gradually becomes mild and chronic. In slight infections there may be no pronounced symptoms, except for occasional coughing and expectoration of rusty sputum, in which the eggs of the parasite, eosinophil leucocytes and Charcot-Leyden crystals are found. In heavy infections the picture is similar to that of tuberculosis; there may be dyspnoea, anorexia, fever, malaise and occasionally haemoptysis. It should be noted that, in regions in which paragonimiasis is endemic, the disease is frequently accompanied by tuberculosis. In the course of the disease periodic aggravations set in. Glandular and visceral infection may produce fever, leucocytosis, and adhesions between vital organs. Brain involvement causes neck-stiffness, a Jacksonian type of epilepsy, hemiplegia and impairment of sight, the disease sometimes being mistaken for tuberculous meningitis.

The prognosis depends on the location and number of parasites. When these are few, the process may be quite benign, but if the worms are numerous and if the patient develops frequent haemoptysis, the disease may take a severe course. Brain involvement is often fatal (Chung Huei-Lan, 1956).

Little is known of the clinical pathology of paragonimiasis in animals. Its anatomical pathology is similar to that in man.

The diagnosis can readily be made by recovery of the eggs of the parasite from the sputum or faeces. Chung Huei-Lan (1956) stressed the necessity of repeated examination of the sputum in doubtful cases. In extra-pulmonary involvement or fresh infections of less than 40 days standing, no eggs are to be expected. Even in an advanced stage of pulmonary paragonimiasis, eggs appear in the faeces in no more than 50% of cases (Vajrastira, 1959).

In such cryptic infections, laboratory methods may reveal the causative agent. Complement-fixation and cutaneous tests have been proposed. However, simple extracts used as an antigen produce group reactions with the sera of persons infected with other trematodes. Sadun et al. (1958/59) introduced improved methods, using for the complement-fixation test the purified acid-*insoluble* antigen fraction, and for the intra-dermal test the acid-*soluble* fraction. These tests proved to be reliable, at least in screening out tuberculosis, although a slight reaction may be evoked when clonorchiasis infection is present. The precipitation test has also been proposed as a means of diagnosis (Norio-So, 1959).

Great difficulties arise when differential diagnosis has to be made between paragonimiasis and tuberculosis or histoplasmosis. The X-ray picture sometimes much resembles that of tuberculosis.

The distribution of human paragonimiasis is not exactly known. Heavy endemic distribution is found in certain areas of South-East Asia (Korea and Japan).

References p. 634/635

The infection is common among villagers who usually do not seek medical care, while it is rare among town-dwellers. For this reason rural cases are usually not adequately represented in hospital statistics. Stoll (1947) calculated that over three million people were suffering from paragonimiasis at the time when he made his investigations. Sadun (1958) even believes that this figure represents an underestimation. Recent investigations (Yokogawa et al., 1955) have shown that, in some endemic areas of Japan, up to 20% of the population are infected. In Korea paragonimiasis is endemic in every prefecture, involving 25% in some localities. Sadun (loc. cit.) found that, on the Cheju-Do Island off the coast of Korea, 3 out of every 4 individuals were infected. To a lesser degree paragonimiasis occurs in Central and South China, Thailand (Vajrastira et al., 1955), Formosa, the Philippines, Indonesia and Samoa. Apart from tigers and other wild animals, a high incidence of paragonimiasis has been recorded in dogs in various parts of India (Rao, 1935; Patnaik 1959). However, no information is available about human infection in that country.

Apart from the Asian regions human infections, allegedly caused by *Paragonimus westermani*, have been recorded in Central Africa, e.g. in the Congo and Nigeria. Zahra (1952) believes that at least 4% of the population in certain parts of equatorial Africa are infected *. Human paragonimiasis has also been recorded in tropical South America, but the determination of the parasites in these cases needs verification.

No effective therapy for paragonimiasis is known. Emetine injections are supposed to ameliorate the course of the disease without killing the parasite. The efficacy of chloroquin is a matter of controversy. According to Chen and Yuan (1959), combined treatment with tartar emetic and chloroquin yielded over 80% of favourable results, while Khoo-Oon-Teikh (1957) found little improvement after the administration of chloroquin either alone or in combination with other drugs during several months.

REFERENCES

AMEEL, D. J., *Amer. J. Hyg.*, 19 (1934) 279.
BUCK, A. A., E. H. SADUN, H. LIESKE, B. K. LEE and H. HAAHE, *Z. Tropenmed. Parasit.*, 9 (1958) 328.
CABALLERO, C. E., *Ann. Inst. Biol. Mexic.*, 17 (1946) 187.

---

* Fain et al. (1957) discovered a new trematode, called *Poikilorchis congolensis*, living in retroauricular cysts or abscesses in Central-Africans. The authors noted the similarity of the eggs of the latter parasite to those of *Paragonimus* and suggested that previous records of paragonimiasis in Africans may in fact have been caused by this newly described species.

CHEN, H. T., *Chin. Med. J., Suppl.*, 1 (1936) 368.
FAIN, A. and J. VANDEPITTE, *Ann. Soc. Belg. Méd. Trop.*, 37 (1957) 251.
SADUN, E. H., *6th int. Congr. Trop. Med. and Malaria*, Portugal, 1958, 58; *Amer. J. trop. Med. Hyg.*, 9 (1960) 562.
TANG, C. C., *Chin. Med. J.*, 3 (1950) 267.
VAJRASTHIRA, S., CH. HARINASUTA and CH. MAIPHOOM, *Japan. J. Exp. Med.*, 29 (1959) 159.
ZAHRA, A., *W. Afr. med. J.*, 1 (1952) 75.

ii. Spelotrema infection

In their comprehensive work on extra-intestinal heterophyiasis of man, Africa and associates (1936, 1940) included in the list of causative agents a species which they initially called *Heterophyes brevicaeca*. Subsequently this parasite was found to belong to the genus *Spelotrema* (Fam. *Microphallidae*) for which crustaceans (*e.g. Amphipods, Isopods* and *Brachyures*) serve as intermediate hosts. Ingestion of such crustaceans brings about human infection with the parasitic worm.

Spelotrema brevicaeca is common in sea-birds in the Far East. The adult worms are as small as the heterophyids and like these they provoke both intestinal and extra-intestinal infections in man. The latter are brought about by the tiny eggs, gaining entrance to the tissues.

iii. Euparyphium infections

Euparyphium ilocanum was occasionally discovered by Garrison (1908) in the stools of Philippine prisoners in Manila. Additional cases of human infection have subsequently been reported by several other investigators. Among them, Tubangui (1931) observed this species also in the brown rat *(Rattus norvegicus)* which represents the main host of the parasite.

E. ilocanum lives in the intestine. It measures 2 to 6 mm, and possesses a collar-like thickening, armed with long spines which are inserted in the tissues of the host. A small freshwater snail *(Gyraulus prashadi)* is the first intermediate host. The cercariae escaping from it enter one of several other freshwater snails, including also *G. prashadi*. In this secondary intermediate host they are transformed to metacercariae. When the metacercaria-carrying snails are ingested by the final host, they develop to the adult worm within one week. Besides *rat* and *man*, the adult parasite settles in *cats, dogs* and *monkeys*. However, while in man the worm may live for several years, in the just mentioned animals it survives only one or two weeks. The pathogenicity of the species seems to be slight. *E. ilocanum* infects man in the Philippines (Africa *et al.*, 1940) and Java (Bonne, 1940). As an animal parasite it has been observed in Southern China (Chen, 1934).

iv. Rare invertebrate-borne trematodiases

Occasional human infections with several other trematode species which are usually parasitic in animals, have been reported in the U.S.S.R., Assam, Malaya, Sumatra, India, the Philippines, Formosa, China, Japan, Rumania and America. The recorded human infections are caused by swallowing of insects serving as intermediate hosts of these trematodes. One of the better known species of this sort is *Plagiorchis javensis*, occurring in Indonesia. An other species, *Philophthalmus*, living in the conjunctiva of birds, has been recorded in Ceylon and Yugoslavia (Markovich, 1939). In Java, human infection with a trematode parasite of monkeys, *Phaneropsolus bonnei*, and another, *Paralecithodendrium molenkampi*, living in bats, have been described by Lie Kian Joe (1959).

REFERENCES

AFRICA, C. M. and E. Y. GARCIA, *Philipp. J. Sci.*, 57 (1935) 253.
AFRICA, C. M., W. LEON and E. Y. GARCIA, *Acta Med. Philip., Monogr. I*, 1940, 132 pp.
BONNE, C., G. BRAS and LIE KIAN JOE, *Amer. J. Digest. Dis.*, 20 (1953) 12.
FAUST, E. C. and C. BONNE, *J. Parasit.*, 34 (1948) 124.
SANDGROUND, J. H., *Geneesk. T. Ned.-Ind.*, 79 (1939) 1722.
SKRJABIN, K. I., *Trematodes of animals and man*, 12 (1956) 53.
TUBANGUI, A. and A. M. PASCO, *Philipp. J. Sci.*, 51 (1933) 581.

g. Schistosomiasis

i. General considerations

Schistosomiasis or *bilharziasis* is a chronic disease caused by any of the 6 trematode species of the genus *Schistosoma* (*Sch. haematobium, Sch. mansoni, Sch. intercalatum, Sch. japonicum, Sch. matheei* and *Sch. bovis*). The first 3 species are specific for man and accidentally develop in animals, the last 2 are specific for animals, accidentally developing in man, while

Sch. japonicum causes infection under natural conditions both in man and animals. All these species show much similarity in their biological and morphological characteristics; they live in veins and their life histories are similar. They differ, however, in some anatomical details, the shape of their eggs and the specificity of the intermediate hosts.

Schistosomes are dioecious; they live in pairs in the veins of their hosts where they deposit their eggs. The shape and size of the eggs are specific for every species. The y contain a formed ciliated larva, the miracidium. By a mechanism as yet insufficiently understood, the eggs move in the tissues in the direction of the nearest excretory channel (intestine or urinary tract), from which they are eventually evacuated. The number of eggs laid by a female differs according to the species. Sandground (1956) showed that *Sch. japonicum* lays about 3500 eggs daily in the hamster, while *Sch. mansoni* lays only about 300 in this host. For further development the eggs must reach water, in which the miracidia hatch out.

The miracidia actively penetrate the appropriate kind of snail, and, by polyembryonic multiplication, they develop a large number of cercariae which escape from the snail and swim in the water. The production of cercariae in the infected snail continues for several months. The cercariae are short-lived; even under optimal conditions, they die within 48 hours if they do not succeed in finding a suitable definitive host. When they come into contact with a suitable final host they penetrate its skin within a few minutes and migrate by way of the blood vessels, first to the lungs and then to the liver. They remain in the hepatic veins for about 8 weeks, during which period they develop into adult males or females. Toward the end of that period the worms join in pairs, the wider male embracing the thin female with the side wings of its "gynaecophoric grove" and the paired worms migrate through the blood vessels (against the blood-stream) to their final location, which is specific for each of the species of schistosomes.

The worms are usually long-lived. There are records of infection with *Sch. haematobium* and *Sch. mansoni* which have lasted 30 years.

The presence of a few worms may be unnoticed, but heavier infections gradually cause a characteristic clinical syndrome of varying severity. The course of schistosomiasis (irrespective of the species involved) may be divided into 3 phases: toxaemic, infiltrative and papillomatous (Girges, 1934).

The toxaemic stage corresponds to the period of development of the young parasites in the veins of the portal system. The symptoms are of a general intoxicative and allergic character, *i.e.* malaise, irregularly elevated temperature, transient urticaria, oedema at various parts of the body and a high eosinophilia.

This syndrome disappears when the worms leave the liver and migrate to their specific locations. *Sch. haematobium* migrates chiefly to the veins draining the genital and urinary system, *Sch. mansoni* to the inferior mesenteric venules, and *Sch. japonicum* chiefly to the superior mesenteric venules. These locations are not always strictly specific; single pairs of the worm may settle in unusual locations, such as the genital organs, lungs or heart (Faust, 1948).

On reaching their final location the worms immediately start to lay eggs, and then the second, *i.e.* the infiltrative, phase begins. It is remarkable that location of the parasites in specific sites does not produce vascular obstruction and that even their eggs moving through the tissues do not provoke cellular reaction. This infiltrative phase lasts for a varying period of time, depending mainly on the number of parasites, and during this stage usually only mild symptoms of disease develop. Haematuria or bloody dysenteric stools may appear; they are caused by pinpoint haemorrhages at the sites at which the eggs escaped through the mucosa. Sooner or later, a number of eggs become stranded in the tissues and cease to move, whereupon a specific reaction sets in: the eggs become surrounded by leucocytes, which are transformed into fibroblasts and eventually "pseudotubercles" are formed. Inside these "pseudotubercles" the eggs die, shrink, disintegrate and become partly calcified. As time passes, the "pseudotubercles" accumulate in the tissues and may cause increasingly severe disorders of the parasitized organs. Colicky pains of various intensity frequently occur, causing considerable loss of working ability. Disturbances in micturition or defaecation neither of which can be properly controlled, are due to imperfect functioning of the infected organs; somatic changes (*e.g.* hepatitis, splenomegaly) are presumably caused by metabolic products of the parasites. During this phase there may be complications due to the eggs being swept away by the blood current, instead of directly penetrating the tissue at the site of oviposition. Such eggs are usually filtered off by the liver, but may occasionally reach the lungs, kidneys or brain, in which organs they cause the formation of "pseudotubercles" and consequent pathological disturbances. According to Chan *et al.* (1957) 4.3% of cases of *schistosomiasis japonica* show acute or chronic cerebral involvement, including epileptic seizures.

In cases in which the progress of schistosomiasis is intensive and remains untreated, serious illness may result. During the long-lasting second phase, damage caused by the worms is incompletely repaired by regenerative processes. In the course of years, during which the regenerative capacity of the tissues declines, degenerative processes and their consequences develop, such as sclerosis of the organs, hyperplasia of the submucosa and its epithelial lining, hypertrophy of the spleen, cirrhosis of the liver and ascites. Especially serious are polypoid growths of the submucosa of the affected organs into the lumen of the intestine or urinary tract giving rise to ulcers and fistulae which may become secondarily infected. In a certain percentage of cases primary carcinoma of the liver or other organs may arise.

Every form of schistosomiasis is predominantely a rural occupational disease of field workers. It also affects other people coming into contact with water containing cercariae, such as fishermen, persons engaged in building bridges or clearing river-banks, as well as children bathing in streams and women washing clothes in open waters.

Schistosomiasis in its various forms is widespread and endemic in many subtropical and tropical regions. It is estimated that at least 150 million persons are affected by any of its forms. The disease saps the health, and therefore the working capacity of large population groups and for this reason if indeed merits the name *world scourge* which has been given to it (Shoushe Pasha, 1947).

The epidemiological situation must not, however, be regarded as static. The increasing use of irrigation in agriculture and fish-breeding is bound to increase the number of snails which carry schistosomes and, as a consequence, the human incidence of schistosomiasis is increased.

There are 3 geographic regions heavily affected by schistosomiasis, *viz.* the Far East which is exclusively affected by *Sch. japonicum,* Central America which is exclusively affected by *Sch. mansoni,* and Africa and the Near East in which *Sch. haematobium* and *Sch. mansoni* both occur, either alone or together. In addition, there are strains, the taxonomic position of which is as yet not settled.

Difficulties in the evaluation of the geographic distribution of schistosomiasis became apparent when the existence of geographical strains of widely distributed species was demonstrated. It appeared that such strains differ from each other in their adaptation to the final or definitive host, in their physiological characteristics, and in the sizes of the adult worms and of the eggs. Such strains exist within the taxonomic frame of well established species, and those of in *Sch. japonicum.* are especially significant. Variation in adaptation of schistosomes to the different regional strains of the same snail species has also been observed in *Schistosoma mansoni* (Files and Cram, 1948–49; Abdel Malek, 1950; Barbosa and Coelho, 1954) and *Sch. haematobium* (Cowper, 1947; McCullough, 1955; Witenberg and Saliternik, 1957). It is evident that in order to clarify the epidemiology of schistosimiasis it is not always sufficient to indicate the species of the parasite. The differentiation of the strains is equally important.

ii. Japanese schistosomiasis

Schistosomiasis japonica or so-called *Katayama disease* is caused by *Schistosoma japonicum*, which lives mainly in the veins of the large intestine. This parasite produces almost round eggs with a small lateral spine. It is very pathogenic to man and its public health significance is great. It is estimated that 30 million people suffer from this infection, mainly in the Yangtze basin. In Japan it is confined to several localities, but isolated foci are found in neighbouring regions (Philippines, Java, Celebes, Thailand). Its spread is enhanced by several factors, of which two are most important: first, the causative agent is not strictly specific to man, as practically all domesticated and numerous wild animals are susceptible and serve as reservoir of the disease; secondly, the intermediate hosts, several species of the snail genus *Oncomelania*, are sturdy, though small, amphibious animals, which live on the edges of swamps and irrigation ditches and in rice-fields, so that agricultural workers are inevitably exposed to them.

Recent investigations have shown that *Schistosoma japonicum* is represented by at least 4 geographical strains (Chinese, Japanese, Formosa and Philippine) each of which is characterised by different adaptations to both the intermediate and definitive hosts (De Witt, 1952, 1954; Hsu *et al.*, 1956–1960). While the Japanese and Chinese strains are highly infective for man, this is not true of the Formosan strain, which is predominantly zoophilic, developing mainly in buffaloes and dogs. Man is only slightly and briefly infected by the initial larval stages, which disappear before they have reached maturity. This strain fails to develop in local macaques, although it readily does so in Japanese and Philippine monkeys. In laboratory infected mice each of the four strains of *Sch. japonicum* manifests a different prepatent period. The size-index of the eggs of these strains has statistically different limits.

Japanese schistosomiasis is the most serious form of this disease because of the incapacitating damage it produces in man (Fig. 89a). Farooq (1960) estimated that, in the Philippines, the disease causes damage which, in the term of economic loss alone, equals $ 26.00 per infected person yearly, so that it is even a heavier economic burden than that due to malaria.

Destruction of the *Oncomelania* vector, which breeds under natural conditions almost all the year round, cannot be achieved by ordinary molluscicides, because this amphibious snail lives in the mud on the water edge. Therefore, dusting the shoreline with Paris green (copper arsenite and acetate) or calcium arsenate, is employed, whenever it is economically easible. In some instances burial of the soil, or burning off the shore grasses, have been found effective.

The presence of reservoir hosts, which include the water buffalo, cow, pig, dog, cat, rat and field mouse, is the most serious problem. The buffalo, which is the chief domesticated animal in the endemic areas, is of the greatest importance as a source of the dissemination of human schistosomiasis.

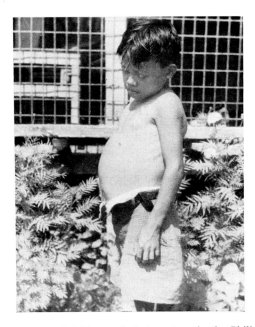

Fig. 89a.   Advanced case of *Schistosomiasis japonicum* in the Philippines (courtesy, World Health Organization, Geneva, No. 882).

iii. Schistosomiasis mansoni

Schistosomiasis mansoni is caused by *Schistosoma mansoni*, a species which lives in the veins of the large intestine and produces elongated eggs with a large lateral spine. This species uses freshwater snails of the genus *Biomphalaria* (also called *Australorbis* or *Taphius*) as intermediate hosts. *Sch. mansoni* is widespread all over Africa, Yemen, Central America, including the West Indies, and the northern belt of South

America. Its occurrence is patchy and is adapted to the distribution of
the snails just mentioned, which breed in stagnant or sluggish waters
The pathological effects of this species are similar to those of *Sch.*
japonicum, and like the latter it creates problems of public health of
prime importance. Fortunately enough, however, *Sch. mansoni*, unlike
Sch. japonicum, uses animal reservoir hosts only to a very limited extent
and cannot, therefore, be regarded as the cause of a true zoonosis.

Schistosoma mansoni was once considered a specifically human parasite. In experimental infection, it appears that, although mice and hamsters are susceptible, rabbits,
rats and domesticated animals, such as dogs, cats, pigs, goats and cows, are poor hosts.
They may be infected, but they do not eliminate the eggs of the parasite.

Cameron (1928) was the first to record a natural infection by *Sch. mansoni* in an
imported African monkey, *Cercopithecus sabaeus*, in the Island of St. Kitts (West
Indies). A number of recently published records indicate that wild rodents and shrews
may require infection with *S. mansoni* under natural conditions. Baretto (1959) found
7 out of 12 sewer rats in Bahia (Brazil) infected. *Gerbillus pyramidum* in Egypt, *Mastomys*
sp. and *Otomys sp.* in South Africa, *Dasymys helukus* in Kenya, *Eonomys hypoxanthus*
in the Congo, *Crocidura luna* in the Congo and *Crocidura olivieri* in Egypt have been
also found infected in nature. An important finding was that recorded by Miller (1959)
and Nelson (1960), who discovered that almost 24 % of the baboons *(Papio doguera)*
in Kenya were infected with *S. mansoni*. This record is the only one which probably
has epidemiological significance, because the distribution of the eggs and the pathological changes in the baboon are similar to those occurring in man, and this animal
retains the infection for years.

Similarly scanty data about natural animal reservoirs of *S. mansoni* have been reported from Brazil. Travassos, 1953, recorded infection in *Didelphys marsupialis*.
Barbosa *et al.* (1953, 1954, 1958) reported natural infection of *Rattus frugivorus, Cavia*
asperea and *Didelphys paraguayensis*. A most important record was published by
Pimentel de Amorim *et al.* (1953, 1954), who found the following 5 rodent species
naturally infected in the wooded region of the state Alagoas in Brazil: *Nectomys*
(45 %), *Oxynycterus angularis* (11 %), *Holochilus sciureus* (25 %), *Zygodontomys pixuna*
(2 %) and *Oryzomys subflavus* (1 %). In view of the high infection-rate of the first
3 species, and of the fact that the infected rodents were found in a locality with a high
incidence in man, it seems very probable that these animals serve as an important
reservoir of human schistosomiasis.

Biological and geographical strains of *S. mansoni* have been described. Files (1951)
summarized observations on several strains of this species in connection with the
unequal susceptibility of reputed vectors of *S. mansoni* present in different endemic
localities. One observation of this sort may be quoted. About 20 years ago there was in
Israel a focus of *Schistosomiasis mansoni* along the Yarkon River (now eliminated), in
which the majority of the infected persons showed eggs of the parasite, not in the faeces,
as is typical for this species, but in the urine.

In addition to typical *S. mansoni,* 2 other forms, which are regarded as species by some authors, or as strains by others (Nelson, 1960), occur in limited localities in Africa. These are *Sch. mansoni var. rodentorum*, discovered by Schwetz (1953) and *Sch. rodhaini*, described by Brumpt (1931), both in Congo rodents. Of these *Sch. rodhaini* has also been found in man and in the dog. The significance of these forms as human parasites is not yet clear.

iv. *Haematobium-group schistosomiasis*

The following is devoted to a group of schistosome species which produce eggs with a terminal spine. The adult stages of these species are very similar; they differ chiefly in their affinity to particular hosts, and partly in the shape and size of their eggs.

The typical representative of this group, *Sch. haematobium*, is a specific human parasite, which has been recorded on rare occasions as an accidental parasite of animals. It produces elongated, oval eggs. In contrast to all other schistosomes it lives in man, not in the veins of the digestive tract, but in those of the urinary system.

At the other extreme is *Sch. bovis,* which is a strictly specific parasite of domestic and wild ruminants (all over Africa, in Iraq, Israel, Sicily and Corsica). Its eggs are distinctly spindle-shaped with attenuated poles.

Eggs resembling those of *Sch. bovis* have been found in human excretions on numerous occasions, but there is a controversy as to their specific identity. Pitchford (1959), who found them in up to 23% of the human population and in 85% of cattle in some villages of the Eastern Transvaal, believes that they are the result of hybridisation between *Sch. haematobium* and *Sch. bovis.*

The adult worms of two other species of this group, *Sch. mattheei* and *Sch. intercalatum*, are morphologically indistinguishable from *Sch. haematobium*, but are intermediate between this species and *Sch. bovis* in the shape and size of the eggs. *Sch. mattheei* was described by Veglia and Le Roux (1929) as a parasite of sheep in South Africa and it has been subsequently found in man and in a baboon *(Papio porcarius)* by Blacke (1932) as well as in rodents. *Sch. intercalatum* was discovered by Fisher (1934) as parasites of the human intestines of persons in the Congo. Subsequent authors stressed the similarity of these two species, but no decisive conclusion as to their identity has been reached. The problem of taxonomical identity and zoonotic significance of the *intercalatum–mattheei* complex remains thus unsolved for the present.

The diagnosis of schistosomiasis may be made by the clinical symptoms, the discovery of the eggs in the excreta or by cystoscopy or rectoscopy, including the examination of snips of the mucosa, or by serological and skin tests.

In endemic areas the diagnosis can often be readily made by clinical examination as early as the third or fourth week of the infection, when other methods still fail to reveal the initial stages of the disease.

Examination of the excreta for the presence of eggs may be useful after the third month of the infection and subsequently. Negative results, however, are not conclusive. It should not be forgotten that in every case of schistosomiasis the number of excreted eggs is subject to considerable fluctuation, and temporary cessation of the appearance of eggs may occur at every stage of the disease. Therefore, examination of excreta in suspected cases should be made at least three times before a negative conclusion is drawn.

Examination of the excreta for the presence of eggs does not permit exact evaluation of the intensity of infection. This is especially true of chronic schistosomiasis, in which few eggs are produced and only some of these are eliminated from the diseased tissues. Examination for the eggs of the parasite is also of little value shortly after treatment, because treatment may result in temporary sterilisation of the worms, which, however, survive and eventually regain the egg producing capacity after a variable period of time.

Direct cystoscopy or rectoscopy may be useful in advanced cases, in which typical pathological changes have developed. Examination of snips taken from the mucosa of the bladder or the rectum during such examinations is of proved value, and often reveals infections which could not be diagnosed by other methods.

Numerous serologic and allergic tests have been proposed, and their techniques are continually being improved. Many methods of preparation of the antigens required for these tests have been introduced, including the use of extracts from adult worms or cercariae or of the livers of infected snails.

The complement-fixation test with an antigen prepared from adult worms, the slide-flocculation test with cercarial antigen (Anderson, 1960) and the fluorescent antibody test (Sadun *et al.*, 1960, 1961) are among the most practical methods for mass examination. The intradermal test might be used for presumptive diagnosis. Additional methods, such as X-ray examination or liver biopsy can be helpful in individual cases, but they are not as reliable as biopsy or immunological tests.

There are a number of drugs which kill schistosomes in the human body, but none of them is absolutely effective. Susceptibility to drugs varies with the species. The most sensitive is *Sch. haematobium*, while *Sch. japonicum* is much less affected. Most potent drugs are organic trivalent antimony compounds. A method of choice is repeated intravenous injection with potassium antimony tartrate (tartar emetic, introduced by Christopherson in 1918). Disadvantages of this treatment are the necessity for careful administration and the appearance of unpleasant side effects. This drug is contraindicated in cases in which the myocardium, kidneys or liver are affected. Unfortunately this precludes its use in advanced schistosomiasis when it would be most useful. Stibophen (Fuadin), the antimonial which is commonly given intramuscularly, is inferior to tartar emetic. The recently introduced TWSt (Friedheim) gave encouraging results in experimental trials and will possibly prove to be a useful addition to the antischistosome drugs. It is much less toxic than tartar emetic and can be given intramuscularly. The less effective Miracil D (= Thioxantone, Nilodin) is given by the mouth and is not toxic; it may therefore be indicated for the treatment of children.

Schistosomiasis is one of the most serious of public health problems, not only because of its detrimental effect on the health of the individual, but mainly because it is widespread in heavily populated areas in tropical and subtropical regions in the Old and New World. Furthermore, it causes enormous economic losses. Control of this disease is, therefore, a task of major public health importance. However, in many endemic regions attempts to control schistosomiasis have not given satisfactory results. The control of this disease still remains an unsolved problem.

By attacking any phase of the life cycle of *Schistosoma* its further development may be upset and the occurrence of schistosomiasis may thus be made impossible. The principal lines of control measures are: educational propaganda, mass treatment of infected populations, the control of vectors (by topographical amelioration, application of molluscicides or by biological methods) and individual protection. Destruction or isolation of animal reservoir-hosts, which would be desirable, especially in Japanese schistosomiasis, is not feasible in practice.

Prophylaxis by means of education and propaganda is possible in a well organised and disciplined community, but illiteracy, together with the low standard of hygiene prevalent in agricultural populations exposed to infection in the tropics, often nullify the preventive measures. The conditions of tropical climates bring about additional difficulties, while there is strong temptation to bathe in infested waters and methods of irrigation (*e.g.* of rice or cotton fields) lead to inevitable exposure to infection. Snail control is only effective when it is continuously applied. Experience has shown that the eradication of the snails has usually only temporary effect, because repopulation recreates the previous situation. Nevertheless the diminution of snail populations by means of molluscicides may significantly reduce the danger of infection.

Topographical control consists in the drainage of swamps, the regulation of streams and ditches, the construction of snail-proof irrigation systems (lined with concrete and conduction of water in pipes instead of in open ditches), the frequent periodical drying of infested water basins and streams, and other measures.

The control of vectors by means of molluscicides and through clearance of vegetation gives the best results hitherto attainable. These measures are not always successful and results depend on various factors, not all of which are known, *e.g.* the species sensitivity of the snails, the chemical composition of the water and the influence of vegetations. The drawback to the use of molluscicides is their high cost and the limited period of their action, even under favourable conditions. They are quickly removed by currents and their application must be repeated at appropriate intervals. Most versatile and inexpensive is copper sulphate which, in an appropriate dilution may in some instances exterminate the snail population. Sodium pentachlorophenate is equally useful. The recently introduced proprietary compound "Bayer 73" has shown properties which may surpass those of other molluscicides.

The efficiency of the biological control of vectors by the introduction of predators or infections of snails is still under investigation. The methods tried are: introduction of the voracious snail, *Marisa cornuarietis* (proposed by Chernin, Ferguson, and others; 1956–1960) to exterminate the eggs and young of the vector of *Sch. mansoni* in Central America; the inoculation of waters with *Bacillus pinotti*, which attacks *Bulinus*, the vector of *Sch. haematobium* in Egypt (Dias *et al.*, 1955); and keeping ducks in irrigation ditches, which is practised in Japan.

Schistosomiasis is an occupational risk to construction-labourers, soldiers, boatmen, fishermen and other persons exposed to infected water. In such employment temporary protection may be achieved by application of cercariae-repelling compounds to the exposed parts of the body. On the other hand the provision of uninfected water for bathing and laundry can afford protection to those who otherwise would have to use infested water.

In order to obtain maximum effectiveness all the methods mentioned above should be applied simultaneously. Control cannot usually be carried out by individuals but must be organised by the authorities.

v. Cercarial dermatitis

Apart from infection by specific adult schistosomes, man is liable to suffer from infection by the cercariae of several schistosomes of animals.

Cercariae of about two dozen species belonging to the genera *Austrobil-harzia, Bilharziella, Gigantobilharzia, Heterobilharzia, Ornithobilharzia, Schistosomatium* and *Trichobilharzia,* have been identified as capable of invading man. These species normally live in birds or mammals, among them in cattle *(Sch. bovis* and *Sch. spindale).* Their life cycles are similar to those of the "human schistosomes".

Although these cercariae are unable to develop to the adult stage in the human body, they can nevertheless penetrate through the skin and move about at the site of their entrance. They do not migrate to the internal organs, but die and desintegrate within a few days. In persons subjected to such invasion for the first time, the infection gives rise to a slight local cutaneous reaction, consisting of small transient maculae, and often also allergic hypersensitivity. If reinfection occurs, a sensitised person responds with an acute skin-reaction characterized by the appearance of papules, pustules or oedema, a condition known as *cercarial dermatitis, swimmers' itch, koganbyo* or *kabure* in Japan, and *sawa-itch* in the Malayan rice fields (Fig. 89b). It is accompanied by severe itching and slight elevation of temperature, but its course is benign and of short duration.

The adult form of the incriminated species of schistosomes normally

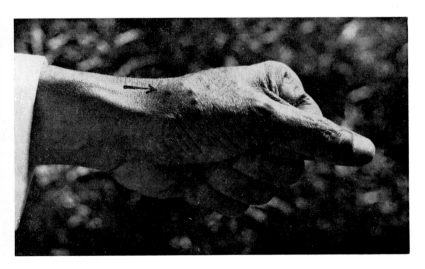

Fig. 89b.   Experimental infection of the skin after exposure to cercariae of *Schistosoma spindale.* (Photo: Dr. M. Anantaraman; courtesy of the *Indian J. Helminth.,* 1958).

References p. 648

develops in water-birds or mammals living near the water, while their cercariae are carried by freshwater or marine snails, according to the species. Cases of cercarial dermatitis have been reported in all parts of the world. Some localities are well-known for the occurrence of this type of dermatitis in bathers or people whose occupation brings them in contact with water frequented by infected birds or mammals, as, for instance, fishermen, workers in rice fields, and persons employed in antimalaria campaigns. Outbreaks involving simultaneous infection in large numbers of people have been recorded.

Control of cercarial dermatitis may be accomplished by eradication of the cercariae-carrying snails by molluscicides.

REFERENCES

AMBERSON, J. M. and E. SCHWARZ, *Trans. roy. Soc. trop. Med. Hyg.*, 47 (1953) 451.
CORT, W. W., *Amer. J. Hyg.*, 52 (1950) 251.
DeWITT, W. B., *J. Parasit.*, 40 (1954) 453.
FAROOQ, M., *Wld Hlth Org. Monogr. Ser., African Bilharziosis*, 3,1960, 22 pp.
FAUST, E. C., *Amer. J. trop. Med.*, 28 (1948) 175.
FILES, V. S., *J. Parasit.*, 35 (1949) 555.
GIRGES, R., *Schistosomiasis*, John Bale and Danielson, London, 1934.
HSU, H. F. and S. Y. LI HSU, *Amer. J. trop. Med. Hyg.*, 5 (1956) 521; *Trans. roy. Soc. trop. Med. Hyg.*, 52 (1958) 363.
KUNTZ, R., *Amer. J. trop. Med. Hyg.*, 4 (1955) 383.
NELSON, G. S., *Trans. roy. Soc. trop. Med. Hyg.*, 54 (1960) 301.
STRONG, J. P., H. C. McGILL and J. H. MILLER, *Amer. J. trop. Med. Hyg.*, 10 (1961) 25.

3

G. G. WITENBERG

Cestodiases

a. Taeniases

Tapeworms of the genus *Taenia* were among the first parasitic worms which were recognized in man. Hippocrates (460–377 B.C.) gave a description of *Taenia saginata* and established its connection with the excreted segments.

Two centuries ago it was determined that 2 species of *Taenia* may be found in man, namely *T. solium* and *T. saginata,* which are similar in many respects, but differ in details of their anatomy, life-cycle and geographical distribution. Both are large worms, usually 4–5 meters long, sometimes attaining up to 10 meters in length. They consist of thousands of segments (proglottids) arranged in a chain (strobila). In the mature stage both species live in the small intestine of man, but they never infect animals. Man acquires the infection on ingesting meat containing the bladder-like larvae, called *cysticerci. Cysticercus bovis,* the larva of *T. saginata,* develops in the muscles of cattle, and *Cysticercus cellulosae,* the larva of *T. solium,* in the muscles of pigs. *Taenia saginata* (the "beef-tapeworm") is the commoner species. According to Stoll's estimate (1947) about 39 million people throughout the world were infected, while *T. solium* (the pork-tapeworm") was harboured by 2.5 million people. The latter species is clinically the more harmful.

One of the prominent differences between the two species is the structure of the scolex, which in *T. saginata* carries 4 suckers while in *T. solium* it has a protrusible rostellum armed with 2 rows of strong sclerotised hooks in addition to the suckers. The scolices of both these species firmly attach the worms to the intestinal mucosa and the parasites remain in this situation, often massed in coils, and unperturbed by the constant peristaltic movements of the intestine. The segments originate by budding from the neck of the worm. The youngest segments, nearest to the head, are very small, but they grow larger and larger as they are pushed further from the scolex by the newly formed segments. Up to 2 dozen new segments are produced daily. The segments in the posterior part of the worm are mature and relatively large (up to 3 cm) and are filled with eggs. These ripe segments become detached from the chain and are eliminated from the host with the faeces. The eggs are dispersed in pastures, where they may be picked up by cattle or pigs respectively; otherwise they perish. In the intestines of cattle and pigs the eggs pass through the stomach, where they are macerated, and then to the intestine where the larvae (oncosphaeres) hatch. Here the oncosphaeres burrow into the blood vessels and eventually enter the blood circulation. Finally they settle down in the muscles and in the course of about 3 months develop into vesicle-like cysticerci, about the size of a pea, each of which contains a formed scolex. The cysticerci remain unchanged and are viable for years until they are ingested by man with insufficiently cooked (fired or smoked) meat. In the intestine of man the vesicle dissolves, the scolex attaches itself to the mucosa and at once starts the production of segments which in the course of $2\frac{1}{2}$ to 3 months grow into a complete chain. This life-cycle was first discovered by Küchenmeister and Leuckart about 100 years ago. Recently the cycle of *T. saginata* has been experimentally reproduced by self infections (Strom, 1939; Talysin, 1947, 1949). The worm ripened on the 91st and 75th day respectively. Every detached segment contained about 120 thousand eggs, so that about 2 million eggs were produced and eliminated daily in the faeces of the host.

Usually only one specimen of *Taenia* is harboured by an individual host. It is presumed that an established worm confers immunity against super-infection. When, however, many cysticerci are ingested at one meal, multiple infections may arise. Cases are known in which tens of adult worms established themselves in one individual. Once he had been infected, man can carry the *taenia* for years. Sandground (1936) noted that untreated taeniasis may last 20 to 35 years.

In general, taenia is not a very toxic parasite, but it may cause fluctuating gastrointestinal discomfort, loss of weight and disturbed sleep. In many instances infected individuals do not suffer from obvious symptoms and tolerate the parasites well over years. In endemic areas the appearance of tapeworm segments in the faeces is often regarded as quite a normal occurrence. The pathological significance of *Taenia saginata* is minor, but its incidence is high. On the other hand *T. solium* plays an important role, in spite of its comparative rarity, because of its association with human cysticercosis (to be discussed in the following chapter).

The diagnosis in man is simple: apart from the finding of eggs by microscopic examination of the faeces, the appearance of the rather large proglottids is definite evidence of taeniasis.

Taeniasis is common in regions where people are accustomed to eat insufficiently cooked or smoked meat, or where poor sanitary conditions favour the dispersal of human faeces in fields or courtyards and where there is insufficient meat inspection for the elimination of infested meat from the market.

Taenia saginata is particularly common in undeveloped countries where cattle breeding is an important occupation and infected herdsmen disperse the eggs in their faeces on the pastures. Ethiopia, South-East Africa, Argentina and Central Asia are important endemic regions of *taeniasis saginata*. Abassov (1958) recorded a 60% incidence in some localities in Soviet Armenia. This species is not found among the Hindus in India, but its incidence reaches 80% in some Nepalese tribes. It is very rare in Australia.

Taenia solium occurs mainly in Europe, in some populations of South-Asia and Africa and in the Western Hemisphere south of Mexico (according to Faiguenbaum, 1961, 15% of pigs in Chile harbour *C. cellulosae*). Apparently it is also common in Madagascar, where Merle (1958) found 10% of pigs infected with these cysticerci. The mainstay of infection with this species are small farms with poor sanitation where the corners of the courtyard serve as places for defecation, so that roaming pigs have ample opportunity to ingest human faeces containing the eggs of the parasite. Because of the ritual prohibition of pork consumption, Moslem populations and orthodox Jewish communities are free from *T. solium*.

The control of taeniasis on a country-wide scale is feasible, but the following conditions must be satisfied if it is to be effective: (a) meat inspection, (b) treatment of infected persons, (c) public education, and (d) proper sanitation.

Adequate meat inspection is possible in well organized countries in which the slaughter of meat-animals may be channelled through properly run slaughterhouses. In countries where slaughtering is practised under domestic conditions, especially on small farms, endemic taeniasis cannot be eradicated. In slaughter-houses meat inspectors eliminate the danger of infection either by destroying infected meat or by cooking or prolonged chilling according to established standards. The presence of *Cysticercus bovis* is recognized in cuts of the thigh muscles, heart or masseters, and that of *C. cellulosae* in cuts of the heart or the tongue. By this method mild infections may be overlooked but for practical purposes these may be ignored. Some countries, especially those which produce meat for

export, may suffer substantial losses through the condemnation of infected carcasses.

Hay (1950) reported 2 cases of cysticercosis in swine (in Poland), in
which cysticerci were found in all the lymph nodes, including the abdominal and cervical nodes, while none were recovered in the muscles.
Up to 7 cysts were observed in single nodes.

Apart from the pig, *Cysticercus cellulosae* also occurs in the dog and in
man *. In dogs it may involve the muscles and brain, but its incidence is
very low and it therefore has practically no importance for human
pathology. Java is perhaps an exception, for here Meyer in 1933 (quoted
by Brumpt, 1936) found that 0.6 % of the dogs which were used for human
consumption harboured *Cysticercus cellulosae.*

The treatment of taeniasis in individual patients is comparatively easy.
Although there is no method which will expel the worm with certainty, a
number of efficient drugs will do so on first application. Best known is the
time honored extract of male fern, but it may cause side effects in man,
i.e. cardiac symptoms and nausea. Other drugs can be used when male
fern is contra-indicated, *e.g.* tetrachlorethylene, hexylresorcinol, acridine
drugs (*e.g.* Mepacrin and Atebrin), or a mixture of metallic tin and
stannous chloride or stannous oxide.

Adequate public education serves to facilitate the introduction of the
control measures just mentioned. Unfortunately the public is often
ignorant of the life history of the *Taenia,* while the butcher regards the
high slaughtering fees as a burden. Thus meat containing cysticerci is
sometimes served at meals even in culturally advanced countries, as is
proved by the continued appearance of new cases of taeniasis.

The ignorance of infected stock attendants is another difficulty. Most
of them are primitive people who indiscriminately discharge their faeces
in places within reach of foraging or grazing animals and thus contribute
to the continuity of the life-cycle of the parasite. One herdsman who is a
carrier of *Taenia* may infect a high proportion of the cattle in his charge.

In some instances the artificial irrigation of pastures with sewage water
is responsible for the spread of infection among the animals.

It should be noted that the eggs of both the species of *Taenia* are thick-
shelled and may withstand desiccation to some degree. Silverman and

---

* Human cysticercosis is discussed in the following chapter.

quiver (1960) found that the eggs of *T. saginata* die after 5 days in sewage sludge kept at a temperature of 35°, while they remain alive up to 20 days at 4°. A possibly insignificant role in the spread of the eggs has been ascribed to birds, which pick up the proglottids of *Taenia* from human faeces left in the open and disseminate the eggs of the parasite in the field with their own faeces. Insects, notably flies, also contribute to the dispersal of the eggs of Taenia.

REFERENCES

ABASSOV, KH. D., *Med. Parazit. (Mosk.)*, 27 (1958) 157.
DIGITASHVILI, M. S., *Med. Parazit. (Mosk.)*, 27 (1958) 218.
EPSEN, A. and H. ROTH, *Rept. XIV Internat. Vet. Congr. (London)*, 2 (1952) 43.
JOYEUX, CH., E. GENDRE and J. G. BAER, *Colloq. Soc. Path. exot.*, Monogr. 2, (1928) 120.
SILVERMAN, P. H. and K. GUIVER, *J. Proc. Inst. Sewage Purific.*, 3 (1960) 345.

b. Human cysticercosis

Adult taenias parasitic in man are strictly specific to this host and never occur in animals. However, their larvae (cysticerci) are less selective and may also develop in other host species; *Cysticercus cellulosae* is more likely to do this than is *C. bovis*. A point of special significance in this phenomenon is that both these cysticerci may use man either as a final or as an intermediate host. This is an important fact, because cysticercosis, unlike taeniasis, may be a dangerous human disease.

Cysticercosis of man was known in the ancient world, but the cysticerci were regarded as foreign bodies until Redi discovered their animal nature and identified them as the larvae of tape-worms.

C. bovis occurs very rarely in man; only a few cases have been recorded (Tanasescu and Repeiuk, 1939; Mazzotti, 1944). Infections with *C. cellulosae* on the other hand, although not very common, are observed wherever *T. solium* is endemic. The incidence of *T. solium* infection has become lower during the last few decades. Even so human cysticercosis has not visibly diminished in incidence and is observed in localities in which infection with the adult worm is extremely rare. It is possible, however, that in these instances the cysticerci of other tapeworms have been confused with those of *T. solium* (Beaver, 1961).

Man becomes infested with *C. cellulosae* in two different ways, *i.e.*

either as in pigs, by ingestion of the eggs of the *Taenia* which have bee
excreted by an infected individual (possibly himself) or by auto-infectio
within the intestine.

The ova of the *Taenia* contain an infective larva (oncosphere), but they cannot hatch i
the intestine. In order to hatch they must first be subjected to the enzymes of tr
stomach. They are usually excreted intact, even when they have already been separate
from the enclosing worm segment. However, sometimes antiperistaltic movemen
of the intestine may drive some eggs or ripe worm-segments back into the stomac
If this happens the eggs are exposed to the digestive juices and, when they return to th
intestine, they behave like eggs which have been swallowed. Massive infections in som
individuals indicate the latter way of infection.

The released oncospheres burrow into the intestinal wall and enter the bloo
circulation by which they are carried to various parts of the body where they develo
into cysticerci. Occasionally the cysticerci are so numerous that they produce a gene
alized infection; sometimes they show predilection for particular organs in whic
they are concentrated.

Statistics regarding the distribution of cysticerci in various organs ar
reliable only if they are based on detailed dissections. Most of the avail
able statistics are, however, founded on clinical observation and therefor
include mainly massive infections or infections which affect vital organs
while light infections remain unnoticed.

As in pigs, the commonest site of cysticerci in the human body appear
to be the skeletal muscles (Fig. 90). However, infections restricted to th
muscles are rarely observed clinically, even when thousands of cysts ar
present, because they do not produce overt symptoms of disease.

Evans (1939) recorded a massive cysticercosis in an athlete, which was accidentall
detected in an X-ray picture (Fig. 91), although there were no complaints of illnes
(except for periodical eruptions on the skin) and eosinophilia amounted only to 1 %
The infection did not prevent the man from winning several medals and cups fo
running and jumping.

A serious situation is created when the central nervous system or the eye
are involved. This is primarily due to mechanical pressure by the parasite
on the neighbouring tissues. These forms of cysticercosis occur mos
frequently in cases of generalised infection.

Sometimes single organs become infected, as for instance, in a cas
reported by Limpscomb (1935), in which 150 cysts were found scattered
throughout the brain, while none appeared elsewhere.

The clinical response of cerebral involvement may be manifold and i
unpredictable. The following symptoms have been recorded: genera

nalaise, anorexia, headache, dizziness, nausea and vomiting, transient motor aphasia, loss of sphincter control, blurred vision, numbness and paresis. Epilepsy of the Jacksonian type, in which there is a tendency to loss of consciousness, is most characteristic of cysticercosis of the brain MacArthur, 1957). The presence of cysticerci in the cerebral ventricles

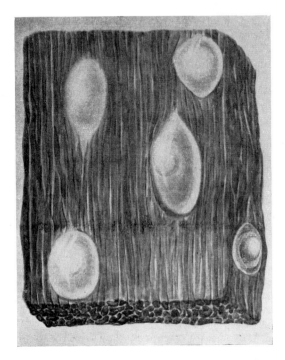

Fig. 90.   Cysticercus bovis in muscle of a cow (original drawing; enlarged 4×).

(Fig. 92) interferes with the circulation of the cerebro-spinal fluid, causing severe symptoms of basal meningitis. Multiple infections of the brain are usually fatal and are most often discovered on post mortem examination. However, cases have been recorded in which timely surgical extirpation of the parasites restored the patient to normal.

It is remarkable that the majority of cases of cerebral cysticercosis have been reported from Great Britain and India. MacArthur (1933) admits that an average of 97 soldiers have been invalided yearly from the British

Army, during a period of 5 years on account of epilepsy caused b cysticerci.

Cysticercosis of the nervous system is no more rare in certain American regions. Mazzotti (1944), in a statistical study in Mexico, recorded 13 case among 450 autopsies in a leading hospital; 25 out of 100 patients operated on for cerebral tumor proved to have cysticercosis of the brain. Busta

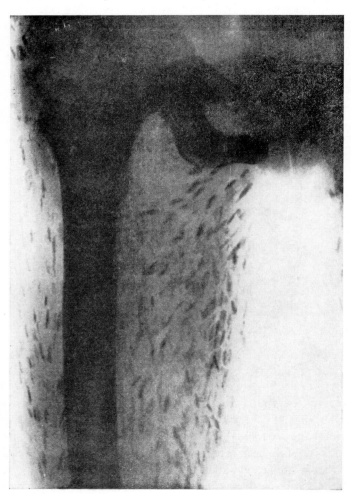

Fig. 91.   Numerous calcified cysticerci in the thigh of a man (courtesy
Dr. R. R. Evans, Trans. roy. Soc. trop. Med. Hyg., 1939).

ᴉonte (1950) recorded cysticerci in the nervous system in 1.5% of his ·atients in Chile.

The longevity of cysticerci in man is not definitely known, but their

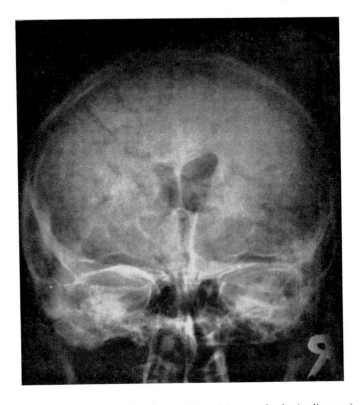

Fig. 92. Cysticerci in fourth ventricle of human brain (radiogram) (courtesy Dr. Owen and Dr. Lenczer, Canad. Med. Ass. J., 1956).

survival for several years has been proved. Eventually they die, shrink and become calcified.

The most reliable diagnostic procedure is by biopsy. This also applies to their localisation in the brain. Young cysticerci are completely transparant to X-rays, but old cysts with a thick outer wall, and especially those which are calcified, can be detected in this manner.

In some cases the Weinberg and Casoni tests may be successfully

applied in diagnosis. Pessoa *et al.* (1926) found the fluid of *C. bovis* an
C. cellulosae suitable as antigens for the complement-fixation tes
In a large proportion of cases of generalised human cysticercosis th
eyes are involved. The cysticerci being most often in the vitreous body an
subretina. Visual troubles betray the initial stages of the growing cys
Ablatio retinae and unilateral cataract may subsequently develop. Th
prognosis of ocular cysticercosis depends on the location of the parasit
When it is removed from the anterior chamber, the restitution of sig
may be complete. Cysticerci in the vitreous body or under the retina ofte
necessitate enucleation of the eye.

The preventive measures against cysticercosis are the same as tho
used against taeniasis.

REFERENCES

ARAMA, R. and A. ASENJO, *J. Neurosurg.*, 2 (1945) 151.
CHUNG, H. L. and C. U. LEE, *Chinese Med. J.*, 49 (1935) 429.
DIXON, H. B. F. and W. H. HARGREAVES, *Quart. J. Med.*, 13 (1944) 107.
EVANS, R. R., *Trans. roy. Soc. trop. Med. Hyg.*, 32 (1939) 549.
EWING, C. W., *Brit. Med. J.*, II (1941) 263.
FAIGUENBAUM, J., *Bol. Chil. Parasitol.*, 16 (1961) 71.
MACARTHUR, W. P., *Trans. roy. Soc. trop. Med. Hyg.*, 26 (1933) 525; 27 (1934) 342.
MAZZOTTI, L., *Rev. Inst. Salubridad Enfermedades Trop.*, 5 (1944) 283.
MENON, T. B. and G. D. VELIATH, *Trans. roy. Soc. trop. Med. Hyg.*, 33 (1940) 537.
TANASESCU, L. and E. REPEINE, *Virchow's Arch. path. Anat.*, 304 (1939) 555.

c. Coenuriasis

The term *coenurus* indicates a bladder-like larva belonging to any of abou
a dozen species of tapeworms of the genus *Multiceps* (related to *Taenia*
which produce numerous large scolices. The adult worms of these specie
which are up to 1 metre in length, live in the intestine of canines (dog
wolves, jackals and others). The eggs of the parasite are excreted in th
faeces of these final hosts, which disseminate the infection. When the
are swallowed by the intermediate hosts (which are various species o
mammals, including man), they develop coenuri in various organs an
tissues of these hosts. Preference for particular organs depends on th
species of the parasite. Within about 3 months a stage is reached which i
infective for dogs. Human infection occurs accidentally and rarely.

The *coenurus* bladder which has a diameter of 1–5 cm, may be single and globular, it may be divided into several lobes or its shape may be irregular. It consists of a thin, transparent membrane filled, but usually not distended, by a clear fluid. A varying number of oval, inverted scolices, sometimes up to hundreds, each about 2 mm long, are irregularly dispersed in several clusters on the inner or outer surface of the bladder membrane. Rarely daughter bladders are formed inside the primary one. The scolices develop into adult worms when swallowed by a suitable final host.

The classification of this genus is still imperfect. The identification of species, in both the adult and the larval stage, is based chiefly on the dimensions of the rostellar hooks. These dimensions, however, overlap in several species, so that some authors express doubt as to their suitability as a specific taxonomic criterion (Baylis, 1932; Sandground, 1937; Clapham, 1942). The two most important species, *Multiceps multiceps* and *M. serialis* are to be considered as biologically different, because they occur in different intermediate hosts (sheep and rabbit respectively) and have specific locations in these hosts (Baillet, 1863; Baylis, 1932).

Larvae of 4 species of the genus *Multiceps* have been recorded in man viz. *M. multiceps, M. serialis, M. glomeratus* and *M. brauni.*

M. multiceps is the most dangerous parasite, for its larva, *Coenurus cerebralis,* has a special affinity for the brain and spinal cord, and is therefore associated with a grave prognosis. It occurs in many parts of the world. Typically it affects *sheep,* in which it sometimes appears in epidemics with high mortality rate (Shumakovitch, 1958). In sheep the presence of a coenurus causes a disease called "gid" or "staggers", which is characterised by incoordination of movement, running in circles, or stupor; it usually ends in the death of the animal. Clinical symptoms in lambs can appear as early as the third week of the infection. The main source of the parasite is shepherds' *dogs* which had acquired the adult worm by eating parts, especially the heads (brain), of infected sheep which have died of the infection or have been slaughtered.

It has been observed in many parts of the world that shepherds have, out of curiosity, removed the bladder-worms from the sheep's skull, and thrown them to the dogs, not realizing the danger of creating additional sources of the disease. Bondarieva (1954) recorded an extreme case in which 267 specimens of adult worms were found in one single dog in Kasakhstan. This experience can be compared with a case of human coenuriasis described by Clapham (1941), in which over 700 scolices were found in one bladder.

Wild carnivores, for instance, the *wolf* and *jackal,* may harbour the adult worm and contribute to the distribution of the infection. However, Bondarieva *(loc. cit.)* demonstrated in experiments that the fox is a poor host.

The experiments of Bondarieva *et al.* (1960) showed that only a small proportion of the onchospheres (eggs) swallowed reached the brain. Less than 70% of lambs, which are the most susceptible hosts, acquired the infection when 500 infective eggs were administered, and the number of coenuri which developed in individual animals was small. It should be noted, however, that Pukhov *et al.* (1953) obtained 30 coenuri in a lamb artificially infected with 70 oncospheres of *M. multiceps.*

Bondarieva *et al.* showed that certain wild ruminants *(Capra sibirica, Ovis ammon* and *Gazella subgutturosa)* can readily be infected with *Coenurus cerebralis,* while deer *(Cervus elaphus)* and the roe-buck *(Capreolus capreolus)* are apparently refractory. Horses, cattle and swine have rarely been found to be infected.

Man is an accidental host of *Coenurus cerebralis* and constitutes a blind alley for the parasite. Yet the infection causes a serious disease. Coenuriasis produces in man varying cerebral manifestations, which resemble those of brain tumor, *e.g.* headache, aphasia, epileptiform seizures and partial paralysis. Several cases of intraocular coenuriasis occurring in Africa have been attributed to this species (Epstein *et al.,* 1959).

Owing to the rarity of coenuriasis in man, human infection is usually diagnosed only incidentally during an operation or at post mortem examination. The diagnosis of the cerebral involvement in man is difficult. The Weinberg test may be indicative, but since it reacts positively in various cestode infections its value for the specific diagnosis of coenuriasis is limited.

The larva of *Multiceps serialis,* called *Coenurus serialis,* typically develops in the connective tissues of rodents, mostly in *rabbits* (but also in squirrels, coypu, monkeys and other animals). The bladder is usually oval and about 5 cm long. Human cases, including infants 1 year old (Johnstone and Jones, 1950) in whom the coenuri are chiefly subcutaneous, have been recorded in all continents, except Australia. In spite of the frequency of both the adults and larvae of this parasite in animals, it is rare in man. The *dog* is the main source of human infection. Man is often responsible for the infection of dogs, particularly hunting dogs, by offering them the offal of rabbits as a reward.

Coenurus glomeratus is the rarest of the human coenuri. It appears in the form of small cysts in the internal organs of small rodents. 3 human cases have been recorded in Africa. The adult worm is unknown. Presumably it is parasitic in some wild carnivore. It is thought that small rodents serve as intermediate hosts in nature. Sandground (1937) and Clapham and Peters (1941) expressed doubt as to the identity of this species, regarding it as an incompletely developed specimen of one of the 2 species mentioned above.

Fain (1956) presumes that at least some cases of human coenuriasis in East Africa are due to the larvae of *Taenia brauni,* a tapeworm common in the dog in this region. The normal intermediate hosts of this tapeworm are small rodents and monkeys, in which tiny bladder-like larvae of the parasite are found in various organs, including the brain.

The only prospect for recovery may be in surgical removal of the coenurus. This is not always favourable, because the chronic granulomatous inflammation influences the functional capacity of the infected organ adversely (Landels, 1949).

The best method of prevention against both human and animal coenuriasis consists in denying dogs offal containing the coenurus cysts. This measure should be supported by the periodic deworming of sheepdogs.

REFERENCES

BAYLIS, H. A., *Ann. Mag. Nat. Hist.,* 14 (1934) 412.
BONDARIEVA, V. I., *Jubil. Vol. Prof. E. N. Pavlovsky,* 1954, 197.
BONDARIEVA, V. I., S. N. BOYEV and I. B. SOKOLOVA, *Trans. 10th Meeting Paras. Probl. Nat. Reservoirs (Moscow),* 2 (1959) 150.
BUCKLEY, J. J. C., *Trans. roy. Soc. trop. Med. Hyg.,* 41 (1947) 7.
CLAPHAM, P. A., *J. Helminthol.,* 19 (1941) 84.
EPSTEIN, E., N. S. F. PROCTOR and H. J. HEONZ, *S. Afr. Med. J.,* 33 (1959) 602.
JOHNSTONE, H. G. and O. W. JONES, *Amer. J. trop. Med. Hyg.,* 30 (1950) 431.
LANDELS, J. W., *J. Clin. Pathol.,* 30 (1949) 60.
NAGATY, H. F. and A. E. EZZAT, *Proc. helminthol. Soc. Wash.,* 13 (1946) 33.

d. Echinococcosis

i. Introduction

Echinococcosis or hydatid disease is one of the most important helminthiases transmitted from animals to man. It is caused by the larval stage of two closely related tapeworm species of the genus *Echinococcus,* of which one, *E. granulosus,* is cosmopolitan, while the other, *E. multilocularis,* is limited in its geographical distribution and has only recently been recognised as a separate species.*

---

* Six more species of the genus *Echinococcus* have been described as parasites of wild carnivores. Their specific validity and their role in human pathology is, however, insufficiently known.

The pathological process caused by the former species is known by the terms "vesicular" or "unilocular echinococcosis" or simply "echino-coccosis", while the process caused by the latter is called "multilocular" or "alveolar echinococcosis". Hydatid disease is summarised in several renowned publications, the most important of which are those of Dew (1928), Dévé (1946, 1948, 1949), Leikina (1957) and Vogel (1957, 1960).

Hydatids, the bladder-shaped larvae of *E. granulosus,* have been known from time immemorial, but until the sixteenth century they were regarded as concrements or malignant tumors. They were recognised about 200 years ago as animal parasites by Goeze (1782).

Investigation of the life history of *Echinococcus* was initiated by Siebold in 1852, and subsequently the connection between human and cattle hydatids on the one hand and the adult worm living in the dog on the other was established by Leuckart (1862) and Krabbe (1865).

It was also observed that in some localities in Europe, especially in Bavaria and Tyrol, hydatids in man and cattle do not appear in the usual form of large single bladders, but rather as clusters of closely packed minute chambers. Virchow (1855) regarded this kind of echinococcosis as an anomalous, pathological occurrence, but Leuckart (1863) decided that the parasite responsible for it is a separate species which he called *Echinococccus multilocularis,* to distinguish it from the species which produces unilocular hydatids. The differentiation of these species was the subject of controversy among scientists for about a century. The plural-istic view, which insists on the differentiation of two species is that now accepted (Rausch, Schiller, Vogel, *et al*).

Apart from the unilocular and alveolar types of hydatids, a third, intermediate type has been observed in rare instances. It occurs mainly in the liver of cattle as a con-glomeration of numerous small cysts, crowded into a limited area and divided by dense fibrous trabeculae, as to acquire a spongy appearance. It has, however, no tendency towards proliferation of the host's tissues which is characteristic of the alveolar hydatid. Dew (1953) called this type of hydatid "multicystic"; Vogel (1960) called it "pseudo-alveolar", and both these authors regarded it as an aberrant form of the conventional unilocular hydatid. It has been found in Europe, but has lately been observed also in New Zealand and Tasmania, where alveolar hydatids are not known to occur.

ii. Unilocular echinococcosis.

Echinococcus granulosus is the more important of the two species because of its cosmopolitan distribution and the frequency of occurrence, and also because enormous losses are incurred through condemnation of infected organs of meat-stock, and the frequency of human infection.

The adult tapeworms live attached to the mucosa, primarily that of the anterior part of the small intestine of the *dog*, wolf and some other wild canines. In very intensive infections the parasites may occupy the whole length of the small intestine (Fig. 93). *E. granulosus* is a very small worm (4–6 mm long); it has, in addition to a scolex

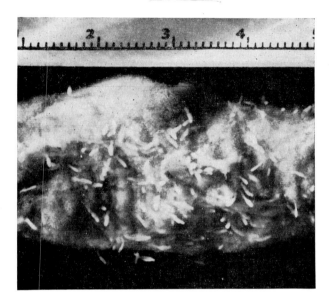

Fig. 93. Echinococcus granulosus; adult tapeworms attached to the mucosa of dog's intestine (original photo).

and neck, only 3 or 4 segments. The scolex is provided with 4 suckers and a protrusible rostellum, armed with a double crown of about 30 hooks. The last segment, which is as long, or longer, than the rest of the worm, contains several hundred eggs and, when it is ripe, it becomes detached from the worm and is eliminated from the host with the faeces. The first ripe segment appears on the 7th to 8th week of infection. Initially the segments are formed slowly but subsequently they develop more rapidly, so that a host infected with only one worm may eliminate several of them daily. In cases of multiple infection the host passes enormous numbers of eggs every day. Outside the host, and often even while they are still in its intestine, the segments disintegrate and the eggs become dispersed in the faeces. Each egg contains a fully developed oncosphere. The latter is about 40 microns in diameter, hatches in the intestine of the intermediate host, penetrates through the intestinal wall and is carried by the blood along the branches of the portal vein to the liver. Most of the oncospheres settle in this organ, but a smaller number pass through the capillaries and are carried with the blood to the lungs and other parts of the body, where they develop into hydatids (Fig. 94). In man and cattle the majority of the oncospheres are lodged in the liver less than 20% in the lungs and the rest in any other part of the hosts' organism, *i.e.* in the brain, kidney, bones, and wall of the urinary bladder; there is practically no organ in which the cysts cannot settle.

The hydatid consists of a friable membrane ½–1 mm thick, filled with transparent fluid. The membrane is composed of two layers, an outer, non-nucleated and laminated one and an inner nucleated germinative one. The hydatid cyst is enclosed in a sheath

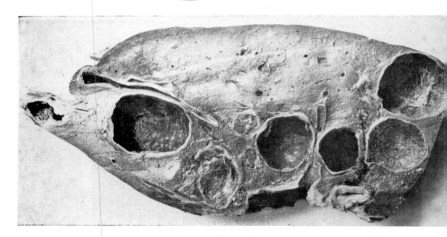

Fig. 94.   Hydatid cysts in liver of cow (Photo: Institute for Veterinary Pathology, State University, Utrecht).

made of vascularized connective tissue produced by the host. On its inner side, the germinative layer gives rise, through budding, to microscopic scolices which are fully developed about 4 months after the infection. The scolices, attached by peduncles to the germinative sheath, are globular or slightly oval structures, containing an inverted rostellum with its hooklets and suckers. Several of them may become detached and float freely in the fluid or they may collect at the bottom of the hydatid. The number of scolices varies; there may be thousands of them but sometimes, especially in cattle, there are none *(sterile cysts, acephalocysts)*. Often, so-called brood-capsules are formed. These are small vesicles, which originate from the germinative membrane, and each of them encloses numerous scolices. Such "brood-capsules" sometimes develop into daughter bladders of various sizes, floating in the cyst's fluid, each of them constructed like the mother bladder and containing a number of scolices of its own. There may be only a few daughter cysts, but sometimes the original bladders are tightly filled up with them.

The hydatids are usually globular. Their shapes may, however, be irregular because unequal pressures may be exerted on them by the surrounding tissues; this is especially pronounced in hydatids which develop in bones. Hydatids may remain unchanged for a very long period (29 years, Coutela *et al.*, 1950), but frequently they die and become calcified, suppurate or disintegrate. Individual hydatids usually grow singly, but numerous hydatids may form a complex cluster of variable size. Usually they cease growing when they have reached 5 to 10 cm in diameter, but exceptionally,

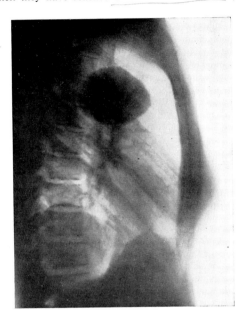

Fig. 95.   Röntgenphoto showing two hydatid cysts in human lung
(Photo: Dr. A. Druckmann, Jerusalem).

growth may cease when the diameter measures only a few millimetres. On the other hand, they sometimes continue to grow so large as to contain as much as 50 litres of fluid (Barnett, 1927, 1944; Dungal, 1946; Oulié, 1924).

   Every scolex represents a single larval parasite and gives rise to an adult worm when ingested by a dog or a similar suitable final host. In the intestine of the final host the scolex evaginates, attaches itself to the mucosa of the small intestine and grows within 5 to 7 weeks to maturity. In this manner, a dog may acquire many thousands of worms through the ingestion of a single hydatid. The life-span of an adult *E. granulosus* is limited to about 6 months.

E. granulosus cannot normally develop in the fox or in the cat (Witenberg, 1933). The hydatids of *E. granulosus* normally develop in domestic or wild *herbivores* and in *pigs*, occasionally also in other animals. The list of intermediate hosts compiled by Llanos (1953) comprises 5 species of *marsupials*, 7 species of *primates*, 11 species of *artiodactyls*, and the *elephant*. On a few occasions hydatids have been found in *rodents* (in *Microcavia australis* by De le Barrera, 1948, and in *Octodon degus degus* by Negme, 1958, both in South America). *Man* is only an accidental intermediate host; he constitutes a dead end for the parasite and does not play any part in its propagation.

The life-cycle of *Echinococcus granulosus* may proceed along three courses (as in trichinelliasis) according to the hosts involved: (1) A *sylvatic* course, involving wild carnivores and wild herbivores, (2) a *pastoral* course, involving wild or domestic carnivores and domestic stock (or man) and (3) a *synanthropic* course, mainly affecting dogs and other domestic animals or man. These courses may either constitute closed circles or they may merge transgress one into one another.

Sylvatic echinococcosis exists in sparsely populated regions and seldom plays a significant role in the direct transmission of hydatid disease to man. It has been best investigated in the northern part of North America where the *wolf* and to a lesser extent the *coyote,* on the one hand, and *caribou, moose* and *deer* on the other, figure in the life-cycle (Rausch and Schiller *et al.*, 1951, 1959; Miller, 1953). The wolf may be infected up to the rate of almost 70% (Sweatman, 1952; Ritcey and Edwards, 1958). Wild-life infection may reach man through the intermediary of the dog. The aborigines, who are largely dependent on the meat of game, feed and thus infect their dogs with the game's viscera. Wolfgang and Poole (1956) found 25% of the dogs of North Canadian Indians infected, while between 13 and 41% of the human population reacted positively in the cutaneous test. The same is true of regions populated by Eskimos.

Recent research (Miller, Wolfgang and Poole) has shown that the epidemiological picture of hydatid disease in North Canada differs from that in Europe. Cameron (1960) summarized these observations and showed that: (a) on the Canadian mainland the hydatids, although not different in structure from the ordinary cysts, occur in man mostly and in animals exclusively in the lungs; (b) they are found in larger deer (caribou, moose, wapiti), but not in other wild or domestic herbivores; experimentally it has so far been impossible to infect sheep, pigs, cattle or rodents; (c) the sera of man or animals infected with the North Canadian strain of *Echinococcus* show properties different from those of ordinary cases and in diagnostic tests a specific antigen made of local material is required. It was therefore concluded that the North

Canadian strain of *Echinococcus*, which is mainly propagated in the sylvatic life-cycle (*i.e.*, deer–wolf–deer with a side-branch to dog–man) is a peculiar variety for which Cameron proposed the name *Echinococcus granulosus var. canadensis*.

Sylvatic echinococcosis is also common in East Europe and some parts of Asia. Paramanathan and Dissanaike (1961) reported that in Ceylon the sylvatic form of hydatid disease involves *jackal* and *deer*, in addition to the ordinary domestic hosts, dog and cattle. In Australia Dew (1952) and Durie and Rick (1952) noticed a sylvatic cycle comprising the *dingo wallaby*.

Echinococcus infection of wild animals, caused either by the adult worm or by the larval cysts, is encountered in many regions and is closely linked with pastoral hydatidosis in which the parasite infests domestic animals. Thus, in South America where the dog is the only carrier of the adult *Echinococcus* in the widespread pastoral course of hydatidosis, cysts have been found in naturally infected rodents and wild ruminants. In Tadjikistan (Asiatic Soviet Union) natural infection of the boar has been recorded (Mielnikova, 1960), while in Israel, where no wild hydatid vectors were found, the author (1933) established a high incidence in jackals naturally infected with *E. granulosus*. Even in Central Europe, involvement of wild animals in the pastoral cycle has been reported, as for instance in Holland, where, according to Jansen (1961), infection in 4% of red deer was recorded.

The mainstay of hydatid disease is the pastoral cycle. This depends principally on the presence of large sheep flocks, though cattle, camels, horses and reindeer may also be involved. The sheep-dogs guarding the herds not only eat the offal of slaughtered sheep, but also devour the bodies of dead sheep left in the field. The exchange of the parasite between sheep and dog is perpetual and, as a result of this, the incidence is usually high in both. The infected dog disseminates eggs of the parasite not only on the field but also in the immediate surroundings of human habitations, thus introducing the infection into a synanthropic cycle in which man may easily be included.

Hydatid disease exists among animals in all parts of the world, although its prevalence varies in different regions. Almost everywhere it involves also man, but the incidence of human infection represents only a fraction of that in animals. The spread of hydatid disease depends on various circumstances, some of them natural, as in the sylvatic life cycle, others conditioned by man. The factors facilitating the endemicity of echinococcosis are not static and, therefore, the prevalence of infection may change, even radically.

The presence of infected dogs is a prerequisite for the synanthropic course of hydatidosis. The main source of infection for the dog are sheep. The importance of sheep as an intermediate host is due, not only to its susceptibility to infection, but also to the fact that hydatids developing in sheep are almost always fertile, in contrast to those found in pigs and cattle. An average of only 20% of those found in pigs and of only 10% of those found in cattle contain infective scolices. The primitive conditions of slaughtering in many undeveloped parts of the world are another important factor in the spread of echinococcosis. Even in certain well organized countries proper meat inspection in carried out only in the cities, whereas in the rural regions slaughter practices are often inadequate to protect local dogs from infection.

Climatic conditions play only a limited role in the spread of echinococcosis. The eggs of *Echinococcus* are covered with a tough protective shell which renders them resistant to adverse environmental conditions. Whereas extreme heat and insolation soon kill the exposed eggs, in damp, shaded places they may withstand months of outdoor influences. They are dispersed by the wind or through flies, and can reach man or animals with soiled food (Clunies-Ross, 1929; Schiller, 1954).

There are no reliable statistics which would provide a full picture of the distribution of human echinococcosis in any geographical region. Available knowledge as to its distribution is fragmentary, since it is based on incidental reports, for the most part from towns or limited districts comprising either clinical or surgical cases or observations made at autopsies. Yet these incomplete data permit us roughly to mark out certain areas of high density of infection.

Although echinococcosis in Europe has been studied for decades, the picture of its incidence is not equally clear in every country. The island of Iceland which, a century ago, was the most heavily afflicted region in the world, with 30% of the population showing hydatid cysts on autopsy, presents a striking example of almost total eradication of hydatid disease (Ofeigson, 1937; Dungal, 1957). The data collected at postmortem examination carried out in that country between 1930 and 1956 showed an incidence of hydatid disease of 3.6%, the majority of cases involving persons over 50 years of age, in whom infection could be traced back to the unfortunate past, while no persons under 20 years of age showed infection. This improvement is due to the enforcement of such control measures as are described in the following pages.

Though it varies in frequency, human hydatidosis is found in practically all regions of Europe. It is rare in northern countries, except in northern Scandinavia where it follows the cycle of reindeer–dog (–man). In France it occurs mainly in the Landes, Languedoc and Province districts, as well as in Sardinia and Corsica. Sardinia where nearly 50% of the dogs are infected (Medda and Ladeivaia, 1960), is one of the most severely affected regions. In Poland hundreds of human cases are observed every year (Kozar, 1957). The infection is prominent in Hungary and grows in intensity farther south, notably in the Balkan countries.

In Hungary, Boray (1954) quoted the human incidence of hydatidosis, based on autopsies, as 170 per 100,000 in selected localities, as compared with 12% infection in sheep, up to 55% in pigs, and 8% tapeworm infection of dogs (caught in the residential quarters of Budapest).

According to the estimate of Suic (1957) and Navenic (1957) 0.32% of autopsies (320 per 100,000) showed hydatid infection of man in Yugoslavia. The incidence in domestic animals is also high, although it varies according to districts: 15–72% in sheep, 12–90% in cattle, 8–70% in pigs, 18% in goats and up to 35% in dogs. In Bulgaria, Stoianov (1936) recorded a human incidence of 0.7% on admission in hospitals during the preceding 15 years, while 660 per 100,000 of autopsies showed hydatid cysts.

According to Maccas (1951) 455 to 706 cases of hydatidosis had been operated upon annually during the preceeding 5 years in hospitals in Greece, which represents 0.95% of all hospitalised patients. The incidence in animals in that country is also very high (24%). On an average of 20% of the dogs are infected.

Information on hydatidosis in the vast regions of Asia is incomplete. Only data obtained from casual observations in a few localities are available and these do not permit drawing any general conclusions. However, considering the widespread raising of cattle and sheep, unlimited propagation of dogs and inadequate sanitary conditions in vast areas, a high prevalence of hydatidosis is to be expected.

Israel is one of the countries in which hydatidosis is kept under control. Rakover (1960) estimated that about 100 cases are diagnosed yearly, of which 40 are of local origin. This makes an incidence of 2 per 100,000. It must, however, be remembered that almost all the cases in Israel occur in a few districts only, among immigrants from Oriental countries who practise the primitive system of sheep breeding native to their regions of origin. In 1933 the present author found 20% of stray dogs and 10% of jackals in the vicinity of Jerusalem carrying adult *E. granulosus*. Recently the incidence has been considerably reduced by enforced destruction of these animals.

In neighbouring Beirut (Lebanon) Pipkin *et al.* (1951) found over 30% of dogs infected with *Echinococcus* and accordingly human hydatidosis is very common in that country (Makhlouf, 1957). Cyprus likewise shows a high incidence in man (about 13 per 100,000 of admissions (Maccas, 1951), while cattle are severely affected.

Hydatidosis is also widespread in Turkey. According to Oytun (1957), 220 hospital admissions were recorded in one year in the hospitals of the country. In the Istanbul clinics for internal diseases these infections comprise 0.32% of the annual overall admissions and 300 per 100,000 (among 3945) of autopsies. Livestock are severely affected, with an incidence of no less than 50% in sheep and goats.

Gazenko (1958) reports a high incidence of hydatidosis in the Altai Region (Central Siberia), where cases of this affliction constitute 0.45 to 3.9 % of all hospital admissions In Ulan-Bator (Outer Mongolia) Dudkievitch (1959) recorded many cases of hydati dosis (5.2 % of all surgical treatments), with 26 % of stray dogs harbouring the tape worm. Human hydatidosis is possibly prevalent in East Caucasus where *Echino coccus* infection was recorded in 50 to 60 % of dogs (Yarubin, 1960; Nikitin, 1958)

Little information is available about hydatidosis in Africa. According to Seneve (1951) human cases are rare in North Africa, despite the high incidence in cattle an sheep in districts rich in water; the disease may be absent from desert settlements. N statistics are available as to hydatidosis in the population of Egypt where, accordin to Halawani (1949) the *camel* is the most infected animal (over 80 % infection i camels, 1.5 % in sheep and an intermediate figure in *buffaloes*). Abdel-Azim (1938 found 2 to 3 % of infected dogs in Cairo and about 10 % in Upper Egypt.

In the Americas there are two areas of endemic unilocular echinococcosis: one i the Far North, comprising the Boreal regions of Canada and Alaska and the other i South America, with Argentina and Uruguay as the most affected countries.

In Canada and adjoining territories there exist peculiar conditions of spread o hydatid disease; here a sylvatic cycle, involving the wolf and wild herbivores (reindeer caribou, moose) overlaps a synanthropic one, involving the dog and man. Sweatmar (1952) found 62 % of wolves and 68 % of moose infected in Ontario. Numerous dogs ar kept in direct association with the aboriginal population and are fed the viscera o hunted animals which often contain hydatids. Thus, these dogs are heavily infectec (up to 50 %, according to Miller, 1953). Under the primitive conditions prevailing ir Polar regions, the food cannot be guarded from contamination and consequently human infection is easily acquired. Since the skinning of hunted animals is usually carried out by women, they are more often infected than men are. Recent surveys showed a very high prevalence of hydatid disease among the Canadian Indians and Eskimos in whom the Casoni test or X-ray examination revealed an incidence varying from 10–45 % (Wolfgang and Poole, 1956; Cameron, 1957).

There is a conspicuous difference in the frequency of echinococcosis in Canada and the United States. In the latter country, human echinococcosis is rare. In the Mayo Clinics only one case is observed in about every 25,000 patients; 95 % of about 650 cases recorded in North America until 1952 were immigrants who had acquired the infection in the countries of their origin (Magath, 1952, 1953). The infection among dogs is even rarer. In the State of Mississippi which appears to be more affected than other States, Hutchinson (1960) observed echinococci in 6 dogs and hydatid cysts in 0.9 % of swine. Riley (1933), after finding 6 of 13 wild moose in Northern Minnesota carrying hydatids and 3 timber wolves in the same locality harbouring the adult worm, suggested that these hosts were the possible sources of the infections.

South America, with its vast cattle and sheep breeding areas and its multitude of uncontrolled dogs, is one of the most severely affected areas. Besides a very high incidence of infection in animals, the number of recorded human cases within the last two decades is counted in the thousands. According to available records Uruguay and Chile are the countries most affected. Sporadic echinococcosis in man has been re corded in the American tropics (Venezuela, Colombia, Ecuador, etc.).

In Uruguay the index of human infection amounts to 15.2 per 100,000 (Parachristophilou, 1957), while 40% of cattle and 60% of sheep harbour hydatid-cysts.
About 600 new human cases are diagnosed yearly in Chile, the mortality rate being more than 8 per 100,000. The disease is most frequent in the Central and Southern parts of the country, which corresponds to the frequency of hydatidosis in cattle (Fig. 96).

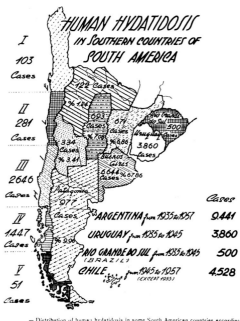

— Distribution of human hydatidosis in some South American countries according to data of Perez Fontana (1949), Ferro (1957), and Neghme and Silva (1958)

Fig. 96. Distribution of human hydatidosis in some South American countries, according to data of Perez Fontana (1949), Ferro (1957) and Neghme and Silva (1958) (Courtesy Prof. A. Neghme, Santiago, Proc. Sixth Internat. Congr. trop. med. and Malaria, Lisbon, 1958).

Neghme *et al.* (1955) examined two groups of stray dogs in Santiago. Those captured in the grounds of the slaughterhouse showed 27% infection, while 4.6% of the dogs captured in the streets were found infected. The incidence in domestic ruminants varied from 10–30%. Parachristophilou gives the incidence of hydatidosis in Argentina as 3.08 per 100,000. That country is an example of successful control of hydatidosis, showing a slow but constant decline: 687 cases in 1947 as against 236 in 1953 (Maccas).
Paraguay is, as Gines (1949) reported, noteworthy for its low incidence (0.034% in cattle).
Extensive cattle and sheep breeding coupled with the traditional use of dogs, makes Australia most suitable for continual spread of hydatid disease. In view of the exten-

siveness of the territory domestic slaughtering without meat inspection is inevitable. Dew (1953) recorded that 20–90% of the adult sheep and 49 to 100% of the cattle in the South-Eastern part of the continent were infected. The infection of dogs in Australia varies from 5.6% on farms on which precautions are being taken to 37.3% where no control measures are adopted (Gemmell, 1958).

Hydatids rarely occur in *rabbits* in Australia. Wallabies are infected at a rate of 20–50%, *kangaroos* to a lesser degree. These animals are the main source of the infection of dingoes, so that a true sylvatic life-cycle of the parasite is thus maintained (Durie and Rick, 1952; Gemmell, 1959).

Although the Australian Government has passed measures designed to prevent the spread of hydatid disease, the local conditions make it difficult to enforce the campaign. Thus, the incidence of echinococcosis in New South Wales has not altered appreciably during the last 30 years, mainly because of the persistent feeding of raw offal to dogs.

The situation in New Zealand approaches that in Australia. Foster (1958) maintains that proportionally New Zealand is one of the most affected countries in the world, having more than 80 new human cases each year. The infection is comparatively rare in urban dogs, but rural dogs show a 10 to 60% infection rate. Laing (1956) recorded the infection in 90% of sheep, 80% of lambs, 60% of cattle and 20% of pigs. Here again, farmers are to be blamed for not taking adequate precautions against the spread of the infection.

Even in localities in which hydatidosis occurs comparatively frequently, it is still a sporadic disease in man. Nevertheless, in view of the hazard to life it presents, its importance in public health is great.

As has been stated above, no organ or tissue of the human body is resistant to the development of hydatids. The severity of the infection depends on the location, size and number of the cysts. Accordingly the clinical manifestations are manifold.

The hydatid of *Echinococcus granulosus* is not a particularly toxic parasite; its growth, though unpredictable, may be slow and benign. In some instances the presence of a cyst remains symptomless for years, especially when it dies, shrinks or becomes calcified. The harm caused by a growing hydatid is mainly due to pressure upon and mechanical destruction of the surrounding tissues. The host's reaction to the cyst is similar to that towards any other foreign body. A pericystic layer (adventitia) is formed around the cyst, which is partly composed of neutrophilic leucocytes and plasma-cells.

The distribution of hydatid cysts in various organs and tissues of the human body is not uniform. Usually approximately 70% of the cysts develop in the liver, 20% in the lungs and the remaining few which develop from the scolices enter the greater circulation and settle in a variety of tissues or organs. Hydatid-cysts may be formed in such sites as the orbit, pericardium, prostate or thyroid. In young people there is a predilection for involvement of the lung. Dévé estimated that up to one third of the patients harbour more than one cyst. Perez Fontana (1949) stated that usually a single cyst develops in children. The youngest recorded child to show hydatid infection was 3 years old. *Echinococcus* cysts usually stop growing when they reach 5 to 8 cm in diameter; in some cases they do not increase in size after they have reached a few millimetres in diameter; sometimes, however, they continue to grow until they contain several liters of content (fluid and daughter cysts).

The pathogenicity of hydatid disease is related to the site in which the cyst develops. In the liver or in the lung a single cyst may not cause any symptoms unless it grows exceedingly large or ruptures. A ruptured cyst presents two risks. In the first place, it sets free an unusually large amount of antigen which, when it is rapidly absorbed (in the bronchi or in the peritoneal or pleural cavity), may cause an alarming, sometimes fatal, allergic reaction. Anaphylactic shock with ensuing pulmonary oedema may cause instantaneous death. Mild anaphylactic symptoms, such as localized urticaria or eosinophilia, may appear as a result of partial absorption of the hydatid fluid. When the fragments of the ruptured cyst are swept into the bronchial, biliary or urinary passages and are quickly eliminated from the tissues, the infection comes to a favourable end.

However, at times these fragments may clog the passages and cause serious complications, for instance, bronchial or biliary abscess and retention of urine. Apart from the anaphylactic effects, most serious sequelae may arise when the cyst ruptures into the abdominal or pleural cavity. In such cases the fragments of the cyst membrane, the scolices or the brood-capsules which possess a remarkable capacity of regeneration often give rise to new complete cysts in these cavities or in neighbouring tissues. In extreme cases, hundreds of cysts may develop and expand the abdomen to enormous proportions. When this happens, the so-called disseminated hydatidosis results and requires repeated surgical intervention to remove the numerous cysts that may grow in unequal succession over a number of years. There are records of such secondary cysts becoming apparent many years after incomplete removal or rupture of the primary cyst.

Another sequela of a rupturing *Echinococcus* cyst may be embolism of arteries, ordinarily in the lungs, but sometimes in distant organs, caused by the scattered debris of the cyst which gain entrance to the blood vessels.

References p. 682

Hydatid disease of vital organs, such as, for instance, the brain, kidney and heart, may have grave consequences if the cysts are not diagnosed and removed in time. Cerebral echinococcosis invariably causes the deformation of brain tissue; yet a cyst in the frontal lobe may sometimes grow to large size before producing symptoms. Echinococcosis of the spinal column always bears a serious prognosis. In several cases the cyst cannot be surgically removed because it erodes the vertebrae in all directions. Moreover, the diagnosis is difficult, and even when it is made, the damage is often already irreparable.

Apart from injury to health, hydatidosis causes serious material losses. Neghme *et al.* (1956) calculated that each afflicted person has to spend on the average 50 days in hospital. Human hydatidosis costs the *"Beneficiencia Publica"* in Chile several millions every year.

In animals, hydatid cysts are considerably less pathogenic than in man. Frequently numerous cysts occupying a large volume are found in the lungs of cattle, sheep or wild ruminants, obviously without affecting the animals's health. Equally remarkable is the fact that many thousands of adult echinococci may cover the intestinal mucosa of an apparently perfectly healthy dog. On the other hand, hydatidosis of domestic ruminants presents one of the most important of the diseases which affect animal industry. Because of its high incidence and continuous lowering of the meat, milk and wool production it inflicts enormous economic damage. In New Zealand, for example, the annual loss through condemnation of infected organs alone amounts to £ 1,500,000 (Begg *et al.,* 1957).

Despite decades of scientific endeavour, the diagnosis of hydatid disease in man is often a perplexing task. Four lines of diagnostic approach involving clinical, radiological, microscopical and serological methods, are usually applied.

Clinical observation is usually of little avail. The cysts are concealed in the tissues and, when clinical signs occur, they cannot usually be interpreted without additional laboratory investigation. Although eosinophilia appears in hydatid disease, it is inconstant, irregular and not specific, thus also of limited diagnostic value.

On the other hand, X-ray examination is most valuable and it is often decisive. The characteristic globular shadow of a solitary cyst is sometimes unmistakable, but often it provides no more than a suggestion.

The differentiation of complicated, dead or multiple cysts from tumours or various other pathological processes is not always possible. In cases of difficulty in the diagnosis of a hydatid in the liver choleangiography and portography are the modern methods of investigation. Microscopical examination is the simplest method, but its application is very limited. Diagnosis is effectively established by recovery of the scolices or their hooklets. This may occasionally succeed in cases in which fragments of ruptured hydatid cysts are evacuated in the urine, sputum or ascitic or pleural fluids.

In some cases serological tests may provide the desired clue, although their value is limited. Authors do not agree on the reliability and relative value of any of these tests. This is mainly due to lack of standardization of the antigen. In addition to the lack of uniformity of the antigens prepared in various laboratories, they are group-specific, so that they also react with antibodies against species of the genus *Taenia*.

The nature of the hydatid antigen is still insufficiently known. It is contained in varying strength in the hydatid fluid and in extracts of scolices or the germinative membrane. It is believed that it is highly diluted in or even absent from sterile cysts which lack scolices. Various methods of purification of the antigen have been proposed, but none has been universally accepted. Most laboratory workers think that the fluid of a living fertile cyst developing in the lung or liver of a man, sheep, horse or pig is most suitable. This fluid, preserved in 0.5% phenol or 1:10,000 merthiolate, may be kept for years without losing strength.

The serological test most frequently used is the complement–fixation reaction first proposed by Ghedini in 1906 and properly evaluated and described by Weinberg (1908–1909), under whose name it became popular. Performed with a suitable antigen this test reveals about 80% of infections; it becomes negative a few months after surgical removal of the hydatid. It does, however, show a certain number of false positive reactions.

The intradermal test, first described by Puntoni (1910) and elaborated by Casoni (1912), is next most commonly used. There is much controversy as to its diagnostic value. Some authors are sceptical about it because frequently it gives false-positive and false-negative reactions. The test is of the immediate-reaction type and is convenient in use. It has, however, the disadvantage in that it remains positive for years, possibly for the rest of the patient's life, even after the cyst has become calcified or suppurative or has been removed (Magath, 1953).

The haemagglutination test which is the latest diagnostic innovation is said to be superior to both of the methods mentioned above (Kagan *et al.*, 1959; Garabedian *et al.*, 1959; Cameron, 1960). The bentonite-flocculation test (Norman *et al.*, 1959) and the collodion-flocculation test (Coudert and Coly, 1956) are very sensitive, but require prolonged and complicated preparation of the antigen. Both of these tests are still in the experimental stage.

Unfortunately there is no effective chemotherapy for hydatid disease. Numerous efforts to kill hydatid cysts in the human body by means of drugs, vaccines or physical methods (diathermy, X-rays, etc.) have failed to give beneficial results. The only treatment which may be expected to provide radical cure is the surgical removal of the hydatid. However, this is possible only in cases in which the cysts are favourably located. Most difficult to remove are hydatids in the bones. In every case the aim of the operation is to remove, or mortify the total of the parasitic tissue, in order to prevent its regeneration or dissemination. It is, therefore, imperative in every operation to sterilize the cyst-ridden cavity by swabbing it with 2% formalin or iodine.

Since not all cysts develop simultaneously, it frequently occurs that some time after an initial operation a new cyst which was not apparent originally appears in the same or neighbouring organ. Gayenko (1958) quoted a case in which for this reason a patient had to be operated upon three times during a period of 4 years and each time a cyst as large as child's head was removed.

Although the progress of surgical technique resulted in considerable decrease of mortality due to hydatid disease, even treated hydatid disease still causes a 2 to 6% mortality.

In cases of inoperable hydatid disease, the so-called "biological treatment" has been proposed (Calgano; Turner *et al.,* Faiguenbaum and Fanta). This entails the repeated intradermal injection of very small doses of the hydatid antigen or of its albuminoid fraction. It does not kill the hydatid but results in allergic desensitization of the patient and thus prevents complications if the cyst should rupture. It is presumed that "biological treatment" arrests the development of the hydatid and, by lessening reaction of the host's tissues, improves his general state of health. However, this method has not yet progressed beyond the experimental stage.

Experience shows that, if left unchecked, hydatid disease in endemic localities will not disappear spontaneously. In order to reduce the spread of the infection, control measures must be vigorously applied. The anti-hydatidosis campaign carried through in Iceland may serve as a model. The remarkable success in the almost complete eradication of hydatid disease in that country is due to relentless enforcement of the control measures (described by Dungall, 1957).

It is evident that, if it is to be successful, any control system must have the cooperation of the public. Essential, therefore, is the education of the local population, particularly of farmers and butchers, concerning the life history of the parasite and the dangers connected with the indiscriminate feeding of dogs with entrails of sheep or cattle.

In Iceland, as long ago as 1863, the government distributed to every family in the country a pamphlet on the nature of hydatid disease in which were described and explained the precautionary measures to be taken, the greatest emphasis being placed on the prevention of dogs from reaching the organs of slaughtered sheep or cattle. A powerful propaganda campaign was waged in the schools and the story of the life cycle of *Echinococcus* was incorporated in the text-books.

It is of primary importance to make slaughterhouses or slaughter-places inaccessible to dogs by thorough fencing. Not only must infected organs be condemned but special stress should be laid on their destruction by boiling or by dumping into dog-proof pits. It should be noted that offal, thoroughly heated to at least 55° is rendered safe for dogs.

The elimination of stray dogs is the next important measure. In some regions in which wild animals such as jackals or wolves participate in the life-cycle of the parasite, they too should be subject to eradication.

A dog infected or suspected of infection with *Echinococcus* is often a cause for embarrassment at home. It should be stressed that the identification of *Echinococcus* eggs in canine excrements is by no means simple. These eggs are so similar to those of any of half a dozen other species of tapeworms parasitic in dogs that differentiation is possible only in fresh stool evacuated by purgative, which contains the entire undigested segments of *Echinococcus*. Serological tests are impracticable in dogs in which *Echinococcus* infection may be masked by the presence of infection with various species of *Taenia*.

As there are no simple means of diagnosing echinococcosis in the dog, all domestic dogs in endemic regions should be regarded as potential carriers of the worm. They must be registered and should undergo anthelminthic treatment at least twice a year. Although this treatment is not always satisfactory, it may bring about a substantial reduction of the infestation. The most popular drug is *Arecoline hydrobromide* which in a dose of 4 mg/kg body weight not only kills most or all of the worms but also immediately eliminates them by its strong purgative action. Deworming should be carried out either in a special building or in a tightly-fenced place, in which the dogs may be kept chained for several hours until the worms have been eliminated. Great care should then be taken to destroy the highly infective stools of the dogs. However effective the measures enumerated may be, only a few contries can boast success in the eradication of hydatid disease.

Another aspect of *Echinococcus* control is the disposal of the eggs of the parasite. This is a serious problem when the life-cyle of the parasite is synanthropic, *i.e.,* when it occurs near to human habitations. Unfortunately, little has been done to prevent infection originating from pet dogs in urban areas. A dog owner "excercising" his pet on the sidewalk and letting its excrements be dispersed by the feet of pedestrians is a common sight, even in modern towns. Wind and flies transport the viable *Echinococcus* eggs from the street to the home and deposit them on human food. It should be noted that the eggs of *Echinococcus* are rather resistant to outdoor conditions. They may remain viable for two years in water at 2°C and may survive for short periods at a temperature as low as —50° (Leikina, 1957). Fortunately enough, prolonged dryness is detrimental to the eggs. Conventional desinfectants do not kill them even after extended contact. When there is need to disinfect soiled objects or floors, a 5% solution of hypochlorite can be used successfully.

Attempts have been made to vaccinate dogs against echinococcosis, but the practical utility of this has still to be established. Turner *et al.* (1936), Forsek and Rukavina (1959), and others, have shown that the number of worms in immunized dogs was distinctly lower and that the longevity of the worms was shorter than it was in control animals. Full immunity, however, has not been achieved.

iii. Alveolar echinococcosis
For almost a century, the validity of the species that causes alveolar echinococcosis was a subject of controversy among scientists, because the diversity of *Echinococcus* species could not be proved by morphological differences in the adult worms. The multilocular species has, therefore, for a long time been regarded merely as a peculiar race which differs from the common *Echinococcus granulosus* in the shape of the larval stage. In 1951 Rausch and Schiller, conducting research on St. Lawrence Island, off the West coast of Alaska, published the observation that multilocular *Echinococcus* occurs in small rodents, while the corresponding adult stage, distinguishable from *E. granulosus*, lives in the polar fox *(Alopex lagopus)* as well as in the dog. Subsequently, Vogel (1957) showed that the Alaskan species is identical with the European alveolar *Echinococcus (E. multilocularis)*. This investigator found, in a

reputedly endemic region in Southern Germany, the larval stage of the parasite in about 1 % of voles *(Microtus arvalis)* and the adult stage in 40 % of common foxes *(Vulpes vulpes)*. In feeding experiments Vogel proved that the fox, as well as the dog and cat (the latter being refractory to infection with *E. granulosus*), may serve as definitive hosts of the adult *E. multilocularis*, while several species of small wild rodents in Europe *(Microtus agrestis, Clethrionomys glareolus* and *Arvicola terrestris)* and also the *domestic mouse* are receptive as intermediate hosts.

The anatomy and life history of the adult form of the two species of *Echinococcus* are rather similar, yet show distinct differences in details (the number of the segments, rostellar hooks and testes; the length of the body and of the ripe segments; the position of the testes, ovary and genital pore; the structure of the uterus; the development in the fox and cat and the time of the first appearance of the eggs).

The life cycle of *E. multilocularis* is predominantly sylvatic. Unlike *E. granulosus* its most suitable hosts are red and polar foxes. Under natural conditions 40 to 100 % of arctic foxes were found to be infected. *E. multilocularis* also matures in the dog, cat and wolf. Many small rodents, some herbivores and man may serve as its intermediate hosts, while voles are the most suitable. The incidence of natural infection in the Tundra vole *(Microtus economus)* amounts to 50 %, but usually it varies greatly, depending on the locality and season.

The oncospheres of *E. multilocularis* predominantly settle in the liver. As a rule a small vesicle develops initially and soon, through both exogenous and endogenous budding of the germinative membrane, new small cysts are given off in every direction until finally the hydatid becomes a tight cluster of small vesicles *(alveolar echinococcus* or *alveolar hydatid)*.

In *man* the alveolar hydatid may be necrotic at the center and filled with a putrid content; it is often surrounded by a thick capsule of connective tissue. In such cysts scolices are rare. Growth is slow and may continue for several years, but metastases can be given off and secondary cysts of identical character may appear in various parts of the body. Dardel (1927, as cited by Vogel, 1957) found cerebral involvement in over 5 % of cases of human alveolar echinococcosis in Switzerland. If it is not checked, this hydatid infection is invariably fatal. In the early stages its recognition is difficult. As the growth of the cystic structure progresses, enlargement of the liver, ascites and icterus appear, these symptoms indicating intrahepatic portal hypertension. On clinical and X-ray examination, alveolar *Echinococcus* may be easily confused with malignant tumour. The usual immunological diagnosis (Weinberg's or Casoni's test) seems to be unreliable (Rausch, 1958). Kagan *et al.* (1959) found that the haemagglutination and flocculation tests are not satisfactory in the differentiation of unilocular and alveolar hydatids.

The incidence of alveolar hydatidosis in Eskimos is mostly due to the prevailing fox-trapping practices. Soiling of the hands and consequently of the food is inevitable during skinning.

The eggs of multiocular *Echinococcus* are very resistant to low temperature and may survive for several years in the extreme cold of Arctic regions. According to Leikina (1957), viable eggs were found in the carcass of a polar fox which had lain for several years under snow in the Tundra. Schiller (1955) found eggs which were still infective after exposure in the laboratory to temperatures as low as $-56°$.

In microtine rodents (and some other suitable hosts) the alveolar hydatid causes a fulminating disease which results in the deaths of these animals in about 5 to 6 weeks. The growth of the cyst is malignant in character and invades the tissues until almost the entire liver is destroyed. Necrosis does not develop, but, as in man, fragments of the germinative membrane are carried with the blood to various parts of the body and thus start metastatic clusters of cysts.

Sheep, pigs, golden hamsters, albino rats and albino mice are unsuitable as intermediate hosts and cannot be infected. However, cotton-rats proved to be very susceptible; they die of the infection within 30 to 75 days.

Knowledge about the geographical distribution (Fig. 97) of *Echinococcus multilocularis* has been widened since the clarification of its life history.

Previously it had been known mainly from Central Europe (Tyrol, Bavaria, Switzerland), but now the presence of this parasite has also been established in East Europe, as well as in the northern half of the Asiatic continent. Euzeby (1960) found infected foxes in the Upper Savoie. Cases were also reported from Yugoslavia. Petrov *et al.* (1960) gave a summary of the distribution of alveolar *Echinococcus* in the Soviet Union. They recognized 20 endemic zones, of which the most important are: the whole of the European and Asiatic northern Tundra zone, Central Siberia, the Central

Asiatic republics* and some European parts of the Soviet Union (Bielorussia, the Stalingrad region, the Ukraine, East Caucasus). Additional findings were reported from Turkey, the Mongolian Republic, the Kurile and Komandorski Islands and limited locations in Japan (the Rebun Island; Rausch and Yamashita, 1957). In some of these zones *Echinococcus multilocularis* has been found in the adult stage in polar or red foxes, the wolf and dog, and, in the larval stage, in numerous species of small rodents and in the wild boar. Also appreciable numbers of human cases have been recorded.

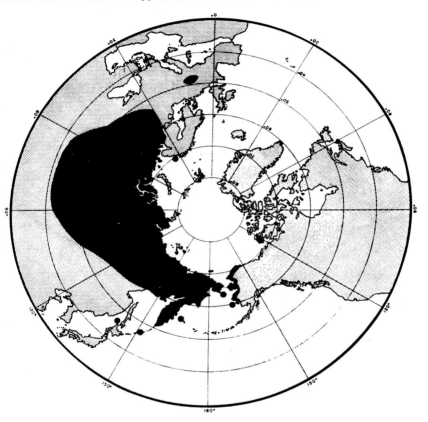

Fig. 97.   Approximate distribution (dark areas and circles) of Echinococcus multi-lulocaris, based on records in the literature (courtesy Dr. R. L. Rausch, Anchorage Alaska, Proc. Sixth Internat. Congr. trop. med. and Malaria, Lisbon, 1958).

---

* In Kazakhstan alveolar *echinococcus* made up 1/3 of all cases of human hydatid disease (Arslanova, 1960). In the Barabinsk steppe Lukashenko (1960) found *E. multiolocularis* in 43% of red foxes, in 80% of wolves and in 2% of dogs. Kadenazi (1959) recorded up to 40% of foxes and 16% of wolves infected in the Omsk region.

St. Lawrence Island, where Rausch and Schiller found a widespread incidence of alveolar echinococcosis (in 40–100% of polar foxes), may be regarded as a continuation of the vast north-Asiatic area of endemicity, comprising also the Kurile Islands and, as an offshoot, the Japanese island of Rebun.

The only possible course of treatment is surgical resection of the affected hepatic lobe, but the chances of recovery are slim, especially in advanced cases. Semionov (1954) summarized data on 152 cases of alveolar echinococcosis recorded in the Soviet Union. Of these 71% were inoperable, 14% terminated fatally after treatment and 8% were cured (for the remaining 7% the result is not given).

REFERENCES

BORAY, J. *Acta vet. Acad. Sci. hung.*, 4 (1954) 93.
DÉVÉ, F. *L'échinococcose secondaire*, Paris, 1946, 288 pp.; *L'échinococcose osseuse*, Montevideo, 1948, 235 pp.; *L'échinococcose primitive*, Paris, 1949, 362 pp.
DEW, H. R. *Hydatid disease*, Sydney, Austral. Med. Publ., 1928, 429 pp.; *Arch. intern. Hidatidosis*, 13 (1953) 319.
DUNGAL, N. *N. Z. med. J.*, 56 (1957) 213.
FANTA, E., J. FAIGUENBAUM and A. NEGHME, *Arch. intern. Hidatidosis*, 11 (1950) 319.
FERRO, A. and A. CHIO, *Pren. med. argent.*, (1950) 1.
GEMMELL, M. A., *Aust. Vet. J.*, 36 (1960) 73.
HEUSCHEN, C. and R. BIRCHER, *Bull. schweiz. Akad. med. Wiss.*, 1 (1945) 209.
HUTCHISON, W. F., *Amer. J. trop. Med. Hyg.*, 9 (1960) 612.
JACKSON-DAVIS, H. *Arch. intern. Hidatidosis*, 7 (1947) 219.
JORGE, J. M., *Arch. intern. Hidatidosis*, 11 (1950) 231.
KAGAN, J. G., L. NORMAN and D. S. ALLAIN, *Amer. J. trop. Med. Hyg.*, 9 (1960) 248.
MAGATH, J. B., *Arch. intern. Hidatidosis*, 11 (1950) 193; ibid., 13 (1952) 218.
MILLER, M. J. *Arch. intern. Hidatidosis*, 13 (1953) 333.
NEGHME, A. and R. SILVA, *Bull. Chileno Parasit.*, 16 (1961) 27.
NORMAN, L., E. H. SADUN and D. S. ALLAIN, *Am. J. trop. Med. Hyg.*, 8 (1959) 46.
PEREZ-FONTANA, V., *Arch. intern. Hidatidosis*, 5 (1941) 18, 421, 596.
PETROV, A. M., A. S. GORINA and R. S. DELIANOVA, *Trans. 12th Meeting All Soviet Union Helm. Soc.*, 1958, p. 105.
RAUSCH, R. and E. L. SCHILLER, *Parasitology*, 46 (1956) 395.
SCHILLER, E. L., *Ann. intern. Med.*, 52 (1960) 464.
VOGEL, H., *Dtsch. med. Wschr.*, 80 (1955) 931; *Z. Tropenmed. Parasit.*, 8 (1957) 404.
WOLFGANG, W. and J. B POOLE, *Amer. J. trop. Med. Hyg.*, 5 (1956) 869.

e. Diphyllobothriasis

i. Introduction

Numerous species of the cestode genera *Diphyllobothrium* (called in the earlier literature *Dibothriocephalus* or *Bothriocephalus*) are parasites of man, mammals or birds which feed on fish or other vertebrates serving as vectors of the larval stage. Some of these species are specific to their final hosts, others may establish themselves in phylogenetically distant hosts, including man.

Diphyllobothriid tapeworms are characterised by their mace-shaped scolex, provided with two slit-like suckers which serve as holdfast-organs by which the worm is attached to the intestinal mucosa of the final host.

At present, the nomenclature of the cestodes in question is still in a state of controversy. Faust, Campbell and Kellog (1929) divided this genus in two subgenera: one, *Diphyllobothrium*, in which the loops of the uterus show a rosette-like pattern, and the second, *Spirometra*, in which the uterus is spirally twisted. Mueller (1937) has raised these subgenera to the status of genera. The species belonging to the genus *Diphyllobothrium* are parasites of man in their adult stage, while the species of the genus *Spirometra* are found in man only in their larval stage, which is called *Sparganum*.

Man shares with animals the infection caused by either the larval or adult stage of several species of these tapeworms. Numerous species belonging to this group have been incriminated as parasites of both man and animals. Recent investigations, however, cast doubt on the validity of some of these species.

There is still less certainty about the species of plerocercoids found in fish. Plerocercoids of most species are so similar in their simple structure that the only method of differentiating between them is to conduct feeding experiments on proper hosts. This has usually not been done and it is therefore difficult to assess the existing statistics regarding the infection of fish.

ii. *Diphyllobothrium latum infection*

The best known species of the group is *D. latum* *, also called the "broad tapeworm" or "fish tapeworm" of man. With respect to anatomy and life history it may serve as a model for other species. It is specific to man, but can also develop in several other mammals in which it apparently does not thrive as well as in man. Yet, in some instances these animals may serve as reservoirs from which the infection spreads to man. *D. latum* is the longest known cestode (and the longest known animal). Usually it is about 10 metres long, but may rarely be as long as 20 metres).

The adult worm lives in the middle part of the small intestine where it is held in the form of a bundle fastened to the intestinal mucosa by means of the two suckers on its scolex. The worm, which may contain several thousand segments, moves slowly but constantly, opposing the pressure

---

* According to Magath (1937) Thaddeus Dunus of Locarno gave a suggestive description of the worm as early as 1592.

References p. 691

of the peristaltic movement of the intestine. In the anterior part of the chain the segments are short and wide, in the posterior part they are almost square.

Attempts to decipher the life history of *D. latum* were made by several early investigators. Although Braun, as early as 1882, showed that infection with *D. latum* is connected with the eating of fish, a further 46 years were needed until Janicki and Rosen (1918) elucidated the complicated life cycle of this parasite, establishing that it requires at least two obligatory intermediate hosts.

The ovoid operculated eggs, which are about 70 microns long, contain a zygote, surrounded by a mass of yolk cells. Some of them are discharged from the ripe segments before these are cast off the chain. Eventually a number of proglottids containing uteri filled with eggs are detached from the posterior extremity of the worm either singly or in short chains. Thus both eggs and proglottids appear in the faeces. A single worm may discharge as many as a million eggs every day. When the eggs reach fresh water, under summer conditions, the first-stage larva *(coracidium)* develops inside them within 10 to 14 days. At low temperatures (about 1° C) the eggs keep alive for several months without developing. Each densely ciliated and actively swimming *coracidium* contains an *onchosphere*, which must be eaten by copepods of the genera *Diaptomus* or *Cyclops*. In every endemic region *D. latum* is adapted to some particular species of these copepods. When a *coracidium* is swallowed by this intermediate host the oncosphere is released in the stomach and wanders into the body cavity, where it develops in about 2 weeks into the next larval stage, the *procercoid*. The procercoid, which is still microscopic in size, consists of an elongated body and a globular appendage. Several procercoids may be harboured by one, almost microscopic, copepod. When the infected copepods are eaten by certain kinds of fish the procercoids are set free, penetrate through the wall of the stomach or intestine of the fish and migrate to various visceral organs (the liver, ovaries, mesentery, etc.) or to the muscles. In these organs they remain free and develop into the third stage, called *plerocercoid*, which eventually grows to a length of several centimeters. The plerocercoid is infective for the definitive host. Under normal circumstances the copepods are eaten by small fishes which do not serve as food for man and thus the plerocercoids are not in a position to reach man. However, these small infected fish are in their turn eaten by certain predatory fish and the plerocerdoids, liberated in the intestines, are not digested but again traverse the stomach wall and migrate to the viscera of the fish-host, in which they continue life at the same stage as that in which they existed in the fish from which they were derived*. As the predator eats more and more small fish it can acquire a great number of plerocercoids. Plerocercoids of every species of diphyllobothriid tapeworms require

---

* French authors have given this process the rather misleading name "re-encapsulation". As a matter of fact, the plerocercoids do not become encapsulated but move freely and erratically in the tissues of the fish.

particular species of fish as hosts. The most suitable fish species for *D. latum* are: pike (*Esox* sp., *Schizostedion* sp.), perch (*Perca* sp.) and burbot (*Lota* sp.).

Plerocercoids found in other species of fish, notably in salmonids, belong to other diphyllobothriid species which develop to the adult stage in fish-eating birds or mammals. A large number of species of fish have been reported as harbouring the plerocercoids of *D. latum*, but subsequent researches have shown that some of these plerocercoids belonged to different species of the same tapeworm group. The morphology of plerocercoids of different species of *Diphyllobothrium* is similar, and identification of the plerocercoids of various species of *diphyllobothriid* tapeworms is not always possible.

When the flesh of fish infected with the plerocercoids of *D. latum* is eaten by man, dog or another suitable host, the parasites reach the small intestine of this host and extrude the scolex by which they attach themselves to the mucosa; they then develop to the adult stage in the course of a few weeks. The minimum age at which the plerocercoid becomes infective for the final host is not known. Kuhlow (1950) presumes that it is approximately 2–3 months and that this period may vary according to the species of fish.

D. latum remains alive in man for a very long time. Riley (1919) recorded the case of a patient in whom this tapeworm was still found alive after 29 years. In another case its longevity (in a person 100 years old) was estimated at 40 years. Often several specimens establish themselves in the human intestine. Yaldigina (1960) recorded a case in which 201 worms were expelled from a single person; Tarassov (1936) described a 23 year old patient from whom 143 worms, with a total length of 117 metres were expelled, the longest of them measuring 17 metres.

Although *man* is the most suitable definitive host of the adult *D. latum*, this worm may also develop in many other mammals, among them the domestic *pig, dog* and *cat*. All these animals may be infected to a high degree in localities (*e.g.* Finland, Alaska, and Siberia) where fish constitute the habitual human food and the offal is accessible to domesticated animals. Tarassov (1935) found 100% of pigs infected in some of the villages north of Leningrad.

The most important source of dissemination of *D. latum* is the *dog*, not only because this animal itself may serve as a final host, but mainly because of its close connection with man's habitation, its habit of feeding on offal and dispersing indiscriminately of its faeces. Saunders (1949) recorded the infection of 34–47% in dogs in Canada (Alberta). Kuhlow (1950) has shown that infection with *D. latum* may possibly be maintained without the participation of man. He found infected fish in regions near Hamburg where local human infection is unknown.

However, the part played by mammals as reservoirs of human infection with *D. latum* is still a matter of controversy. Some contemporary investigators tend to attach to these animals only a limited significance.

Kuhlow (1955), and Petrov and Dubnitzky (1959) found that up to 100% of the plerocercoids may reach full development in the dog, while the lengths of the adult worms do not surpass 6.5 metres and their longevity is about 1 year. On the other hand, the assertion of Essex and Magath (1931), supported by Tarassov (1934), that only a proportion of *Diphyllobothrium* eggs discharged by the dog are capable of development, contradicts the observation of Hobmaier (1927) and Kuhlow (1955), who found that the eggs discharged by dogs were all viable.

Le Bas (1924), Ward (1929) and Podyapolskaya (1958) *et al.* expressed the opinion that the *cat* is not a suitable host of *D. latum*. It was shown that the development of the worm in a cat requires 3 months, while in man it is completed within 4–6 weeks. Moreover, the worm remains alive in the cat several months only as compared with many years in man.

Next in importance in the epidemiology of diphyllobothriasis is the *fox*, although it is a poor host. In the red fox, *D. latum* may reach 1.60 metres, but it survives for only about 100 days. In the polar fox the worm reaches only 0.5 metre in length.

Age and race apparently play no part in human infection. In endemic regions all the inhabitants are liable to infection. Zachokke *et al.* (1932) recorded the infection in a child under 2 years of age in East Germany.

In spite of the complexity of the life history of *D. latum*, which might be expected to limit its distribution, this parasite has been recorded in diverse regions, all of them temperate or cool. The exact geographical distribution of the parasite cannot, however, be assessed with accuracy at present, because many of the existing records are based on inadequate observation of the anatomy of the worms found, so that the validity of the identification of their species is uncertain.

The maintenance of human infection is the result of several factors, *i.e.* (a) the presence of human and or animal reservoirs, (b) the presence of suitable intermediate hosts, (c) the feeding habits of the population, chiefly the ingestion of inadequately cooked fish products, and (d) the extent of the pollution of natural waters. Changes in any one of these factors, usually in the feeding habits, may drastically change the incidence of human infection.

For instance, in 1932 Zschokke *et al.* found that up to 34% of the German population of the Kurisches Haff (which then was a part of East Prussia) were infected with *D. latum*. As Vogel (1929) explained, the infection was maintained by the custom of eating raw fish liver. Gervel *et al.* did not find a single case among 679 persons of the new population of this region, examined in 1957. In some countries, as in Yugoslavia, *Diphyllobothrium* does not occur, although the natural conditions and the availability of suitable intermediate hosts would seem to favour spread of the infection (Simitch and Petrovitch, 1955).

Lack of sanitary habits and the pollution of water basins with sewage are important factors in the spread of the infection. When human excreta are introduced into open waters the coracidia become available to the copepod hosts and when fish offal is disposed of indiscriminately the plerocercoids are put at the disposal of scavenging mammals.

The highest incidence of infection with *D. latum* is found in the countries bordering the Baltic Sea (Finland, Sweden, Lithuania, etc.) where the abundance of lake-fish facilitates spread of the parasite. This region is followed in importance by North Russia, Central Siberia, the lower Volga region, Switzerland and North America. Records of other localities, such as Australia, Africa and South America are *sub judice* until the specific identity of the locally prevailing species has been adequately investgated. Vik and Muroma (1956) estimated that almost 1 million people of Finland's population of 4.5 millions harbour this parasite. Records have been published (Holander, 1945) which show that 20–25% of the inhabitants of certain parishes near the coast of Finland and up to 50% of those in the eastern parts of the country are infected. According to Fagerstrom (1952) 100,000 cases of *Diphyllobothrium* infection are treated every year in that country.

Tarassov (1933, 1936) found that more than 40% of the population in the villages north of Petrozavodsk (north-west Russia) were infected. In some places the infection rate of the population rose to 78%, while 100% of burbot *(Lota lota)*, 88% of pike *(Esox lucius)*, and 35% of perch *(Perca fluviatilis)* were infected with the plerocercoids of *D. latum*. According to Shmielova (1955), the plerocercoids are most abundant in the abdominal cavities of the fish or under the serous coats of the stomach and intestine; in the muscles their incidence was lower. The organ most important for the transmission of the infection to man is the roe, which provides the "ikra" (caviar), which is eaten raw or slightly salted soon after its preparation. Usually a few plerocercoids are found in a single fish, but sometimes as many as 1000 may be counted (Petruchevsky, 1951).

There is little information on the presence of *D. latum* in the Far East. An endemic focus on the Sakhalin Islands has been mentioned, in which, according to Bombelo (1960), 20% of the aborigines harbour a species that may be *D. latum*.

The cases of infection with *D. latum* recorded in North America during the first quarter of the present century occurred mostly among immigrants from Scandinavian countries. As Magath (1931, 1937) and others have shown, *D. latum* is present in the northern United States. In certain lakes, which drain into Canada, up to 100% of the fish suitable as hosts harbour the plerocercoids of *D. latum*. The relevant fish-species are: pike *(Schizostedion* sp.), perch *(Perca flavescens)* and burbot *(Lota maculosa)*. According to Cameron (1936), in Central Canada the plerocercoids of *D. latum* develop in pike, pickerel, sanger and perch. However, in 1945 this author expressed some doubt as to whether the species concerned is really identical with *D. latum*. Saunders (1949) recorded that 14 to 60% of the aborigines of Alberta carry *D. latum*. Vergeer (1928, 1930) suggested that dogs play a prominent role in disseminating this parasite. However, in the light of recent reports on the species of *Diphyllobothrium* occurring in North America, the identity of worms mentioned by this author must possibly be revaluated. Barron (1929) called attention to the fact that many infections occur in Jewish women. He explained this by the custom of preparing so called "gefüllte Fisch", which is made of minced fish meat tasted for flavour before it is cooked.

There is apparently no age limit to infection with *D. latum*. The course of the pathogenic process is similar in men and women. In most cases infection with *D. latum* is benign and people can often ignore slight symptoms for years. In a few instances, however, a most severe sequela develops in the form of pernicious anaemia.

This appears as a consequence of the megaloblastic hyperplasia of the bone-marrow and its effect on the patient closely resembles the so-called Addison's or Biermer's (also called idiopathic or cryptogenetic) anaemia. Cryptogenetic anaemia is due to a constitutional atrophy of the mucous lining of the stomach, resulting in the arrest or reduction of the gastric secretion containing the *intrinsic factor* of Castle. The mechanism of the appearance of *Diphyllobothrium*-anaemia is not yet fully clear. Usually the gastric secretion of *Diphyllobothrium* carriers corresponds to that of non-infected people and the intrinsic factor is not reduced (Hellander, 1945). Von Bonsdorf (1948) and Chandler (1950) suggested the explanation that this anaemia is caused chiefly by the intensive absorption of vitamin B_{12} by the worm, whereby an insufficient quantity of this substance is left to the human organism. The fact that not every infected man develops anaemia is explained by the different location of the worm. *D. latum* is most frequently located in the ileum, rarely in the jejunum or in the colon. When it is in the ileum, the worm absorbs vitamin B_{12} before it can be absorbed by the intestinal mucosa and thus gives rise to anaemia, whereas, when the worm is lower down the alimentary canal, the vitamin has already been absorbed by the intestinal mucosa before it could reach the worm and therefore anaemia does not occur. The causative influence of *Diphyllobothrium* on the genesis of anaemia is evident when the symptoms dramatically disappear with the expulsion of the worm.

Exact statistics about the incidence of anaemia occurring as a result of *Diphyllobothrium* infection are available for only a few investigated localities. The frequency of clinically observed morbidity is still a matter of controversy. It is generally accepted that it occurs only in one of several hundreds or even thousands of infected persons. Yet Bazhenova (1960) found pernicious anaemia in 7% of infected people; however, in 40% of them macrocytosis was the only symptom. In persons from whom the worms had been previously expelled, slight macrocytosis and hypochromia lasted for up to 3 years after treatment. The incidence apparently depends largely on the constitution of the individual concerned and on the nutritional habits of the population. The syndrome develops gradually and the patients usually do not apply to the doctor before the symptoms become disturbing.

The complaints consist of fatigue, dizziness or nausea, anorexia, rarely abdominal pain or diarrhoea, palpitation, paraesthesia of the fingers and toes, and sometimes soreness of the tongue. In later stages glossitis occurs accompanied with more or less marked atrophy of the papillae. Loss of weight is usually not marked. The patient often looks pale, with subicteric shade, and sometimes shows oedema of the ankles. The erythrocyte-count may fall to 500,000–1,000,000, and the haemoglobin index to less than 20%. The colour-index may be increased. Poikilocytosis, anisocytosis with a preponderance of macrocytes, polychromasia, basophilic stippling and nuclear fragmentation occur in most cases to varying degrees. Occasionally normoblasts or megaloblasts are found. The leucocyte-count is usually normal, but a decrease to a figure as low as 2,000 has been observed. The white cell picture is, as a rule, characterised by lymphocytosis, the appearance of hypersegmented neutrophils and occasionally by eosinophilia. The thrombocyte count may be reduced to a value below 20,000 and the prothrombin value is lowered (Tötterman, 1939, 1944; von Bonsdorf, 1956). The bone-marrow shows hyperplasia of the erythrocytic stem cells, mainly of the promegaloblasts and megaloblasts, and numerous immature cells and giant leucocytes.

The amount of gastric juice (in the Ewald and Boas test) is normal; free hydrochloric acid is often present as well as Castle's intrinsic factor; uropepsin is excreted at a normal rate in about 50% of cases.

Neurological symptoms rarely develop only in neglected cases when anaemia has persisted for years. Severe sequelae may appear such as, for instance, spinal cord disturbances, degeneration of peripheral nerves and atrophy of the tongue. The following symptoms can thus become evident (Björkenheim, 1957): paraesthesia in the form of numbness and formication of the fingers and lower extremities; impairment of tactile sensation; markedly diminished muscle tone in the lower extremities; stiffness of the fingers, the patient not being able to button his coat; difficulty in walking and ataxia.

In some cases of *Diphyllobothrium* infection a slight hyperchromic anaemia occurs with normal gastric acidity. In 6 cases out of 12 treatment

with liver preparations (Tötterman, 1944) had no effect, while the expulsion of the parasite was effective. This author supposed that the two
types of tapeworm anaemia, pernicious and hyperchromic, are not different stages of the same blood disease; it is presumed that the hyperchromic
anaemia is caused by resorption of tapeworm toxins.

The diagnosis of diphyllobothriasis is made by finding in the faeces the characteristic
ova and segments of *Diphyllobothrium*; in repeated stool examinations they are invariably detected. When the diagnosis is doubtful, differential diagnosis of the anaemia
should be made, by taking into consideration Addison's anaemia, which chiefly affects
elderly persons, the absence of Castle's intrinsic factor and a diminished amount of
free acid in the stomach.

In many instances the presence of *Diphyllobothrium* is discovered by chance during
routine examinations of stools, or even of the *oxyuris* anal swab.

Treatment should be twofold: causative and symptomatic. Fern-root
preparations or acridin compounds have a specific effect. In refractory
cases the drugs will act if they are administered through a duodenal sound.
Improvement may follow within 2 or 3 days after the treatment, provided
that the patient is given sufficient extrinsic factor. To attain this it is
advisable to provide a suitable diet rich in this element, such as, for instance, meat and milk and to administer vitamin B_{12} or liver extract. Folic
acid may be helpful, except when neurological symptoms are evident, in
which event it may, on the contrary, aggravate the condition.

The best single means of preventing the spread of *Diphyllobothrium*
infection is to teach the population to abstain from eating insufficiently
cooked fish. Wherever local conditions contradict this, other measures
may effectively alleviate the situation. Systematic treatment of people, including even those who do not show symptoms of the disease, would
diminish the chance of spreading the infection. Destruction of the
domestic offal to prevent it becoming accessible to dogs, is no less
important. Rational sewage disposal may also contribute to reduction of
the spread of the infection. When fish is stored, the following observations
should be noted: the plerocercoids of *Diphyllobothrium latum* die at $-6°$
after 7 days, at $-18°$ in 5 days and in 10% brine after 2 to 6 days,
according to the size of the fish (Titova, 1955).

In addition to the broad (fish) tapeworm, *D. latum,* which in its adult form commonly
occurs in endemic regions in man and secondarily or incidentally in other mammals,
several other species of the genus *Diphyllobothrium,* which normally are parasites of

mammals or birds, have been recorded as secondary or incidental parasites of man. Their plerocercoid stages, like that of *D. latum,* develop in fish. Podyapolskaya (1958) listed 7 species of this group as occurring in man in the Soviet Union alone: *D. giliaticum* (Rutkievich, 1937; Sakhalin Island), *D. luxi* (Rutkievich, 1937), *D. minus* (Cholodkovsky, 1916), *D. nenzi* (Petrov, 1938), *D. skrjabini,* Plotnikov, 1933, *D. strictum* Talysin, 1932 *D. tungussicum* Podyapolskaya and Gniedina, 1932. The latter species were found in 28% of *Tungus* and *Yakut aborigines* in central Siberia. In one case 477 worms were expelled from a single patient. The following additional species of this group have been recorded from other parts of the world: *D. norvegicum* (Vick, 1957, experimental infection), *D. parvum* (Stephens, 1908), *D. taenioides* (Leon, 1916), *D. cordatum* (Leuckart, 1863). The identification of most of these species was made at a time when the specific characteristics of diphyllobothriid worms were insufficiently known. When more information about these species is available, some of them will doubtless prove to be synonyms and the list may consequently be reduced. Magath (1937) stated that records of the endemic occurrence of this parasite outside the Northern temperate zone are not reliable. A number of human infections with *D. latum,* reported in literature between 1890 and 1959, were observed outside the established endemic areas. Several of these were solitary cases in which the identification of the parasite was not certain. Cameron (1957) stated that the bear is the true host of diphyllobothriids which commonly occur in man and the dog in some parts in Canada. As a matter of fact, *D. ursi* Rausch, 1954, is the species found in the North American bear. In South Wales and Eire, several cases were quoted by Baylis (1945), whereas in this locality 2 bird-inhabiting species have been found, *viz. D. dendriticum* and *D. ditremum.* which by experimental infection in mammals can develop into adult worms.

REFERENCES

BONSDORFF, B. VON, *Acta med. scand.,* 129 (1947) 213; *Exp. Parasit.,* 5 (1956) 207.
JANICKI, C. and F. ROSEN, *Korresp. Bl. schweiz. Ärz.,* 45 (1917) 1505.
KUHLOW, F., *Z. Parasitenk.,* 16 (1953) 1; *Z. Tropenmed. Parasit.,* 6 (1953) 213.
MAGATH, T. B. and H. E. ESSEX, *J. prev. Med.,* 5 (1931) 227.
TALYSIN, TH., *Z. Parasitenk.,* 2 (1930) 535; 4 (1932) 722.
TARASSOV, V. A., *Ann. Parasit.,* 14 (1936) 472.
TOETTERMAN, G., *Acta med. scand.,* 118 (1944) 422.
VIK, R., *Ny Mag. Zool.,* 5 (1957) 25.
VOGEL, H., *Dtsch. med. Wschr.,* 55 (1929) 1631.

iii. Sparganosis

In 1882 Manson, during a post mortem examination on a human subject, recovered from the perirenal tissue several larval worms which were identified by Cobbold (1883) as a new species, called *Ligula mansoni.* This species was subsequently allocated by Stiles (1902) to the group-name *Sparganum,* which merely refers to a peculiar type of cestode larvae. The Japanese investigator Ijima (1905) discovered similar larvae in a human body but these showed fission and lateral budding. These worms were regarded as a new species and were called *Sparganum proliferum*. Later, in several geographical regions of the world similar spargana were frequently found in the connective tissue and various organs of numerous animals (frogs, snakes, chicken, hedgehogs, monkeys, hogs, etc.). At that time the adult forms of these larvae were unknown and no specific correlations between the observations were made.

Eventually it was proved that spargana are plerocercoids, possibly of several species of tapeworms related to *Diphyllobothrium latum,* which develop like the latter, but differ from it by not requiring fish, but other vertebrates or, accidentally, man as hosts in their plerocercoid stage. Adult worms have been recovered from cats and dogs after experimental feeding with plerocercoids taken from other animals or from man. Infection with these worms under natural conditions has also been recorded in wild carnivores, such as the lion, tiger and fox. Subsequently it was found that the dog and domestic or wild cat *(Felis viverrina, Felis serval)* sometimes harbour the adult worms and also spargana of apparently the same species as well.

According to Wardle and McLeod (1952) at least 14 species belong to this group, but their taxonomy is still a subject of controversy. Faust, Campbell and Kellogg (1929) proposed to classify in the subgenus *Spirometra* the species which produce spargana in animals other than fishes and in this manner to separate them from the species of the genus *Diphyllobothrium*. Mueller (1936) subsequently suggested raising this subgenus *Spirometra* to generic rank *. According to Stunkard (1949) it is premature, in the present state of knowledge, to define exactly the borderline between the genera *Diphyllobothrium* and *Spirometra*. However, various biological characteristics between these two groups of worms, of which one requires fish, the other land or amphibious animals as intermediate hosts, suggest a definite taxonomic difference, and for this reason the genus *Spirometra* is adopted here.

There is also disagreement about the specific names of spargana, based on principles of zoological nomenclature, mainly that of priority. Because differentiation between species which produce spargana in different geographical regions has been inadequate, these species have been given different names according to these regions. Thus, the name *Spirometra mansoni* has been preferentially used in records from the Far East, whereas *S. erinacei europaei* (or simply *erinacei*) and *S. ranarum* are mentioned in European records, and *S. mansonoides* in the North-American records. According to Iwata (1933) spargana from various animals (hedgehogs, weasels, frogs, snakes, etc.) or from man in the Far East, develop in cats and dogs into the same adult species. Iwata reduced most of the species producing spargana *(D. decipiens, D. felis, D. houghtoni, D. mansoni, D. mansonoides, D. okumurai, D. ranarum, D. reptans)* to one species which he called *Diphyllobothrium erinacei*.

In the present chapter the specific name *S. mansoni* which is traditionally used in literature, is adopted for the Old World species, while *S. mansonoides* is retained for the North-American species.

---

* Baer and Fain (1955) suggested that the creation of a genus *Spirometra* is not justified, but if it is to be distinguished, the name *Lueheella* Baer, 1924, should have priority. Yet the generic name *Spirometra* is widely used in modern literature.

It should be stressed, however, that the synonyms of spargana and the corresponding adult worms are accepted here only as a temporary measure to provide a workable terminology. Most species of *Spirometra* are insufficiently known and the range of variations within each of them is not precisely defined. Proper names of the species of the genus *Spirometra* will be established when this deficiency has been removed.

The life history of *Spirometra* is now well established. It appears that the coracidia hatch after 12 to 14 days, and after they have been swallowed by copepods of the genus *Cyclops*, they develop into procercoids. The latter become plerocercoids (= spargana) (Fig. 98) in a wide range of hosts, including Amphibia, snakes, mammals (among them rats and monkeys) and birds (including chickens and the Guinea fowl). The size of spargana varies from a few millimeters to 40 centimeters. They are lodged in various

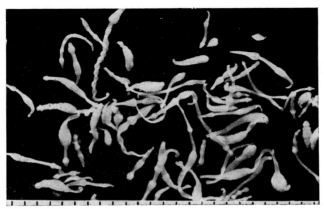

Fig. 98. Plerocercoids (spargana) of Spirometra mansonoides showing characteristic contractions (courtesy Prof. J. F. Mueller, Syracuse, N.Y., J. Parasit., 1959).

parts and organs of the body, and have been found under the skin, between the skeletal muscles, under the peritoneum and in the scrotum. The adult worms develop in domesticated and wild carnivores within 10–30 days. The incidence may be high. The adult worm superficially resembles *D. latum*, but is much smaller, its length varying between 60 and 200 cm, while it may be up to 11 mm wide; the convolutions of the uterus are not rosette-like, but resemble a spiral with 2–8 bends.

Although man is a suitable host for spargana, he becomes infected only accidentally and in fact represents a "blind alley" in the life cycle of the parasite. The mechanism of human infection is not clear. The presence of spargana in animals does not necessarily indicate the existence of sparganosis in man; animals may be heavily infected in localities in which no human sparganosis has been recorded. On the other hand, the establishment of spargana in man in localities in which adult species of *Spirometra* are known to occur in animals, suggests that the human spargana represent the larvae of these local species. It has been proved that, like the plerocercoids of *Diphyllobothrium latum*, the spargana ingested by an unsuitable host may gain entrance to the tissues and continue their existence unchanged. These facts suggest that man may become infected by ingesting spargana which have developed in animals. Although it has not been proved experimentally that this can occur, there are indications that it does happen. Weinstein *et al.* (1954) have produced evidence that cases of human sparganosis in Korea followed the eating of raw, infected watersnakes. Another possible mode of infection is suggested by the fact that oriental natives treat wounds, and particularly eye diseases, by applying to the parts of the body affected poultices made of the fresh flesh of lower animals, mainly frogs. In these cases the sparganum, stimulated by warmth, migrates from the "medicine" material into the human tissue and settles in it as a parasite (Casaux, 1924). Such transmission of spargana has been reproduced experimentally in monkeys by Evanno (1927) and in dogs by Faust (1932).

A third possible mode of human infection may be by the ingestion of infected copepods, in the same manner as occurs in lower animals. This mode of infection, however, has not yet been proved.

Sparganum is usually not highly pathogenic to man; it is to be regarded rather as a nuisance. In some cases, the parasite causes discomfort or at least an uneasy feeling while it is migrating under the skin. Occasionally abscesses may be formed at the site in which the sparganum is located (Faust, 1928). Orbital sparganosis is a serious condition well known in South-East Asiatic countries as a consequence to the "treatment", mentioned above, of eye diseases with muscle tissue of freshly killed frogs (Joyeux and Houdemer, 1925).

Sparganosis, both animal and human, is commonest in the Far Eastern countries, notably in Japan and China. In some villages in Japan as many as 95% of cats and 20% of dogs harbour the adult worms (Ando, 1925). In the Philippines, India and Burma it is known only in animals. However, successful implantation of a sparganum, removed from a snake, into a human volunteer in Burma (Meggitt, 1924), suggests that, under suitable conditions, local sparganosis may also occur spontaneously in man.

It is presumed that there is only one species of Sparganum (or *Spirometra*) in the Far East although this species has been variously called *mansoni, erinacei, decipiens* and otherwise. Its commonest denomination is *Spirometra* (or *Sparganum*) *mansoni*,

According to Gaillard and Ngu (1946) this species requires, under natural conditions, two vertebrate intermediate hosts, of which the first is a tadpole. In some places frogs may be heavily infected with spargana which they acquire by preying on infected tadpoles, whereas the latter become infected by eating copepods infected with procercoids. The full life cycle requires about three months.

Another species of sparganum which occurs rarely in man in the Far East is *Sparganum proliferum* (Ijima, 1905). It is found dispersed in various organs and tissues of man, and may be 2 cm long; it is often enclosed in oval cysts. In structure it resembles the plerocercoid of *Diphyllobothrium*, but it is characterised by a tendency to branching and multiplication by fission. Its specific nature is not known. Mueller (1937) considers *S. proliferum* to be a teratological larva of an ordinary sparganum which branches indefinitely. Yoshida (1914) described a case of serious illness caused by a large number of these spargana.

Cases of human sparganosis have been recorded also in North America: one of the ordinary *mansoni* type (in Florida, by Stiles, 1908) and the other of the *proliferum* type (in Texas, by Moore, 1914). Mueller suggested that these cases were caused by *Spirometra mansonoides*. Since then additional cases have been reported in Texas (Read, 1952) and in Mississippi (Brooke *et al.*, 1960).

Animal spargana are known to occur in some of the eastern and southeastern states of the United States, mainly in water-snakes, 50–90% of which are infected in certain localities (Florida). The parasite reaches 8 mm in length. Its life history has been worked out by J. F. Mueller (1935–1959) who recognised two species: one very rare, occurring in the south, resembling *S. mansoni* and the other *S. mansonoides*. The natural final host of *S. mansonoides* is the bobcat *(Lynx rufus)*, while in human habitations it occurs in domestic cats. The dog, too, may be infected, but is not as favourable a host as the cat and it loses the parasite spontaneously after a few weeks. The domestic cat develops immunity against the worm in the course of infection. In this host the eggs appear on the tenth day and are abundant at the end of the third week. After repeated infection the adult worms become stunted in their development, and may remain only 30 cm long.

In cats the parasite causes general illness and loss of weight. Among laboratory animals, only mice become regularly infected with these plerocercoids; 4 days after infection with the plerocercoids, rodents are infective for cats. The results of the infection are emaciation during the acute initial stage, and sometimes death. In mice which survive this phase of the infection the sparganum may be encapsulated and the host recovers.

References p. 698

The rat is inferior as a host of spargana and supports the infection well. Occasionally experimental infections of guinea pigs and monkeys have been successful. The monkey reacted with chronic inflammation and swelling around the site of infection.

The spargana of *Spirometra mansonoides* can be artificially transferred to other hosts and they then continue their normal development. Mueller *et al.* (1939, 1941) succeeded in transplanting spargana from animals to human volunteers. A plerocercoid 2 mm long grew in 2 months to a length of 60 mm. Symptoms associated with the infection were: local induration, periodic diffused urticaria, oedema, chills, eosinophilia (at the fourth to fifth week after infection) and malaise.

The ease with which monkeys can be infected by the mouth with spargana suggests that also man can probably be infected by this route. In an effort to explain the rarity of the human cases of sparganosis reported in North America, Mueller (1938) pointed out that infection may easily escape recognition, because the spargana, so long as they do not settle in vital organs, provoke only insignificant reactions.

Numerous cases of the infection of various animals with spargana were already known in Latin America when Diesing established the group-name *Sparganum*. Subsequently additional cases have been recorded from the continent and the West Indies (Cameron, 1936). Adult worms have been recovered from dogs, and cats (domestic and wild), which were fed with locally collected spargana; their exact species-identification is unknown. According to Kouri in certain districts of Cuba 100% of the cats harbour *Diphyllobothrium mansoni*.

So far there is no record of sparganosis of man in South America.

There is evidence that *Spirometra mansoni* is established in Australia, especially in the eastern districts of the country.

Sandars (1953, 1954) presented a summary of Australian records among which 3 autochthonous cases of human sparganosis are mentioned. Sparganosis is common in animals in Australia. In some areas (for instance around Brisbane) one fourth of the frogs *(Hyla coeruela)* have been found to be infected. Spargana were found in numerous species of lizards, snakes and mammals (among them the wild boar and two species of marsupials as well as foxes). In one instance about 300 spargana were recovered from a single water-snake. Sparganosis of the wild pigs which are fattened in Australia for human consumption presents a serious

problem. Bearup (1953) quotes an example in which all of 49 pigs of this
kind were condemned as unsuitable for human consumption because of
widespread sparganosis, and another instance in which 24 out of 38 pork
carcasses were condemned for the same reason.

Specimens of spargana resembling those reported from the Far East,
were recovered from man and animals in tropical and South Africa. A
summary of human cases has been published by Fain and Piraux (1959).

Spargana were found in *Genetta genetta*, the *serval*, the *okapi*, a monkey *(Cercopithecus
mitis)* and a rodent *(Lophyzomus aquillus)*. Two species of adult *Spirometra* are known
from Africa: *Diphyllobothrium pretoriensis* recorded in the wild canines *Otocyon
megalotis*, *Lycaon pictus* and *Thos adustus* and *D. theileri* in the wild felids: the lion,
Felis serval, *F. caffra* and *F. pardus*. It is not known to which of these species the
recorded spargana belong and whether domestic animals take part in the maintenance
of these parasites.

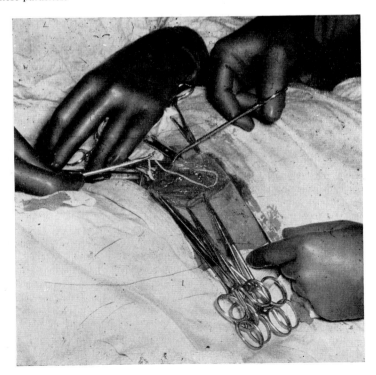

Fig. 99.   Surgical removal of sparganum from a man in Korea (courtesy Drs.
Weinstein, Krawczyk and Peers, Amer. J. trop. med. Hyg., 1954).

References p. 698

The first records of sparganosis of animals in Europe were compiled by Rudolphi, who in 1810 mentioned *Vermis (dubius) ranarum* from frogs and in 1819 *Dubium erinacei europaei* from the hedgehog. Records of spargana in snakes, frogs and pigs were published subsequently under a variety of names, mainly in Italy. In 1923 Kotlán obtained adult worms by feeding cats with *Sparganum raillieti* which had been discovered by Ratz (1912) in pigs in Hungary. The exact identity of this species has not been determined, and it is not known whether it is similar to any Far Eastern or American species. Apparently the same spargana were subsequently found in Serbia. Dubinina (1951) recorded the presence of spargana in frogs, water-snakes (100%), rodents and crows in the Volga Delta. These spargana developed into adult worms in dogs, cats and foxes.

No case of human sparganosis has so far been recorded in Europe.

The only treatment of human sparganosis occasionally practicable is surgical removal of the parasite (Fig. 99).

REFERENCES

BAER, J. G. and A. FAIN, *Exp. Parc. Nat. Upemba*, 36 (1955) 38.
BEARUP, A. J., *Aust. J. Sci.*, 10 (1948) 183; *Aust. vet. J.*, 29 (1953) 217.
DUBININA, M. N., *Zool. Zh.*, 30 (1951) 421.
FAIN, A. and A. PIRAUX, *Bull. Soc. Path. exot.*, 52 (1960) 804.
FAUST, E. C., *Proc. exp. Biol. (N.Y.)*, 26 (1928) 252; *J. trop. Med. Hyg.*, 32 (1929) 76.
FAUST, E. C., CAMPBELL and KELLOGG, *Amer. J. Hyg.*, 9 (1929) 560.
GALLIARD, H., *Ann. Parasit. hum. comp.*, 23 (1948) 23.
MUELLER, J. F., *J. Parasit.*, 22 (1936) 471; 23 (1937) 568.
MUELLER, J. F. and F. COULSTON, *Amer. J. trop. Med.*, 21 (1941) 399.
SANDARS, D., *Proc. roy. Soc. Queensland*, 63 (1951) 65.
SANDARS, D. F., *Aust. Med. J.*, 41 (1954) 817.

f. Hymenolepidiases

i. Hymenolepis nana infection

Hymenolepis nana * is the smallest and the commonest of the tapeworms of man. The adult worm is usually 25–50 mm long, but specimens as small as 10 mm and as long as 240 mm occur. The worm is very narrow, almost filiform and is provided with a

---

* The most frequently used synonyms of this species are: *Taenia nana, Hymenolepis fraterna, H. murina, Rodentolepis fraterna*. Its vernacular name is the dwarf tapeworm

minute scolex, about 0.3 mm wide which has 4 suckers and a proboscis, armed with a crown of hooks. The mature segments are shorter than 1 mm. They rarely appear in the faeces because they easily disintegrate in the intestine and liberate the eggs. These are colourless, almost globular, 40–50 microns in diameter, and have 2 shells, the space between which is filled with a semi-transparent fluid. The eggs eliminated with the faeces of the final host contain a fully-formed oncosphere.

On the basis of observations in laboratory animals the development of the worm may proceed in different ways. It may occur directly (when the eggs are ingested by the proper final host) or indirectly (when an insect acts as intermediate host); mice may serve as intermediate hosts, or (as is presumed, but not definitely proved) auto-infection may take place. Direct development is presumably the most common one. Eggs ingested by suitable hosts (man or mouse) are initially macerated in the stomach; they open in the intestine and the escaping oncosphere burrows into the mucosa of the jejunum where it develops into a microscopic cysticercoid within about 5 days. This form returns to the lumen of the intestines and matures within 10–12 days.

The cysticercoids may develop within the body of an insect or its larva which have ingested the eggs of *H. nana*. Experimentally this mode of development has been reproduced in the larvae of fleas and mealworms *(Tenebrio molitor, Tribolium consufum)*. Up to 230 cysticercoids have been found in a single beetle of the species *T. molitor*. This development requires 14–30 days, depending on the temperature. The cysticercoids remain dormant until the insect-host has in turn been swallowed by man or by a rodent, and they then develop in the intestines of the mammalian host into mature tape worms (Bacigalupo, 1928–1932).

A third mode of development has been demonstrated by Garkavi (1956–1959) and Heyneman *et al.* (1958). They found that in more than 80% of white mice some cysticercoids do not develop in or under the intestinal mucosa, but in the lymph nodes, in which they sometimes remain for more than a month. Mice harbouring such cysticercoids can be regarded as intermediate hosts which give rise to infection when they are eaten by a suitable final host (cannibalistic rat, monkey).

Obviously insects are the most suitable intermediate hosts for this parasite, because in them a much greater proportion of eggs develops to the cysticercoid stage than in direct development.

H. nana is a cosmopolitan parasite but it is usually commoner in warm and dry climates in temperate zones. There is no adequate explanation for this phenomenon. Although it is chiefly a parasite of children, it also occurs in adults.

A cestode which is morphologically indistinguishable from *H. nana* occurs in domestic *rats* and *mice*, in laboratory rodents *(guinea pig, hamster)* and in certain small, wild rodents *(chinchilla)*. Under experimental conditions, it may infect monkeys (Saeki, 1925). There is a controversy among investigators as to the specific identity of these worms which are parasitic in such unrelated hosts. Some authors propose to regard the parasites of rodents and man as different subspecies, adapted to their respective hosts; this may explain the fact that their geographic distribution does not always coincide. Some strains develop better in mice than in rats, or better in the ordinary domestic mouse than in the white laboratory mouse (Shorb, 1933). These adaptations are emphasized by their faster development, larger size and longer life span, but rarely by total exclusion of development in a non-adapted host. Thus, cross-infection of reciprocal hosts with human and rodent parasites has been successfully produced. Recent opinion tends, therefore, to the existence of various strains of a single species, *H. nana*, each of which is physiologically adapted to particular hosts, but still able to invade other hosts.

The incidence of human infection varies greatly, not only in different geographical regions, but also in various localities in these regions. In most instances it does not affect more than 5 % of the population, although in particular instances it may increase to 40 % (according to Simich and Petrovitch, 1955, recorded in Macedonia). Moreover, the intensity of infection varies considerably. Usually it is slight, but rare cases have been reported in which thousands of worms were counted in one individual (Schnell, 1919; Gigitashvili, 1958).

It is noteworthy that *H. nana* is usually more commonly found in towns than in villages. Pessoa and Correre (1926) established in the State of Sao Paulo an average incidence of 5.9 %, while in the town of Sao Paulo it amounted to 9.5 % and in the provincial fazendas 0.5 to 1 %. In the town Mogi Das Cruzes 29.5 % of the population were found infected.

There is controversy about the longevity of *H. nana* in man. Headlee (1941) observed uninterrupted infection in an individual lasting 7 years; it was terminated by treatment, after which the worm did not reappear for more than a year.

Infection with *H. nana* is not always accompanied by clinical symptoms. Adults are usually more tolerant than young people, and cases have been recorded in which the infection was entirely masked. The symptoms attributed to the infection in children are restlessness, irritability, diarrhoea, abdominal pain and disturbed sleep. Eosinophilia does not always occur, although Doncaster and Habibe (1958) noted it in a third of their patients, while in 7 % of the cases it rose to over 11 %. Rarely, nervous symptoms appear, of which the most distressing are epileptic attacks in various forms, including cyanosis, loss of consciousness and convulsions (Gorodadze and Gigitashvili, 1958). The frequency and duration of these attacks vary in different cases; usually their duration is brief. In half of the cases the fits were preceded by aura, mostly in the form of accentuated abdominal symptoms, dizziness or headache. Specific treatment halts the symptoms and thus demonstrates their etiology.

The epidemiology of *H. nana* is insufficiently understood and is beset with contradictory phenomena.

The high incidence of infection in man and animals would suggest a high degree of resistance and infectivity of the eggs, but the contrary seems to be true. According to Shorb (1933) the eggs of *H. nana* die within 11 days, even under optimal conditions. They are very susceptible to heat and dryness which quickly kill them. Yet examples of very high incidence have been recorded in hot and dry regions, for instance 20% in Teheran (Biocca, 1959); 12–20% in Chile (Neghme *et al.*, 1955); 15% in Egypt (Wells and Blagg, 1937). Even in such hot and dry areas as the Kharga Oasis in the Sahara, Nagaty and Rifaat (1957) recorded a 6% infection rate.

The most paradoxical phenomenon in the epidemiology of *H. nana* is the low infectivity of its eggs for animal hosts, which is clearly demonstrated by the investigations of Shorb (1938) and Hunninen (1935). The percentage of successful infections is disproportionate to the number of eggs ingested. Thus 1500 eggs per rat (using a rat strain) produced a 100% infection rate, whereas only a few of the rats became infected when more or less than this quantity were administered. A similar picture was obtained when mice were infected with a mouse strain. Using a dose of 55,000 eggs given to mice, only about 4% developed into adult worms; almost one third of the eggs were eliminated in the faeces during the first two days.

Unfortunately, the infectivity of *H. nana* eggs to man is unknown. Authors differ in their opinion on the question whether infection in man and animals produces immunity to super-infection.

Another unsolved problem in the epidemiology of *H. nana* is the role of animals in the spread of human infections. Although cross-infection with human and animal strains of the parasite have been produced experimentally, it is not definitely known to what extent animals serve as disseminators of human infection under natural conditions. Investigators are divided on two theories, the unitarian and dualistic. According to the former theory there exists only one species, *H. nana,* which lives in both man and rodents, while environmental conditions determine the intensity of their infections. According to the dualistic theory, the parasites of rodents constitute a distinct biological variety *(H. nana fraterna)* which does not infect man under natural conditions. The protagonists of the latter theory base

References p. 702

their opinion on a conspicuous disparity of the infection rate in both categories of hosts. According to Joyeux (1929), for instance, more than 20% of rats were infected in Paris at a time when there were no human infections. The reverse condition was recorded by Gorodilova (1944), who found among children living in a settlement under insanitary conditions an incidence of up to 58%, while only 0.9% of the local mice were found infected.

Thus, while the unitarists believe that animals are the main disseminators, the dualists maintain that man is the principal culprit. However, although facts indicate that domestic rodents may serve as source of human infection with *H. nana*, in the majority of instances man himself seems to be the main source, and it is the human strain that is spread.

No anthelmintic will invariably and effectively expel *H. nana*, but reduction of the number of parasites and sometimes their total elimination may be attained by several drugs. Atebrin and other acridin derivatives are regarded as the most convenient drugs. Gentian violet and methylene blue are also effective (Maplestone and Mukerji, 1939). Fern extract showed an average efficacy of 25%. It is claimed that hexylresorcinol, hexachlorethylene and Dichlorophen (May and Baker) are efficacious against *H. nana* in man, while Halawani (1948) found that Nivaquin and Camoquin yielded satisfactory results.

In view of the present conception of the spread of infection with *H. nana*, it is conceivable that improved hygienic conditions and the destruction of rodents are imperative for the reduction of its incidence.

REFERENCES

BIACIGALUPO, J., *Rev. chil.-Hist. nat.*, 36 (1932) 144.
BADALIAN, A. L., *Skryabin 80 Years Jubil. Vol.*, 1958, p. 50.
BAYLIS, H. A., *Parasitology*, 16 (1924) 415.
BRUMT, E. J. A., *Arch. Zool. Exp. et Gen.*, 75 (1933) 235.
CORT, W. W., *J. Parasit.*, 9 (1922) 48.
GALYAMINA, V. D., *Med. Parazit. (Mosk.)*, 28 (1959) 733.
GARKAVI, B. L., *Dokl. Akad. Nauk U.S.S.R.*, 111 (1959) 240.
GORDADZE, G. N. and M. S. GIGITASHVILI, *Skryabin 80 Years Jubil. Vol.*, 1958, p. 114.
GORODILOVA, L. I., *Med. Parazit. (Mosk.)*, 13 (1944) 18.
HARANT, H., J. GIROUX and M. BRAUN-BLANQUET, *Bull. Soc. Path. exot.*, 40 (1947) 89.
HEADLEE, W. H., *J. Parasit.*, Suppl. 27 (1941) 23.
LARSH, J. E. Jr., *J. Parasit.*, 32 (1946) 477.
OTTO, G. F., *J. Parasit.*, 21 (1935) 443.
PESSOA, S. B. and C. CORREA, *Folha méd.*, 7 (1926) 37.
WOODLAND, W. N. F., *Parasitology*, 16 (1924) 424.

ii. Hymenolepis diminuta infection

Hymenolepis diminuta is another species of the tapeworm-genus *Hymeno-lepis*, which usually lives in the intestine of small rodents. Different from *H. nana*, which seems not to have any preference as to the host, *H. diminuta* infects man only accidentally. Domestic *rats* are most receptive, but various wild and laboratory rodents may serve as hosts as well. It has very rarely been encountered in dogs.

H. diminuta is usually 40–60 cm long and from 2.5–4 mm wide. It is characterised by the absence of hooks from the scolex and by a sac-shaped uterus in the terminal segments. After detachment from the chain, the proglottids quickly desintegrate, liberating the eggs which are eliminated with the faeces. The eggs resemble those of *H. nana* in that they have two membranelike shells, the innermost one (the embryophore) being separated from the outer one by a gelatinous substance. The eggs measure 70–80 microns. When dried they do not survive for longer than one week, and in water at a temperature of 20–23° they do not survive for longer than one month.

H. diminuta requires an arthropod intermediate host in which the cysticercoid develops in a manner similar to that described for *H. nana*. Various arthropods are suitable as intermediate host. These include, as far as is known at present, 11 species of *Coleoptera* (among them flour-eating beetles, fleas and cockroaches), 5 species of *Lepidoptera,* 6 species of *Aphaniptera,* 1 species of *Dermaptera* and 1 of *My iapoda* (Roman, 1937). The development of the cysticercoid in the arthropod lasts from 1 week to 2 months depending on the temperature which must not be lower than 20° (Narihara, 1937),

H. diminuta is a common parasite of rodents all over the world. An incidence up to 20% has been found in domestic rats. The lifespan in rats seems to be rather brief. The parasite is more abundantly present in the summer than in autumn. Its pathogenic action in animals is insufficiently known.

H. diminuta is also a cosmopolitan parasite of man, but infections are sporadic and are never heavy. Exceptionally numerous specimens were present in one person, as, for instance, in a case reported by Yonina (1943), in which 35 worms were found. The infection is seldom epidemic. In one instance 9.6% of children in a village in Southern Italy were found to be infected (Le Nigro *et al.*, 1961). Man may be host of this parasite at any age; infection has been observed in a baby 6 months old as well as in old people.

Infection with *H. diminuta* is often symptomless. In cases of heavy infection or in highly sensitive persons, nausea, restlessness, weakness, abdominal pain and loss of appetite may appear.

The worms can be eliminated by means of the anthelmintics normally used for the treatment of cestode infections, among which male-fern is the most effective.

REFERENCES

BACIGALUPO, J., *Rev. Soc. Ent. argent.*, 15 (1952) 263.
BASNUEVO, L. G., *Rev. Rub. Med. trop. Parasit.*, 5 (1949) 58.
MORENAS, L. and J. COUDERT, *Arch. Mal. Appar. dig.*, 38 (1949) 496.
NARIHARA, N., *J. med. Ass. Formosa*, 33 (1934) 148.
POTAPIENKO, N. A. and A. Y. GUTZEVITCH, *Trop. Med. Vet.*, 8/9 (1930) 28.
ROMAN, E., *C. R. Soc. Biol. (Paris)*, 126 (1937) 26.
SCHEID, G. and H. MENDHEIM, *Z. Kinderheilk.*, 65 (1948) 587.
SPINDLER, L. A., *J. Parasit.*, 16 (1930) 38.

g. *Rare zoonotic cestode infections*

i. *Inermicapsifer- and Railletina infections*

Two genera of cestodes occurring in man, *Inermicapsifer* and *Railletina*, are so similar to each other that they are easily confused. Both are specific for animals but may also occur in man. The chief difference is the scolex, that of *Inermicapsifer* being unarmed, while that of *Railletina* is armed. Thus the genus can not be identified by fragments of the worms which lack the scolex or by ripe segments eliminated with the faeces. The segments contain eggs which are enclosed in numerous cocoons (capsules).

The genus *Inermicapsifer* is represented in man by a species, *I. arvicanthidis* which is common in rodents and in *Procavia* in Africa and Madagascar. Some investigators regard *I. cubensis,* which occurs in Cuba and Venezuela, as a synonym of *I. arvicanthidis.*

The life history of this species is as yet unknown. The worm may be more than 40 cm long; its gravid segments measure 3 by 1 or 2 mm and contain 50 to 180 cocoons, each enclosing 4–15 eggs. According to Baer *et al.* the worm had been recorded in Cuba in more than 100 cases up to 1954, mainly in children, 1 to 5 years old.

The pathogenicity of the parasite is slight. It can easily be expelled not only by anthelminthics but also by ordinary castor oil or any other cathartic. Numerous species of the genus *Railletina* are known as parasites of birds and mammals. Several of these have been recorded as accidental human parasites but in many cases their specific identification is a matter of controversy. Lately some investigators have recognized a large number of supposedly valid species, while others tend to classify these under fewer names or even under one single name, regarding the other names as synonyms.

To sum up the recently published evidence, it appears that 3 species out of those recorded from man may tentatively be retained. These are: *R. celebensis* (up to 600 mm long), occurring in *rodents* and *man* in South-East Asia, the Philippines, Indonesia and East Australia; *R. demerarensis* (120 mm long), found in man and rodents in Tropical America; and *R. siriraji* (260 mm long) known only from man in Thailand. The life histories of these species are as yet obscure. Most of the infections were sporadic. Endemic occurrence has been recorded only by Leon (1949), who observed more than 100 cases of infection with species of *Railletina* in Equador. A survey of 866 children in the endemic rural area showed an infection rate of 3.1%. Apparently these worms are not markedly pathogenic.

The incidence in rodents may be high. Thus, Narihara (1935) recorded a 54% infection rate in water rats and 8% in brown rats in Formosa. Miyazaki (1950) found an incidence of up to 14% of *R. celebensis (R. madagascariensis)* in brown rats in Kagoshima City (Japan), where human infections have never been observed. At all events, the geographical distribution of these parasites seems to be wide.

ii. Dipylidium infection

Dipylidium caninum, the commonest cestode of dogs and cats, is a cosmopolitan parasite. It may be up to 50 cm long, but usually it is shorter. The pinkish gravid segments have the shape of cucumber seeds. They are expelled, sometimes in large numbers, with the faeces and soon disintegrate to liberate the eggs encased in cocoons. For further development these cocoons must be ingested by the larvae of the flea of the dog or cat, in which the cysticercoids are formed. When the larvae are transformed into adult fleas, they contain infective cysticercoids of *Dipylidium*. The dog and cat become infected by swallowing these fleas.

References p. 706/707

When an infected flea is accidentally swallowed by man, the cysticercoids may settle in this unusual host and develop to adult worms. Such an event has not infrequently been observed in children all over the world.

Dipylidium is not very pathogenic for man and may easily be eliminated by any conventional anticestode anthelmintic drug.

iii. Bertiella infection

Bertiella studeri is a common parasite of various species of African and Asiatic monkeys, among them chimpanzees and orang utans. It has been found only once in a dog but several times in man in Kenya, Mauritius, India, Indonesia and the Philippines. The maximum length of the worm is about 30 cm, its width 1 cm, the terminal segments being much broader than they are long.

Bertiella requires a coprophagous mite as intermediate host, which must be swallowed by the final host in order to let the larva develop to the adult stage.

B. studeri causes intestinal discomfort. It can be eliminated by tetrachlorethylene or extract of male fern.

iv. Drepanidotaenia and Moniezia infections

Drepanidotaenia lanceolata is often found in ducks and geese, while species of *Moniezia* are parasites of sheep. These species have been recorded as rare accidental human parasites. The former requires a copepod *(Cyclops,* sp.), the latter a coprophagous mite as intermediate host, and both must be swallowed by the final host for further development.

REFERENCES

General:

GRADWOHL, R. B. H. and P. KOURI, *Clinical Laboratory Methods and Diagnosis,* Vol. 3, C. V. Mosby Publ., St. Louis, 5. ed., 1956.

PODYAPOLSKAYA, V. P. and V. F. KAPUSTIN, *Helm. Diseases of Man,* Moscow, 1958, p. 423.

Inermicapsifer infections:

BAER, J. G., P. KOURI and F. SOTOLONGO, *Acta trop.,* 6 (1949) 120.

CALVO FONSECA, R., *Rev. Cuba. Med. trop. Parasit.,* 5 (1949) 8.

FAIN, A., *Bull. soc. Path. exot.,* 43 (1950) 438.

OYEUX, CH. and J. G. BAER, *Bull. soc. Path. exot.*, 42 (1949) 581.
OTOLENGO, F., *Rev. Cuba. Lab. clin.*, 3 (1949) 131.

Railletina infections:
BAER, J. G. and D. F. SANDARS, *J. Helminth.*, 30 (1956) 173.
CHANDLER, A. and A. PRADATSUNDARASAR, *J. Parasit.*, 43 (1957) 81.
DOLLFUS, R. P., *Ann. Parasit.*, 17 (1940) 415; 542.
OYEUX, CH. and J. G. BAER, *Bull. soc. Path. exot.*, 22 (1929) 114.
EON, L. A., *Rev. cuba. Med. trop. Parasit.*, 5 (1949) 1.
PRADATSUNDARASAR, A., *J. med. Ass. Thailand*, 43 (1960) 56.
TUNKARD, H. W., *J. Parasit.*, 39 (1953) 272.

Dipylidium infection:
EARUP, A. J. and G. L. MORGAN, *Med. J. Aust.*, 1 (1939) 104.
MOORE, D., *Amer. J. trop. Med. Hyg.*, 9 (1960) 604.

Bertiella infection:
DAMS, A. R. D. and L. WEBB, *Ann. trop. Med. Parasit.*, 27 (1933) 471.
BLANCHARD, R., *Bull. Acad. Méd. (Paris)*, 69 (1913) 286.
RAM, E. B., *Amer. J. trop. Med.*, 8 (1928) 339.
TUNKARD, H. W., *Amer. J. trop. Med.*, 20 (1940) 305.

G. G. WITENBERG

Acanthocephala infections

Worms of the phylum *Acanthocephala* are exclusively parasitic, but none of them is specific for man. Yet, on rare occasions man can serve as a facultative host for 2 species which are ordinarily parasites of animals namely *Macracanthorhynchus hirudinaceus* (syn. *Echinorhynchus gigas* and *Moniliformis moniliformis*.

Macracanthorhynchus hirudinaceus (the *thornyheaded worm*) is a universally encountered specific parasite of the pig and wild boar. The female of this worm measures 20 to 40 cm, the male about half that length. They live in the small intestine, where they are attached to the mucosa by a strong proboscis armed with 6 rows of hooks and cause trauma and the formation of a nodule about 6 mm in diameter on the serous side of the intestine. When several of these worms are present, they cause unthriftiness of the animal. Apart from direct toxic injury, the worm may do harm by introducing pathogenic microorganisms into the intestinal wall. Besides swine, in other animals such as squirrels and chipmunk it may develop as an accidental parasite. Insect larvae serve as vectors.

Only 2 cases of human infection have been recorded, one in the Ukraine (Skrinnik, 1957) and another *("Echinorrhynchus hominis")* in Prague (Lambl, 1859).

Moniliformis moniliformis is a specific parasite of several species of murine rodents.

The female reaches a length of about 35 cm, the male that of approximately 8 cm. The whole body is beset with bead-like swellings which give the worms a segmented appearance. The strong proboscis with which they are firmly anchored to the in estinal wall is armed with 15 or more rows of hooks. The eggs are passed in the host's faeces and, when ingested by cockroaches or coprophagous beetles, they give rise to infective larvae *(acanthellae)*. The final host becomes infected by the ingestion of these infected insects.

M. moniliformis is cosmopolitan. In some localities it is harboured by 50% or more of the domestic rats. Hoffman (1930) reported infection of a rat with 167 specimens of the parasite which completely occluded the intestine and caused starvation of the animal. Apart from rodents, this worm may accidentally develop in dogs, foxes or man.

Human infections are rare. They have been recorded from Italy, the United States, Sudan, Java and Israel (Witenberg, 1951). Most of them were slight infections involving only a few worms which caused intestinal discomfort. The infection can be diagnosed by the detection of the characteristic eggs in the faeces.

A most interesting case of experimental human infection was recorded by the eminent parasitologist Grassi who, while investigating the life history of this parasite (1888), swallowed its larvae which had developed in a beetle *(Blaps mucronata)*. Three weeks later rather heavy symptoms, including intestinal pains, diarrhoea, tinnitus and general weakness, appeared. Eggs of the parasite were found in the stools on the 35th day after ingestion. After treatment with male-fern, 53 worms were eliminated.

REFERENCES

BECK, J. W., *J. Parasit.*, 45 (1959) 510.
MOOR, D., *J. Parasit.*, 32 (1946) 257.
RAUSCH, R., *J. Parasit.*, 32 (1946) 94.
SKRINNIK, M. R., *Med. Parazit. (Mosk.)*, 27 (1958) 450.
WITENBERG, G., *Harefuah*, 41 (1951) 180.

5

G. G. WITENBERG

Hirudiniases

a. Introduction

Leeches are annelid worms, known from time immemorial as symbols of parasitism because of their ability to suck blood. However, it is not always realised that only some species of leeches are blood suckers, while others are predators feeding on small animals which they swallow.

The body of the leech is very elastic and capable of extreme contraction and extension (Fig. 100). Every leech has 2 suckers, a smaller anterior one connected with the oral opening and a larger posterior one, serving only for attachment. Leeches are hermaphrodite, but cross fertilisation between two specimens usually occurs to produce eggs, which are deposited in groups, often encased in a capsule (cocoon).

The leeches which feed on the blood of animals are usually not partic-

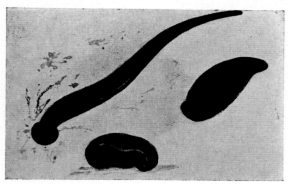

Fig. 100. Limnatis nilotica in various stages of contraction (courtesy Dr. Seyfart, Zentralbl. Bakteriol., 1917).

ular about their victims; man is rather often attacked. It should be borne in mind, however, that man is only accidentally affected and animals are the primary hosts of leeches.

The blood sucking leeches are divided in two groups: *Gnathobdellae*, provided with toothed jaws, which cut a triradiate wound in the host's skin or mucosa, and *Rhynchobdellae*, which introduce into the body of the host an extrusible "siphon" through which they suck. The latter group are parasites of lower animals and seldom attack man, while the *Gnathobdellae* attack him at any opportunity.

The blood sucking property of leeches was known in early history and its application for medical purposes is an ancient tradition. However, the mechanism of this blood sucking has long been misinterpreted. Nowadays we know that the effect of a leeches' bite is not due to the removal of blood, but to the introduction of certain substances into the blood. Before it sucks blood, the leech, like other parasites which feed on blood, introduces its saliva into the wound. This contains *hirudin*, which causes local hyperaemia, prevents the clotting of the blood, dissolves the erythrocytes, and serves as a digestive agent. The anticoagulating property of hirudin is demonstrated by continued bleeding at the site of the bite, until its action is exhausted. Thus, the victim suffers considerable loss of blood in addition to the amount taken by the leech itself.

Leeches are temporary ectoparasites, because they attack a host only when they are hungry and drop off when they are engorged. The leech then withdraws for a prolonged period to a sheltered place, slowly digesting the accumulated food.

Most leeches live in water, but there are several species which live on land, mainly in tropical forests. Blood sucking leeches are a serious pest of domesticated animals and are annoying or sometimes dangerous parasites of man.

According to the mode of parasitism on man leeches have been divided in 3 groups: (a) aquatic leeches, which attack the skin, (b) aquatic leeches which attack mucous membranes, and (c) land leeches.

b. Aquatic leeches which attack the skin

Several species of leeches are used for medicinal purposes. The best known is the European medicinal leech, *Hirudo medicinalis*.

This leech, when relaxed and unfed, is up to 12 cm long; when it is fully engorged, it is up to 20 cm long and weighs 15 g. The pattern on its dorsal side varies in numerous local races. It is preponderantly dark and usually possesses three double, interrupted, yellowish lines running along the body, over which are distributed numerous small black spots. In most specimens, the ventral side is uniformly pale, sometimes with black dots.

The medicinal leech lays, usually once a year, about 10 eggs which are enclosed in an oval cocoon, fastened to some object in the water. The young, which resemble the adults in shape, hatch 4–8 weeks after their appearance and grow slowly. Feeding is a casual process for the leech. They feed on frogs, but medium sized leeches need mammalian blood for development. Sometimes long periods of starvation separate two feedings. Under optimum conditions the medicinal leech lives up to 20 years. It was once common in the wild state all over Europe. Intensive catching for about 2 centuries has brought about its disappearance from many localities. According to Lukin (1951), it still may be found in nature in the southern part of the Soviet Union and in the Caucasus. The leeches now in medical use come from artificial breeding establishments, especially advanced in Hungary and the U.S.S.R.

Nowadays leeches are no longer universally used for medicinal purposes, because the progress of modern physiology and therapy has rendered them unnecessary. Nevertheless, leech therapy is still applied to a certain degree, and some medical specialists still believe that leech therapy is useful for certain ailments, e.g. thrombosis and embolism. According to Bottenberg (1935), one of the leading leech-trading firms in Germany sold 34,000 leeches in 1934, while breeding establishments in Hungary profitably export medicinal leeches to many parts of the world.

Hungry leeches are activated by a sudden stir of water. People and animals entering the water presumably attract leeches by the concussion they produce.

A controversy exists concerning the ability of leeches to transmit pathogens. Numerous pathogenic organisms survive for several days in the digestive tract of the leech. Shevkunova and Ptchelkina (1958) have shown that the medicinal leech can maintain the rickettsiae of Q-fever alive in its gut for as long as 53 days and can infect an animal during the repeated acts of sucking. It is advisable, therefore, to discard a leech after it has been used for a therapeutic purpose.

In addition to *Hirudo medicinalis* several other species of leeches have been employed for medicinal treatment, *e.g. Hirudo troctina* in North Africa and southern Europe, *Poecilobdella granulosa, P. javanica* and *P. manilensis* in South Asia, *Liostomum officinalis* in Mexico, *Hirudo nipponia* in Japan, and *Macrobdella decora* in the United States.

The three species of the genus *Poecilobdella* (syn. *Hirudinaria*) mentioned above, viciously attack man and beast under natural conditions.

These leeches are similar in appearance, have a black-spotted dorsal and light-rusty ventral side with black stripes along the ventro-lateral margin of the body. They differ, however, in geographic distribution: *P. granulosa* occurs in the upper plains of India, *P. manilensis* in the lowlands of the whole tropical South-West of Asia, while *P. javanica* is found in the Sunda Islands and Burma. *P. manilensis* and *P. javanica* are large and robust and may be 15 cm long; they are common in rice fields and swamps where they attack buffaloes and carabaos (hence the name carabao-leech) and are able to pierce the thickest skin. Rice field workers suffer much from these leeches. Ducks and fish are used for the control of this pest.

c. *Aquatic leeches which attack mucous membranes*

There exists a group of gnathobdellid leeches, the piercing organ of which is too weak to cut the skin, but they are perfectly adapted to cutting thin mucous membranes. The instincts of these worms are directed to locating and reaching these membranes.

These leeches, which are common in the regions of early civilization, were possibly known to ancient man before the skin biting leeches. Herodotus mentions them as occurring in the mouths of crocodiles. The Arab writer Quadi Abu Ali (9th century) described a case of pharyngeal hirudiniasis in man (Cameron, 1950). Savigny, who accompanied Napoleon's army in Egypt, described the torments which these leeches caused to the soldiers.

The best known leech of this group is *Limnatis nilotica,* which occurs in the countries surrounding the Mediterranean and extends as far east as Persia and Tadjikistan. It is especially well-known in North Africa, the Balkans and Levant countries and it frequently attacks man. Thus, Marshak (1958) recorded 110 cases which he observed in northern Israel during 24 years of laryngological practice; this author quoted another 100 cases observed by Summerfeld (1949) in the same country. Kotz (1951, quoted by Shevkunova, 1958) recorded 147 cases observed during his 7 years of practice in the Caucasus.

Limnatis nilotica reaches 15 cm in length and is almost black, with a greenish tinge and has narrow orange stripes along the ridges of the body. It lives in springs and water holes, rarely in marshes. These leeches usually crawl on the bottom or are attached to stones or plants; when a man or animal enters the water they swiftly swim in a snake-like fashion towards the prospective victim. *Limnatis* rarely bites the skin; it usually reaches the mouth or nostrils of drinking animals or man, attaching itself to the mucosa.

Limnatis nilotica is not particular with respect to the host, although it normally attacks mammals, including the domestic species. It also sucks the skin of frogs but under natural conditions it would eventually be swallowed and digested by this host. Wild mammals are the natural carriers which disseminate these leeches in the locality.

Limnatis attaches itself with its anterior sucker to the soft parts of the mouth or to the bucco-pharyngeal cavities, its body flopping freely. The leeches are mostly lodged in the pharynx, larynx, palate, uvula or vocal cords, but when they are numerous, especially in cattle, they attach themselves to the gums, under the tongue or the upper parts of the respiratory tracts as well. Sometimes they remain attached close to the vocal cords for many days, during which time their weight may be increased almost tenfold. This increase is partly due to the stored blood, but partly to the growth of the body, which is very rapid during the sojourn of the leech in the host (Shevkunova, 1955).

Thanks to its remarkable ability to distend, the leech can enter very narrow ducts, such as the urethra of man and animals or the teats of a cow. Cases are known of attachment of *Limnatis* to the eye (Fig. 101). When swallowed, the leech soon dies in the stomach.

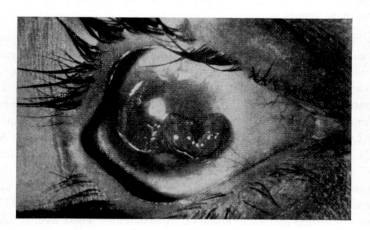

Fig. 101.   Limnatis nilotica attacking a human eye (courtesy Dr. Gilkes, Brit. J. Ophthal., 1957).

L. nilotica is able to attack at all times during its life; even the smallest individuals which have just left the eggs can attach themselves to the mucosae of mammals and suck blood. The parasite does not fill its digestive tract in one feeding (as does *Hirudo medicinalis*), but does this by stages, with intervals during which it remains fixed. The digestive organs of *L. nilotica* are empty 3 to 4 weeks after the meal. Even so, the leech may survive long periods of starvation.

Cattle using pools for drinking often suffer greatly from this parasite; as many as 30 leeches may be lodged in the mouth cavity (Fig. 102).

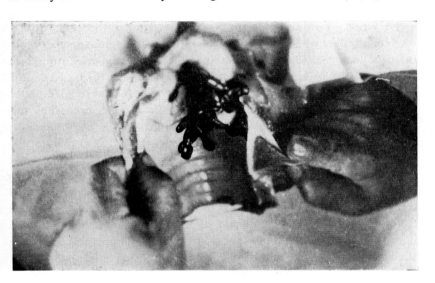

Fig. 102.   Multiple *Limnatis nilotica* in larynx of a cow causing asphyxia.
(Photo: Dr. M. Moses, Jerusalem).

When fully engorged the leeches detach themselves as the animal starts drinking again and thus escape to the outer water, where they hide in crevices or under stones to digest the accumulated blood meal.

In man, usually a single specimen of *Limnatis* settles in the pharynx or in the upper part of the respiratory tract, although cases are known in which as many as 10 leeches had attacked 1 man (Seyfart, 1917). The leech remains in the host for periods varying from several days to several weeks. The attached parasite causes twofold harm: mechanical injury and anaemia. The irritation caused by the mechanical action of the leech may result in swelling of the invaded organs and interference with swallowing or breathing. Especially dangerous are cases in which the leeches are lodged near the vocal cords or have been inhaled into the trachea or into a bronchus. Paroxysmal cough, change of voice or disphony caused by oedema of the throat are then the commonest symptoms. On the other hand, in some instances a leech may remain in the throat for days without provoking any symptoms.

As the worm persists in its location, anaemia develops and this is especially conspicuous when the host has been invaded by several leeches. Haemorrhages invariably occur bringing about increasing anaemia. The loss of blood is only partly due to the sucking action of the leech. Most of the blood is lost when the leech changes its place of attachment, which frequently happens. Because of the widening of the capillaries around the wound and the lowered capacity of blood coagulation, the blood continues to exude from the abandoned site, sometimes for an extended period of time, and if the process is repeated, the host may suffer irreparable loss of blood, which may eventually lead to death.

When the leech is fully engorged it may be detached with pincers; but at the beginning of sucking it is attached so firmly that attempts to remove it often cause it to tear apart, so that its separated anterior sucker is left in place and continues to suck, while the blood runs from its torn end. A special method to induce the leech to leave the site of attachment must therefore be employed, e.g. by the application of anaesthetics (for instance cocaine) or of acrid substances (strong salt solution, tobacco, iodine, alcohol). Sometimes, even these methods do not bring immediate success.

A specific laryngo-pharyngitis in man caused by worms is known in Lebanon by the name of "Halzoun". This Arabic word means snail, and it refers to the fact that the incriminated worm often has a coiled appearance. Three kinds of parasites have been mentioned as a cause of this syndrome. Khouri (1951) as well as Watson and Kerim (1956) blamed the cattle liver-fluke, *Fasciola hepatica*, which is supposed to infect man when he eats infected lamb liver which has been insufficiently cooked. Brumpt (1936), however, unsuccessfully tried to reproduce "Halzoun" experimentally by feeding dogs for more than a month with raw liver containing numerous *F. hepatica*. Witenberg (1944) showed that, in some rare instances, a parasitic trematode of fish-eating birds, *Clinostomum*, may be the culprit, but in most cases the causative agent is the leech *Limnatis nilotica*.

In Central Asia, *Limnatis nilotica* is replaced by a species, *L. paluda*, which lacks the lateral orange stripes and lives in stagnant pools. Its behaviour is similar to that of the preceding species. In West Africa the genus *Limnatis* is represented by *L. africana*, in Argentina by *L. viatrix*, in Central America by *L. cubensis*. In the northern United States it is replaced by *Macrobdella decora* and in the southern States by *M. ditetra*, which attacks the mucous membranes of man and animals (Mayer, 1959).

d. Land leeches

Several genera of land leeches united in the family *Haemadipsidae* occur in tropical regions, particularly in those surrounding the Indian Ocean (Madagascar, Ceylon, Malaya, Japan). They are characterised by peculiar anatomical structures and by the fact that they live in rain forests. Best known are representatives of the genera *Haemadipsa* and *Philaemon*. The former prevail in Asia and the Sunda Islands, the latter in Australia, including Tasmania and in South America. These are leeches usually not more than 3 cm long, and mostly dark colored. They may be found moving along grasses with characteristic "measuring" strides, or standing erect on their posterior sucker and waving their bodies. They are very efficient in reaching a passing beast or man. People walking in infested places during the day may quite unexpectedly discover the leeches dangling on their skin on any part of the body (mostly on the legs), or may experience a faint feeling of chill caused by the trickling of blood from the incisions, after the leeches have fallen off. These leeches are able to creep on to their victim even when it is in motion, swiftly crawling between the fur of animals, or between the tight clothes of man, and even through the holes of the shoe laces in order to reach the skin, which they pierce painlessly.

Some observers assert that land leeches climb on to the lower branches of trees or shrubs to a height of some 4 feet and await the victim on the edges of the leaves. When a man or animal is passing and happens to brush up against them, the leeches may fasten on to the clothing or the body. Sometimes hundreds of specimens attack a man within a short time. During the second world war the pest of land leeches was a cause of severe strain to armies fighting in the jungles of Burma and Malaya. In localities where there is a periodic rainy season, land leeches disappear during the dry season, burrowing into the soil or creeping under logs, to reappear when the damp conditions have returned.

References p. 718/719

The land leech sucks for 40–120 minutes and then drops off. After that, blood continues to flow slowly from the wound for some 30 minutes until the hirudin is washed away and the wound is closed by a clot. A small haemorrhage in the skin around the wound remains for 4 to 8 days. Usually the wound heals by itself, but, sometimes, if the affected place is not properly attended to, secondary infection may aggravate the condition. In cases of massive infection the loss of blood may be considerable and in animals it may sometimes even cause death. Land leeches may attach themselves to the eye, and horses, cattle and dogs (as well as snakes and frogs) are sometimes blinded by such invasions. The harm which land leeches cause to man and domestic animals may be such that certain districts dominated by these parasites become almost uninhabitable (Moore, 1927).

The most common land leech is *Haemadipsa zeylanica*, which occurs in most of the tropical regions of South East Asia. *Haemadipsa sylvestris* is the largest species of the genus; it occurs in the forests of Assam. When it is fully stretched it may reach 3 inches in length. In Japan the genus is represented by *H. japonica*.

Garments, however tight, do not afford sufficient protection in a locality where land leeches abound. Repellents may be indicated, either in the form of an ointment applied on the exposed parts of the body, or by impregnation of the clothes. Ointments containing 25–50% of dimethylphthalate (according to Ribbands, 1946, dibutylphthalate is almost useless), ethyl phenyl hydracrylate, 2-ethylhexanediol or dimethyl carbamate may provide protection for several hours (these compounds, however, do not act against aquatic leeches). The insecticides Lindane, Aldrin and Dieldrin are not effective in the concentrations recommended for the control of insects. According to Petru (1950) Gammexane is highly toxic to leeches. Apparently spraying a solution of this substance around camps or similar settlements in the jungle may provide temporary protection against invasion by land leeches.

REFERENCES

BOTTENBERG, H., *Die Blutegelbehandlung,* etc., Hippocrates Verl., Stuttgart, 1953, pp. 128.
CHIN, TA-HSIUNG, *J. Parasit.,* 35 (1949) 215.
FUKUOKA, G., *Physiol. Ecol. Contr. Otsu Hydrobiol. Exp. Sta. Kyoto Univ.,* 27 (1945) 1.
GILKES, M., *Brit. J. Ophthal.,* 41 (1957) 124.

HARDING, W. A. and J. P. MOORE, *The Fauna Britisch India*, Hirudinea, London, 1927, pp. 302.

HARRISON, J. L., J. R. AUDY and R. TRAUB, *Med. J. Malaya,* 9 (1954) 61.

MARSCHAK, A., *Harefuah*, 54 (1958) 47.

RIBBANDS, C. R., *Ann. trop. Med. Parasit.,* 40 (1946) 314.

EYFART, C., *Zbl. Bakt., I. Abt. Ref.,* 79 (1917) 89.

SHEVKUNOVA, E. A., *Tr. Inst. Zool. Akad. Nauk Kazakh S.S.R.,* 9 (1958) 247.

SINEVA, M. V., *Zool. Zh.,* 28 (1949) 213.

STAMMERS, F. M. G., *Parasitology,* 40 (1950) 237.

WITENBERG, G., *Acta med. orient. (Tel-Aviv),* 3 (1944) 191.

B. Pathological conditions caused by arthropod parasites

1

O. THEODOR

Introduction

There are no specific ectoparasites of man except the human louse. Even the human flea, *Pulex irritans*, is primarily a parasite of a number of mammals. Of 400 records in Hopkins and Rothschild's catalogue of the Siphonaptera of which the host is given, less than a third are from humans. Some of the hosts of *Pulex irritans* live in caves in which man probably came into contact with them and thus the flea passed on to humans. All arthropods, insects, ticks and mites which attack man, are primarily parasites of animals and it would serve no useful purpose to enumerate them here. Some of them attack man because they are not specific in their choice of a host, others because their normal hosts are not available (for instance, the mass attacks of dog and cat fleas on man in abandoned houses or the attacks of Argasid ticks, such as *Argas reflexus*, which may enter human dwellings when the pigeon cotes are removed). The attacks of most of them cause only temporary inconvenience, in fact, no more than the proverbial "flea bite".

In some cases, however, the disturbances are more severe and may have serious or even fatal consequences. Only these cases are dealt with here. Some arthropods transmit disease and these are treated in their respective chapters, as far as they are zoonoses. In some instances arthropods transmit purely human parasites, such as the *Plasmodia* of human malaria, although the mosquitoes concerned are parasitic on animals to the same degree as they are on humans.

The arthropods which transmit zoonoses are the following:
Simulium (onchocerciasis in Africa and America) (p. 582).

Phlebotomus (the various forms of leishmaniasis, papataci fever and verruga peruana or Oroya fever) (p. 475).

Aedes aegypti and various other species of the genus (yellow fever) (p. 375).

Mosquitoes, various species of which transmit Western Equine and St. Louis encephalitis (p. 359, 369).

Glossina (African trypanosomiasis) (p. 505).

Fleas (plague and murine typhus) (p. 68, 278).

Reduviid bugs (Chagas' disease or South American trypanosomiasis) (p. 516).

Ixodid ticks (the various forms of tick typhus, Q-fever, Russian tick-borne encephalitis and tularaemia) (p. 74, 302, 380).

Argasid ticks (the spirochaetes of endemic or tick relapsing fever).

Trombiculid mites (scrub typhus in East Asia) and a *Dermanyssid Mite* (rickettsial pox) (p. 296, p.300).

Dermanyssus gallinae (St. Louis encephalitis among chickens) (p. 369).

2

O. THEODOR

Diptera (Myiases)

a. Phlebotominae

The role of species of *Phlebotomus* in the transmission of the leishmaniases has been mentioned above. The reaction to their bites may assume the clinical picture of a generalized papular or vesicular dermatitis. This is particularly common in young children or in newcomers to a country who were not exposed to *Phlebotomus* bites in their home country.

The picture is that of an allergic reaction, a sensitization to the bites of *Phlebotomus*. The first bites cause papules, which appear several days after the bite. After repeated bites the papules appear earlier, begin to itch and become inflamed. In some persons blisters appear instead of papules. At the stage of strongest inflammation of the papules old bites are reactivated. Scratching causes secondary infection and a generalized dermatitis results from it. In the further course of the sensitization the papule-reaction changes into an immediate wheal-reaction, which may last for a long time. Later on desensitization ensues (Theodor, 1935). This condition is known as "Harara" in the southern Mediterranean countries. Dostrovski gives a detailed description with illustrations in the *Handbook of Tropical Dermatology*.

b. Simuliidae (Black Flies, Buffalo Gnats)

These are small, humpbacked flies which develop in running water in which the larvae live attached to submerged stones, roots of trees, etc. They are widely distributed throughout the world, from the Arctic and

Antarctic circles to the tropics. In Africa and South America they transmit Onchocerciasis (p. 582). In some areas they appear in enormous numbers and make the neighbourhood of their breeding places uninhabitable during the season of their appearance. Such mass appearances are reported from the Balkans (Columbacz district), and from some localities in North America (Mississippi, Arkansas). Attacks by *Simuliidae* may cause the deaths of large numbers of animals. Thus, in 1923 they killed in Roumania 16,474 domestic animals, among them about 10,000 head of cattle. No deaths of humans were reported from these attacks, but many cases of illness.

Their bites are painful and cause itching papules or vesicles, which may become confluent in mass attacks. There may be fever and lymphangitis. In people constantly exposed to the bites of *Simuliidae* immunity may eventually develop. The pathological conditions caused by their bites are oedema, with serous and bloody infiltration of the skin reaching into the adjacent muscles, and haemorrhages in the skin and internal organs.

Myiasis

Myiasis is a pathological condition due to infestation with the larvae of cyclorrhaphous flies, most of which belong to the families *Calliphoridae,* including the *Sarcophaginae,* and *Oestridae.*

The larvae of most of these flies develop in decomposing organic matter, especially in dead animals. A number of species have become accustomed to lay eggs in purulent wounds, which apparently attract them just as a dead body does. In some of these flies the affinity to living organisms has become so strong that they parasitize them by preference, always, however, being attracted by wounds or discharges from body cavities. In the family *Oestridae* this development has gone a step further and these flies attack healthy animals belonging to a certain species or group of species. They undergo in them a more or less complicated development and complete it in a specific organ or tissue of the host animal. Thus, *Gasterophilus* develops in the stomach of horses and donkeys, and *Oestrus ovis* in the nasal cavity of sheep and goats. With this high specificity in the choice of host and organ, they cause relatively little damage. Their low pathogenicity combined with their inability to develop in any hosts other than their natural hosts, indicates a high degree of adaptation between parasite and host.

From the medical or veterinary point of view the various forms of myiasis have been classified according to the localization of the parasites in the host: traumatic, enteric, ocular etc. From the biological point of view, however, the classification proposed by Patton in 1921 seems more satisfactory, because it takes into account the degree to which the parasitic mode of life has become necessary for the fly. Patton distinguished three groups, *viz.* (1) accidental, (2) semi-specific or facultative, and (3) specific or obligatory myiasis-producing *Diptera*.

The first group contains a number of species of different families which are found occasionally in the intestinal tract and are as a rule, ingested with food.

In *semi-specific or facultative myiasis* most of the flies belong to the family *Calliphoridae*. They normally breed in dead animals and may infect wounds or body cavities, such as the ears, or nose, with evil-smelling discharges. Some of them feed only on necrotic tissues on the surface of wounds and by removal of this tissue, by mechanical stimulation of new growth, by alkalinizing the wound and by their secretion of allantoin and thus of urea derived from this, they may influence the healing process favourably. They have been introduced artificially with good therapeutic results into slowly healing lesions, such as those of chronic osteomyelitis. The larvae of *Lucilia caesar* and those of some strains of *Lucilia sericata* have been used for this purpose. Today, treatment with living larvae has been superseded by the direct use of urea.

Other species, however, pass from the wound into the living adjacent tissue. They behave in the living organism in the same manner as in a dead body, without regard to the limits of organs or the type of tissue they destroy. They may even attack cartilage and bone. Thus, they often cause serious tissue-destruction, which sometimes results in death.

A number of species cause serious damage to *sheep* breeding (blow flies). Most of these develop primarily in dead animals, but they are often attracted to wool soiled with faeces and pass from the wool into irritated and wounded skin. But even the species which attack living animals by preference lay their eggs or larvae in or near wounds or organs with evil smelling discharges and apparently do not attack normal skin. The most important of these blow flies are:

Wohlfahrtia magnifica in Southern Russia,
Lcilia sericata in England,

Lucilia cuprina in Australia,
Callitroga hominivorax (The Screw Worm Fly) and *Phormia regina* in North America.
Chrysomyia bezziana in Africa and India,
Chrysomyia chloropyga in South Africa.

Some of these species, and others in addition, attack *man* occasionally. Thus, *Wohlfahrtia magnifica* and *Lucilia sericata* are known to cause myiasis of wounds and of the ears, eyes and nose in the Mediterranean region. In cases in which the infestation was allowed to progress un-

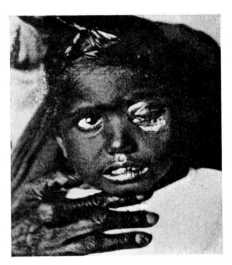

Fig. 103. Myiasis of the orbital sinus caused by larvae of *Chrysomyia bezziana* and *Sarcophaga fuscicauda* (From: W. S. Patton and A. M. Evans, Insects, Ticks, Mites and Venomous animals (1929), courtesy H. R. Grubb Ltd, Croydon).

checked, loss of the inner ear and loss of an eye have ensued (Fig. 103). Herms (1961) quotes a fatal case of infestation with *Callitroga hominivorax* in the nasal cavity, with perforation of the soft palate and the nasal septa. In some of these species this semi-specific, destructive behaviour is combined with a clearly marked tendency to attack living animals and healthy tissue. Some of them, such as *Chrysomyia bezziana* in India, according to Patton (1922), are unable to develop in dead tissue. Others, such as *Callitroga hominivorax*, can be reared in meat when the larvae are transferred to it at the age of 24 hours, but they have never been found in dead animals in nature. These flies do not as a rule attack healthy

References p. 739

animals. Several cases have however been reported from Canada (Ford, 1936), in which *Wohlfahrtia vigil* deposited larvae on the normal skin of young children. These larvae penetrated the skin and caused myiasis. Ford also records the attack of this fly on normal guinea pigs in which the larvae were deposited near the eye, as well as infestation of newborn and 5 day old mice.

This group of species, which combines destructive behaviour with a marked tendency to attack living or even healthy animals, has to be considered as transitional between the semi-specific and the specific myiasis-producing Diptera.

In *specific or obligatory myiasis*, all members of the family *Oestridae* but only a few *Calliphoridae* belong to this group. Most flies of this group are highly specific in their choice of a host, others *(Cordylobia, Dermatobia)* attack a number of different animals, but always show a definite preference for a certain host. As stated above, they become localized in a certain organ or tissue and cause relatively little damage. Thus, the mucosa in the stomach of a horse or donkey may be literally covered with hundreds of the larvae of *Gasterophilus* without the animal showing any indication of serious damage or discomfort. There is no destruction of tissue. These flies always attack normal hosts.

c. Calliphoridae

Cordylobia anthropophaga (Tumbu Fly, Ver de Cayor) is a parasite of the skin of various wild *rats* in Africa, but it also attacks other animals. *Dogs* and *man* are commonly infested. The eggs are deposited on ground soiled with urine or faeces. The young larvae actively bore into the skin and form a localized, painful, inflamed swelling, which resembles a furuncle, but has a small opening through which the larva breathes. After about 10 days, the larva leaves through this opening and pupates in the ground.

A specialized development is that of some *Calliphoridae,* the larvae of which are blood suckers. Some of these *(Protocalliphora)* parasitize the nestlings of birds.

Auchmeromyia luteola (Congo floor maggot). The larvae of this species are commonly found in or near human dwellings where they hide in the cracks of walls or in the ground during the day. Like bugs or Argasid ticks, they attack persons sleeping on the floor and suck their blood, gorging themselves in 15–20 minutes and leaving the host after feeding. They feed every 1 or 2 days, but are able to stand dryness and starvation for a long time. Their bite is not painful and has no serious consequences. *Auchmeromyia* frequently attacks cattle, but its natural hosts are probably warthogs *(Phacochoerus)* and *Orycteropus,* in the burrows of which the flies are often found (Lewis, 1933).

d. Oestridae

All species of this family are narrowly specific and restrict their activities to a certain organ or tissue of their host. The adults have rudimentary mouthparts and do not feed. They live only a short time and are seldom seen. Some of them attack man occasionally.

Oestrus ovis (Sheep nose-bot). This species is almost cosmopolitan, being found wherever sheep and goats occur. Its larvae are normally parasitic in the nasal cavity, and in the maxillary, ethmoidal and frontal sinuses of *sheep* and *goats,* and may cause a purulent discharge and serious disturbances if the larvae are numerous. The larvae live attached to the mucosa and leave through the nostrils or are sneezed out when they are mature. They pupate in the ground. Other related genera parasitize the nasal cavity and sinuses of horses and other ungulates *(Rhinoestrus)* or camels *(Cephalopina)*.

Oestrus deposits its larvae in a milky fluid, sometimes into the eyes, more rarely into the nose or mouth of *humans,* generally shepherds near their flocks. Most cases are reported from areas, such as the highlands of Algeria, in which the sheep population is small in comparison to the human population. In Australia, where the sheep population greatly exceeds the human population, human infections are unknown, and only a single case has been reported from New Zealand. Ophthalmomyiasis due to *Oestrus ovis* is most commonly known in the countries bordering the Mediterranean, particularly from Algeria, where the infection is called "thimni" (Sergent, 1952). Isolated cases are known from all over the world.

The larvae cause a painful conjunctivitis, rhinitis or inflammation of the throat, but they are unable to develop to maturity in any but their natural hosts and only the first stage larvae have been found in man.

Cases of ophthalmomyiasis due to *Rhinoestrus purpureus* have been recorded from southern Russia. Some of the cases attributed to *Rhinoestrus* in other countries may have been due to *Oestrus ovis*, as the larvae have often not been correctly identified.

No serious consequences of infestation of the eyes or throat with *Oestrus* or *Rhinoestrus* have been reported. All cases of ophthalmomyiasis with serious tissue destruction have been found to be due to species of either *Hypoderma* or *Wohlfahrtia*.

Hypoderma (Ox warble-flies). The species of this genus are mainly parasites of *cattle*. The eggs are deposited on the hairs of the abdomen or legs. The young larvae bore into the skin and migrate through the body. At one stage, they are found in the wall of the oesophagus, and some of them may enter the spinal canal. Finally they reach the tissues under the skin of the back. Here they cut a hole through the skin through which the larva breathes. It now becomes stationary and completes its development. The hole in the skin is enlarged with the growth of the larva which, when it is mature, leaves through this hole and pupates in the ground. *Hypoderma* causes considerable economic damage by loss of flesh, reduction of milk yield and depreciation of the value of the hides.

A number of cases of infestation of *humans* are known. Herms (1961) described a case in which the larvae migrated from the groin to the knee, and from there to the shoulder, from which it was removed. The larvae have even been found inside the eye ball, causing in some cases the loss of the eye. The larva wanders in the subcutaneous tissue, where its path can be followed by swollen and painful areas, but it is not as easily recognizable as the larvae of *Gasterophilus* (see below), which wanders much closer to the surface. *Hypoderma* may cause serious discomfort, pains and cramps. The larva finally becomes stationary, creates a swelling with a small opening and is then generally removed before it is mature. In most cases the effects of the infestation are not very severe, although James (1947) records a case of infestation with seven larvae of *Hypoderma lineatum* which resulted in nearly complete paralysis of the legs lasting for several months, and a fatal case in which the larvae caused an ulcer in the lower jaw.

Dermatobia hominis (Ver de macaque, Macaw worm) is widely distributed in South and Central America as far north as Mexico. It occurs mainly in, or on the edge of forests, and in river valleys. It is parasitic in a number of mammals and also attacks *man*. *Cattle* are most commonly infested, *pigs* and man to a lesser extent. This species has a unique method of egg deposition. The female catches a mosquito or fly, rarely a tick, and deposits a batch of eggs on its abdomen. When the mosquito seeks a blood meal, or when the fly visits a suitable host, the larvae hatch and enter the skin of the host, according to some authors, through the puncture wound. The larvae do not wander, but create a furuncle-like lesion, lasting 6–10 weeks, in which the larva develops as the larva of *Hypoderma*. The larva breathes through a small opening in the skin. The lesions may be painful and may cause considerable discomfort, but usually they heal well after removal of the larva. Heavy infestation of animals may have fatal results.

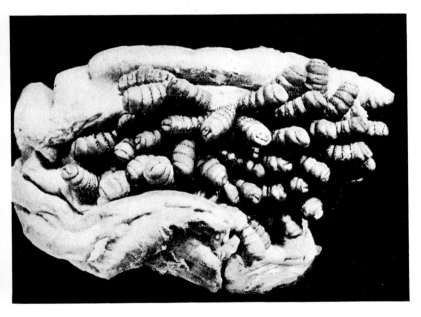

Fig. 104. Part of horse-stomach with larvae of *Gasterophilus intestinalis*. (From: W. S. Patton and A. M. Evans, Insects, Ticks, Mites and Venomous Animals (1929), courtesy H. R. Grubb Ltd., Croydon).

References p. 739

Gasterophilus (Horse stomach bots).

These flies are mainly parasites of the stomach of *horses*. The eggs are laid on the forelegs or on the lips or face. After hatching, which is induced by licking or some other mechanical stimulus, the larvae are either taken up by the lips or make their way over the skin to the mouth. Here they burrow in the mucosa of tongue or cheeks, where they generally remain in the *stratum germinativum* or immediately beneath it. They then migrate to the pharynx and after about 1 month arrive in the stomach, where they attach themselves to the mucosa and complete their development (Fig. 104). The mature larvae pass out with the faeces and pupate in the ground. In most cases no serious damage is caused. *Man* is occasionally infested, but the larvae never develop beyond the first stage. The young larva burrows in the skin at a depth of 2 or 3 mm progressing at the rate of 1 to 2 cm per day and producing a narrow, irregularly winding red line 1 to 3 mm wide. There may be itching and irritation at the point at which the larva burrows. In human cases the larva also remains either in, just beneath, or above the *stratum germinativum* and thus behaves in the same way as it does in its natural host at this stage.

This infestation is called *creeping disease* or *creeping eruption*, larva

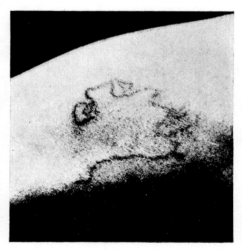

Fig. 105.   Creeping eruption caused by a *Gasterophilus* larva in skin of human arm. (By permission from Riley and Johannsen, Medical Entomology; courtesy McGraw-Hill Book Comp. Inc., New York, 1938).

migrans or (in German) Hautmaulwurf and has to be distinguished from similar conditions caused by larvae of *Ancylostoma*. No serious consequences of infestation with the larvae of *Gasterophilus* have been reported and it is relatively simple to remove the larva after making the skin area concerned transparent with xylol, or oil or defining the position of the larva by marking its progress. The larva, however, may be found some distance ahead of the recognizable end of its path (Fig. 105).

3

O. THEODOR

Siphonaptera (Fleas)

As has been stated above, various fleas of animals (dog, cat, rat) may attack man if their normal hosts are not available. Their role in the transmission of disease is dealt with in preceding chapters.

There is, however, one species of flea which causes serious effects, and may in some cases, by facilitating secondary infection, bring about death

Tunga penetrans (Chigoe, Sandflea). This species is widely distributed in America, from Florida and Mexico in the north nearly to Buenos Aires in the south. Only recently, in the second half of the 19th century, has it

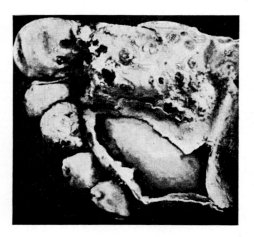

Fig. 106. *Tunga penetrans*. Plantar surface of human foot with chigoes in situ. (From W. S. Patton and A. M. Evans, Insects, Ticks, Mites and Venomous Animals (1929); courtesy H. R. Grubb, Ltd. Inc., Croydon).

nvaded Africa and it is now widely distributed throughout the continent nd Madagascar. When freshly hatched, it is one of the smallest fleas in xistence, being only about 1 mm long. It attacks a great number of nimals, but seems to prefer *man* and *pigs*. The fertilized female burrows nto the skin, as a rule into the sole of the foot, between the toes or under he toe nails. As the eggs develop the female grows to the size of a pea. The posterior tip of the abdomen protrudes from a small opening in the kin through which the flea breathes and through which the eggs are leposited. Its presence causes irritation and inflammation, and a raised welling is formed, which is often filled with pus. In cases in which the leas are numerous, the lesions may become confluent and may, if they re not removed, cause serious ulceration (Fig. 106). Through secondary nfection, gas gangrene and tetanus may develop. A number of deaths lue to this cause have been recorded from Costa Rica.

In one exceptional case, eggs developed in the tissue of the host in he neighbourhood of the burrows of the females (Faust and Maxwell, 1930). This is the only known case of an infestation of man with flea larvae.

Treatment consists in the aseptic removal of the fleas, and prevention in wearing shoes.

4

Hemiptera (Bugs)

A number of bugs of the family *Cimicidae*, which are primarily parasites of various mammals and birds, may attack man and cause dermatitis. Thus, *Haematosiphon inodora,* a parasite of fowls in Mexico, has been reported to cause a vesicular or papular dermatitis with intense itching. It has also been reported that various bugs of bats *(e.g. Cimex pipistrelli)* attack man occasionally.

The role of *Reduviid* bugs in the transmission of Chagas' disease is treated in Chapter V (p. 516).

5

O. THEODOR

Acarina (Ticks and Mites)

Ticks

All ticks are blood suckers in both sexes and in all their early stages (there are a few exceptions in which the males and some of the early stages apparently do not suck blood).

The ticks or *Ixodoidea* contain two families, the *Argasidae* or soft ticks and the *Ixodidae* or hard ticks. The *Argasidae* have a uniform, moderately elastic integument, and lay several groups of eggs, altogether about a thousand, feeding between each oviposition. From the egg hatches a six-legged larva and there are 4 or 5 nymphal stages. Feeding takes place after each moult, so that the whole development takes several months if food is available, and more than a year if temperatures are low and host animals are scarce. These ticks live for several years. They feed like bugs, engorging in 20–40 minutes and leave the host after each feed to hide in cracks in walls or in the ground. Superfluous fluid from the blood meal is excreted through a filtering apparatus which opens between the first and second coxa, often erroneously called the coxal gland.

In the *Ixodidae* part of the body is covered with hard, sclerotised plates, but the rest of the body is covered with a soft, very elastic integument which permits an enormous increase in volume in the female when she gorges with blood; the male can expand much less. There is a six-legged larva as in the *Argasidae*, but only a single nymphal stage. The young larvae are able to starve for a long time. They crawl on to branches of weeds or shrubs and wait for a passing host, to which they attach themselves. The *Ixodidae* remain attached to their host permanently and only stop feeding in order to moult. Moulting may take place on the same host, so that the ticks may spend the whole of their development on a single host individual or they may leave the host for the moult and attack another host. Some species of ticks, like the dog tick *(Rhipicephalus sanguineus)*, may attach themselves to another individual of the same species; others, like some *Hyalommas*, may be parasitic on birds or rodents as larvae and nymphs, and on cattle as adults.

The fully engorged female drops off the host, hides on the ground under stones or branches and lays an enormous number of eggs, in some species up to 15,000 in a single batch, after which she dies.

The *Argasidae* transmit mainly spirochaetes or tick relapsing fever, while the *Ixodidae* transmit the various forms of tick typhus, the virus of some forms of encephalitis and some cattle diseases, such as piroplasmosis, anaplasmosis and theileriasis. They also transmit tularaemia among animals.

All ticks are primarily parasites of a number of animals and show relatively little specificity in the choice of their hosts. Man is attacked only rarely.

The effect of the bite of ticks is reported by various authors, to be harmful. As a rule the bite itself is not painful and one often finds the tick only after it has become firmly attached. Harmful effects of tick bite are generally due to careless removal of the tick, when parts of the mouthparts are left in the wound; secondary infection may follow with resulting ulceration. The bite of Argasid ticks is often not felt at all, but causes local haemorrhage and itching after a longer or shorter interval. On the other hand, repeated bites by Argasid ticks have been reported to cause serious discomfort. *Argas reflexus*, a parasite of pigeons may enter human dwellings after removal of the pigeon cotes. Its bites cause painful inflamed swellings and general symptoms, such as fever and dyspnoea (Mayer and Madel, 1949).

Tick paralysis.

The bite of some Ixodid ticks may cause an ascending motor paralysis which may end fatally. This paralysis has been mainly reported from the North-Western part of the U.S.A. and the adjacent parts of British Columbia, and from the eastern and western coastal areas of Australia. Cases have also been observed in South Africa and the Mediterranean, mainly in domestic animals, most often in sheep and more rarely in dogs and other animals; only a few cases have been recorded in man.

The ticks mainly concerned are: *Ixodes holocyclus* in Australia, *Dermacentor andersoni* and *D. variabilis* in America, *Ixodes rubicundus* in South Africa and *Ixodes ricinus* in the Mediterranean.

The disease is common among *sheep* in South Africa, North America and Crete. Outbreaks among *cattle* have been reported from Montana in the U.S.A., from British Columbia and from Yugoslavia. In Australia a number of cases have been recorded in *man* (22 cases up to 1945), and in various animals, but apparently not in sheep. In North America most cases seem to be concentrated in a relatively small area to the East of Vancouver and Seattle. 170 cases were reported from there by Jellison and Gregson (1950); this region corresponds with a part of the area of distribution of the tick mainly responsible for the disease, *Dermacentor andersoni*.

As a rule a single tick, in most cases a fully engorged female, is found attached on the head or near the neck. Children between 2 and 5 years are most commonly affected. Weakness of the legs appears on the first day, and paralysis develops which is often complete in 48 hours. Reflexes are absent. Respiratory difficulties follow, and death takes place by respiratory paralysis, often preceded by convulsions. If the tick is removed, improvement is prompt within a few hours and the patient recovers completely without any residual disability, which is characteristic for poliomyelitis. Sensory involvement is rare.

The course of the disease in animals is similar to that in man. Thus, a completely paralysed Hereford yearling from which 36 ticks *(D. andersoni)* were removed, recovered completely within 4 days without any residual effects (Jellison *et al.*, 1951).

The cause of the disease is still unknown. It is apparently not due to a living agent, because it cannot be transmitted from affected animals, and recovery regularly and promptly follows the removal of the tick. It thus seems that a toxin is injected by the parasite. A toxin which gives similar results experimentally has been demonstrated in the eggs of *Rhipicephalus sanguineus* (Regendanz and Reichenow, 1935). This toxin, however, is present in many species of ticks, and not only in those which cause paralysis. It has been suggested that the toxin is produced by the female during the development of the eggs, but recently a case of paralysis caused by a male *Hyalomma* was reported from South Africa. Ross (quoted by Theiler, 1949) reported the presence of a toxin which produces paralysis, in the salivary glands of *Ixodes holocyclus* in Australia, and Oxer (ibid.) found that engorging larvae too can cause paralysis. Murnaghan (1960) showed that "the paralysis produced in the dog by *D. andersoni* is due to the failure to liberate acetylcholine at the neuromuscular junction, because of a conduction block in the somatic motor fibres, produced by the tick toxin".

It is not clear why only a few specimens of a species of tick produce this toxin, while the majority do not, nor why *D. andersoni* produces paralysis only in a small part of its area of distribution. Theiler thinks that the production of the toxin may be due to a pathological condition in the females.

Paralysis due to Argasid ticks has rarely been recorded. Thus, *Ornithodorus lahorensis* in Central Asia causes paralysis in *sheep* (Rastegaieff, 1936). A paralysis of a different type has been reported for *Argas persicus* in *ducks* and *geese*. Here the paralysis appears about 5 days after the feeding, and the injury is permanent, leading in most cases to death (Coles, quoted by Theiler, 1949).

No human cases of paralysis due to Argasid ticks are known.

Mites

A number of parasitic mites transmit disease to man. Thus, scrub typhus (tsutsugamushi disease) is transmitted in eastern Asia by various species of *Trombicula* (p. 296) and the virus of Western Equine and St. Louis encephalitis is transmitted among chickens by *Dermanyssus gallinae*, but this virus is conveyed to man by mosquitoes. *Allodermanyssus sanguineus* transmits *Rickettsia akari*, the causative organism of Rickettsial pox, which is primarily an infection of house mice.

A number of mites may cause a more or less serious dermatitis in man. Some of these mites are parasitic, others are inhabitants of various store products and may attack man when he comes into contact with them.

Dermanyssus gallinae and allied species are parasites of wild and domestic birds. They usually attack man when their normal hosts are not available or when the mite population becomes very numerous. The attack causes a papular or vesicular dermatitis with severe irritation.

Various species of *Ornithonyssus* (= *Liponyssus*), which are parasites of rats and fowls, may cause a similar dermatitis.

Trombiculidae (Chiggers or harvest mites). The larvae only of these mites are parasitic on a large number of animals. The nymphs and adults are not parasitic. The larvae appear in some localities in temperate climates in enormous numbers, during late summer. Their attack causes a severe dermatitis and may make it impossible to remain in the infested area. The larvae do not suck blood, but inject a proteolytic enzyme with their saliva. They suck lymph and the liquefied tissue. Their saliva creates in the skin a feeding tube ("histiosiphon"), which is a canal formed as a reaction by the tissue of the host. This is a hyaline, hardened tube which sometimes extends through the epithelium into the dermis and through which the fluid is sucked up. The bites cause a papular or vesicular dermatitis, which itches intensely.

The mites mainly concerned are *Trombicula* (syn. *Leptus*) *autumnalis* in Europe and *T. alfreddugesi* and *T. batatas* in America. *T. akamushi* and *T. deliensis,* the main vectors of scrub typhus in East Asia, do not cause dermatitis, and their bites are, as a rule, not noticed. Other species of *Trombicula* and *Schoengastia* cause "scrub itch" in the Oriental and Pacific Region.

Sarcoptes scabiei, the mite causing human scabies is treated in another chapter. Mites morphologically indistinguishable from the mite, causing "mange" in man, also occur in a number of animal species (see pages 740-748).

REFERENCES

Faust, E. C. and J. A. Maxwell, *Arch. Derm. Syph. (Cic.),* 22 (1930) 94.
Ford, N., *J. Parasit.,* 22 (1936) 309.
Herms, W. B., *Medical Entomology,* 5th ed., New York, 1961, 643 pp.
James, M. T., *U.S. Dept. Agric. Misc. Publ. No. 631,* 1947.
Jellison, W. L. and J. D. Gregson, *Rocky Mtn. med. J.,* 47 (1950) 28; *Vet. Med.,* 46 (1951) No. 5.
Lewis, E. A., *Bull. ent. Res.,* 24 (1933) 263.
Mayer, A. and W. Madel, *Desinfektion und Schädlingsbekämpfung.,* 41 (1949) No. 10.
Nuttall, G. H. F. *et al., Ticks, Vol. 1, Argasidae,* Cambridge, 1918, p. 92.
Patton, W. S., *Bull. ent. Res.,* 12 (1921) 239; *Indian J. med. Res.,* 9 (1922) 635.
Rastegaieff, E., *Bull. Soc. Path. exot.,* 29 (1936) 730.
Regendanz, P. and E. Reichenow, *Arch. Schiffs- u. Tropenhyg.,* 35 (1931) 255.
Sergent, Ed., *Arch. Inst. Pasteur Algér.,* 30 (1952) 319.
Theiler, G., *S. Afr. Biol. Soc.,* Pamph. No. 14, 1949.
Theodor, O., *Trans. roy. Soc. trop. Med. Hyg.,* 29 (1935) 273.

6

J. TAS AND J. VAN DER HOEDEN

Scabies

(Acariasis, scab, mange, Räude, Krätze)

The role of mites as the cause of human scabies was established in the nineteenth century, although the parasites had already been observed at least two centuries earlier. They were regarded as being secondary invaders, and the disease itself an expression of ill-health caused by dyscrasia.

The adult mites (Order *Acarina*, Class *Arachnida*) have four pairs of legs, but the larvae have only three pairs. Several genera of the family *Sarcoptidae* ("itch mites") and the family *Demodicidae* ("follicle mites") are pathogenic to different vertebrate hosts. The most important genera which cause scabies of animals are *Sarcoptes*, *Psoroptes* and *Chorioptes*. There are within the genus *Sarcoptes* several subspecies, generally regarded as being varieties or biological races which are adapted to different host species. Each of these varieties may maintain itself on other hosts for a much more limited time.

Sarcoptes scabiei is barely visible by the unaided eye. The female, which is practically the only form distinguished in routine examinations, is about 0.45 mm long and 0.35 mm in width, the male being smaller (0.23 and 0.19 mm). The thorax and abdomen are united, the mite bearing some resemblance to a turtle.

S. scabiei of man cannot be differentiated morphologically from the varieties encountered in animals. Their differences are of a biological nature. *Notoedres cati* of cats and rabbits (formerly called *Sarcoptes minor*) is smaller than *S. scabiei* and cannot be seen without magnification.

Sarcoptic mites burrow in the skin and live very superficially in the *stratum corneum*. Copulation takes place in the burrow, where the males join the females, which lay about 20 eggs, 2 at a time, prolonging the burrow as successive eggs are laid. This accounts for the zig-zag line which can be seen in the skin in cases of human scabies.

Three nymphal stages precede the adult stage, which is reached after about 3 weeks.

The species of *Psoroptes* have a more oval form and are the largest of the scabies mites; they are 0.5 to 0.8 mm long. They do not burrow, but live on the skin, subsisting on serum and pus which they obtain by introducing their heads after perforating the epidermis.

The species of *Chorioptes* are 0.3 to 0.6 mm long; they live on scales on the surface and do not penetrate into the skin.

The species of *Demodex* are elongated and have a worm-like shape; they are 0.25 mm long and live in the hair follicles of different species of animals.

Two methods may be used for the demonstration of these parasites. Material (scraped off the epidermis and epidermal crusts) is gently warmed to about body temperature. If live mites are present, they will be seen crawling about on a dark background and then can readily be picked up with a needle and put on a slide for microscopic examination.

By the other method the addition of a 10% solution of potassium hydroxide to the material gives good results, even when no live mites are present. The elements of the skin are dissolved by the caustic, but the mites and their eggs are more resistant (chitin) and may be clearly seen under the microscope.

There is a marked difference between the clinical appearances of animal and human scabies. While animal scabies is generally characterized by scales, crusts and alopecia on various parts of the body, the different species of mites causing different effects, human scabies shows specific lesions on selected parts of the body.

There is, however, a rare form of human scabies, which bears some resemblance with animal scabies. This form, called "Norwegian scabies", was first described by Danielssen and Boeck (1847) in leprosy patients in Norway. It is characterized by scales and crusts that may cover the human body wholly or partially without specific preference as to localization. The peculiarity of the clinical picture was ascribed to the anaesthesia of the skin of these leprosy patients. It was assumed that the fact that they did not scratch encouraged undisturbed development of the parasites, a situation similar to that in animals which also cannot scratch freely.

The appearance of scabies in farm animals is mostly seasonal. The mites tend to spread and produce skin lesions in the autumn, winter and spring, whereas, during the summer season, on pasture, the disease as a rule disappears spontaneously. During the hot months several mites remain dormant, cool weather causing recurrence of the lesions.

Long-lasting and disseminated scabies may seriously impair the general physical condition of the animals suffering from it, this being the result of the intense itching, irritation and restlessness; it is perhaps also partly due to inadequate functioning of the skin.

The mites are conveyed from animal to animal by direct contact or, indirectly through the common use of covers, brushes and other equipment, or during transport of the animals in contaminated trucks. In cool and humid weather and when they are separated from their hosts, the parasites survive for about 3 weeks, but are destroyed within 2 days by exposure to direct sunlight in a dry atmosphere.

Sarcoptic scabies is caused by the several varieties of *S. scabiei* which are adapted to different animal species. These are called var. *bovis, -equi, -ovis, -caprae,* etc.

In *cattle* the manifestation may quickly spread from animal to animal affecting a large area of the body, but mostly the parts on which the skin is thin and those thickly covered with hair. The skin becomes toughened, wrinkled and is covered with crusts and scabs that leave bleeding patches on becoming detached.

In the *horse, donkey* and *mule, S. scabiei* var. *equi* burrows deeply into the skin, causing intense irritation and itching, from which the animals seek relief by energetic rubbing. The skin is swollen and inflamed and

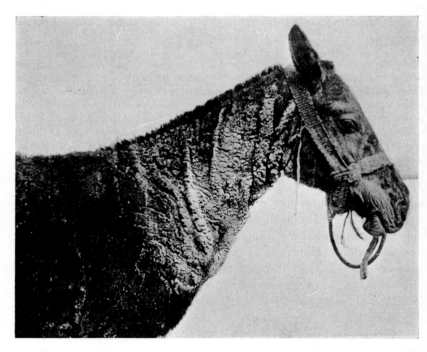

Fig. 107.   Sarcoptes scabies in a horse (Courtesy Prof. D. Swierstra, Institute for Veterinary Parasitology, State University, Utrecht).

shows blisters, lumps, ridges and ruptures. The discharged tissue fluid, mixed with debris, builds up dry scabs in the leathery thickened, wrinkled skin (Fig. 107). Rapid dissemination over the entire body is favoured by lowered general resistance of the animal.

Sarcoptic scabies in *sheep,* localized on the head ("black muzzle"), is

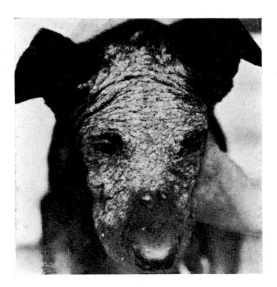

Fig. 108.   Sarcoptes scabies in a dog.
(Photo: Department of Small Animal Diseases, Veterinary Faculty, State University, Utrecht).

common in certain regions of the Old World, but has not been observed in America.

Sarcoptes scabiei var. *suis* affects mainly young *pigs,* the infestation beginning on the head, whence it may spread over the body and cause severe itching.

Mange in *dogs* (Fig. 108) caused by *Sarcoptes scabiei* var. *canis* and *Notoedres cati* infestation in *cats* (Fig. 109) may involve the entire skin and may then severely impair the health of these animals.

In the U.S.A. "common scab" in cattle is caused by *Psoroptes equi* var. *bovis.* The mites prick the skin and the dried oozing tissue fluid, together with foreign materials, forms thick rough crusts on the hardened and thickened skin.

References p. 748

In horses and sheep the equine and ovine varieties of *Ps. equi* cause intense itching. Great economic loss may be incurred from the shedding of large parts of the wool. In goats, the caprine variety of *Psoroptes* provokes scabies especially in the ears.

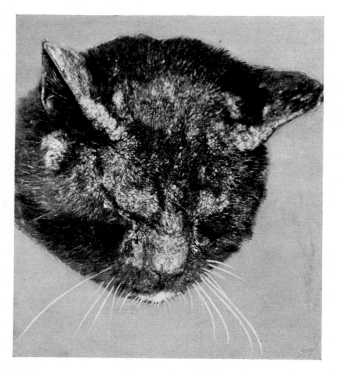

Fig. 109.   Sarcoptes scabies in a cat (Courtesy Prof. M. Ruyter, Dermatological Clinic, State University, Groningen).

Chorioptes ("leg mange") spreads slowly among cattle, progressing after several months from the legs to different parts of the body. As a rule, the lesions are not very noticeable; the skin is raw and bleeds easily.

Chorioptes ("foot mange") of equines generally affects the skin below the hocks and knees; it resembles psoroptic scab in appearance. Among small ruminants "foot scabies" is much commoner in goats than in sheep. *Chorioptes* very seldom affects cats and dogs.

Intensely itching scabies of the ears is often observed in rabbits. The mite, *Notoedres cati* var. *cuniculi*, causes severe otitis externa with thick masses of doughy crusts consisting of dried exudate, epithelium and mites.

In a variety of other domesticated and wild animals and birds mange can also be encountered ("scaly leg" in poultry).

Demodex folliculorum is often found in the animal skin. In swine, it causes a tenacious folliculitis with pustules and ulceration. "Follicular red mange" caused by the same parasite in young dogs, often takes a very serious, sometimes lethal, course with intense emaciation.

Under certain conditions, animals may be affected by a variety of scabies mites which are not particularly adapted to this host-species. Usually this occurs only when the infestation is massive.

The regular form of *human* scabies, caused by *S. scabiei* var. *hominis*, is characterized by burrows in the skin, 2 to 3 cm in length, situated in particular on the hands, wrists, elbows, anterior axillary fold, the area around the mammary nipples and the navel, the penis and buttocks. Often the primary burrow cannot be found, but, secondary papules, vesicles, pustules and eczematization will have developed. In such cases the diagnosis may be based on the localization of these secondary lesions.

Irritation and pruritus do not develop until several weeks after infection with ovigerous mites. Scratching may then cause a secondary pyoderma, which is detrimental to the mites and causes a marked decrease of their number.

Scabies transmitted from animals to man is self limited in its course and, as a rule, it readily disappears, leaving a transient pigmentation. A more protracted course has occasionally been recorded. In such cases it is probable that repeated invasions by the mites occurred as a result of prolonged contact with scabby animals thus simulating persistence of the original infestation.

Very few records of human infestation by *Psoroptes* or *Chorioptes* have been recorded in the literature. The incidence of it is extremely low and, when it occurs, the skin affection is transitory.

Although *Demodex folliculorum* is often found in the hair follicles and comedones of human beings, it never produces scabies. Transmission of the parasite from animals to man has not been observed.

In some regions of the world sarcoptic scabies of animals is still a frequent hazard to farmers and other people engaged in occupations that bring them into close contact with domestic animals. (Fig. 110). In contrast to "human scabies", infestations of animal origin do not usually cause secondary eczema or pyoderma, and burrows are usually absent.

The sarcoptes mite of dogs is easily transmitted to human beings and sometimes it can maintain itself in man for a considerable time. *Notoedres cati* generally abandons the human skin more readily.

Mange of swine and sheep is rarely conveyed to man. On the other hand several reports mention human scabies derived from goats and camels.

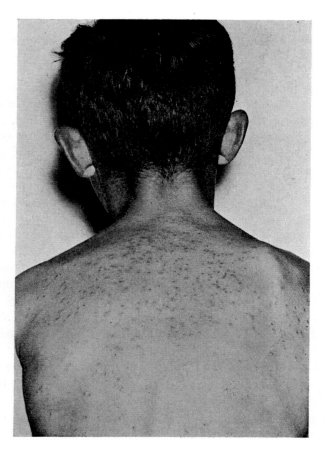

Fig. 110.   Sarcoptes scabies in an 11-year old boy; source of infection was the cat pictured in Fig. 109 (Courtesy Prof. M. Ruyter, Dermatological Clinic, State University, Groningen).

Widespread scabies occurred among the soldiers of the British Camel Corps who were fighting against the Turkish army during the First World War.

Formerly, scabies was very frequent in war time among horses which were insufficiently tended and exposed to adverse hygienic conditions. Its high incidence caused the German economy during the years 1917–1918, a loss of a billion Gold Marks (Koegel). One consequence of this high incidence was a frequent occurrence of scabies of equine origin among the German cavalry soldiers. They complained of severe itching, with redness and papules on parts of their bodies which came into direct contact with the skin of the horses, or with saddles and objects used for cleaning the animals.

Scabies is not seldom observed among the personnel of zoological gardens, who tend various kinds of wild animals.

In an enquiry into the occupational infectious diseases in the Netherlands (Van der Hoeden, 1939) it was established that entire farmers' families and 89 out of 641 veterinarians had suffered from animal-borne scabies, several of them repeatedly. Among veterinary surgeons engaged in general rural practice, about one third had been affected. The source was traced to cattle in 77, to dogs in 6 and to horses in 3 of them. Meanwhile, as a result of the much lower incidence of mange in domestic animals, the disease has become in later years much less frequent in occupationally exposed persons.

For the prevention of the spread of scabies among animals, and from these to man, it is essential to maintain strict cleanliness and to remove the infested animals until they have been cured by specific treatment. Cure is effected by the application of chemical substances which will destroy the parasites without damaging the skin of the hosts. Earlier treatment with lime-sulphur and nicotine sulphate often injured the animals. Since 1948, benzene hexachloride and lindane or toxaphene are used in dips, or, when dipping is not possible, by spraying.

Blankets covering scabby animals, leatherware and other objects or equipment which come into close contact with the skin of the animals should be thoroughly cleansed.

Human sufferers of scabies are usually treated with an emulsion of benzyl benzoate.

References p. 748

REFERENCES

BAKER, E. W., T. M. EVANS and others, *A manual of parasitic mites of medical and* *economic importance,* National Pest Control Association, New York, 1956, pp. 170.

EMDE, R. N., *Arch. Derm.,* 84 (1961) 633.

ERSHOV, V. S., *Parasitology and parasitic diseases of livestock,* State Publishing House for Agricultural Literature, Moscow, 1956, p. 310.

NEVEU-LEMAIRE, M., *Traité d'Entomologie Médicale et Vétérinaire,* 1938, pp. 1339.

SANDERINK, J. F. H. and F. H. OSTWALD, *Documenta Med. geogr. trop. (Amst.),* 9 (1957) 255.

Yearbook of Agriculture, 1942, Keeping Livestock Healthy, U. S. Government Printing Office, p. 38, 62, 476, 590, 735, 1174, 1237.

Yearbook of Agriculture, 1956, Animal Diseases, p. 292, 347, 349, 517, 555, 565.

CHAPTER VII

DISEASES OF MAN TRANSMISSIBLE THROUGH ANIMALS

A. MICHAEL DAVIES

1. Introduction

In addition to the agents causing zoonoses there are a number of human pathogenic organisms which may infect animals and so form a reservoir for their further transmission to man. The animals may be suffering from these "human diseases" or the organisms may be merely non-pathogenic commensals.

The more important members of this group are:

1. True infections of animals with human disease (sometimes indicated as *zooanthroponoses*), amongst which may be mentioned tuberculosis of dogs, cows, pigs, monkeys and parrots due to the human-type of *Mycobacterium tuberculosis* and infection of cows with cowpox from a recently vaccinated individual. They have partly been considered in foregoing chapters. *2.* Streptococcal infections, septic sore throat and scarlet fever; *3.* diphtheria; *4.* staphylococcal infections; *5.* enterobacteria, pathogenic *E. coli* and *Salmonella* infections; *6.* enteroviruses; *7.* parasitic worms.

Some of these conditions will be considered in more detail here.

2. Streptococcal infections (Septic sore throat. Scarlet fever)

Mastitis, acute or chronic, is a common affliction of the cow. The most common cause of this condition is *Streptococcus agalactiae,* which is not pathogenic to man. Occasionally, the udder is infected with *Str. pyogenes* from the hand of a milker who is a healthy carrier or who suffers from a sore throat or a discharging ear. In such a case, the milk may be contaminated with the *Streptococcus,* which is pathogenic for man.

The consumption of unpasteurized milk infected with *Str. pyogenes* has given rise to many widespread epidemics of septic sore throat and scarlet fever in several countries in Europe and in North America. At first it was believed that *Str. agalactiae* (formerly also called *Str. mastiditis*) from

TABLE XXXI

(after Wilson, 1932)

| Organism | Infection | | Mode of infection of milk |
	Disease in the cow	Disease in man	
Streptococcus pyogenes	very rarely mastitis	septic sore throat, scarlet fever	1. droplet infection from the milker or in dairy 2. udder of cow infected from a human source is the main factor in large epidemics
Coryne-bacterium diphtheriae	very rarely on ulcerated teats	diphtheria	1. droplet infection from the milker or in dairy 2. ulcerated teat of cow infected from a human source is the main factor in large epidemics
Staphylococcus pyogenes	mastitis	acute food poisoning due to staphylococcal toxin	1. infected udder of cow 2. hands or droplet infection of milker or in dairy
Salmonella enteritidis, S. typhi-murium, other salmonellae	enteritis and septicaemia, especially in older cattle	acute food poisoning and salmonellosis	1. faeces of infected cattle 2. occasionally, infected udder 3. urine and faeces of rodents 4. possibly from hands of human carrier
Salmonella dublin	enteritis: calf diarrhoea	salmonellosis	1. faeces of infected cattle 2. possibly from hands of human carrier
Salmonella typhosa, S. schottmülleri, Shigellae	no disease?	typhoid; para-typhoid; bacillary dysentery	1. hands of human carrier 2. contaminated water used in cleaning milk utensils or added to the milk

bovine mastitis was the causative organism, but Savage (1911) swabbed his own throat with large numbers of a recently isolated strain of these cocci and showed that they are harmless to man. He went on to establish that cows which caused epidemics of septic sore throat were infected with a "human" strain of *Streptococcus* and his conclusions were confirmed by Frost and Carr (1927) and subsequently by many other workers.

Acute tonsillitis and septic sore throat in man are mainly due to infection with *Streptococcus pyogenes* (Table XXXI). Certain strains of this streptococcus produce an erythrogenic toxin and are thus capable of causing scarlet fever in susceptible persons. In most populations susceptible persons are in a minority, so that epidemic infection may produce many cases of streptococcal sore throat, of whom only a proportion will have the typical rash of scarlet fever. The division between the two diseases is clinical, the aetiology and mode of spread being identical.

The earleast recorded outbreak probably occurred in Kensington, London, in 1875, when there were several cases of sore throat and scarlet fever among people who had eaten cream coming from a district where many cases of sore throat had been reported. Better authenticated was the Aberdeen outbreak of 1881 with 300 cases among 90 of 110 families supplied with infected milk. A large outbreak of 548 cases took place in Christiana in 1908 and the first outbreak in the United States was in the Boston area in 1911 (Winslow, 1912). In this last epidemic over 2,000 cases of septic sore throat were reported with 48 deaths. A single dairy, which provided only 1 to 2% of the milk of Boston and Cambridge, Mass., was responsible for infection in 93% of the milk-consuming families. Cases of septic sore throat were discovered in the families of a farmer and a milk handler on the farms which supplied the milk.

The U.S. Public Health Service reported 103 outbreaks of milk-borne septic sore throat and 105 outbreaks of milk-borne scarlet fever in the United States between 1920 and 1944. The cause of the outbreak was investigated in 61 epidemics of septic sore throat and 65 epidemics of scarlet fever, which involved 11,657 persons and caused 144 deaths during the period 1928–1944. Cattle were held responsible for 54% of the cases and 71% of the deaths. 57 outbreaks of septic sore throat in New York State (excluding New York City) were reported by Dublin *et al.* (1943) for the years 1917–1941. Of 9 outbreaks investigated by these authors, 5 were of scarlet fever and 4 of mixed scarlet fever and sore throat. All but one were due to consumption of milk from cows with infected udders. Similarly, outbreaks have been reported from Denmark, Iceland, Germany and the United Kingdom. Among the more notable ones was that in Copenhagen in 1935 which involved 10,000 people (Madsen and Kalbak, 1940). 450 persons who fell ill with scarlatina in Pinneberg (Germany) had taken raw milk from one and the same source. Part of the milk had come from cows milked by the mother of a child with scarlatinal nephritis (Pels Leusen, 1937). In the 1936-Doncaster outbreak there were 135 cases of scarlet fever and 229 of sore throat, all due to *Str. pyogenes*-

type 2, excreted by a cow with induration of the udder caused by the same organism (Watson, 1937).

A number of the recorded epidemics of milk-borne streptococcal infection have undoubtedly been due to contamination of the milk by a handler excreting *Str. pyogenes* from an infected throat or ear. More and more however, the evidence points to infection of the cow's udder as the source of massive contamination of the milk (Wilson and Miles, 1955). The epidemiological evidence is strengthened by the fact that *Str. pyogenes* introduced into milk, multiplies only slowly at room temperature (Jones 1928: Pullinger and Kemp, 1937). Many of the known outbreaks were spread by milk from small farms with poor hygienic practices and only in 7 of the 208 epidemics reported by the U.S. Public Health Service was the milk pasteurized and infected later. Prevention of milkborne streptococcal infection demands therefore veterinary and medical inspection of the cow and her milker, hygienic milking techniques and pasteurization of milk

There are a number of reports in the literature of infection of cattle by *Str. pneumoniae* (pneumococci) frequently of type III, which is also pathogenic for man. Both pneumonia and pneumococcal mastitis in calves have been reported, but there is no record of infection of man from this source. The subject is summarised by Römer (1959).

3. Diphtheria

The early bacteriological literature is rich in descriptions of the isolation of the human diphtheria organism, *Corynebacterium diphtheriae,* from a variety of animals (dogs, cats, hens, horses and cows). It is clear, however that several diphtheria-like organisms exist both in man and animals and that many of the earlier reports lack objective proof of the identity of the *Corynebacterium* involved.

From an epidemiological point of view, the most important animal to be infected with *C. diphtheriae* is the *cow.* In spite of early reports to the contrary, the cow does not naturally suffer from diphtheria infection. The lesion is a mild ulceration or abrasion of the skin of the udder, which becomes secondarily contaminated with the *Corynebacterium* from the hands of a carrier or from a manifest case of diphtheria. The importance of such a lesion in infecting milk with large numbers of these organisms was first demonstrated by Dean and Todd (1902) and was more recently confirmed by Wilson and Miles (1955). It would seem that most epidemics of milk-borne diphtheria are caused in this way, although in some cases the milk was infected later, either in the dairy or by a human carrier. The U.S. Public Health Service reported 24 outbreaks of diphtheria involving 488 cases during the years 1907–1954, which were due to infected milk. Wilson and Miles pointed out that most of the early reports on milk-borne outbreaks of diphtheria depended solely on epidemiological evidence, because of the technical difficulties of isolating *C. diphtheriae* from the milk and because of the fact that the milk causing the outbreak was usually not available for bacteriological examination. Thus only in the case of continued contamination of a milk supply is there a good chance of finding the source. That it is possible to isolate diphtheria organisms from infected milk was shown by Goldie and Maddock (1943), who used selective media containing tellurite. In their case, a small out-break was due to infection of the milk by the producer's wife, while she was nursing a child sick with diphtheria.

In every suspected case of milk-borne diphtheria there is need for the most stringent tests to prove the identity of the organism. No organism derived from such a source should be reported as *C. diphtheriae* until its character has been established by a properly controlled virulence test.

These remarks on the identity of the organism also apply to reports on diphtheria infections in other animals. *Cats,* for example, are very resistent to infection of the mucous membrane with human diphtheria (Savage, 1919–20), although there are a few convincing records in the literature. Simmons (1920) isolated *C. diphtheriae* from two cats, one of which slept with a woman who developed fatal diphtheria a week later. The organisms, both those taken from the cat and the woman, were virulent for guinea pigs. Amongst other oddities may be mentioned the isolation of virulent diphtheria organisms from the *horse* (Minett, 1920; Ramon and Erber, 1934) and the *monkey* (Dold and Weigmann, 1934).

Litterer (1925) isolated virulent diphtheria organisms from *fowls* in two flocks owned by families with a child sick with diphtheria in each. While this example is authenticated, other authors have confused the diphtheria-like disease of fowls, which is due to a pox virus, with infections by *Corynebacterium.* "It seems improbable that these birds, even if they do occasionally become infected from human sources, play any serious part in the epidemiology of the disease" (Wilson and Miles, 1955).

4. Staphylococcal infections

Like man, nearly all domestic and laboratory animals are susceptible to infection with *Staphylococcus pyogenes* and because this organism is ubiquitous, it is usually impossible to determine the source of the infection with it. Several outbreaks of staphylococcal food poisoning due to infected milk have been described in the literature and chronic staphylococcal mastitis is rather common in cows.

Staphylococci were originally classified according to the pigmentation of their colonies on agar medium, *i.e. albus, aureus* and *citreus,* but in recent years, the classification has come to be based more on biochemical properties. Most human pathogens produce an α-haemolysin, which is active against rabbit and sheep erythrocytes, while many animal and some human pathogens produce a β-haemolysin, which lyses sheep and bovine red cells. The secretion of coagulase, an enzyme capable of clotting plasma, indicates pathogenicity and pus production. Such coagulase-positive strains are grouped generically under the heading *Staphylococcus pyogenes.* Certain strains of *S. pyogenes,* usually those belonging to bacteriophage group 3, are capable of producing a heat resistant enterotoxin and this enterotoxin is one of the common causes of food poisoning. There is no certain way of differentiating enterotoxin-producing, from other pathogenic strains of staphylococci; at the present time, any coagulase-positive staphylococcus found in food, might be considered a potential pathogen. Heating of the food may kill the germs without rendering it harmless, because the preformed enterotoxin can withstand 100° for 30 minutes.

Staphylococci do not multiply extensively in raw milk kept at ordinary temperatures, but they may do so if they are exposed to higher ones. Possibly the first classical outbreak was described by Barber (1914), who isolated *Staphylococcus* from the milk of a particular cow. When it was consumed immediately, the milk was harmless, but after standing for a few hours at room temperature (28–30°), it caused typical food poisoning. Cultures of the organism gave rise to acute food poisoning in volunteers after an incubation period of 2 hours. Drysdale (1950) reported another outbreak in which 30 members of a club became ill within an hour of drinking coffee with boiled milk supplied by an Arab goatherd. One of the goats suffered from mastitis and the raw milk contained coagulase-positive *Staph. aureus.* The boiled milk caused vomiting and diarrhoea when it was fed to a monkey.

In most of the reported cases of staphylococcal food poisoning, the food handler, rather than the animal, is the source of the disease. A high proportion of mankind carry pathogenic staphylococci in their noses, whence they may easily reach foodstuffs. Should the food be a suitable

:ulture medium for the staphylococcus (milk and its products such as :ottage cheese, cream and ice cream are particularly suitable) then only a few hours in a warm room are needed for the production of enterotoxin and hence, of food poisoning. Animals are sometimes the source however, as in the case of the goat and cow with mastitis cited above.

The author has observed an outbreak of food poisoning affecting 160 people in which the source was minced meat. The mince contained the offal of several animals, among them a calf with suspected lung abscess. The meat had been well ground and mixed and had been left for several hours in a warm kitchen before it had been placed in the refrigerator. Subsequent cooking destroyed the rich growth of staphylococci, but not the enterotoxin, and two thirds of the people who ate the meat were attacked, within 1–2 hours, with violent vomiting and diarrhoea.

5. Enterobacteriae

In an examination of household pets, Mian (1959) found serotypes of pathogenic E. coli in 14% of dogs and 8% of cats. In one instance he found the same serotype (O 55, B 5) in a child with diarrhoea and in a dog in the same house. The possibility must be considered that the baby infected the dog and not necessarily, vice versa. It is known that many of the pathogenic E. coli cause diarrhoea in infants, calves, lambs and piglets (Rees, 1958; 1959), but the interrelationships and epidemiology of these infections remain to be elucidated. Buxton (1955) observed that "pets can contract salmonellosis from members of the household who may be themselves infected; so that in cases of mixed human and animal infections, care must be taken in deciding the primary source of infection within the household".

45 out of 103 cats examined by Mackel and his co-workers (1960) yielded recognized or suspected types of E. coli pathogenic to man.

Peters (1949) recorded the case of a keeper in the Rotterdam Zoo who contracted bacillary dysentery during an outbreak of this disease among the monkeys he was nursing. Chronic bacillary dysentery has been demonstrated in monkeys living in zoological gardens, as well as in newly captured monkeys.

6. Enteroviruses

Koprowsky (1958) has reported the isolation of poliovirus type 1 from the stools of 1 out of 5 calves, two months old, which had been under observation since the age of 4 weeks; but he did not comment on the possible human source of the infection. Similarly, neutralizing antibodies have been discovered in the sera of cows to poliovirus (Bartell and Klein, 1955), coxsackie viruses (Klein, 1958) and adenoviruses (Gold and Ginsberg, 1957). The question whether these antibodies are the result of infection with these viruses (as they seem to be) is meanwhile unanswered.

REFERENCES

BARTELL, P. and M. KLEIN, Proc. Soc. exp. Biol. (N.Y.), 90 (1955) 597.
BUXTON, A., Proc. roy. Soc. Med., 48 (1955) 636.
DOLD, H. and F. WEIGMANN, Z. Hyg. Infekt-Kr., 116 (1934) 154.
DRYSDALE, A., J. trop. Med. Hyg., 53 (1950) 12.
DUBLIN, I. D., E. F. H. ROGERS, J. E. PERKINS and F. W. GRAVES, Amer. J. publ. Hlth.
    33 (1943) 157.
GOLD, E. and H. S. GINSBERG, Fed. Proc., 16 (1957) 414.
GOLDIE, W. and E. C. G. MADDOCK, Lancet, 1 (1943) 285.
JONES, S. F., J. exp. Med., 47 (1928)) 965.
KLEIN, M., Ann. N.Y. Acad. Sci., 70 (1958) 362.
KOPROWSKY, H., Ann. N.Y. Acad. Sci., 70 (1958) 369.
LEUSEN, F. P., Zbl. Bakt., I Orig., 140 (1937) 90.
MACKEL, D. C., R. E. WEAVER, L. F. LANGLEY and T. M. DE CAPITO, Amer. J. Hyg., 71
    (1960) 176.
MADSEN, TH. and K. KALBAK, Acta path. microbiol. scand., 17 (1940) 305.
MIAN, K. A., J. Amer. med. Ass., 171 (1959) 1957.
PETERS, J. C., Vet. Rec., 61 (1949) 659.
RAMON, G. and B. ERBER, C. R. Soc. Biol. (Paris), 116 (1934) 726.
REES, T. A., J. comp. Path., 68 (1958) 388; 69 (1959) 334.
RÖMER, O., Nord. Vet.-Med., 11 (1959) 361.
WATSON, R., Brit. med. J., (1937 I) 1189.
WILSON, G. S. and A. A. MILES, Topley and Wilson's Principles of Bacteriology and
    Immunity, 4th ed., London, 1955.

INDEX

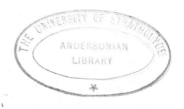
PRINTED IN THE NETHERLANDS